FDG-PET/CT and PET/MR
in Cardiovascular Diseases

Matthieu Pelletier-Galarneau
Patrick Martineau

Editors

FDG-PET/CT and PET/MR in Cardiovascular Diseases

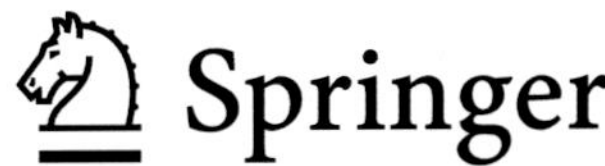 Springer

Editors
Matthieu Pelletier-Galarneau
Montreal Heart Institute
Montréal, QC, Canada

Patrick Martineau
BC Cancer Agency
Vancouver, BC, Canada

ISBN 978-3-031-09809-3   ISBN 978-3-031-09807-9   (eBook)
https://doi.org/10.1007/978-3-031-09807-9

This Springer imprint is published by the registered company Springer Nature Switzerland AG
The registered company address is: Gewerbestrasse 11, 6330 Cham, Switzerland

To Melanie, Parker, and Ella
—Patrick Martineau

To Marie-Michèle, Simone, Mathilde, Claire, and Clémence
—Matthieu Pelletier-Galarneau

Preface

For decades now, molecular imaging has played a foundational role in the evaluation of cardiovascular pathology focusing primarily on the assessment of coronary artery disease and systolic function. More recently, the increasing availability of PET imaging has led to significant evolution in the field of molecular cardiovascular imaging. In particular, FDG-PET, which had long been used for the imaging of noncardiac infection, inflammation, and malignancy, has revealed itself to be immensely useful in a number of cardiovascular applications. Today, many centers offer routine cardiovascular PET imaging for a number of indications, ranging from the evaluation of infection (e.g., endocarditis), inflammatory processes (e.g., cardiac sarcoidosis), cardiac malignancy, as well as other applications such as viability imaging. Furthermore, technological advances have brought forth a new imaging modality, PET/MR, for which the implications for cardiac imaging are still being determined.

Molecular imaging has embraced the opportunities that PET imaging has provided; however, with new roles come new challenges. The rapid growing body of literature and the broad variety of pathologies that can now be routinely encountered pose a challenge for clinicians. This can be especially true in nonspecialist centers where studies for such indications are less frequently performed. With this in mind, the purpose of this book is to present a clinically oriented, up-to-date, and in-depth review of the various applications of FDG-PET/CT and FDG-PET/MR in cardiovascular diseases, along with high-quality clinical cases with emphasis on the current available evidence. We envisioned creating a reference textbook that will be useful to nuclear medicine physicians, radiologists, cardiologists, residents, postgraduate fellows, and technologists. The first section reviews the technical basis of cardiovascular PET/CT and PET/MR imaging as well as those aspects of cardiac metabolism relevant to cardiac PET imaging. The following chapters present specific pathologies or indications, supported by clinical cases. The last two chapters are collections of cases including common pitfalls and interesting cases.

The contributing authors constitute a group of internationally recognized experts in the field of molecular imaging stemming from North America and Europe. To them, we are deeply indebted. We cannot adequately express our sincere gratitude to each who volunteered their time and effort to provide what we believe to be a thorough yet concise textbook. We thank our mentors who have guided us at each step of our careers. Most importantly, we dedicate this book to our families who have shown unflagging support, and infinite patience, while we spent our evenings and weekends in offices, eschewing family activities so we could make a little bit more headway on "the book."

Montréal, QC, Canada   Matthieu Pelletier-Galarneau
Vancouver, BC, Canada   Patrick Martineau

Contents

Part VI Variants and Cases

Part I

Instrumentation and Metabolism

Cardiac Positron Emission Tomography Basics

Chad R. R. N. Hunter and Robert A. deKemp

Introduction

Positron emission tomography (PET) is an imaging modality that uses the physics of positron annihilation to sort photons into parallel arrays without the need for a collimator, thus greatly increasing sensitivity. Imaging begins after injection of a small amount of a positron emitting radioactive isotope, often bound to an organic moiety, called a radiotracer. The radiotracer will distribute itself throughout the body according to its unique biochemistry, with regions of higher uptake indicating a higher degree of a specific biochemical process. Thus, what is imaged is the biochemical uptake and extraction of a tracer in various tissues. This distinguishes PET imaging from anatomical imaging modalities such as CT or MRI since it is the biochemical function of the patient being imaged, which is why it is rightly called "functional imaging."

After injection, a ring of detectors arranged around the patient will passively detect the photons emitted from positron annihilation events (this will be covered in greater detail in section "Basic Radiation Physics in PET Imaging"). Events are recorded over time and binned and reconstructed into separate consecutive time frames. Each reconstructed time frame is a three-dimensional representation of the tracer distribution within the patient for that time frame. For a given organ, the change in activity over time for the whole time series is known as a time activity curve. Time activity curves in various tissues and organs can be used in kinetic modeling to perform quantitative analysis of the metabolic function in the organ or tissue. For example, the time activity curves in the blood pool region and the myocardium can be used for kinetic modeling of blood flow to the myocardium to aid in the detection of coronary artery disease.

Detection of positron annihilation photons is accomplished with scintillation crystal detectors combined with photon multipliers to amplify the signal detected. Scintillation is a process whereby the deposited photon energy is converted into a large number of lower energy (usually blue light) photons called scintillation photons. The intensity of the scintillation light is proportional to the energy of the photon that was converted and can be used to discriminate legitimate photons from noise, this is covered in detail in section "Radiation Detection and PET Detector Systems". One of the earliest PET scanners was the Donner 280-Crystal tomograph which used NaI(Tl) scintillation crystals [1]. As technology improved, the NaI(Tl) crystals were gradually replaced with the bismuth germanate oxide (BGO) crystals which were more dense than NaI(Tl) and thus the crystal detectors could be

C. R. R. N. Hunter · R. A. deKemp (✉)
Department of Cardiac Imaging, University of Ottawa Heart Institute, Ottawa, ON, Canada
e-mail: chunter@ottawaheart.ca;
radekemp@ottawaheart.ca

M. Pelletier-Galarneau, P. Martineau (eds.), *FDG-PET/CT and PET/MR in Cardiovascular Diseases*, https://doi.org/10.1007/978-3-031-09807-9_1

made smaller resulting in improved image resolution. Bismuth germanate oxide (BGO) crystals were the dominant scintillation crystal used in the 1980–1990s. In the late 1990s the lutetium oxyorthosilicate (LSO) crystal detector was developed for PET, with superior light emission properties compared to BGO. Currently lutetium-yttrium oxyorthosilicate scintillation crystals (LYSO) are also in use for PET detector systems, with very similar properties to LSO [2].

The light output from scintillation crystals is too low to be measured directly and must be amplified. In the early development of PET scanners, photomultiplier tubes (PMTs) were used to amplify the scintillation light. One of the limitations of PMTs is that they are sensitive to magnetic fields, thus are unsuitable to applications that combine PET with MRI. In addition, due to their size, many crystals must be coupled to a single PMT. In the early 2000s advances in semiconductor technology resulted in the development of silicon photomultiplier tubes (SiPMs) for PET. Since SiPMs are not sensitive to magnetic fields they can be used in PET/MRI systems. In addition, due to their small size each crystal could be individually coupled to a unique SiPM.

In this chapter, basic radiation physics important to PET detector systems such as radioactive decay, positron annihilation, and photon scattering will be discussed. In addition, the physics and engineering related to photon detection (scintillation and photomultiplication) and image reconstruction will also be discussed.

Basic Radiation Physics in PET Imaging

Radioactive Decay by Positron Emission and Electron Capture

An unstable nucleus will stabilize by undergoing radioactive decay. In the case of PET isotopes, this is through a process of either positron annihilation or electron capture. The existence of the positron was first predicted by Paul Dirac in the 1930s when he noticed the wave equation contained negative solutions [3]. Shorty after this prediction these particles were detected by Carl

D. Anderson [4]. Positrons are a form of antimatter that have the same properties as electrons (spin and mass) but with the opposite coulomb charge. The process whereby an element X will decay via positron (β^+) emission to element Y is given in Eq. (1.1). During this process a proton becomes a neutron, and a positron is emitted

$$_A^Z X \rightarrow {}_A^{Z-1}Y + \beta^+ + v_e \tag{1.1}$$

where A is the number of nucleons, Z is the number of protons, and v_e is an electron neutrino. Positron emission can only occur if the energy-equivalent of the mass difference between the daughter and parent atom is at least 1.022 MeV or twice the rest mass energy of an electron. The neutrino and positron are emitted with some initial kinetic energy with most of the energy of emission going to the positron. Since the amount of energy shared between the two particles varies, there is a characteristic energy emission spectrum for the positron. If the minimum energy threshold is not reached, the decay mode will be electron capture instead of positron emission.

The Positron Annihilation Process

PET detectors take advantage of the physics or positron annihilation for imaging purposes, in this section the physics of positron decay and annihilation are covered. Positrons are emitted with some initial kinetic energy as mentioned above. Since positrons rarely annihilate in transit, they must first slow down until they no longer have enough kinetic energy to overcome the Coulomb potential. As positrons travel, they gradually lose energy through positron–electron interactions known as Bhabha scattering. The distance traveled by the positron before annihilation varies according to the positron energy and has a stochastic distribution that decreases as a bi-exponential function of distance from the point of annihilation. The representative distance is called the positron range and is typically expressed as the root mean square (RMS) of the distribution—for example, see Table 1.1. Once sufficient energy is lost and the positron cannot overcome the Coulomb potential, the positron will combine with an electron and undergo an

Table 1.1 Common isotopes used in PET imaging [5–12]

Isotope	Source	Positron abundance Fraction	E_{MAX} MeV	E_{MEAN} MeV	Decay half-life Min	Range (RMS) mm	Range[a] (FWHM) mm
C-11	Cyclotron	0.99	0.96	0.39	20.4	1.2	2.8
N-13	Cyclotron	1.00	1.19	0.49	9.96	1.8	4.2
O-15	Cyclotron	1.00	1.72	0.74	2.07	3.0	7.1
F-18	Cyclotron	0.97	0.64	0.250	109.8	0.6	1.4
Cu-62	Generator	0.98	2.91	1.280	9.76	6.1	14
Cu-64	Cyclotron or reactor	0.19	0.653	0.278	762	0.7	1.7
Ga-68	Generator or cyclotron	0.89	1.90	0.83	67.7	2.9	6.8
Rb-82	Generator	0.96	3.35	1.40	1.26	2.6	6.1
Zr-89	Cyclotron	0.23	0.897	0.397	4740	1.3	3.1

[a]Approximate Gaussian FWHM = 2.355 × RMS

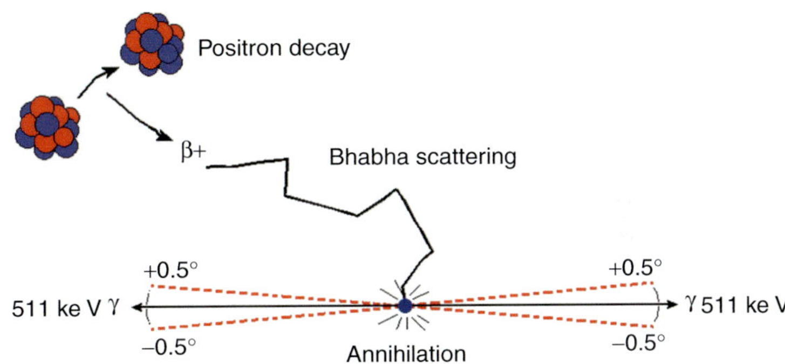

Fig. 1.1 Schematic of the positron decay and annihilation process

annihilation reaction whereby both particles are transformed into electromagnetic waves (photons). Most of the time the positron and electron have very little kinetic energy compared to their respective rest mass energy; thus, in order to conserve momentum, two photons with equal but opposite momentum are produced. This process is illustrated in Fig. 1.1.

Since the positron and electron may not be totally at rest when they annihilate, the photons will have a small angular deviation of about ±0.5° [13]. PET detectors rely on the collinearity of these two photons, which will be covered in detail in section "Radiation Detection and PET Detector Systems".

Important Isotopes Used in PET Imaging

One of the important advantages of PET imaging is that most of the positron emitting isotopes are the same (or similar to) elements commonly found in biology. Thus, PET tracers made from these isotopes can be made to perfectly reflect the biological function under investigation. Additionally, most PET isotopes have short half-lives compared to longer lived SPECT isotopes (e.g. technetium-99m has a 6-h half-life). This shortens the imaging time, the time between consecutive imaging studies (important for rest/ stress studies in cardiology), and improves dosimetry. A list of isotopes commonly used for PET imaging can be found in Table 1.1.

The isotopes C-11, N-13, and O-15 are limited to facilities with an on-site cyclotron due to their short half-lives. Other isotopes like F-18, Cu-64, and Zr-89 have half-lives that are long enough to be transported, and thus facilities that are within driving or flying distance of an off-site cyclotron can make use of these radioisotopes [14, 15].

The most common tracer with F-18 is made by replacing a hydroxyl (OH⁻) group in a deoxy-glucose molecule with F-18 to form 2-deoxy-2-[F-18]fluoro-D-glucose (FDG). The FDG tracer acts as an analogue of glucose and is useful for characterizing tissues with increased glucose uptake such as fast-growing tumor cells or ischemic tissues which have switched to anaerobic glycolysis.

Radiation Detection and PET Detector Systems

The goal of nuclear medicine imaging is to assess a particular biochemical process occurring within a patient. This can be used to measure abnormal tissue growth for oncology, blood flow to the heart for cardiac imaging, uptake in regions of the brain to look for cerebral diseases, and many more biochemical processes. All this is accomplished by measuring the radiative emissions from an unstable isotope within a patient. The source is a radioactive isotope-labeled molecule or radiopharmaceutical (called a radiotracer) that has the necessary chemical properties to follow the biological process under investigation and is injected into the patient in small amounts. In order to put these radiative emissions in a usable format, the angular information of the photons must be quantized (i.e. grouping all photons at the same angle together, also known as collimating) to form projection information, the details of which will be discussed later in this chapter. Various tomographic image reconstruction algorithms can then be used to produce a 3D representation of the tracer distribution throughout the patient for a particular time period. To collimate the incident photons, a physical collimator such as those used in single-photon emission tomography (SPECT) can be used. Physical collimation works by using a dense material like lead or tungsten to reject (through absorption) photons that have too high an incident angle. Since the rejected photons are absorbed by the collimator, they are lost forever which has a detrimental impact on sensitivity.

PET detectors take advantage of the physics of positron annihilation. Positron annihilation produces two photons with a 180° angular separation; thus, "electronic" collimation is naturally built into the imaging physics for PET. Older 2D PET systems included physical collimation between axially adjacent detector rings. To collimate the emissions within the trans-axial planes, detectors placed around the radiation source only need to look for coincident events. The angular information needed to form the projection information is determined from the line of response connecting two detectors, thus collimation is inherently built into the PET detector system.

Scintillation Detectors

All modern PET scanners use a system of crystal detectors arranged as a ring around the patient. The detectors have important properties for detecting and discriminating photons that emanate from the patient. Early PET detectors consisted of an array of NaI(Tl) crystals. These were gradually replaced with BGO, then LSO and LYSO scintillation crystal radiation detectors [2, 16]. Regardless of what crystal detector is used, all have some common properties. That is, all detector crystals used for PET imaging have high stopping power for the 511 keV photons emitted from a positron annihilation event and all are scintillation crystals.

Scintillation is a process whereby a higher energy photon is absorbed and converted into a number of lower energy photons called scintillation photons or scintillation light. The total energy of all the low energy photons will be proportional to the total energy deposited by the high energy photon assuming no losses. Therefore, the energy of the incident high energy photon can be measured by the amount of scintillation light generated. Thus, the ideal detector would convert all the incident photon energy into scintillation light. To facilitate this, scintillation crystals are chosen from materials that are transparent to scintillation light, in order to collimate the scintillation light, and have a high probability for 511 keV photons to interact via the photoelectric effect to absorb all the photon energy. Accurate measurement of the energy of the incident photon is necessary in order to remove noise from spurious photons (photons not originating from an annihilation event) interacting with the detector.

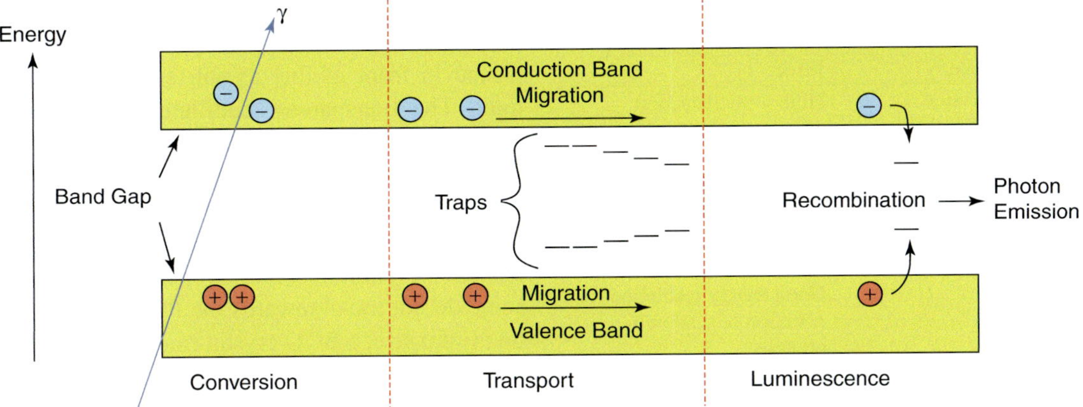

Fig. 1.2 Diagram of band-gap structure, production of electron–hole pairs during conversion, migration of electron–hole pairs during transport, and recombination resulting in emission of photon

Scintillation is a three-stage process: conversion, transport, and luminescence [17, 18]. Scintillation crystals have a band-gap structure similar to a semiconductor consisting of a valence band, conduction band, and a forbidden region (band-gap)—see Fig. 1.2. During the conversion process an incident photon (γ) interacts with the scintillation crystal, the energy is deposited in the crystal through interactions such as Compton scatter and the photoelectric effect. Compton scatter results in only part of the energy of the incident photon deposited, whereas with the photoelectric effect the entire photon is absorbed. This process produces an electron–hole pair in the crystal lattice, with the electron promoted to the conduction band and the valence band is left with a deficit of charge. In the case of the photoelectric effect, the deficit will be in the innermost shell of the atom, leaving the atom in an unstable state. This atom will stabilize when an electron in the outer shell falls to the inner shell and will produce a characteristic X-ray and/or auger electrons. These characteristic X-rays then go on to interact with the scintillator and can excite loosely bound electrons to form additional electron–hole pairs in the crystal lattice. High energy electrons also interact with other electrons via scatter and promote some to the conduction band. The culmination of these effects can result in multiple electrons being promoted to the valence shell resulting in multiple electron–hole pairs, in a process called conversion. Due to the band-gap structure of the crystal, only electrons that absorb the minimum energy defined by the band-gap energy will be promoted from the valence band to the conduction band. Electron–hole pairs will migrate through the crystal and lose some energy due to non-radiative re-combinations (quenching) during the transport stage which reduces the efficiency of the crystal. Doping agents are added to the crystal in order to produce multiple traps within the crystal lattice with energy levels in the forbidden region (band-gap) range. During the luminescence stage, electron–hole pairs within the traps recombine and photons with the characteristic scintillation light are produced. This process is illustrated in Fig. 1.2 [17, 18].

The properties of scintillation crystals that are important to PET imaging are summarized in Table 1.2 [19]. The detector efficiency describes how well the crystal converts the deposited photon energy into electron–hole pairs. Having a scintillator with high efficiency will improve energy resolution and make detection of the photon more accurate. The process from conversion to luminescence takes a finite amount of time. If a second photon interacts during this process, the light from the second event will be added to the first causing a pile-up effect. Since this process is very fast ($\approx$40 ns for LYSO) this effect is only important for high count rates. If the crystals have a high light output, the physical sizes of the crystals can be made smaller, which increases spatial resolution. In addition, it is easier to man-

Table 1.2 Desirable characteristics of a PET scintillation crystal [19]

Crystal property	Effect
High conversion efficiency for electron–hole pair production	High γ-ray detection efficiency
Fast light decay time	Low pile-up/good coincidence timing
High light output	Large number of crystals per PMT Good energy resolution for rejection of scattered photons
Scintillation light wavelength near PMT response	High detection quantum efficiency for collection of scintillation photons
Transparent to scintillation light	Good transport of light output to PMT
Same index of refraction as PMT coupling	Good optical coupling to PMT
Resistant to radiation	Stable response over time
Non-hygroscopic	Easier to package crystals
Physically rugged	Easier to produce smaller crystal elements

ufacture small crystals if the material is more rugged. The energy resolution for the 511 keV photons should be as high as possible; thus, scintillation crystals tend to be dense so they primarily interact via the photoelectric effect to fully absorb the energy of the incident photon. It is important that the scintillation light has a wavelength matched to the PMT response, the PMT coupling has the same index of refraction as the crystal, and that the crystal is transparent to the scintillation light to avoid optical losses. Materials exposed to radiation degrade over time; therefore, it is important for scintillation crystals to be radiation resistant to increase stability and longevity. Since some crystals such as NaI(Tl) deteriorate when exposed to moisture (hygroscopic), non-hygroscopic crystals are more desirable since they do not need an air-tight seal.

Scintillation crystals such as BGO can be sensitive to damage by ultraviolet (UV) light and must be shielded, and the ambient temperature can change the detector efficiency. In addition, scintillation light is in the visible (blue) spectrum, thus ambient light would interfere with the measurement of radiation. Therefore, scintilla-

tion crystals are packaged to protect them from the environment and typically a mylar sheet is placed in front of the crystal to block ambient light. The transparent scintillation crystals act like optical light guides which carry the scintillation photons to the photomultiplier tubes (PMT). This relies on total internal reflection; however, some photons escape the crystal and due to fact that the emission of scintillation light is isotropic some do not travel towards the PMT. Depending on crystal size, a BGO crystal can lose up to 40% of the scintillation light and for LYSO it can be up to 50% [16]. Typically, a detector is formed from crystal arrays each made from a single block of crystal with grooves cut to form a 2D array of crystals. The grooves are not cut entirely through the crystal block and are filled with Teflon to protect the crystal arrays. A typical arrangement involves coupling 4 PMTs to a single crystal detector (2D array) block [20]. Since the grooves are not cut entirely through the crystal some crosstalk between the PMTs is allowed and used for position determination.

Photomultiplier Tubes (PMTs)

The light output from the scintillation process is too low to be measured directly and must be amplified prior to being quantified. Scintillation photons are directed by the crystal to the photomultiplier tube (PMT) where they interact with the photo-cathode. When scintillation photons interact with the photo-cathode they liberate an electron which is ejected through a focusing electrode and accelerated towards the first dynode. There are a series of successive dynodes held at ever-increasing voltage potentials which causes more electrons to be accelerated and thus greatly amplifies the signal. The final signal is measured by an electric circuit to record the amplitude of the pulse, the whole process is illustrated in Fig. 1.3 [21].

One of the limitations of PMTs is that they cannot be used in an environment where high magnetic fields are present such as those utilized in magnetic resonance imaging (MRI). In addi-

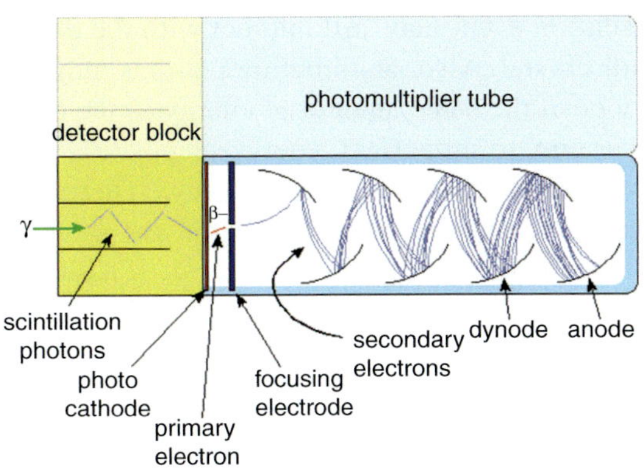

Fig. 1.3 Schematic of a photomultiplier tube with detector block attached

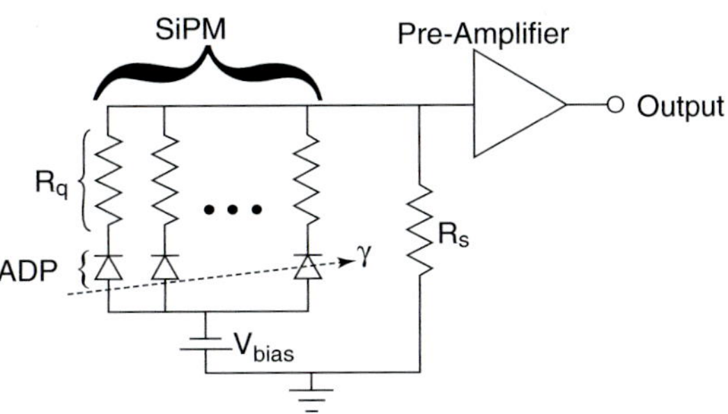

Fig. 1.4 SiPM photomultiplier circuit diagram. The SiPM is made up of an array of ADP semiconductors operated in the Geiger-Muller mode. Gamma rays deposit energy into the ADP semiconductors producing electron–hole pairs [25]

tion, PMTs are expensive relative to their surface area which increases the cost of PET detector systems. Due to the fact that PMTs are bulky it would be impractical to couple a PMT to individual crystal detectors which is why detector blocks are used instead. Finally, PMTs have limited detection quantum efficiency (~35% for PMTs vs. 80% for SiPM) which is the proportion of incident light photos converted into electrons [22–24]. Therefore, to improve PET imaging and couple PET with MRI a different method of signal amplification is required. Recent developments in semiconductor technology have offered a solution in the form of silicon photomultipliers (SiPMs). SiPMs are also commonly called single-photon avalanche diode (SPAD) arrays, but are also known by the following terms: solid-state photomultiplier (SSPM), pixelated Geiger-mode avalanche photon detector (PPD), multipixel Geiger-mode avalanche photodiode (GM-APD or G-APD), or multipixel photon counter (MPPC). SiPMs are made up of an array of single-photon avalanche photodiodes (APD) operating in the Geiger-muller mode. When a sufficient voltage is applied to an ADP a large electric field is generated. When a photon interacts with the ADP a charge is created and due to the electric field any charges in this field will be accelerated; this creates more electron–hole pairs and multiplies the signal via this "avalanche" of charges. These charges then produce an output pulse that is proportional to the number of scintillation photons that interacted with the APD. The gain of an ADP (and thus SiPM) varies as a function of the temperature and must be temperature controlled; however, SiPMs are insensitive to magnetic fields which is useful for PET/MRI applications and have excellent timing characteristics for time-of-flight PET imaging [25, 26].

A circuit diagram for a SiPM is shown in Fig. 1.4. The SiPM is made up of a parallel array of a large number (10^2 to 10^5) of ADP semiconductors with a voltage applied in the reverse bias direction (V_{bias}) [25]. This reverse bias voltage (typically <100 V) puts the ADP in a Geiger-Muller mode as discussed previously [22]. Each ADP is in series with a quenching resistor (R_q) which sets the restoration time for the SiPM to return back to the Geiger-Muller mode following detection of scintillation light. The output voltage from the SiPM is read across a shunt resistor (R_s) and the final signal is amplified with a pre-amplifier.

The PET Camera

In a vacuum, photons travel at the speed of light ($\approx 3 \times 10^8$ m/s or 30 cm/ns). Thus, a photon would take 2 ns to travel the distance for a PET detector system with a diameter of 60 cm. Positron annihilation produces two gamma rays of equal energy (511 keV) but opposite direction (with 180° separation) as previously discussed. These photons are highly penetrating to human tissues due to their high energy, so we expect them to escape the body. Due to their fast speed, it is expected that if both photons interact with the detector, they will interact at roughly the same time.

Radioactive tracers produce many decay events within the patient that occur simultaneously. This in turn produces many photon detections per second depending on the activity within the field of view. The measured coincident signals are then amplified with photomultiplier tubes and checked for coincident timing as illustrated in Fig. 1.5—recreated from [27].

Signals from the PMT are transformed by a pulse generator into a sharp pulse with an amplitude proportional to the deposited energy. Photons that arise from events like electron capture and other interactions within the body and photons that do not correspond to an anni-

hilation event may still interact with the detector crystal. Also, annihilation photons may not deposit the same amount of energy in the crystal due to imperfect energy deposition and variations in detector efficiency. Therefore, pulses from the pulse generator are selected using an energy threshold to decide if a photon is likely due to an annihilation event as shown in Fig. 1.6 [21].

If the pulses are accepted, they are then fed into a gate-pulse generator, which transforms the pulses into a square wave which has a width that is twice the coincident timing window (2τ), but preserves the timing difference between the two peaks. Since there is no way to discriminate between the emission of two separate annihilation events, a coincidence timing window is used to reject or accept a measured coincidence as shown in Fig. 1.7 [21]. The final detected events are then recorded and stored.

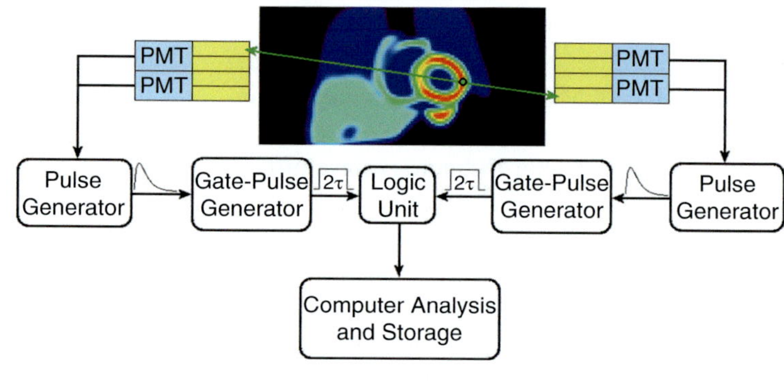

Fig. 1.5 Coincident timing circuitry

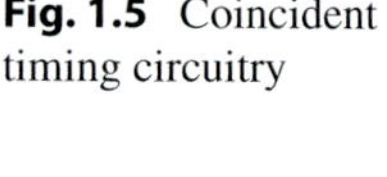

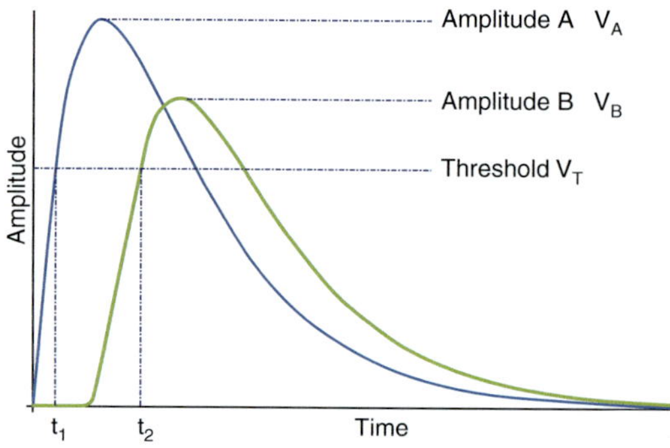

Fig. 1.6 Example pulses from the pulse generator. These pulses are within the energy window and are accepted as coincident events [21]

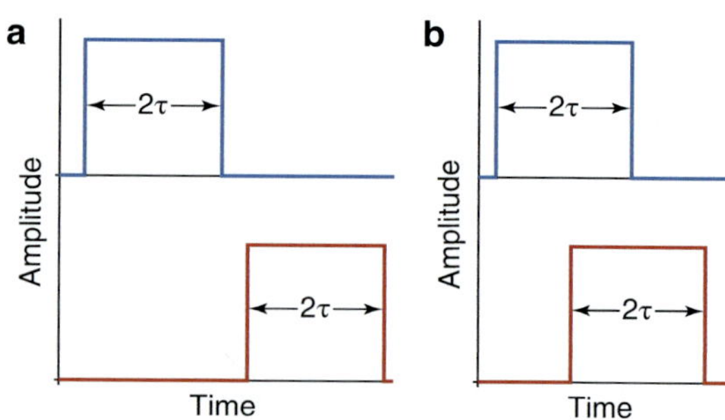

Fig. 1.7 Prompt coincident timing window showing two cases: (**a**) example pulses are not in coincidence and are rejected and (**b**) example of pulses in prompt coincidence [21]

Data Acquisition, Projections, and Sinograms

A small point source in the field of view will produce several emission lines from coincident events at various angles. If we restrict observation to a single trans-axial plane and plot the displacement from the center of the scanner as a function of angle from the horizontal, the displacement will trace out a sinusoidal function as shown in Fig. 1.8—recreated from [28]. Collection of these displacements grouped by angle and stacked is therefore called sinograms and will be described later.

The detector block and thus the rings in a PET scanner are stacked axially as shown in Fig. 1.9—recreated from [21]. Older 2D-mode scanners had thin tungsten septa between the detector rings for attenuation of photons between the trans-axial planes. 2D reconstruction limited the axial angles for coincidence detection to these separate trans-axial planes. This design helped to reduce scatter between image planes but at the cost of lower sensitivity since photons are highly absorbed in dense tungsten. Due to advancements in 3D image reconstruction (e.g. Fourier re-binning, iterative statistical methods, and

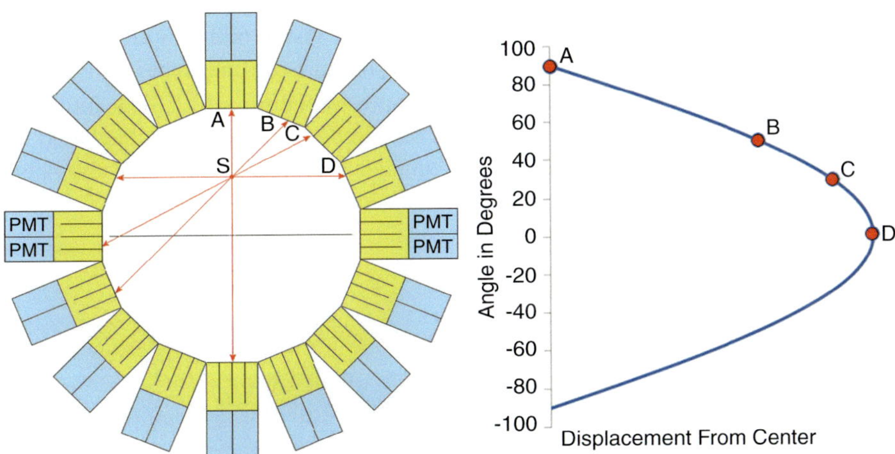

Fig. 1.8 Sinogram of a point source "S." Lines of response A, B, C and D from the point source are plotted on the displacement graph tracing out a sinusoidal function [28]

Fig. 1.9 Example of some lines of response (**a**) with the septa in place, restricting the coincident events to the trans-axial planes only for 2D reconstruction in older scanners and (**b**) the septa are removed allowing a larger angular acceptance between trans-axial planes along the scanner axis

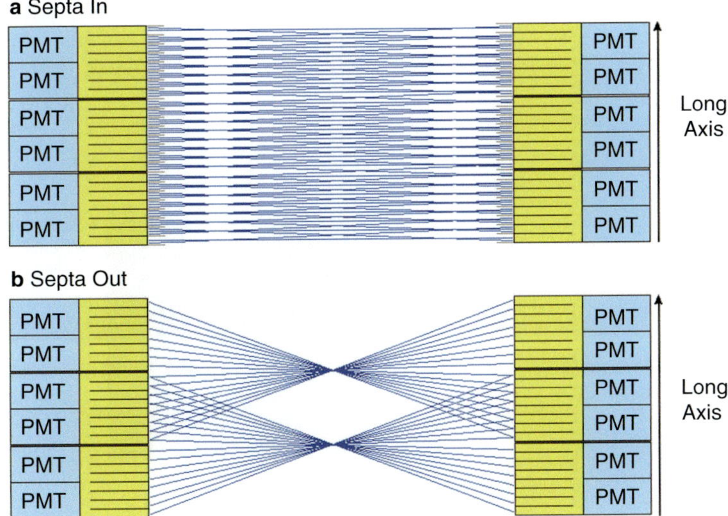

model-based scatter correction) physical collimation has become unnecessary and modern PET scanners no longer have any tungsten septa.

Each line of response has an axial and transaxial angle determined by the crystal geometry. Lines of response with a common angle (parallel lines of response) are grouped together into a projection. Projections can then be stacked in increasing angular displacement along the radial axis into a data structure called a sinogram as shown in Fig. 1.10 (recreated from [29, 30]). A 1D projection is a summation of all counts (coincident events) for all lines of response at the same angle. In Fig. 1.10, part A shows 1D projections at 0° and −45°. A full sinogram is made up of all projections for all angles (full 180° from −90° to +90°) and contains all projection information for a single slice (or plane) within the axial length of the scanner. Sinograms for all slices (including the oblique angles) are stacked in a 3D matrix for

form a 3D sinogram. An angular projection as shown in Fig. 1.10, part B is formed by stacking all 1D projections for all slices at a common angle, where the heart wall is clearly visible in the projection image as a horse-shoe or donut shape.

In Fig. 1.10, part A shows this function with lateral displacement "L" along an angular vector ℓ at angles at 0° and −45°. An example of the projection profile is also shown.

A summary of various scanner geometries is given in Table 1.3, which shows scanners using BGO, LSO, and LYSO scintillation crystals. The GEHC Advance and Discovery 690 (D690) scanners both use PMTs, whereas the Siemens Biograph Vision 600 (V600) uses the newer silicon photon multiplier tubes (SiPMs). Due to the superior properties of LYSO scintillation crystals compared to BGO crystals, the D690 scanner has smaller crystal elements than the Advance. The

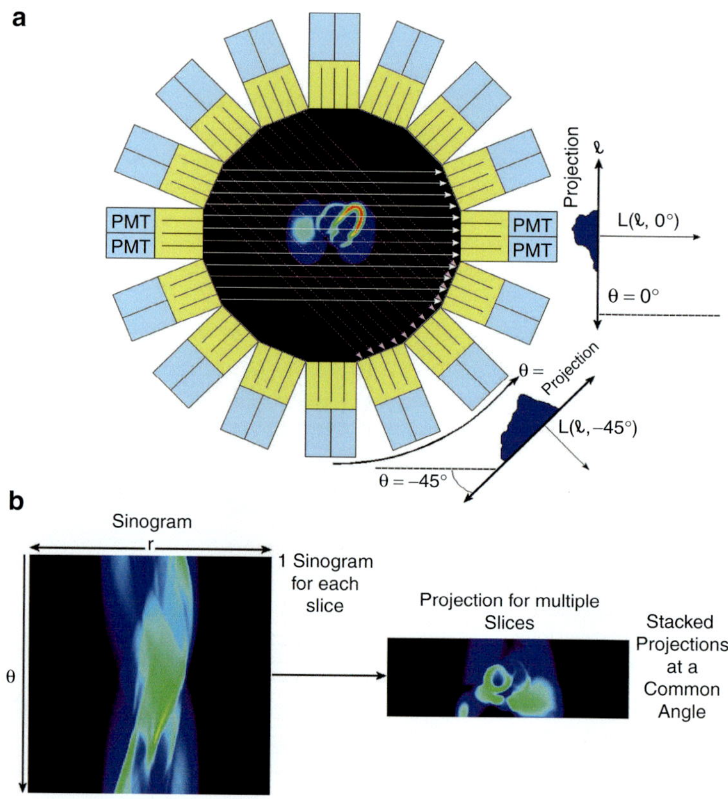

Fig. 1.10 Lines of response at the same angle grouped together at 0° and −45° shown in (**a**). Stacking all the grouped sinograms by angle forms a single sinogram, as shown in (**b**). If we take a single projection at an angle for all trans-axial slices we get the stacked projection view (right side of (**b**))

Table 1.3 Example PET scanner designs

Model	GEHC Advance [30]	GEHC Discovery 690 [31]	Siemens Vision 600 [32, 33]
Approximate year	1995	2010	2020
Crystal block arrangement (trans-axial × axial)	6 × 6	9 × 6	5 × 5
Detector crystal size (mm^3) (trans-axial × axial × depth)	4.0 × 8.1 × 30	4.2 × 6.3 × 25	3.2 × 3.2 × 20
Number of detector rings	18	24	80
Detector crystals/ring	672	572	760
Axial FOV (cm)	15.2	15.7	26.3
Ring diameter (cm)	92.7	81.0	82.0
Detector crystal material	BGO	LYSO	LSO
Photodetector type	PMT	PMT	SiPM

V600 scanner has even smaller crystal sizes than either the Advance or D690 due to further advances in technology such as SiPM photodetectors. Typical reconstructed image matrix sizes range from 128 to 880 pixels, for example, on the V600, with the Advance having 35 trans-axial slices, the D690 having 47 slices, and the V600 having 159 slices.

Correction for Physical Effects and Image Reconstruction

When positron annihilation results in two (unscattered) photons being detected by the PET system this is known as a true coincidence, as shown in Fig. 1.5. However, the physical effects of photon scatter, absorption, and unpaired (accidental or chance) detection will lead to false coincidences such as scatter, random, and cascade gamma coincident events. Any two photons detected within the prompt coincidence time window (Fig. 1.7b) are called prompt coincident events and include all the true, random, scatter, and cascade gamma events. Ideally, the recorded true events count rate should be directly proportional to the isotope activity concentration. However, because the PET scanner records all photon pairs in the prompt coincidence window, the contaminating effects of attenuation, scatter, randoms, and prompt-gamma coincidences must be removed for accurate measurements of isotope concentration.

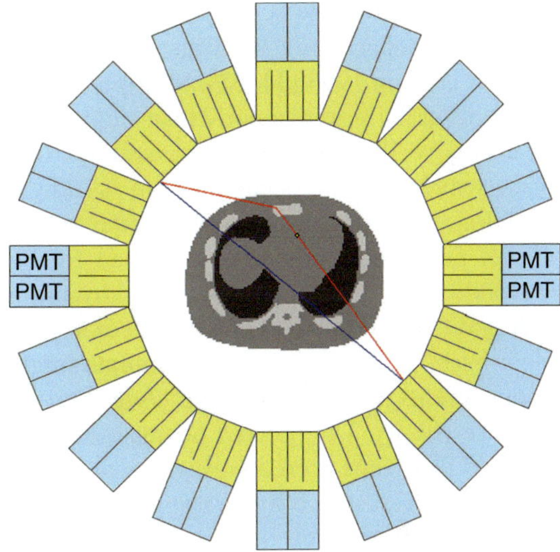

Fig. 1.11 Representation of a scatter coincidence. Emission occurs at a point within the heart (blue circle) and one of the 511 keV photons scatters in the bone of a rib. The recorded line of response (blue) is mispositioned as it does not intersect with the point of annihilation

Correction for Scatter Coincident Events

When one of the annihilation photons undergoes Compton scatter but both photons are detected as valid annihilation photons, it produces a line of response that does not intersect the point of annihilation as shown in Fig. 1.11. We call this a scatter coincidence and, depending on the object size and acquisition mode (2D vs. 3D), scatter events can make up 20–80% of all measured prompt events. Therefore, scatter events are a significant source of noise for PET imaging.

High angle scatter events (approaching 90°) would produce photons that approach half their initial energy (255.5 keV) and would therefore be outside the energy window of the detector and are rejected. Therefore, most scattered coincidences result from relatively small angle scatter events and therefore only produce a small offset from the true annihilation position. A narrower energy window can be used to reject more scatter, but at the expense of reduced sensitivity to true (i.e. unscattered) photons.

The most common scatter correction method is the simulated single scatter (SSS) algorithm proposed independently by Watson et al. and Ollinger et al. in 1996 [34, 35]. Multiple scatter events occur far less frequently than single scatter events so the SSS algorithm assumes that most scatter events occur due to a single Compton interaction. Since multi-scatter events are not negligible, these are accounted for by convolution of the single-scatter distribution with a one-dimensional Gaussian kernel. The Klein-Nishina formula is used to simulate single scatter events that occur along each line of response (LOR). The process begins after random and dead time corrections where an initial estimate of the scatter is made using a back-projection of the emission data at low resolution (sometimes as low as 1 cm^3 voxel volume). To scale the images to the true activity concentration, a normalization factor is estimated from the tails of the scatter outside the body contour, this is illustrated in Fig. 1.12. Typically, the initial estimate is used in conjunction with iterative reconstruction (to be discussed later in this chapter) by incorporating the SSS estimate in the forward projection component of the reconstruction.

Accurately modeling and determining scatter in the patient requires a priori knowledge of both the scattering medium and the emission distribution making scatter correction one of the most difficult PET corrections to implement.

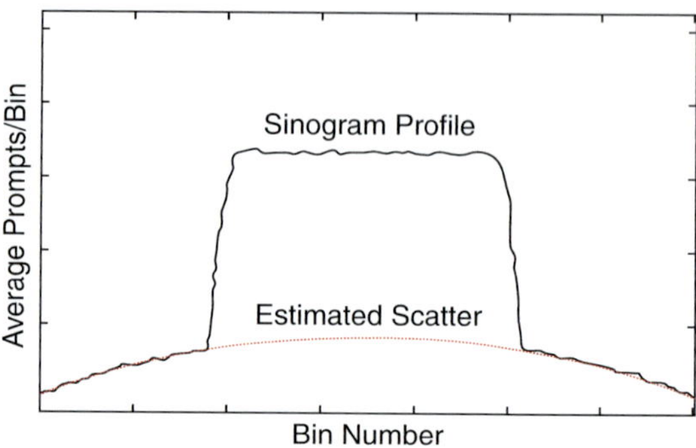

Fig. 1.12 Example of a sinogram profile (black solid line) and estimated scatter from the tails of data (red dotted line) outside the object used in the SSS estimate for scatter correction

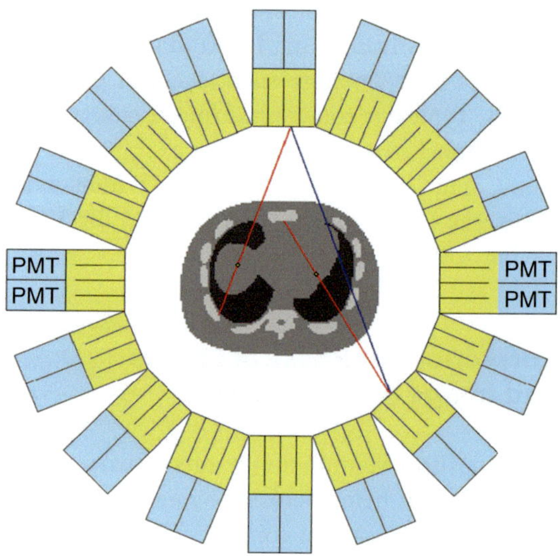

Fig. 1.13 Representation of a random coincidence. The blue line is the recorded line of response which is mispositioned as it does not intersect with either point of annihilation

Correction for Random Coincident Events

When two photons from different annihilation events are detected by the system and recorded as a coincident event, the line of response does not correspond to the point of annihilation as shown in Fig. 1.13. These events are known as random coincident events and have a nearly uniform distribution for objects centered in the field of view.

The probability of a random coincidence increases with higher levels of activity. The delayed coincidence method is the most commonly used method used to correct for random coincidences. This method uses a dual coincidence circuit where a second circuit has a delay in the coincidence timing to measure the delayed coincidences. The timing of the delay is set such that true coincidences will not be detected and only randoms are measured in the delayed window. Random events cannot be removed from the scan data and create a background noise in the final images. However, the bias in the measured activity concentration of the image can be corrected to produce quantitative images in units of activity concentration.

Correction for Cascade Gamma Coincident Events

Some radioactive isotopes produce a high energy gamma ray called a cascade gamma simultaneously with the emission of a positron, and this cascade gamma may be detected by the PET detector system. For example, about 15% of the time Rb-82 will emit a 776.5 keV gamma ray (in addition to the positron), which can scatter and fall within the energy window for acceptance [36]. Cascade gammas (sometimes called prompt gammas) are emitted from the nucleus, whereas annihilation photons are emitted from the site of annihilation which could be some distance away from the decay event due to the positron range. If a cascade gamma is detected in coincidence with another photon, it is called a cascade gamma coincident event, as illustrated in Fig. 1.14.

While random coincidences occur due to two separate decay events with some temporal separation, cascade coincidences will be correlated in time with the positron annihilation gamma photons since they occur at nearly the same time; thus, the delayed window random correction technique does not correct for cascade events. The line of response from cascade gamma coinci-

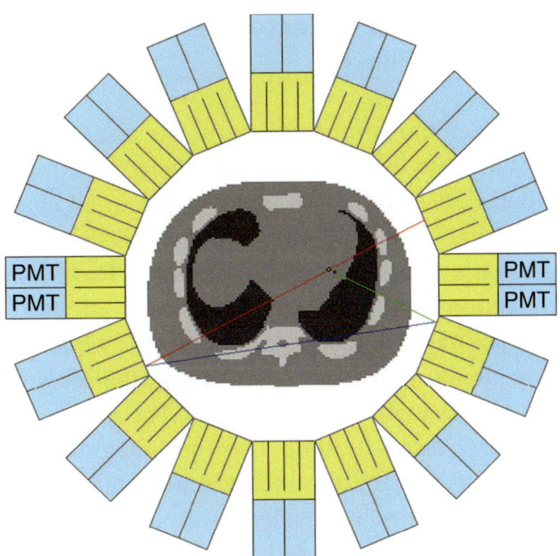

Fig. 1.14 Representation of a cascade gamma coincidence. The green line is the cascade gamma ray, the red line represents the colinear annihilation gamma rays, and the blue line is the recorded line of response which is mispositioned as it does not intersect with the point of annihilation

dences is shifted from the true annihilation location and has a uniform noise distribution similar to random coincidences and thus needs to be corrected. The uniform distribution is a result of the fact that cascade emissions are isotropic and not correlated with the annihilation photon orientation [36].

Cascade gamma correction is often combined with scatter correction. Sinograms are first corrected for randoms, attenuation, and dead time, then the shape of the cascade gamma distribution is estimated from a cascade gamma compensation (CGC) kernel and the shape of the SSS distribution is determined. Sinograms are masked to select activity outside the body contour which is assumed to contain only scatter and cascade gamma coincident events. Data outside the body is then fit to a combination of the CGC and SSS distributions, and after scaling these are subtracted from the data to produce a sinogram corrected for scatter and cascade gamma coincidences [36].

Correction for Detector Dead Time and Pulse Pile-Up

After a photon interacts with the scintillation crystal there is a time interval where the scintillation light is produced, converted into an electronic pulse, and finally into the square wave gate-pulse as shown in section "Radiation Detection and PET Detector Systems". If a second photon interacts with the detector while the first photon is still being processed, the secondary photon will not be detected. The electronic circuitry takes a finite time to integrate the incoming signal from the detector. During this time, any subsequent signals from the PMTs cannot be processed and the detector is effectively "dead" for a period of time known as the detector dead time. If the second photon occurs early during the detection process (before integration) the second photon is indistinguishable from the first photon and both photons are integrated together, according to the total energy absorbed. This combines the signal of the first photon to the signal of the second and is known as pulse pile-up.

The conversion time in scintillation takes <1 ps and is not a significant source of pile-up; however, there is a significant delay from transport to luminescence due to the time it takes to recapture the electron–hole pairs. The total decay time from conversion to luminescence (also known as the crystal response time) for BGO scintillation crystals is 300 ns and 40 ns for LYSO [37–39].

To illustrate the effect of detector dead time, Fig. 1.15 shows the ideal (true coincidences) count rate vs. the measured count rate. At low activities there are very few dead time or pile-up events; thus, the measured count rate and ideal count rate are almost the same and behave like a linear function. The ideal detector would have a linear response for all levels of activity, but due to events lost to detector dead time and to increase in random events, the coincidence count rate drops off at high activity levels. At high count rates the system response can become saturated where any further increase in total activity results in little to no increase in count rate.

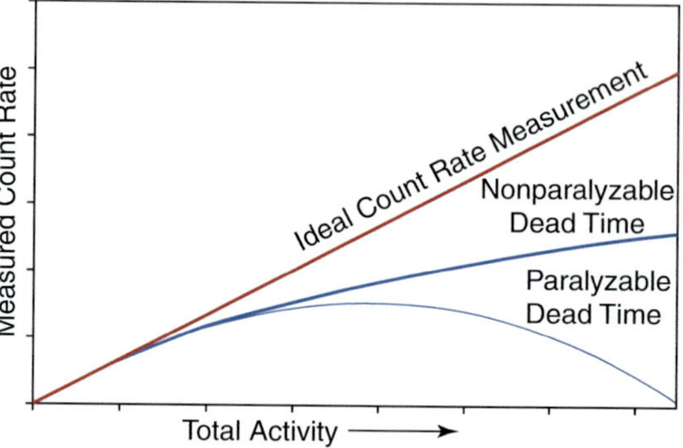

Fig. 1.15 Coincident count rate measurement as a function of activity in the scanner field of view, according to paralyzable and non-paralyzable dead time models. The ideal count rate (no dead time losses) would be linear increasing in proportion to total activity

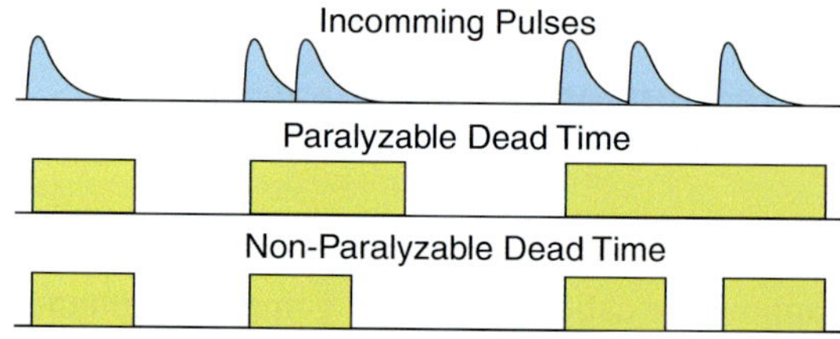

Fig. 1.16 Examples of paralyzable and non-paralyzable dead time responses. Length of dead time is extended for the paralyzable case when subsequent pulses arrive close enough together

Dead time effects are classified as paralyzable or non-paralyzable and illustrated in Fig. 1.16. The circuitry used for coincidence detection needs time to reset which creates non-paralyzable dead time. During non-paralyzable dead time the detector is insensitive to photon interactions for a fixed period of time, and any pulses arriving during this time are discarded. Paralyzable dead time is more complex since pulses arriving during the dead time effectively reset the integration clock, extending the length of the dead time. This process can continue to increase to a point where no additional photons are detected. All photons detected during this process are integrated together. PET detectors systems often consist of a combination of both paralyzable and non-paralyzable dead time effects.

The prompt coincidences (trues (T) + randoms (R) + scatter (S)) will have the same dead time losses as the randoms in a delayed window since both are acquired from timing windows of the same length. Randoms can be removed using a delayed window leaving just $T + S$ and should be proportional to the activity in the field of view following dead time correction.

The effect of dead time on the true count rate (T), randoms count rate (R), scatter count rate (S), and prompt count rate ($T + R + S$) is shown in Fig. 1.17. At low activity levels the randoms rate is lower than the scatter and/or trues rate and increases linearly with activity. For higher activity levels dead time becomes more significant; therefore, the randoms count rate will dominate. At very high activities, all measured count rates will decline as the system becomes saturated since the system bandwidth is reached.

Scanners can have paralyzable, non-paralyzable, or a combination of both dead time effects. For instance, the older GE Advance can be modeled by two paralyzable dead times, one at the individual crystal level (332 ns) and one at the block level (625 ns), whereas the GE D690 has a 200 ns paralyzable dead time at the block level (where pile-up occurs) followed by 200 ns non-paralyzable dead time required for the detector circuit to reset. Measured data is adjusted according to these system models to produce images where the corrected (trues) count rate is proportional to the isotope activity concentration. Modern scanners take advantage of fast computers and data transfer speeds, enabling high coincidence bandwidth limit (e.g. 1Gbit/s network data transfer rate can support ~15 Mcps using 64-bit event words) [40]. Newer scanners with extended axial field of view such as the EXPLORER (United Medical Imaging) and QUADRA (Siemens) have such high sensitivity that the injected activity must be limited to avoid uncorrectable dead time effects that will occur when the coincidence bandwidth is exceeded.

Correction for Photon Attenuation

As photons travel through the tissue medium some photons are absorbed or scattered out of the scanner field of view. These photons are removed from the detector system which causes a loss of counts. If this loss is not accounted for, the measured activity concentration in the patient would be underestimated. Reconstructed PET images before and after correction for attenuation are shown in Fig. 1.18.

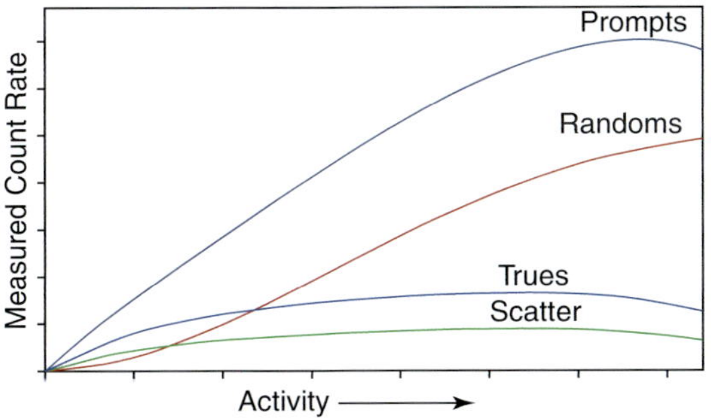

Fig. 1.17 Count rate measurement of true, scatter, and random events as well as total prompt coincident ($T + R + S$) events as a function of activity in the PET field of view

Fig. 1.18 PET images reconstructed without (top) and with (bottom) attenuation correction. The apparent distribution of tracer activity is markedly altered in the uncorrected images

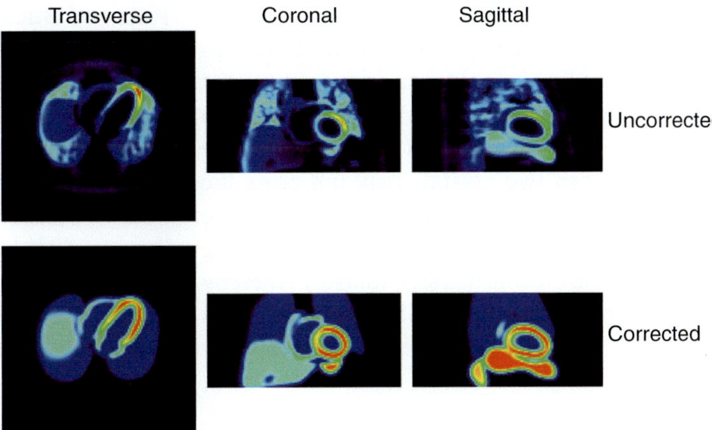

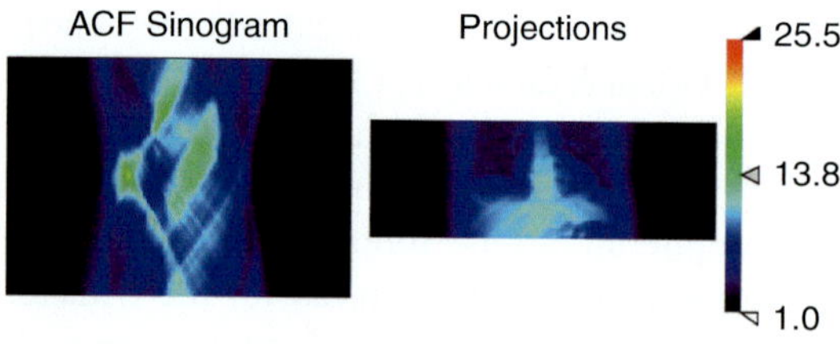

Fig. 1.19 ACF sinogram for a simulated heart scan (left) and projection view at a single angle (right). The ACF values are unit-less scalars used as a multiplicative correction of the recorded true coincidences

Modern PET systems include a computed tomography (CT) scanner for patient positioning and attenuation correction purposes. A secondary use for the CT is to correlate the regions of tracer uptake with the anatomical location of organs in the body. A CT produces a rotating X-ray source around the patient and measures the intensity of the photons that travel through the patient to a detector on the other side. This creates projection images of photon attenuation in Hounsfield units (HU) but can be converted to units of photon attenuation for 511 keV photons. Thus, CT images can be directly used to calculate the attenuation correction factor (ACF). CT projections can be stacked to form a multiplicative ACF sinogram for correction of PET sinograms as shown in Fig. 1.19 [41, 42].

Intrinsic and Reconstructed Spatial Resolution

In imaging, the minimum separation distance between two objects where both objects are distinguishable from each other is known as the spatial resolution. The assumption in PET imaging is that the lines of response correspond to the tracer position (decay events); however, due to positron range the resultant line of response (LOR) between two crystals may not cross the point of decay. This difference between the decay and annihilation positions adds a blurring effect to the reconstructed images, thereby reducing image resolution. Short-lived isotopes have more energetic positrons with correspond-

ingly larger positron ranges and thus lower image resolutions (Table 1.1). In addition, when positrons annihilate there may be some residual angular momentum which causes a ±0.5° angular distribution (non-collinearity) in the emission angles that can cause a small loss in image resolution (Fig. 1.1).

Annihilation photons are highly penetrating and if the incident angle to the crystal is not 90° it may penetrate the initial crystal and deposit some or all of its energy to the adjacent crystal. Crystal penetration causes the LOR to be assigned to the wrong crystal, which causes an asymmetric blurring effect in the radial direction. This effect becomes more pronounced for emissions nearer the edge of the detector ring.

Image Reconstruction from Projections

PET and CT imaging relies on the mathematics of tomographic image reconstruction which takes projection information and reconstructs an estimate of the 2D (or 3D) object. A projection is a collection of LOR at the same angle but with a spatial distribution across the object, i.e. spanning an image plane. In PET, a LOR is a summation of all coincident events that occur between two detectors. Reconstruction of projection information was first proposed by Johan Radon in 1917 and first applied to image reconstruction in 1956 [27, 43].

Filtered Back-Projection

The mathematical principles of image reconstruction start with the radon transform. By extending the radon transform with the projection slice theorem we can develop the inverse Fourier transform that is used to reconstruct the image function called a back-projection. However, this requires filtering and is thus called filtered back-projection [29, 44]. Due to the fact that this is an analytical model, this reconstruc-

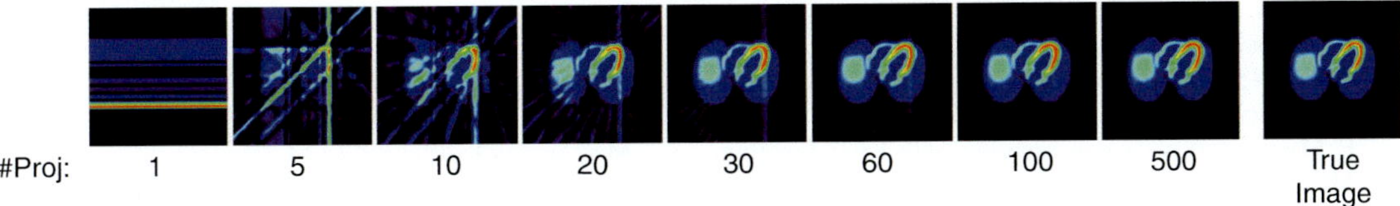

Fig. 1.20 Example of the effect of the number of projection angles on image reconstruction. The image reconstructed using 100 and 500 projections is nearly identical to the original image

tion method is easy to implement and fast to compute. However, back-projection lacks any modeling of the physical characteristics of PET imaging such as noise and sometimes produces negative values in the reconstructed image. Furthermore, insufficient projection information can lead to streaking effects. The effect on the number of projections for a filtered back-projection reconstruction is shown in Fig. 1.20. When a single projection angle is used, there is just one projection back-projected onto a blank matrix. The reconstructed image converges to the true object as the number of projection angles increases, with little improvement beyond 100 projection angles.

Iterative Reconstruction

The probability of detecting a number of events from a radiative process follows a Poisson distribution. By extending the probability of detecting a single event to the sum of all possible events and developing the maximum log-likelihood function from this mathematical framework, an iterative reconstruction algorithm is formed. Since this method takes into account the physics of radiation detection, noise can be accurately modeled as part of the reconstruction, and the reconstructed images do not suffer from streaking effects as seen with back-projection. In addition, a priori knowledge can be applied to remove the possibility of negative values in the reconstructed images. However, the algorithm is necessarily more complex and is therefore computationally expensive. Typically, clinical images are reconstructed using iterative reconstruction due to the advantages highlighted above.

References

1. Derenzo SE, Budinger TF, Huesman RH, Cahoon JL, Vuletich T. Imaging properties of a positron tomograph with 280 Bgo crystals. IEEE Trans Nucl Sci. 1981;28(1):81–9.
2. Jones T, Townsend D. History and future technical innovation in positron emission tomography. J Med Imaging (Bellingham). 2017;4(1):011013.
3. Dirac PAM, Fowler RH. A theory of electrons and protons. Proc R Soc Lond Ser Contain Pap Math Phys Character. 1930;126(801):360–5.
4. Anderson CD. The positive electron. Phys Rev. 1933;43(6):491–4.
5. Cattin P, Harders M, Hug J, Sierra R, Szekely G. Computer-supported segmentation of radiological data. In: Suri JS, Wilson DL, Laxminarayan S, editors. Handbook of biomedical image analysis. Segmentation models part B, vol. 2. Boston, MA: Springer US. p. 753–98. https://doi.org/10.1007/0-306-48606-7_14.
6. Zanzonico P. Positron emission tomography: a review of basic principles, scanner design and performance, and current systems. Semin Nucl Med. 2004;34(2):87–111.
7. Anderson CJ, Ferdani R. Copper-64 radiopharmaceuticals for PET imaging of cancer: advances in preclinical and clinical research. Cancer Biother Radiopharm. 2009;24(4):379–93.
8. Fujibayashi Y, Matsumoto K, Yonekura Y, Konishi J, Yokoyama A. A new zinc-62/copper-62 generator as a copper-62 source for PET radiopharmaceuticals. J Nucl Med. 1989;30(11):1838–42.
9. Zweit J, Goodall R, Cox M, Babich JW, Potter GA, Sharma HL, et al. Development of a high performance zinc-62/copper-62 radionuclide generator for positron emission tomography. Eur J Nucl Med. 1992;19(6):418–25.
10. Jødal L, Le Loirec C, Champion C. Positron range in PET imaging: non-conventional isotopes. Phys Med Biol. 2014;59(23):7419–34.
11. Jødal L, Le Loirec C, Champion C. Positron range in PET imaging: an alternative approach for assessing and correcting the blurring. Phys Med Biol. 2012;57(12):3931–43.
12. Conti M, Eriksson L. Physics of pure and non-pure positron emitters for PET: a review and a discussion. EJNMMI Phys. 2016;3(1):8.

13. Derenzo SE, Budinger TF. Resolution limit for positron-imaging devices. J Nucl Med. 1977;18(5):491.

14. Nakazato R, Berman DS, Alexanderson E, Slomka P. Myocardial perfusion imaging with PET. Imaging Med. 2013;5(1):35–46.

15. Balsara RD, Chapman SE, Sander IM, Donahue DL, Liepert L, Castellino FJ, et al. Non-invasive imaging and analysis of cerebral ischemia in living rats using positron emission tomography with 18F-FDG. J Vis Exp. 2014;94:51495.

16. Ramirez RA, Wong W-H, Kim S, Baghaei H, Li H, Wang Y, et al. A comparison of BGO, GSO, MLS, LGSO, LYSO and LSO scintillation materials for high-spatial-resolution animal PET detectors. In: IEEE nuclear science symposium conference record, vol. 2005; 2005. p. 2835–9.

17. Nikl M. Scintillation detectors for X-rays. Meas Sci Technol. 2006 Feb;10(17):R37.

18. Lecoq P. Scintillation detectors for charged particles and photons. In: Fabjan CW, Schopper H, editors. Particle physics reference library: volume 2: detectors for particles and radiation. Cham: Springer; 2020. p. 45–89. https://doi.org/10.1007/978-3-030-35318-6_3.

19. Melcher CL. Scintillation crystals for PET. J Nucl Med. 2000;41(6):1051–5.

20. Casey ME, Nutt R. A multicrystal two dimensional BGO detector system for positron emission tomography. IEEE Trans Nucl Sci. 1986;33(1):460–3.

21. Herman GT, Carvalho BM. Simultaneous fuzzy segmentation of medical images. In: Suri JS, Wilson DL, Laxminarayan S, editors. Handbook of biomedical image analysis. Segmentation models part B, vol. 2. Boston, MA: Springer; 2005. p. 661–705. https://doi.org/10.1007/0-306-48606-7_12.

22. Roncali E, Cherry SR. Application of silicon photomultipliers to positron emission tomography. Ann Biomed Eng. 2011;39(4):1358–77.

23. Marrocchesi PS, Bagliesi MG, Batkov K, Bigongiari G, Kim MY, Lomtadze T, et al. Active control of the gain of a 3 mm×3 mm silicon PhotoMultiplier. Nucl Instrum Meth Phys Res A. 2009;602:391–5.

24. Mirzoyan R, Laatiaoui M, Teshima M. Very high quantum efficiency PMTs with bialkali photocathode. Nucl Instrum Meth Phys Res Sect Accel Spectr Detect Assoc Equip. 2006;567(1):230–2.

25. Dam H, Vinke R, Dendooven D, Loehner H, Beekman F, Schaart D. A comprehensive model of the response of silicon photomultipliers. Nucl Sci IEEE Trans. 2010;57:2254–66.

26. Jha AK, van Dam HT, Kupinski MA, Clarkson E. Simulating silicon photomultiplier response to scintillation light. IEEE Trans Nucl Sci. 2013;30(1):336–51.

27. Radon J. On the determination of functions from their integral values along certain manifolds. IEEE Trans Med Imaging. 1986;5(4):170–6.

28. Fahey FH. Data Acquisition in PET Imaging. J Nucl Med Technol. 2002;30(2):39–49.

29. Prince JL, Links J. Medical imaging signals and systems. 1st ed. Upper Saddle River, NJ: Prentice Hall; 2005. p. 496.

30. Turkington TG. Introduction to PET instrumentation. J Nucl Med Technol. 2001;29(1):4–11.

31. Bettinardi V, Presotto L, Rapisarda E, Picchio M, Gianolli L, Gilardi MC. Physical performance of the new hybrid PET/CT Discovery-690. Med Phys. 2011;38(10):5394–411.

32. Anna M, Oddbjørn K, Live S, Erik EP. Quantitative comparison of PET performance—Siemens Biograph mCT and mMR. EJNMMI Physics. Goa. 2016;3(1):5. https://doi.org/10.1186/s40658-016-0142-7.

33. Kjærnes S, Birger ØL, Live A, Maria EA. Image quality and detectability in Siemens Biograph PET/MRI and PET/CT systems—a phantom study. EJNMMI Physics. Karlberg. 2019;6(1):16. https://doi.org/10.1186/s40658-019-0251-1.

34. Ollinger JM. Model-based scatter correction for fully 3D PET. Phys Med Biol. 1996;41(1):153–76.

35. Watson CC, Newport D, Casey ME. A single scatter simulation technique for scatter correction in 3D PET. In: Grangeat P, Amans J-L, editors. Three-dimensional image reconstruction in radiology and nuclear medicine. Dordrecht: Springer; 1996. p. 255–68. https://doi.org/10.1007/978-94-015-8749-5_18.

36. Moncayo VM, Garcia EV. Prompt-gamma compensation in Rb-82 myocardial perfusion 3D PET/CT: effect on clinical practice. J Nucl Cardiol. 2018;25(2):606–8.

37. Positron Emission Tomography. Clinical practice. Radiology. 2007;244(2):380.

38. Moszynski M, Kapusta M, Wolski D, Szawlowski M, Klamra W. Energy resolution of scintillation detectors readout with large area avalanche photodiodes and photomultipliers. IEEE Trans Nucl Sci. 1998;45(3):472–7.

39. ter Weele DN, Schaart DR, Dorenbos P. Scintillation detector timing resolution; a study by ray tracing software. IEEE Trans Nucl Sci. 2015;62(5):1972–80.

40. Count rate lost model for D690. GE; 2015.

41. Ostertag H, Kübler WK, Doll J, Lorenz WJ. Measured attenuation correction methods. Eur J Nucl Med. 1989;15(11):722–6.

42. Kinahan PE, Townsend DW, Beyer T, Sashin D. Attenuation correction for a combined 3D PET/CT scanner. Med Phys. 1998;25(10):2046–53.

43. Bracewell RN. Strip integration in radio astronomy. Aust J Phys. 1956;9:198.

44. Scudder HJ. Introduction to computer aided tomography. Proc IEEE. 1978;66(6):628–37.

Yoann Petibon, Chao Ma, Jinsong Ouyang, and Georges El Fakhri

Introduction

Hybrid positron emission tomography (PET) and magnetic resonance (MR) (PET/MR) is rapidly gaining momentum as a powerful imaging modality for both clinical and basic research applications. The first clinical whole-body PET/MR systems were FDA-cleared and installed in 2010. Since then, the number of systems in use worldwide has grown steadily, with ~260 fully integrated PET/MRs installed globally at the end of 2020 (Fig. 2.1a). The expanding base of installed scanners in the last decade has been accompanied with very active research, both fundamental and clinical, with over 4250 articles referencing PET/MR by the end of 2020 (Fig. 2.1b). At its most basic level, PET/MR combines the strengths of each modality, enabling imaging of physiology with the exceptional molecular sensitivity of PET complemented with the high-resolution structural information of MRI and its multitude of complementary functional (e.g., perfusion) and molecular (e.g., spectroscopy) measurements. Besides the superior soft-tissue contrast of MRI as compared to computed tomography (CT) as well as its unique ability to probe tissue composition, the use of MRI as the

anatomical complement to PET comes with the benefit of a lower effective radiation exposure in PET/MR as compared to PET/CT, which is a significant advantage for pediatric applications and protocols that require serial imaging, e.g., for staging and monitoring response to therapy. Furthermore, the intrinsic spatial and temporal alignment of PET and MR data in fully integrated PET/MR machines can be exploited to perform MR-based motion correction of PET [1] and anatomically guided PET reconstruction [2] for partial volume effect correction and noise control, yielding substantial improvements in PET image quality and accuracy. Last but not least, simultaneous PET/MR offers opportunities to quantify physiological processes that would otherwise be difficult to assay with either modality alone as demonstrated in cardiac imaging with quantitative mapping of mitochondrial membrane potential using a voltage-sensitive PET tracer and MRI-based measurement of myocardial extracellular volume fraction [3–5].

PET/MR has been the subject of active interdisciplinary research aimed at developing solutions for many of the physical (e.g., instrumentation) and practical (e.g., attenuation correction) challenges associated with this hybrid imaging modality. Furthermore, thorough research has been undertaken to take full advantage of the unique opportunities (e.g., motion correction) of this imaging technique in specific clinical applications. The aim of this chapter is to

Y. Petibon · C. Ma · J. Ouyang · G. El Fakhri (✉)
Gordon Center for Medical Imaging, Department of Radiology, Harvard Medical School, Massachusetts General Hospital, Boston, MA, USA
e-mail: elfakhri.georges@mgh.harvard.edu

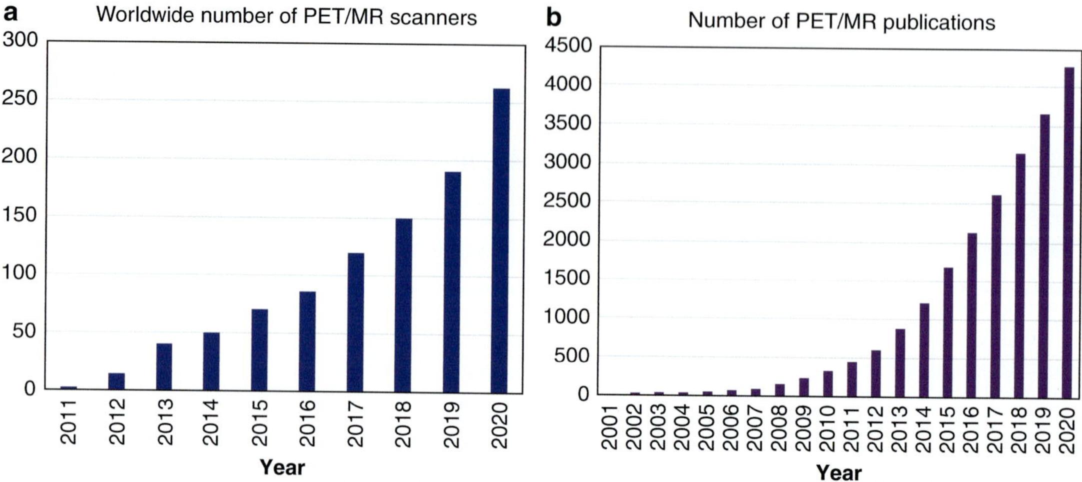

Fig. 2.1 (**a**) Number of PET/MR scanners installed worldwide. (Source: Siemens Healthineers, GE Healthcare, United Imaging). (**b**) Number of PET/MR publications. (Source: PubMed)

provide a brief overview of the challenges and opportunities associated with PET/MR, with a particular emphasis given to cardiac imaging applications. We also briefly present current clinical applications as well as future directions in cardiac MR imaging in the context of PET/MR.

PET/MR Instrumentation

The integration of PET and MRI scanners into a single machine represents a significant engineering achievement owing to the mutual interferences and crosstalk between the two systems [6, 7]. Indeed, all components needed for the formation and acquisition of MR signals (e.g., static main magnetic field (B0), radiofrequency field (B1), and gradient fields) can affect the normal operation of standard PET detectors and electronics, therefore necessitating the development of specific MRI compatible instrumentation for combined PET/MR scanners. For example, the photomultiplier tubes (PMTs) that had traditionally been used in PET detectors for signal amplification cannot be operated in the presence of even small magnetic fields, as electromagnetic forces perturb the movement of electrons down the chain of dynodes in the PMT and significantly impair its amplification power [6]. Integrated PET/MR scanners instead rely on a different type of photodetector technologies such as avalanche

photodiodes (APDs) [8] or silicon photomultipliers (SiPMs) [9], which are largely insensitive to magnetic fields. Likewise, the introduction of PET instrumentation (e.g., scintillation crystals, electronics, shielding) into the bore of the magnet can affect MRI data acquisition by distorting the B_0 and B_1 fields and the linearity of the gradient fields, resulting in image artifacts. For example, PET scintillation crystals that contain gadolinium such as LGSO (lutetium gadolinium orthosilicate) are not suitable for use in PET/MR due to their high magnetic susceptibility [10]. Hybrid PET/MR systems thus employ detectors made with materials such as lutetium-yttrium oxyorthosilicate (LYSO). There are also physical constraints associated with integrating a PET scanner within an MRI gantry since the two systems have outer bores in the range of ~1 m diameter, requiring the PET instrumentation to be very compact in order to fit into the bore. In this regard, APDs and SiPMs are not only MRI compatible but also much less voluminous than PMTs and therefore represent a particularly well-suited technology for PET/MR. Nevertheless, combined PET/MR systems all have narrow bores (about 60 cm diameter), which can cause practical difficulties for studying large or claustrophobic patients.

Four clinical whole-body (WB) PET/MR scanners have been introduced commercially so far. The first WB PET/MR machine was released by Philips Healthcare in 2010 with the TF

Ingenuity [11]. Unlike the systems that followed, the TF Ingenuity PET/MR allowed for sequential—as opposed to simultaneous—PET and MRI scanning, with each system physically separated from the other to minimize interferences, and a rotating bed shuttling the patient between the two gantries. In spite of the physical separation between the two scanners, magnetic shielding still had to be introduced within the design of the PET scanner to allow its detectors—based on conventional PMTs and LYSO crystals (size: 4 ×4 ×22 mm^3)—to properly function. Shortly after, Siemens Healthcare introduced the Biograph mMR, the first fully integrated WB system capable of simultaneous PET and MR acquisition [12]. The Biograph mMR is a hybrid PET/MR system consisting of a 3-T whole-body MRI scanner and a PET gantry installed between the gradient and body coils. The PET detector system employs lutetium oxyorthosilicate (LSO) scintillators (4 ×4 ×20 mm^3) coupled with APD arrays and allows an axial coverage of 25.8-cm, compared to the 18-cm axial FOV of the Ingenuity TF. In 2015, General Electric (GE) released the Signa PET/MR [13, 14] the first integrated PET/MR machine with time-of-flight (TOF) capability. The MRI component of the Signa is based on 3-T Discovery 750w MRI platform and the PET detector system employs lutetium-based scintillators ("LBS," size: 3.95× 5.3× 25 mm^3) coupled to SiPMs, offering a 394 ps TOF timing resolution and a 25 cm axial FOV [14]. The uPMR 790 is another integrated TOF PET/MR system recently introduced by United Imaging Healthcare [15]. The scanner comprises a 3-T superconducting magnet and a PET system consisting of LYSO crystals (size: 2.76× 2.76× 15.5 mm^3) also coupled with SiPMs. The system has a timing resolution at ~540 ps [15] and its axial field of view is 32 cm long, the largest among all currently available commercial PET/MR scanners.

As mentioned above, all integrated clinical WB PET/MR scanners rely on solid-state photodetectors such as APDs or SiPMs. Both devices are silicon semiconductor photodetectors, based on a modified p-n junction with an external bias voltage applied for charge carrier acceleration [9]. Because the distances traveled by the charges in the APD and SiPM are small, these photodetectors are largely insensitive to magnetic fields [6, 16, 17]. Though APDs are MRI compatible and highly compact, their amplification performance strongly depends on the temperature and the strength of the applied voltage [6], which requires very tight control of these parameters for stable operation. Furthermore, APDs have a much lower gain than conventional PMTs as well as a poor timing resolution, precluding measurement of photon TOF. The SiPM is an alternative photodetector technology consisting of a 2-D array of thousands of APDs operated in Geiger mode (i.e., with a bias voltage higher than the breakdown voltage). In the SiPM, each Geiger APD within the detector array effectively operates as a single photon counter and is processed independently and simultaneously with the other ones [6, 9]. SiPMs have a very high gain, equivalent or higher than that of conventional PMTs, as well as an excellent timing resolution, which enables TOF measurement.

Attenuation Correction

Attenuation correction (AC) is critical to obtain quantitatively accurate PET images. Until the introduction of hybrid PET/computed tomography (CT) systems in the early 2000s, standalone PET cameras employed rotating positron-emitting transmission sources to directly measure attenuation of annihilation photons. In PET/CT scanners, attenuation maps are derived from low-dose CT images by exploiting the linear relationships that exist between CT Hounsfield units (HU) and attenuation coefficients at 511 keV [18]. However, none of the commercially available PET/MR systems is equipped with a CT gantry or a transmission source, meaning that attenuation maps must be obtained from MR images [19, 20]. Generating accurate MR-based attenuation maps for human tissues is technically very challenging as there is no direct relationship between the tissue properties measured by MRI (e.g., proton density, relaxation times) and the underlying electron densities which determine the linear attenuation coefficients. For instance, tissues such as bone and lung exhibit drastic differences in the degree to which they attenuate annihilation photons, yet both show very low MRI signals when imaged by conventional pulse sequence because of their ultra-short T_2^* relaxation times (<1 ms) and low proton densities.

MR-based AC (MRAC) in PET/MR has been the subject of extensive research and several approaches have been investigated. The most widely used MRAC method consists in segmenting MR images of the subject into different tissue classes and then to assign a discrete attenuation coefficient to each tissue type [19, 20]. The most commonly used segmentation-based MRAC

method relies on a fast 3D two-point Dixon acquisition for water/fat separation. The acquired in-phase and out-phase images are then used to generate piecewise constant PET attenuation maps with four compartments: air, lung, fat and non-fat soft tissue [19]. Though widely used in PET/MR scanners, this approach has several limitations, the principal one being that it incorrectly assigns the attenuation coefficient of soft tissue to cortical bones. This underestimation of attenuation effects introduces substantial quantitation errors within the bones themselves and in tissues located in their vicinity [21, 22] (Fig. 2.2).

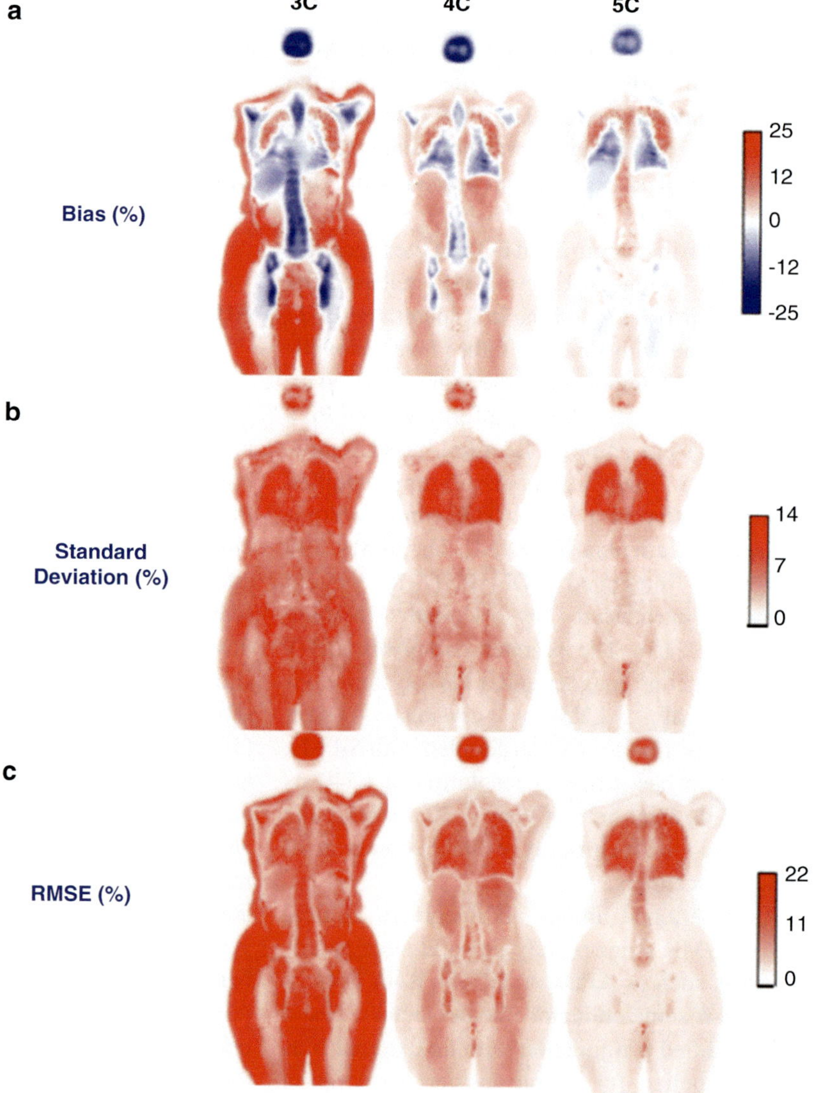

Fig. 2.2 Whole-body atlases of mean (**a**), standard deviation (**b**), and root mean-squared error ("RMSE," **c**) ^{18}F-FDG SUV bias computed based on 23 patient data sets for different segmentation-based attenuation correction methods. 3-classes ("3C": air, lung, soft-tissue), 4-classes ("4C": air, lung, fat, non-fat soft-tissue), and 5-classes ("5C": air, lung, fat, non-fat soft-tissue, bone) attenuation maps. (Reproduced from [24], with permission)

Besides bones, tissue misclassification errors have been reported in other body locations such as the bronchus, causing further image artifacts [23]. Nevertheless, the bias in activity estimates reported within soft tissue organs such as the heart, liver, and kidney remains relatively small with these approaches, in the range of a few percent typically [24]. To obtain bone information for MRAC, methods leveraging special pulse sequences with very short echo times such as UTE (ultrashort-echo-time), ZTE (zero-echo-time), or combination of UTE/ZTE with Dixon acquisitions have been investigated in brain [25–28] and pelvic [29] imaging applications. However, these approaches come at the price of longer acquisition times and often require some level of human intervention, e.g., during bone segmentation [29]. A second type of approach to MRAC generates attenuation maps that can account for bones by registering image data from individual subjects to pre-computed attenuation atlases/templates, as shown in brain [30–32] and whole-body [33] imaging. These methods have been found to offer accurate results in the brain [34]; however, their application in body imaging remains challenging due to the larger subject-to-subject variability in terms of anatomy, body mass index, and/or disease [35]. Furthermore, atlas-based methods are intrinsically limited in their ability to account for subject-specific variations in bone density and structure. A third category of MRAC techniques employs machine learning to synthesize pseudo-CT distributions from MR images in a fully automated fashion [36–40] (Fig. 2.3). These methods usually rely on deep convolutional neural networks (CNNs) to learn a nonlinear mapping between input MRI data (e.g., Dixon data only [36, 40], Dixon-ZTE [37], multi-echo Dixon/UTE [38]) and ground-truth CT attenuation during a training step, using patch- [37] or slice-based [36, 38] approaches. CNNs are a specific kind of artificial neural net-

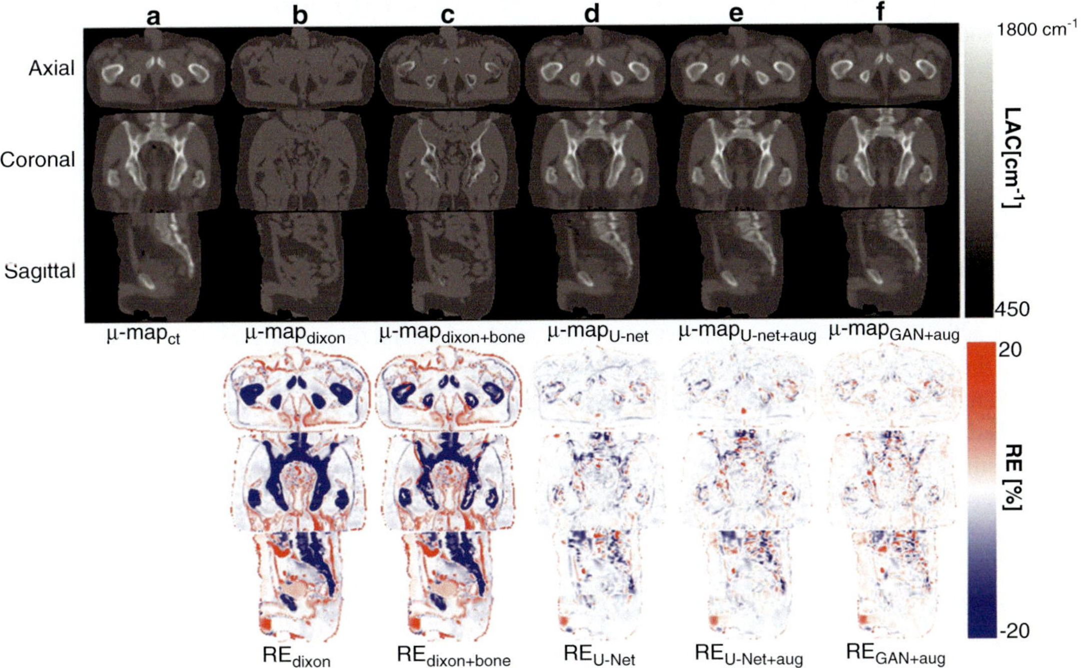

Fig. 2.3 Comparison of attenuation maps in the pelvic region obtained using (**a**): CT (μ-map$_{CT}$); (**b**): the standard Dixon MRI-based method (μ-map$_{dixon}$), (**c**): Dixon MRI with atlas-based bone information (μ-map$_{dixon + bone}$); and (**d–f**): deep learning based algorithms (μ-map$_{U\text{-}net}$, μ-map$_{U\text{-}net + aug}$, and μ-map$_{GAN + aug}$). Overall, there is excellent correlation between CT and the different deep-learning approaches. The lower panel displays images of relative differences between the different attenuation maps and the reference CT. (Reproduced from [40], with permission)

works specialized for the analysis of image data. Deep CNNs typically operate by applying a series of filtering and down/upsampling operations designed to extract the most relevant features of the input data for the task at hand. The parameters of the deep CNN (e.g., filters' coefficients) are learned during a training phase in which a cost-function measuring the discrepancy between outputs of the deep CNN (e.g., "pseudo-CT" image) and the labels (e.g., ground-truth CT image) is minimized. Deep learning based MRAC algorithms have been shown to provide accurate results in the pelvis [36, 37, 40] and brain [38, 39], typically within a few percent of the reference CT-based results. However, their performance has yet to be fully evaluated in large patient cohorts.

The challenge of attenuation correction in PET/MR is further complicated by the so-called truncation artifacts [20]. Indeed, the transaxial FOV of MRI is usually restricted to a sphere of 25 cm radius around the isocenter where the B0 field has the best uniformity, meaning that attenuating tissues positioned toward the edges of the bore cannot be imaged accurately and display severe geometric distortions or even signal voids and truncation [41]. For instance, thoracic PET/MR studies with arms-down often truncate the MR signal from the arms, complicating the estimation of attenuation effects from the truncated tissues. If uncorrected, truncation artifacts in the attenuation maps can lead to bias in the reconstructed activity distributions that extend well beyond the missing tissues. Different methods have been developed to address this problem. PET-based approaches, such as maximum likelihood estimation of activity and attenuation (MLAA) [42, 43], seek to estimate body contours from the emission data themselves. However, the quality of MLAA-based correction depends on the type of tracer used and inaccurate results have been reported with tracers that show low accumulation in the extremities such as ^{68}Ga-PSMA [41]. MR-based methods for truncation correction include "B0 Homogenization Using Gradient Enhancement" (HUGE) [41, 44], which effectively extends the MR FOV beyond its traditional limits. Unlike MLAA, this approach is agnostic

to the radiotracer used during the study and was found to provide more robust performance than (non-TOF) MLAA-based methods across different tracers [41].

Finally, PET/MR scanning of the body often requires the use of flexible radiofrequency (RF) surface coils for MR data acquisition, which are made of various materials such as plastic and rubber as well as high attenuating components such as the hardware used for electronic circuitry [45]. These RF coils are located in the PET FOV during the acquisition but are not accounted for by current attenuation correction schemes since their position and individual geometries are in practice unknown in whole-body scans. Studies have reported PET count losses in the range of 2–5% due to these flexible RF coils and substantial underestimation of the reconstructed activity concentration in the vicinity of the high attenuating electronic hardware components [46].

Motion Correction

Signal-to-noise ratio (SNR) in PET primarily depends on the number of coincidence events acquired during the scan. Consequently, acquisition times typically extend over several minutes for each bed position (and even up to 1 or 2 h for some dynamic studies), making PET particularly susceptible to patient movement, both involuntary (e.g., respiration and cardiac contractions) and voluntary (e.g., body motion). Cardiac PET studies are especially subject to motion effects as the heart undergoes the simultaneous action of respiratory motion, shifting the heart by more than 1 cm along the superior–inferior direction [47], and cardiac contractions, moving the base of the heart toward the apex by an average of ~12 mm [48] while thickening the wall by ~4–6 mm [49]. In addition to these pseudo-cyclic physiologic displacements, subjects may move in a completely unpredictable manner during the PET scan, e.g., due to discomfort, pain, coughing, or deep breathing, and such body movements are more likely to occur during longer acquisitions, e.g., dynamic PET studies. The continuous motion of organs during scanning introduces artifacts that alter quantification of tracer concentration in moving tissues and deteriorate the diagnostic quality of PET images. Two types of image artifacts result from motion. One presents as a spatially dependent smearing (or blurring) of the reconstructed activity distributions, reducing the effective PET spatial resolution and introducing errors in estimates of local radioactivity concentration. The other stems from spatial inconsistencies between the attenuation map—acquired during a breath-hold in standard PET/CT and PET/MR protocols—and the emission data, which can be treated as acquired at an average position over many motion phases, cardiac/respiratory cycles, and body poses. Motion-induced emission/attenuation discrepancies can introduce severe image artifacts primarily in regions adjacent to large attenuation gradients (e.g., heart/lung and liver/lung interfaces), deteriorating the diagnostic value of PET [50, 51].

Integrated PET/MR systems are uniquely capable of providing an accurate and robust solution to the motion problem in PET [1, 52–57]. Indeed, owing to its lack of ionizing radiation, excellent soft-tissue contrast, high SNR, and very good spatiotemporal resolution, MRI has ideal characteristics for measuring organ motion. Furthermore, because of the simultaneity and inherent alignment between the two modalities, MRI-derived motion information can be leveraged to compensate motion effects in PET images. MR-based motion correction of PET has been investigated extensively in recent years, with applications in imaging of the brain [58, 59], thoracic or abdominal malignancies [60–69], and heart [64, 70–79].

MR-based PET motion correction approaches are generally quite complex, involving a coordinated set of MR sequences, PET acquisitions, and data postprocessing steps that often need to be customized depending on the targeted body region (e.g., brain vs. heart) and the type of motion to be corrected (e.g., physiologic vs. bulk motion) [55]. Figure 2.4 presents a general PET/MR data acquisition and processing pipeline for cardiac/respiratory motion correction. The first step is a PET/MR scan involving the acquisition of an attenuation map followed by a special pulse sequence designed to capture organ motion during PET data acquisition in list mode, in which each coincidence event is recorded as to its time of acquisition. Motion measurement sequences are usually customized for capturing the specific motion of the organ or body region of interest. For instance, tagged MRI [80] can be employed to measure contractile motion of the myocardium [81, 82] but it is not practical to use tagging for measuring respiratory motion of the heart as tag patterns fade more rapidly than a typical respiratory cycle. Alternatively, T2-prepared bright blood MRI sequences might be better suited for measuring heart respiratory displacements [77]. Another critical aspect of the PET/MR acquisition scheme pertains to the tracking of motion phases as a function of scan time, such that each coincidence event and MR k-space readout can be gated, i.e., assigned a specific motion phase. Cardiac motion phase tracking can be achieved quite robustly with electrocardiogram (ECG) devices. For respiratory motion, phase tracking can be performed via 1-D navigator echoes [63, 83] or low-resolution 2-D image navigator modules [69, 77] inserted in the motion measurement sequence, or using respiratory bellows or list-mode PET-driven signals [62, 81, 84]. Phase tracking signals are then used to construct motion-resolved MR volumes, i.e., 3D images of the subject's anatomy in the different motion instants, and to bin the PET coincidence events into the different phases. The next step is motion estimation which is typically performed by registering the MR volumes from the different phases to a reference one, although some groups have also investigated registration algorithms that make use of both PET and MR images [79]. This step produces motion vector fields (i.e., dense sets of 3D displacements), describing the voxel-to-voxel spatial coordinate correspondence between each motion phase and the reference phase. A motion-dependent attenuation map can then be synthesized by applying the estimated motion vector fields to the acquired attenuation map after aligning it to the reference MR volume to compensate for potential discrepancies. At last, the motion fields and motion-dependent attenuation maps can be integrated within itera-

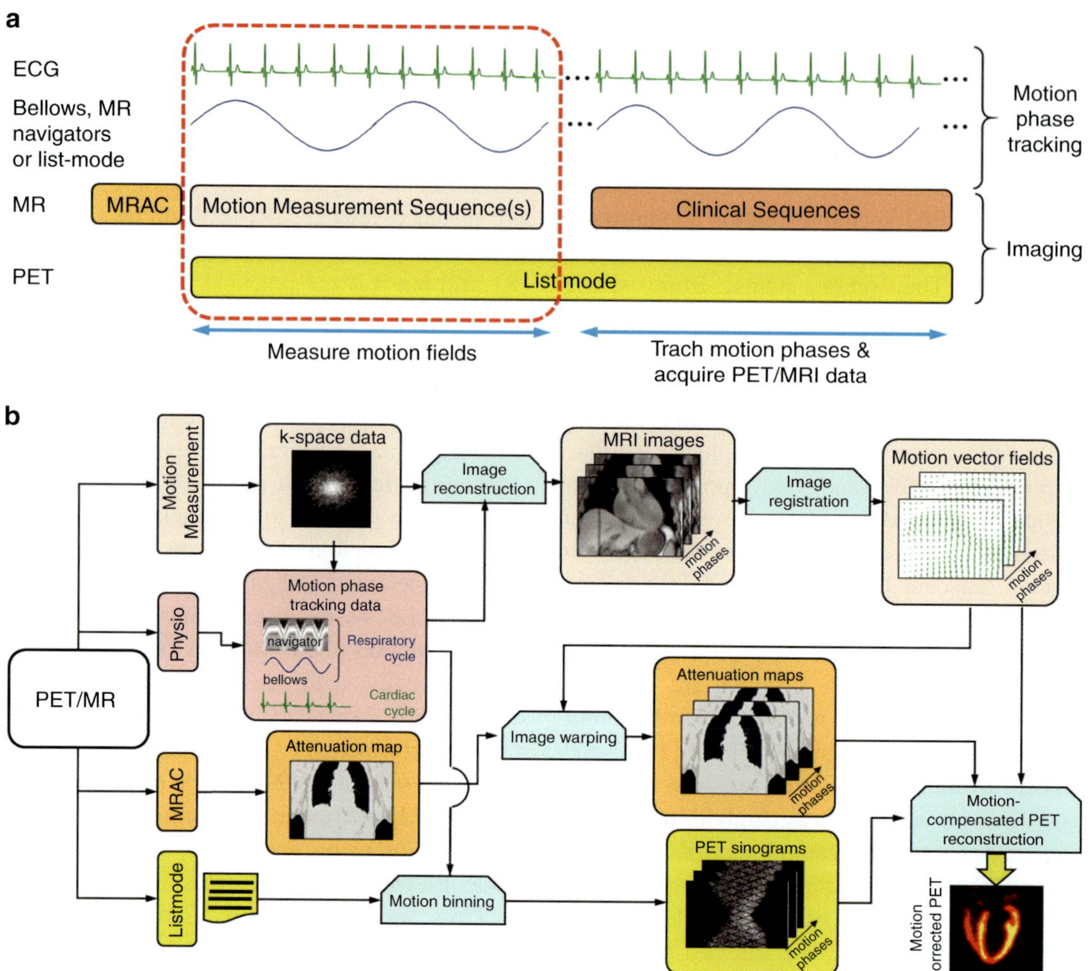

Fig. 2.4 Schematic representation of PET/MR data acquisition (**a**) and processing pipeline (**b**) for MR-based motion correction of PET

tive PET reconstruction [85, 86] to correct motion effects. An alternative approach that is also easier to implement is to independently reconstruct each gated PET volume using standard algorithms and then to apply the estimated motion fields to align them to the reference phase, followed by averaging of the resulting images. Figure 2.5 illustrates the impact of MR-based PET motion correction in myocardial perfusion imaging [82] using ^{18}F-flurpiridaz [87].

It is worth noting that the pulse sequences used for motion field measurement are usually not part of the diagnostic MR protocol and clinical sequences are thus played either before or after these acquisitions. In theory, it is possible

to make use of the PET data acquired during diagnostic MR imaging for motion correction by continuing the acquisition of motion phase tracking signals as illustrated in Fig. 2.4a. As for respiratory motion phase tracking, while it is technically possible to incorporate MR navigators into clinical pulse sequences, modifying every sequence across all manufacturers is impractical; additionally, navigator acquisitions can interfere with the normal operation of other sequences. A more practical approach is to rely on external sensors or methods that do not interfere with the MR or PET acquisition such as respiratory bellows or list-mode driven respiratory gating [84].

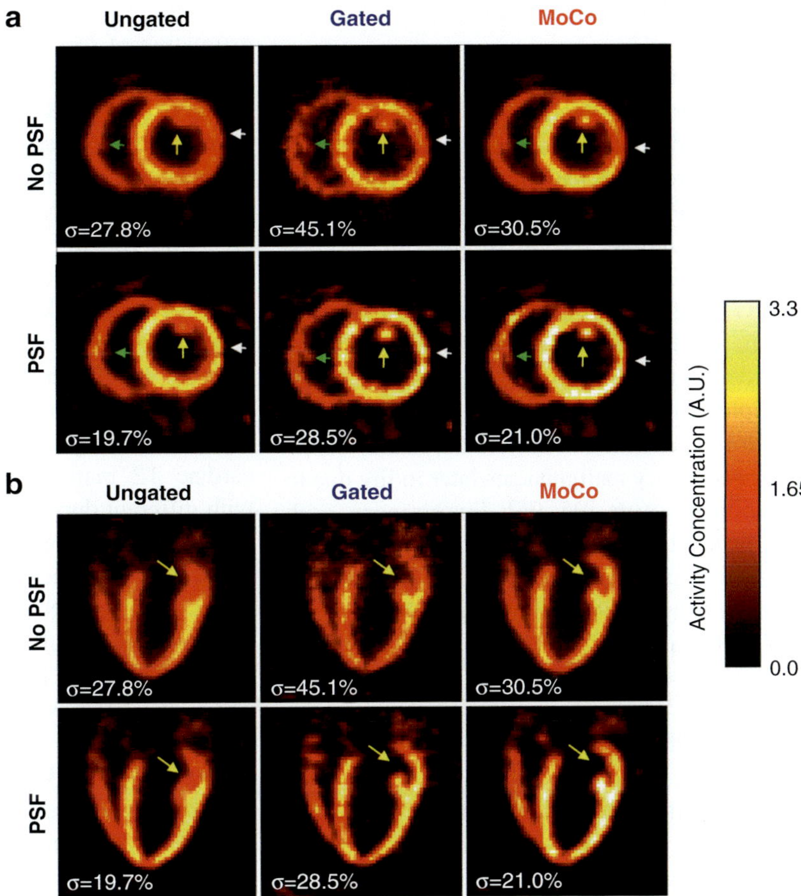

Fig. 2.5 Impact of motion and point spread function (PSF) correction in ^{18}F-Flurpiridaz PET/MR myocardial perfusion imaging (swine model). (**a**) and (**b**), respectively, show short- and long-axis PET images reconstructed without motion correction ("Ungated"), cardiac gating ("Gated," end-diastole), and motion correction ("Moco") based on a tagged MRI acquisition, each without and with PSF modeling. MR-based motion correction leads to higher image resolution as evidenced by improved visibility of the papillary muscles as compared to no motion correction. (Reproduced from [82], with permission)

Owing to the unpredictability of body motion, its tracking and measurement using MRI would effectively require playing a dedicated structural (or navigator) sequence continuously during the PET acquisition [88]. An alternative and arguably more practical strategy is to rely on PET-driven methods [89–91]. One possible approach is to divide the PET list-mode data into temporal frames of relatively short duration (a few seconds, typically) and then to reconstruct the data in each frame using ultra-fast list-mode based reconstruction algorithms [89]. The resulting images can then be used to determine motion fields between each frame and a selected reference one using image registration. In cases where the activity distribution changes rapidly, during a dynamic study, for instance, registration can be performed between temporally adjacent frames to improve motion estimation. Note that the same approach could be used to account for both body and respiration motion if very short time frames (e.g., <1 s) are employed, although PET image noise may degrade the performance of motion estimation and correction. An alternative PET-driven strategy for body motion correction consists in computing the coordinates of the activity distribution's center of mass ("COM") [91] or center of detection [90] ("COD"—if TOF is available) from the list-mode data as a function of scan time. Analysis of the extracted traces can then be used to detect motion under the assumption that body movements cause abrupt changes in COM or COD coordinates. List-mode scan data can then be parsed into frames accordingly, reconstructed and registered for motion estimation and correction [90, 91].

Radiation Dose Reduction

PET/MRI offers a substantially reduced radiation exposure compared with PET/CT owing to the elimination of CT and the associated radiation dose from the patient workup. For whole body examinations, a potential reduction in effective radiation exposure of up to 80% can be achieved with PET/MRI relative to standard PET/CT [92–94]. This represents a significant benefit for children and young adult populations considering the cumulative dose associated with multiple examinations, e.g. for staging, therapy monitoring, and follow-up, and the risk of developing secondary malignancies later in life due to radiation exposure [95, 96]. Furthermore, with MR acquisition protocols generally requiring longer time per bed position, it may also be possible to further reduce the injected tracer dose in PET/MR examinations [95].

Cardiac MRI

Because of its high spatial and temporal resolution and excellent soft-tissue contrast, cardiac MRI is recognized as the reference method for myocardial tissue characterization and ventricular function assessment, providing structural and functional information of the heart complementary to the molecular information from PET [97]. Conventional T1- and T2-contrast weighted cardiac MR sequences, such as late gadolinium enhancement (LGE) and fast spin-echo (FSE), provide qualitative assessment of the myocardium but are limited in their ability to detect and grade diffuse diseases. Cardiac parametric mapping methods, including T1, T2, and T2* mapping, can address these limitations by providing quantitative characterization of myocardial tissue composition [98]. The longitudinal relaxation time (T1) characterizes alterations in the structure and intra/extracellular components of the myocardium. Modified Look-Locker inversion recovery (MOLLI) is a widely used method for cardiac T1 mapping [99]. It utilizes inversion recovery (IR) pulses followed by ECG-gated balanced steady-state free precession (bSSFP)

acquisitions over multiple cardiac cycles to allow estimation of myocardial T1 in a single breath-hold. A variety of inversion- and/or saturation-recovery schemes have been developed to improve the accuracy of T1 mapping [100]. The extracellular volume fraction (ECV), measured from pre- and post-contrast T1 values, is an emerging biomarker for diffuse fibrosis, e.g., in heart failure, dilated cardiomyopathy, and amyloidosis, which is known to be particularly challenging to detect using the conventional LGE method [98]. The transverse relaxation time (T2) is sensitive to changes in water content of the myocardium, e.g. in presence of edema [101]. In cardiac T2 mapping, T2 preparation modules with different durations are inserted in each cardiac cycle followed by ECG-gated bSSFP or spoiled gradient echo (GRE) acquisitions with breath-holding [98]. The T2* relaxation time reflects the decay of the transverse magnetization in the presence of local B0 field inhomogeneity and is used for assessment of myocardial iron load. Cardiac T2* mapping is often performed using ECG-gated GRE acquisitions at different echo times with breath-holding [98]. Finally, cardiac cine MR imaging is the gold standard approach to assessing ventricular function, including ejection fraction, myocardial mass, and myocardial wall motion [102].

All current commercial PET/MR scanners operate at 3 T. Compared to 1.5 T, cardiac MR at 3 T faces several unique challenges. Due to the more severe B0 inhomogeneity at 3 T, sequences using bSSFP acquisitions are prone to the well-known banding artifacts, imposing challenges in B0 shimming and preventing from 3D cardiac imaging. In addition, transmit B1 variations on the order of 30–60% over the left ventricle have been reported [103], causing bias in the estimated T1 values at 3 T. Besides the above hardware-related challenges, cardiac and respiratory motions cause significant difficulties in cardiac MR. As a result, commercially available cardiac parametric mapping sequences are 2D imaging sequences with breath-holding acquisitions, which limit both the resolution and spatial coverage in the slice selective direction. Furthermore, acquiring multiple parametric maps (T1, T2, etc.)

prolongs the total imaging time. Therefore, very active research efforts are being undertaken to achieve 3D, high-resolution, multi-parametric cardiac imaging with free-breathing or even ECG-gating free acquisitions, including respiratory and cardiac gating-based free-breathing methods [104], sparse sampling methods with constrained image reconstruction [105, 106], MR multitasking [107], and MR fingerprinting [108].

References

1. Ouyang J, Li Q, El Fakhri G. Magnetic resonance-based motion correction for positron emission tomography imaging. Semin Nucl Med. 2013;43(1):60–7. https://doi.org/10.1053/j.semnuclmed.2012.08.007.
2. Bai B, Li Q, Leahy RM. Magnetic resonance-guided positron emission tomography image reconstruction. Semin Nucl Med. 2013;43(1):30–44. https://doi.org/10.1053/j.semnuclmed.2012.08.006.
3. Alpert NM, et al. Quantitative in vivo mapping of myocardial mitochondrial membrane potential. PLoS One. 2018;13(1):e0190968.
4. Pelletier-Galarneau M, et al. In vivo quantitative mapping of human mitochondrial cardiac membrane potential: a feasibility study. Eur J Nucl Med Mol Imaging. 2021;48(2):414–20. https://doi.org/10.1007/s00259-020-04878-9.
5. Alpert NM, et al. In-vivo imaging of mitochondrial depolarization of myocardium with positron emission tomography and a proton gradient uncoupler. Front Physiol. 2020;11:11–491. https://doi.org/10.3389/fphys.2020.00491.
6. Vandenberghe S, Marsden PK. PET-MRI: a review of challenges and solutions in the development of integrated multimodality imaging. Phys Med Biol. 2015;60(4):R115–54. https://doi.org/10.1088/0031-9155/60/4/R115.
7. Delso G, Ziegler S. PET/MRI system design. Eur J Nucl Med Mol Imaging. 2009;36(S1):86–92. https://doi.org/10.1007/s00259-008-1008-6.
8. Renker D. New trends on photodetectors. Nucl Instrum Methods Phys Res Sect Accel Spectrometers Detect Assoc Equip. 2007;571(1–2):1–6. https://doi.org/10.1016/j.nima.2006.10.016.
9. Roncali E, Cherry SR. Application of silicon photomultipliers to positron emission tomography. Ann Biomed Eng. 2011;39(4):1358–77. https://doi.org/10.1007/s10439-011-0266-9.
10. Yamamoto S, Kuroda K, Senda M. Scintillator selection for MR-compatible gamma detectors. IEEE Trans Nucl Sci. 2003;50(5):1683–5. https://doi.org/10.1109/TNS.2003.817375.
11. Zaidi H, et al. Design and performance evaluation of a whole-body ingenuity TF PET–MRI system. Phys Med Biol. 2011;56(10):3091–106. https://doi.org/10.1088/0031-9155/56/10/013.
12. Delso G, et al. Performance measurements of the Siemens mMR integrated whole-body PET/MR scanner. J Nucl Med. 2011;52(12):1914–22. https://doi.org/10.2967/jnumed.111.092726.
13. Grant AM, Deller TW, Khalighi MM, Maramraju SH, Delso G, Levin CS. NEMA NU 2-2012 performance studies for the SiPM-based ToF-PET component of the GE SIGNA PET/MR system: PET performance measurements of the GE SIGNA PET/MR. Med Phys. 2016;43(5):2334–43. https://doi.org/10.1118/1.4945416.
14. Levin CS, Maramraju SH, Khalighi MM, Deller TW, Delso G, Jansen F. Design features and mutual compatibility studies of the time-of-flight PET capable GE SIGNA PET/MR system. IEEE Trans Med Imaging. 2016;35(8):1907–14. https://doi.org/10.1109/TMI.2016.2537811.
15. Chen S, et al. NEMA NU2-2012 performance measurements of the united imaging uPMR790: an integrated PET/MR system. Eur J Nucl Med Mol Imaging. 2021;48(6):1726–35. https://doi.org/10.1007/s00259-020-05135-9.
16. Pichler BJ, et al. Performance test of an LSO-APD detector in a 7-T MRI scanner for simultaneous PET/MRI. J Nucl Med. 2006;47(4):639–47.
17. España S, Fraile LM, Herraiz JL, Udías JM, Desco M, Vaquero JJ. Performance evaluation of SiPM photodetectors for PET imaging in the presence of magnetic fields. Nucl Instrum Methods Phys Res Sect Accel Spectrometers Detect Assoc Equip. 2010;613(2):308–16. https://doi.org/10.1016/j.nima.2009.11.066.
18. Kinahan PE, Hasegawa BH, Beyer T. X-ray-based attenuation correction for positron emission tomography/computed tomography scanners. Semin Nucl Med. 2003;33(3):166–79. https://doi.org/10.1053/snuc.2003.127307.
19. Martinez-Möller A, et al. Tissue classification as a potential approach for attenuation correction in whole-body PET/MRI: evaluation with PET/CT data. J Nucl Med. 2009;50(4):520–6. https://doi.org/10.2967/jnumed.108.054726.
20. Keereman V, Mollet P, Berker Y, Schulz V, Vandenberghe S. Challenges and current methods for attenuation correction in PET/MR. Magn Reson Mater Phys Biol Med. 2013;26(1):81–98. https://doi.org/10.1007/s10334-012-0334-7.
21. Samarin A, et al. PET/MR imaging of bone lesions—implications for PET quantification from imperfect attenuation correction. Eur J Nucl Med Mol Imaging. 2012;39(7):1154–60. https://doi.org/10.1007/s00259-012-2113-0.
22. Schulz V, et al. Automatic, three-segment, MR-based attenuation correction for whole-body PET/MR data. Eur J Nucl Med Mol Imaging. 2011;38(1):138–52. https://doi.org/10.1007/s00259-010-1603-1.
23. Robson PM, et al. MR/PET imaging of the cardiovascular system. JACC Cardiovasc Imaging.

2017;10(10 Part A):1165–79. https://doi.org/10.1016/j.jcmg.2017.07.008.

24. Ouyang J, Chun SY, Petibon Y, Bonab AA, Alpert N, El Fakhri G. Bias atlases for segmentation-based PET attenuation correction using PET-CT and MR. IEEE Trans Nucl Sci. 2013;60(5):3373–82. https://doi.org/10.1109/TNS.2013.2278624.

25. Sekine T, et al. Clinical evaluation of zero-Echo-time attenuation correction for brain [18] F-FDG PET/MRI: comparison with atlas attenuation correction. J Nucl Med. 2016;57(12):1927–32. https://doi.org/10.2967/jnumed.116.175398.

26. Cabello J, Lukas M, Förster S, Pyka T, Nekolla SG, Ziegler SI. MR-based attenuation correction using ultrashort-Echo-time pulse sequences in dementia patients. J Nucl Med. 2015;56(3):423–9. https://doi.org/10.2967/jnumed.114.146308.

27. Juttukonda MR, et al. MR-based attenuation correction for PET/MRI neurological studies with continuous-valued attenuation coefficients for bone through a conversion from R2* to CT-Hounsfield units. Neuroimage. 2015;112:160–8. https://doi.org/10.1016/j.neuroimage.2015.03.009.

28. Han PK, et al. MR-based PET attenuation correction using a combined ultrashort echo time/multi-echo Dixon acquisition. Med Phys. 2020;47(7):3064–77. https://doi.org/10.1002/mp.14180.

29. Leynes AP, et al. Hybrid ZTE/Dixon MR-based attenuation correction for quantitative uptake estimation of pelvic lesions in PET/MRI. Med Phys. 2017;44(3):902–13. https://doi.org/10.1002/mp.12122.

30. Izquierdo-Garcia D, et al. An SPM8-based approach for attenuation correction combining segmentation and nonrigid template formation: application to simultaneous PET/MR brain imaging. J Nucl Med. 2014;55(11):1825–30. https://doi.org/10.2967/jnumed.113.136341.

31. Delso G, et al. Anatomic evaluation of 3-dimensional ultrashort-echo-time bone maps for PET/MR attenuation correction. J Nucl Med. 2014;55(5):780–5. https://doi.org/10.2967/jnumed.113.130880.

32. Hofmann M, et al. MRI-based attenuation correction for whole-body PET/MRI: quantitative evaluation of segmentation- and atlas-based methods. J Nucl Med. 2011;52(9):1392–9. https://doi.org/10.2967/jnumed.110.078949.

33. Paulus DH, et al. Whole-body PET/MR imaging: quantitative evaluation of a novel model-based MR attenuation correction method including bone. J Nucl Med. 2015;56(7):1061–6. https://doi.org/10.2967/jnumed.115.156000.

34. Ladefoged CN, et al. A multi-centre evaluation of eleven clinically feasible brain PET/MRI attenuation correction techniques using a large cohort of patients. Neuroimage. 2017;147:346–59. https://doi.org/10.1016/j.neuroimage.2016.12.010.

35. Izquierdo-Garcia D, Catana C. MR imaging–guided attenuation correction of PET data in PET/MR Imaging. PET Clin. 2016;11(2):129–49. https://doi.org/10.1016/j.cpet.2015.10.002.

36. Torrado-Carvajal A, et al. Dixon-VIBE deep learning (DIVIDE) pseudo-CT synthesis for pelvis PET/MR attenuation correction. J Nucl Med. 2019;60(3):429–35. https://doi.org/10.2967/jnumed.118.209288.

37. Leynes AP, et al. Zero-Echo-time and Dixon deep pseudo-CT (ZeDD CT): direct generation of pseudo-CT images for pelvic PET/MRI attenuation correction using deep convolutional neural networks with multiparametric MRI. J Nucl Med. 2018;59(5):852–8. https://doi.org/10.2967/jnumed.117.198051.

38. Gong K, Han PK, Johnson KA, El Fakhri G, Ma C, Li Q. Attenuation correction using deep learning and integrated UTE/multi-echo Dixon sequence: evaluation in amyloid and tau PET imaging. Eur J Nucl Med Mol Imaging. 2021;48(5):1351–61. https://doi.org/10.1007/s00259-020-05061-w.

39. Spuhler KD, Gardus J, Gao Y, DeLorenzo C, Parsey R, Huang C. Synthesis of patient-specific transmission data for PET attenuation correction for PET/MRI neuroimaging using a convolutional neural network. J Nucl Med. 2019;60(4):555–60. https://doi.org/10.2967/jnumed.118.214320.

40. Pozaruk A, et al. Augmented deep learning model for improved quantitative accuracy of MR-based PET attenuation correction in PSMA PET-MRI prostate imaging. Eur J Nucl Med Mol Imaging. 2021;48(1):9–20. https://doi.org/10.1007/s00259-020-04816-9.

41. Grafe H, et al. Evaluation of improved attenuation correction in whole-body PET/MR on patients with bone metastasis using various radiotracers. Eur J Nucl Med Mol Imaging. 2020;47(10):2269–79. https://doi.org/10.1007/s00259-020-04738-6.

42. Nuyts J, Dupont P, Stroobants S, Benninck R, Mortelmans L, Suetens P. Simultaneous maximum a posteriori reconstruction of attenuation and activity distributions from emission sinograms. IEEE Trans Med Imaging. 1999;18(5):393–403. https://doi.org/10.1109/42.774167.

43. Nuyts J, Bal G, Kehren F, Fenchel M, Michel C, Watson C. Completion of a truncated attenuation image from the attenuated PET emission data. IEEE Trans Med Imaging. 2013;32(2):237–46. https://doi.org/10.1109/TMI.2012.2220376.

44. Lindemann ME, Oehmigen M, Blumhagen JO, Gratz M, Quick HH. MR-based truncation and attenuation correction in integrated PET/MR hybrid imaging using HUGE with continuous table motion. Med Phys. 2017;44(9):4559–72. https://doi.org/10.1002/mp.12449.

45. Eldib M, Bini J, Faul DD, Oesingmann N, Tsoumpas C, Fayad ZA. Attenuation correction for magnetic resonance coils in combined PET/MR imaging. PET Clin. 2016;11(2):151–60. https://doi.org/10.1016/j.cpet.2015.10.004.

46. Kartmann R, et al. Integrated PET/MR imaging: automatic attenuation correction of flex-

ible RF coils: AC of flexible RF surface coils. Med Phys. 2013;40(8):082301. https://doi.org/10.1118/1.4812685.

47. Klein GJ, Reutter RW, Huesman RH. Four-dimensional affine registration models for respiratory-gated PET. IEEE Trans Nucl Sci. 2002;48(3):756–60.

48. Rogers WJ, et al. Quantification of and correction for left ventricular systolic long-axis shortening by magnetic resonance tissue tagging and slice isolation. Circulation. 1991;84(2):721–31.

49. Fisher M, von Schulthess G, Higgins C. Multiphasic cardiac magnetic resonance imaging: normal regional left ventricular wall thickening. Am J Roentgenol. 1985;145(1):27–30. https://doi.org/10.2214/ajr.145.1.27.

50. Gould KL, Pan T, Loghin C, Johnson NP, Guha A, Sdringola S. Frequent diagnostic errors in cardiac PET/CT due to misregistration of CT attenuation and emission PET images: a definitive analysis of causes, consequences, and corrections. J Nucl Med. 2007;48(7):1112–21.

51. Loghin C, Sdringola S, Gould KL. Common artifacts in PET myocardial perfusion images due to attenuation-emission misregistration: clinical significance, causes, and solutions. J Nucl Med. 2004;45(6):1029–39.

52. Catana C. Motion correction options in PET/MRI. Semin Nucl Med. 2015;45(3):212–23. https://doi.org/10.1053/j.semnuclmed.2015.01.001.

53. Munoz C, Kolbitsch C, Reader AJ, Marsden P, Schaeffter T, Prieto C. MR-based cardiac and respiratory motion-compensation techniques for PET-MR imaging. PET Clin. 2016;11(2):179–91. https://doi.org/10.1016/j.cpet.2015.09.004.

54. Catana C. PET/MRI: motion correction. In: Iagaru A, Hope T, Veit-Haibach P, editors. PET/MRI in oncology: current clinical applications. Cham: Springer International; 2018. p. 77–96. https://doi.org/10.1007/978-3-319-68517-5_5.

55. Lalush DS. Magnetic resonance–derived improvements in PET imaging. Magn Reson Imaging Clin. 2017;25(2):257–72. https://doi.org/10.1016/j.mric.2016.12.002.

56. Rakvongthai Y, Fakhri GE. Magnetic resonance–based motion correction for quantitative PET in simultaneous PET-MR imaging. PET Clin. 2017;12(3):321–7. https://doi.org/10.1016/j.cpet.2017.02.004.

57. Polycarpou I, Soultanidis G, Tsoumpas C. Synergistic motion compensation strategies for positron emission tomography when acquired simultaneously with magnetic resonance imaging. Philos Trans A Soc Math Phys Eng Sci. 2021;379(2204):20200207. https://doi.org/10.1098/rsta.2020.0207.

58. Catana C, et al. MRI-assisted PET motion correction for neurologic studies in an integrated MR-PET scanner. J Nucl Med. 2011;52(1):154–61.

59. Huang C, et al. Motion compensation for brain PET imaging using wireless MR active markers in simul-taneous PET-MR: phantom and non-human primate studies. Neuroimage. 2014;91:129–37.

60. Chun SY, et al. MRI-based nonrigid motion correction in simultaneous PET/MRI. J Nucl Med. 2012;53(8):1284–91.

61. Guerin B, et al. Nonrigid PET motion compensation in the lower abdomen using simultaneous tagged-MRI and PET imaging. Med Phys. 2011;38:3025.

62. Furst S, et al. Motion correction strategies for integrated PET/MR. J Nucl Med. 2015;56(2):261–9.

63. Petibon Y, et al. Relative role of motion and PSF compensation in whole-body oncologic PET-MR imaging. Med Phys. 2014;41(4):042503. https://doi.org/10.1118/1.4868458.

64. Petibon Y, et al. Impact of motion and partial volume effects correction on PET myocardial perfusion imaging using simultaneous PET-MR. Phys Med Biol. 2016;62(2):326.

65. Rank CM, et al. Respiratory motion compensation for simultaneous PET/MR based on highly undersampled MR data. Med Phys. 2016;43(12):6234–45. https://doi.org/10.1118/1.4966128.

66. Fuin N, et al. Concurrent respiratory motion correction of abdominal PET and dynamic contrast-enhanced–MRI using a compressed sensing approach. J Nucl Med. 2018;59(9):1474–9. https://doi.org/10.2967/jnumed.117.203943.

67. Dutta J, Huang C, Li Q, El Fakhri G. Pulmonary imaging using respiratory motion compensated simultaneous PET/MR. Med Phys. 2015;42(7):4227–40.

68. Fayad H, Schmidt H, Wuerslin C, Visvikis D. Reconstruction-incorporated respiratory motion correction in clinical simultaneous PET/MR imaging for oncology applications. J Nucl Med. 2015;56(6):884–9.

69. Grimm R, et al. Self-gated MRI motion modeling for respiratory motion compensation in integrated PET/MRI. Med Image Anal. 2015;19(1):110–20.

70. Wang X, Rahmim A, Tang J. MRI-assisted dual motion correction for myocardial perfusion defect detection in PET imaging. Med Phys. 2017;44(9):4536–47. https://doi.org/10.1002/mp.12429.

71. Petibon Y, et al. Cardiac motion compensation and resolution modeling in simultaneous PET-MR: a cardiac lesion detection study. Phys Med Biol. 2013;58(7):2085–102. https://doi.org/10.1088/0031-9155/58/7/2085.

72. Küstner T, et al. MR-based respiratory and cardiac motion correction for PET imaging. Med Image Anal. 2017;42:129–44. https://doi.org/10.1016/j.media.2017.08.002.

73. Huang C, et al. Accelerated acquisition of tagged MRI for cardiac motion correction in simultaneous PET-MR: phantom and patient studies. Med Phys. 2015;42(2):1087–97.

74. Robson PM, et al. Correction of respiratory and cardiac motion in cardiac PET/MR using MR-based motion modeling. Phys Med Biol. 2018;63(22):225011. https://doi.org/10.1088/1361-6560/aaea97.

75. Kolbitsch C, et al. Cardiac and respiratory motion correction for simultaneous cardiac PET/MR. J Nucl Med. 2017;58(5):846–52. https://doi.org/10.2967/jnumed.115.171728.

76. Petibon Y, El Fakhri G, Nezafat R, Johnson N, Brady T, Ouyang J. Towards coronary plaque imaging using simultaneous PET-MR: a simulation study. Phys Med Biol. 2014;59(5):1203–22. https://doi.org/10.1088/0031-9155/59/5/1203.

77. Munoz C, et al. Motion-corrected simultaneous cardiac positron emission tomography and coronary MR angiography with high acquisition efficiency. Magn Reson Med. 2018;79(1):339–50. https://doi.org/10.1002/mrm.26690.

78. Munoz C, Neji R, Kunze KP, Nekolla SG, Botnar RM, Prieto C. Respiratory- and cardiac motion-corrected simultaneous whole-heart PET and dual phase coronary MR angiography. Magn Reson Med. 2019;81(3):1671–84. https://doi.org/10.1002/mrm.27517.

79. Mayer J, Jin Y, Wurster T-H, Makowski MR, Kolbitsch C. Evaluation of synergistic image registration for motion-corrected coronary NaF-PET-MR. Philos Trans A Soc Math Phys Eng Sci. 2021;379(2200):20200202. https://doi.org/10.1098/rsta.2020.0202.

80. Axel L, Dougherty L. MR imaging of motion with spatial modulation of magnetization. Radiology. 1989;171(3):841–5. https://doi.org/10.1148/radiology.171.3.2717762.

81. Petibon Y, Sun T, Han PK, Ma C, Fakhri GE, Ouyang J. MR-based cardiac and respiratory motion correction of PET: application to static and dynamic cardiac [18] F-FDG imaging. Phys Med Biol. 2019;64(19):195009. https://doi.org/10.1088/1361-6560/ab39c2.

82. Petibon Y, et al. Impact of motion and partial volume effects correction on PET myocardial perfusion imaging using simultaneous PET-MR. Phys Med Biol. 2017;62(2):326–43. https://doi.org/10.1088/1361-6560/aa5087.

83. Würslin C, et al. Respiratory motion correction in oncologic PET using T1-weighted MR imaging on a simultaneous whole-body PET/MR system. J Nucl Med. 2013;54(3):464–71. https://doi.org/10.2967/jnumed.112.105296.

84. Büther F, et al. List mode-driven cardiac and respiratory gating in pet. J Nucl Med. 2009;50(5):674–81.

85. Qiao F, Pan TS, Clark JWJ, Mawlawi OR. A motion-incorporated reconstruction method for gated PET studies. Phys Med Biol. 2006;51:3769–83.

86. Lamare F, et al. List-mode-based reconstruction for respiratory motion correction in PET using non-rigid body transformations. Phys Med Biol. 2007;52(17):5187–204. https://doi.org/10.1088/0031-9155/52/17/006.

87. Nekolla SG, et al. Evaluation of the novel myocardial perfusion positron-emission tomography tracer [18] F-BMS-747158-02: comparison to [13] N-ammonia and validation with microspheres in a pig model. Circulation. 2009;119(17):2333–42. https://doi.org/10.1161/CIRCULATIONAHA.108.797761.

88. Marin T, et al. Motion correction for PET data using subspace-based real-time MR imaging in simultaneous PET/MR. Phys Med Biol. 2020;65(23):235022. https://doi.org/10.1088/1361-6560/abb31d.

89. Spangler-Bickell MG, Deller TW, Bettinardi V, Jansen F. Ultra-fast list-mode reconstruction of short PET frames and example applications. J Nucl Med. 2021;62(2):287–92. https://doi.org/10.2967/jnumed.120.245597.

90. Lu Y, et al. Data-driven voluntary body motion detection and non-rigid event-by-event correction for static and dynamic PET. Phys Med Biol. 2019;64(6):065002. https://doi.org/10.1088/1361-6560/ab02c2.

91. Sun T, et al. Body motion detection and correction in cardiac PET: phantom and human studies. Med Phys. 2019;46(11):4898–906. https://doi.org/10.1002/mp.13815.

92. Martin O, et al. PET/MRI versus PET/CT for whole-body staging: results from a single-center observational study on 1,003 sequential examinations. J Nucl Med. 2020;61(8):1131–6. https://doi.org/10.2967/jnumed.119.233940.

93. Sher AC, et al. Assessment of sequential PET/MRI in comparison with PET/CT of pediatric lymphoma: a prospective study. Am J Roentgenol. 2016;206(3):623–31. https://doi.org/10.2214/AJR.15.15083.

94. Gatidis S, Bender B, Reimold M, Schäfer JF. PET/MRI in children. Eur J Radiol. 2017;94:A64–70. https://doi.org/10.1016/j.ejrad.2017.01.018.

95. Moradi F, Iagaru A, McConathy J. Clinical applications of PET/MR imaging. Radiol Clin North Am. 2021;59(5):853–74. https://doi.org/10.1016/j.rcl.2021.05.013.

96. Pearce MS, et al. Radiation exposure from CT scans in childhood and subsequent risk of leukaemia and brain tumours: a retrospective cohort study. Lancet. 2012;380(9840):499–505. https://doi.org/10.1016/S0140-6736(12)60815-0.

97. On behalf of the European Society of Cardiovascular Radiology (ESCR), et al. Hybrid cardiac imaging using PET/MRI: a joint position statement by the European Society of Cardiovascular Radiology (ESCR) and the European Association of Nuclear Medicine (EANM). Eur J Hybrid Imaging. 2018;2(1):4086–101. https://doi.org/10.1186/s41824-018-0032-4.

98. Messroghli DR, et al. Clinical recommendations for cardiovascular magnetic resonance mapping of T1, T2, T2 and extracellular volume: a consensus statement by the Society for Cardiovascular Magnetic Resonance (SCMR) endorsed by the European Association for Cardiovascular Imaging (EACVI). J Cardiovasc Magn Reson. 2017;19(1):1–24. https://doi.org/10.1186/s12968-017-0389-8.

99. Messroghli DR, Radjenovic A, Kozerke S, Higgins DM, Sivananthan MU, Ridgway JP. Modified look-locker inversion recovery (MOLLI) for high-resolution T 1 mapping of the heart. Magn Reson Med. 2004;52(1):141–6. https://doi.org/10.1002/mrm.20110.

100. Kellman P, Hansen MS. T1-mapping in the heart: accuracy and precision. J Cardiovasc Magn Reson. 2014;16(2):1–20.

101. Verhaert D, et al. Direct T2 quantification of myocardial edema in acute ischemic injury. JACC Cardiovasc Imaging. 2011;4(3):269–78. https://doi.org/10.1016/j.jcmg.2010.09.023.

102. Kramer CM, Barkhausen J, Bucciarelli-Ducci C, Flamm SD, Kim RJ, Nagel E. Standardized cardiovascular magnetic resonance imaging (CMR) protocols: 2020 update. J Cardiovasc Magn Reson. 2020;22(1):17. https://doi.org/10.1186/s12968-020-00607-1.

103. Sung K, Nayak KS. Measurement and characterization of RF nonuniformity over the heart at 3T using body coil transmission. J Magn Reson Imaging. 2008;27(3):643–8. https://doi.org/10.1002/jmri.21253.

104. Weingärtner S, Roujol S, Akçakaya M, Basha TA, Nezafat R. Free-breathing multislice native myocardial T1 mapping using the slice-interleaved T1 (STONE) sequence. Magn Reson Med. 2015;74(1):115–24. https://doi.org/10.1002/mrm.25387.

105. Qi H, et al. Free-running 3D whole heart myocardial T1 mapping with isotropic spatial resolution. Magn Reson Med. 2019;82(4):1331–42. https://doi.org/10.1002/mrm.27811.

106. Han PK, et al. Free-breathing 3D cardiac T $_1$ mapping with transmit B $_1$ correction at 3T. Magn Reson Med. 2021;87(4):1832–45. https://doi.org/10.1002/mrm.29097.

107. Shaw JL, et al. Free-breathing, non-ECG, continuous myocardial T1 mapping with cardiovascular magnetic resonance multitasking. Magn Reson Med. 2019;81(4):2450–63. https://doi.org/10.1002/mrm.27574.

108. Hamilton JI, Jiang Y, Eck B, Griswold M, Seiberlich N. Cardiac cine magnetic resonance fingerprinting for combined ejection fraction, T1 and T2 quantification. NMR Biomed. 2020;33(8):1–17. https://doi.org/10.1002/nbm.4323.

Review of Cardiac Metabolism and FDG

3

Patrick Martineau
and Matthieu Pelletier-Galarneau

Introduction

The heart is a unique organ. It is the first functional organ developed in embryogenesis and will beat continuously until death. It has been estimated that the human heart will beat an average of 2.5 billion times during an individual's life and pump approximately one million barrels of blood during that time. In order to have the energy to accomplish this under varying physiological and pathological conditions, cardiac metabolism has evolved uniquely from other physiological systems in order to provide a reliable and an adaptable source of energy.

PET has been widely used for in vivo assessment of myocardial metabolism in animals and humans and has proven itself to be an accurate and useful tool able to shed light on different facets of cardiac function. The most commonly utilized radiotracer is 2-deoxy-2-[^{18}F]fluoro-D-glucose (FDG), a glucose analog, while a plethora of additional agents are available for probing different aspects of cardiac metabolism and physiology, including oxygen consumption, fatty acid metabolism, innervation, and perfu-sion [1]. An important limitation of studying cardiac glucose metabolism with FDG is that this technique is unable to assess glucose oxidation in its entirety and can only scratch the surface of this pathway—after transport across the cellular membrane by glucose transporters (GLUT) and phosphorylation by hexokinase, FDG does not undergo any additional metabolic transformations apart from dephosphorylation by glucose-6-phosphatase. Nonetheless, studies have shown FDG-PET to be a useful tool for the assessment of in vivo myocardial metabolism.

In this chapter, we briefly and superficially review the basics of cardiac metabolism, as well as its implications for cardiac imaging with FDG-PET. A complete overview of the intricacies of cardiac metabolism would be beyond the scope of this volume. Nonetheless, we hope the reader gains an appreciation of the complexity and sophistication of the mechanisms involved. In addition, we briefly review the alterations in cardiac metabolism which manifest in various common cardiac pathologies. These are of particular relevance to cardiac imagers as these are frequently encountered on FDG-PET imaging.

P. Martineau (✉)
BC Cancer, Vancouver, BC, Canada
e-mail: patrick.martineau@bccancer.bc.ca

M. Pelletier-Galarneau
Montreal Heart Institute, Montréal, QC, Canada
e-mail: Matthieu.pelletier-galarneau@icm-mhi.org

Cardiac Metabolism in Health

The Basics of Cardiac Metabolism: Free Fatty Acids, Glucose, Ketones

Cardiac metabolism has been a topic of active research since at least the work of Tigerstedt in the early twentieth century [2]. Following that, a number of pioneering discoveries were made concerning cardiac metabolism and function; however, particular attention needs to be cast on the work of Randle et al. who in 1963 proposed the glucose-fatty acid cycle (which has since been known as the eponymous "Randle cycle") as a model describing the dynamic interactions among the basic metabolic substrates of the myocardium [3]. While there still remains much to learn about cardiomyocytes, the Randle cycle provides a useful and accessible paradigm to help understand the relationship between the hormonal milieu, substrate availability, and cardiomyocyte functioning. Central to this concept is the competitive interaction between glucose and free fatty acids (FFAs) as metabolic substrates. Depending on both hormonal factors and availability, these substrates are transported into cardiomyocytes and progress along a series of enzyme-catalyzed steps, ultimately culminating in the production of ATP within the mitochondria (Fig. 3.1).

FFA Metabolism in Myocardium

Of the total energy budget for the heart, approximately 60–70% is derived from the oxidation of FFAs [4]. FFAs enter cardiomyocytes via at least four separate proteins—the fatty acid translocase FAT/CD36 and the fatty acid binding protein (FABPpm), as well as two very-long-chain acyl-CoA synthetases, ACSVL2 and ACSVL4, also known as the FA transport proteins (FATP1 and FATP6) [5–7]. FFA transport into cardiomyocytes is stimulated by both contraction and insulin albeit to a much lower degree than glucose (1.5-fold for FFAs vs. 2–14-fold for glucose) [8–10]. Once within cardiomyocytes, FFAs are transformed into fatty acyl-CoA, through the actions of acy-CoA synthase, and into fatty acyl-carnitine by carnitine palmitoyltransferase I

(CPT-I) β [11]. β-oxidation transforms fatty acyl-CoA to acetyl-CoA providing nicotinamide adenine dinucleotide and hydrogen (NADH) and flavin adenine dinucleotide (FADH$_2$). Within the mitochondria, acetyl-CoA is further oxidized by the tricarboxylic acid (TCA) cycle, producing three NADHs, one FADH$_2$, and one guanosine triphosphate (GTP) per molecule. NADH and FADH$_2$ are subsequently oxidized by the electron transport chain, producing ATP. GTP can be converted to ATP through the action of nucleoside-diphosphate kinase. FFA metabolism provides a large amount of ATP—for example, the complete oxidation of a single palmitate molecule generates 105 ATP molecules [12].

Glucose Metabolism in Myocardium

While FFAs serve as the heart's principal metabolic substrate, carbohydrate metabolism predominates during high workloads (such as during exercise or pressure overload) [13, 14] and in the postprandial state. Roughly 10–40% of myocardial ATP production can be attributed to carbohydrate and lactate metabolism (the latter primarily when exercising), with smaller contributions also arising from amino acid and ketone metabolism (primarily when fasting) [15].

Glucose is either taken up from the circulation or generated by the hydrolysis of intracellular glycogen stores. Glucose transport into the cell is facilitated by glucose transporters (GLUTs) and is the rate-limiting step in myocardial glucose utilization [16]. GLUTs comprise a family of membrane proteins, which are known to exhibit high specificity for glucose molecules; however, it has been shown that glucose analogs such as 2-deoxyglucose and FDG also enter cells via GLUTs. While over a dozen different types of glucose transporters have been described in the literature (in addition to numerous types of sodium-glucose co-transporters), the principal isoforms in the heart are GLUT1 and GLUT4 [17].

GLUT1 was the first of the GLUT family to be discovered and acts as a uniporter glucose protein widely expressed in human tissue [18]. GLUT1 is a membrane spanning glycoprotein with 12 transmembrane domains. Although GLUT1 is

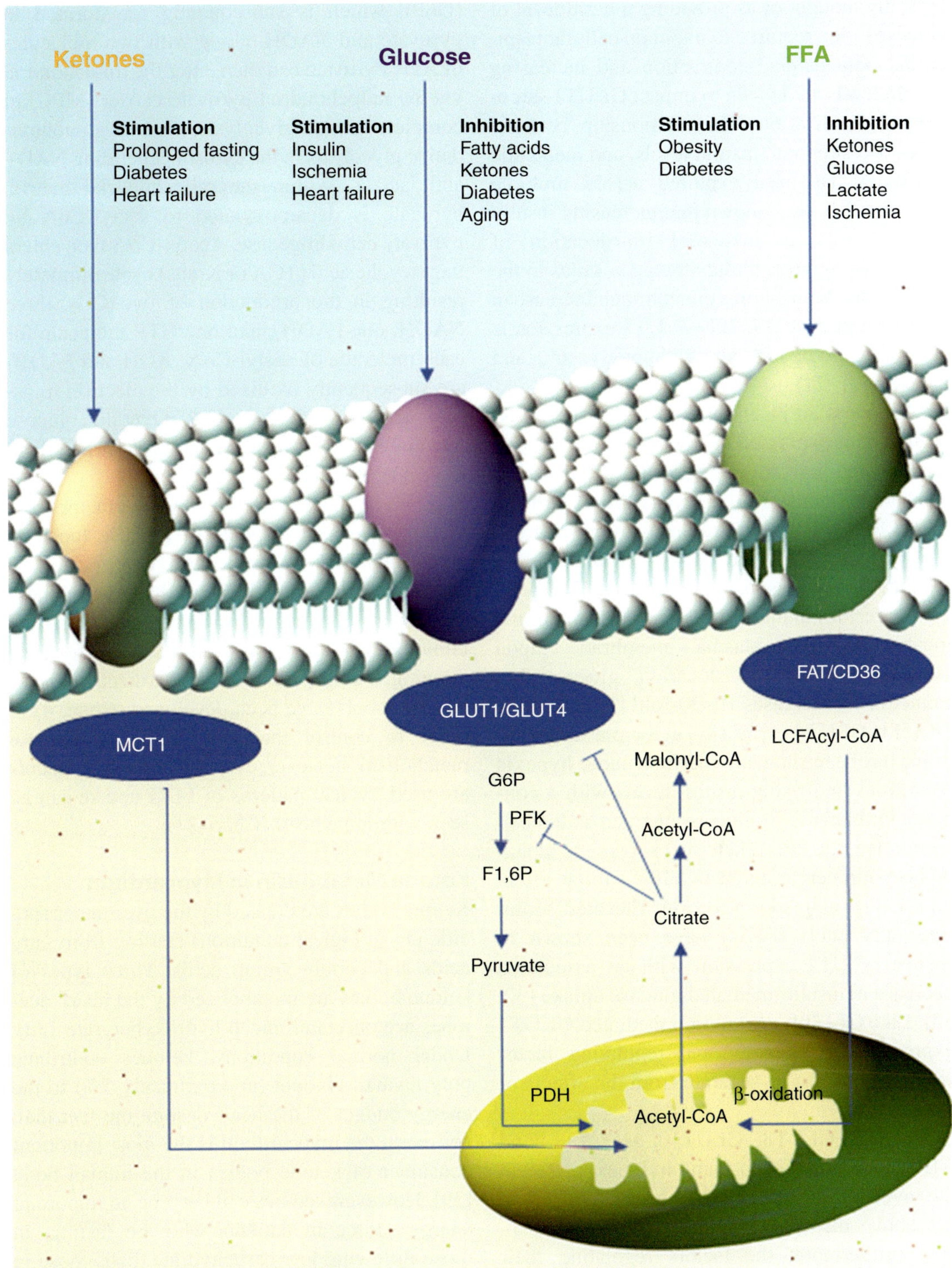

Fig. 3.1 This figure provides a simplified overview of cardiac metabolism with attention to the three main metabolic substrates—free fatty acids (FFA), glucose, and ketones—as well as the clinical factors which stimulate or inhibit their use. *FFA* free fatty acids, *MCT1* monocarboxylate transporter 1, *GLUT* glucose transporter, *FAT/CD36* fatty acid translocase/cluster of differentiation 36, *G6P* glucose-6-phosphatase, *PFK* phosphofructokinase, *F1,6P* fructose-1,6-bisphosphate, *PDH* pyruvate dehydrogenase, *CoA* coenzyme a, *LCF* long chain fatty

typically thought of as providing a basal level of glucose influx required to maintain cellular respiration, both cardiac contraction and increasing insulin levels are known to impact GLUT1 sarcolemmal localization. The relationship between GLUT1 expression, insulin levels, and metabolic substrates has been explored across multiple studies. It has been shown that increasing insulin levels results in increased translocation of GLUT1 from intracellular storage vesicles to the plasma membrane with a concomitant increase in glucose transport [19, 20]. GLUT1 expression is also known to be increased in hypoglycemia and hypoxia [21–24].

GLUT4 is an insulin-sensitive glucose transporter and is expressed in adipose tissue, skeletal muscle, and myocardium [25]. GLUT4 expression predominates in the myocardium with the GLUT1/GLUT4 ratio in rat hearts reported to be 0.1–0.6 [9, 26]. Unlike GLUT1, which mainly localizes to the plasma membrane, GLUT4 principally resides in intracellular vesicles and translocates to the plasma membrane upon stimulation. Upon translocation, glucose flux immediately increases 10–20-fold [27, 28]. Like GLUT1, GLUT4 expression at the plasma membrane has been shown to increase under hypoxic conditions and rising insulin levels with a concomitant increase in glucose flux across the cell membrane [24, 29]. Likewise, exposure to alpha- or beta-adrenergic agonists has a similar effect on GLUT4 as insulin [30, 31]. Elevated serum free fatty acids (FFAs) have been shown to reduce GLUT4 expression with an associated decrease in insulin-mediated glucose uptake [32, 33]. Like GLUT1, contraction mediated GLUT4 expression is an additional regulating factor which appears to be separate from the effects of insulin [34].

GLUT3, GLUT8, GLUT10, GLUT11, and GLUT12 have all been found to be expressed in the myocardium, although to a lesser degree than the above discussed glucose transporters [35–37]; furthermore, the factors regulating their myocardial expression and roles in cardiac glucose metabolism remain unclear.

After entering the cardiomyocyte, hexokinase transforms glucose to glucose-6-phosphate (G6P), which is subsequently transformed to pyruvate and NADH, along with two molecules of ATP. Pyruvate can then enter the mitochondria via the mitochondrial pyruvate carrier (MPC) to complete aerobic glycolysis, or undergo nonoxidative glycolysis in the cytosol generating NAD+ and lactate. Within the mitochondrial matrix, pyruvate is decarboxylated to acetyl-CoA by pyruvate dehydrogenase. Acetyl-CoA then enters the tricyclic acid (TCA or Krebs) cycle ultimately resulting in the production of two CO_2, three NADH, one $FADH_2$, and one GTP molecule for each molecule of acetyl-CoA. ADH and $FADH_2$ are subsequently oxidized by the electron transport chain, producing ATP. Overall, glucose metabolism yields up to 31 molecules of ATP per molecule of glucose [12].

From an imaging perspective, the factors regulating myocardial uptake of glucose (and, by extension, FDG) significantly complicate the assessment of cardiac PET FDG studies as these factors are challenging to ascertain within the clinic but can have drastic implications for PET imaging. For this reason, standardized preparation protocols have been developed (Chap. 4) in order to control the contribution of glucose metabolism; however, even when these protocols are used, typical patterns of FDG uptake can be seen within the heart (Chap. 23).

Ketone Metabolism in Myocardium

Ketone bodies are created by the liver under specific physiological conditions starting from fatty acids and certain amino acids. Three types of ketone bodies are metabolized by the heart: acetone, acetoacetate, and β-hydroxybutyrate [38]. Under normal conditions, ketones contribute only a small amount (approximately 5%) to the energy budget of the heart despite the fact that, per mass, the myocardium is the most important consumer of ketone bodies in the human body [39]. However, ketones can become an important energy source in patients who are fasting, in those following low-carbohydrate diets, those in the post-exercise state, as well as in neonates [38]. In general, plasma ketone body concentrations tend to be elevated in states with low insulin and high fatty acid levels.

Ketones are transported into cardiomyocytes using monocarboxylate transporters MCT1 [40]. Once within cardiomyocytes, ketone bodies are oxidized through a series of reactions to form acetyl-CoA, a substrate for the TCA cycle. Per carbon moiety, oxidation of ketone bodies is more energy efficient than glucose utilization but less efficient that FFA oxidation. Ketone oxidation inhibits myocardial FFA and glucose oxidation [41–43]. This latter observation may have important consequences for FDG-PET preparation protocols which require prolonged patient fasting.

Cardiac Metabolism in Disease

Cardiac Metabolism and Aging

Animal studies have shown that the proportion of energy obtained from fatty acid oxidation in the heart declines with age [44, 45]. These results have been confirmed in humans using PET studies [46]. However, it appears that this reflects an overall decrease in cardiac metabolism seen in the elderly heart rather than a shift in preferred metabolic substrate as concomitant reductions in glucose metabolism have also been reported [47]. Interestingly, an association with increased intramyocardial lipid accumulation in elderly hearts has also been reported—a similar association has also been noted in patients with diabetes and obesity [47–49]—but the significance of this finding remains unclear. This decrease in myocardial fatty acid utilization is associated with lower expression of cardiac peroxisome proliferator-activated receptors (PPAR) α, a nuclear receptor protein associated with cardiac energy metabolism [50].

In addition to decreased fatty acid metabolism, overall glucose oxidation rates appear to decrease with age, although glucose uptake and glycolysis actually increase [44, 46, 47]. The reason for this apparent uncoupling between glucose oxidation and glycolysis remains unclear; however, alterations in both fatty acid and glucose oxidation are known to be associated with

impairments of cardiac function [51–55]. Although the impact of aging on cardiac FDG-PET requires further attention, one study reported lower physiological cardiac uptake in patients older than 30 years of age when compared to younger patients [56].

Cardiac Metabolism and Heart Failure

Heart failure (HF) is a clinical syndrome which develops when cardiac function is inadequate to support an individual's physiological needs. It is a relatively common condition, affecting an estimated 2% of the adult population [57]. It is also well established that the development of HF is often associated with metabolic shifts in the heart.

The hypothesis that heart failure is caused by the heart running out of energy goes back to the 1930s when an association between falling creatine levels and heart failure was noted by Herrman and Decherd [58]. Since that time, the association between alterations in cardiac metabolism and impaired cardiac function has been further reinforced [53–55, 59–64]. Multiple studies have suggested that early heart failure is associated with an increase in glucose consumption, while FFA metabolism remains essentially stable [15, 65–67]. With worsening failure, the heart appears to develop a degree of insulin resistance and a concomitant decline in glucose utilization, accompanied by a decrease in FFA metabolism [68–71]. Mitochondrial oxidative phosphorylation decreases with glycolysis uncoupling from glucose oxidation resulting in energy deficient myocardium reliant largely on glycolysis to supply it with ATP [52]. Interestingly, it has been noted that ketone metabolism is increased in the failing heart although the reasons for this remain unclear [72–75]. Abnormalities of glucose metabolism in patients with heart failure have been confirmed on PET studies [56, 71, 76]. In particular, in the study by Israel et al., patients with heart failure were noted to have increased cardiac FDG uptake compared to normal controls [56].

Cardiac Metabolism in Obesity and Diabetes

The prevalence of obesity and diabetes has drastically increased in the last few decades. The World Health Organization now estimates that over half of the global population is overweight or obese [77]. In addition, close to 10% of adults have diabetes [78]. Both conditions predispose patients to adverse cardiovascular outcomes with diabetic patients having a twofold increased risk of developing heart failure when compared to control subjects [79].

Obesity and type 2 diabetes are associated with elevated plasma FFA levels as well cardiac steatosis [80, 81]. Not surprisingly, FFA uptake is significantly increased in patients with prediabetes when compared to nondiabetic subjects [82]. In addition, there is a reported decrease in myocardial glucose uptake in patients with diabetes, which may be related to downregulation of GLUT4 transporters [9, 83]. This decrease has been observed in FDG-PET studies of diabetic patients [56, 84–87]. These findings suggest an important shift in cardiac metabolism away from glucose metabolism the significance of which becomes clear when one considers the efficiency of cardiac metabolism—while FFAs generally produce more molecules of ATP when compared to glucose, they also require greater amounts of oxygen to metabolize. This implies that a shift away from glucose oxidation reduces the overall efficiency of cardiac metabolism. This, together with a reduced ability of the myocardium to adapt substrate use (i.e. due to insulin insensitivity) may relate to these patient's increased risk of developing heart failure.

Cardiac Metabolism in Ischemia

The effects of acute ischemia on cardiac metabolism are significant as the lack of oxygen drastically impairs oxidative phosphorylation and reduces ATP formation [88, 89]. This results in an increase in myocardial glucose uptake and glycolysis, likely in an effort to maintain ATP production. However, the lack of oxygen prevents pyruvate's oxidation by mitochondria, which instead gets converted to lactate. The result of this is the accumulation of significant amounts of lactate and a concomitant decrease in pH within cardiomyocytes and an associated decrease in myocardial contractility. This reduction in contractility, in turn, has the effect of reducing myocardial oxygen demand and may serve as a protective mechanism [90]. If the degree of ischemia is severe or prolonged but insufficient to cause necrosis, the state of impaired contractility can persist for days to weeks after restoration of blood flow, a condition known as stunning [91].

In the context of chronic ischemia, myocardium can undergo metabolic and functional changes referred to as "hibernation"—in contrast to stunning, hibernating myocardium is a persistent state of impaired functionality associated with reduced resting flow. While the initial hypothesis behind hibernating myocardium was that chronic ischemia would lead to a self-protective decrease in function and metabolic changes to match supply, a review of the evidence suggests that hibernation is more likely to be associated with repeat episodes of ischemia and stunning, as well as an impairment of myocardial flow reserve rather than reduced blood flow per se [92, 93]. A clinically important aspect of hibernating myocardium is that it often shows an improvement in function after revascularization; however, the recovery of function can be prolonged and occur over weeks to months following therapy. A metabolic hallmark of hibernating myocardium is preserved or even increased glucose metabolism compared to other reference areas in the heart [94]. This preserved use of glucose is associated with an increase in intracellular glycogen accumulation within hibernating myocardium and increased expression of GLUT4 [95, 96]. Although the reason for the shift in glucose metabolism by hibernating myocardium remains unclear, this may reflect a protective adaptive mechanism to ensure adequate supply of substrate for anaerobic metabolism during repeat episodes of ischemia. Conversely, FFA metabolism with a relatively higher oxygen requirement would seem to be particularly unsuitable for myocardium with a precarious oxygen supply. From a clinical perspective, the reliance of hibernating myocardium on glucose metabolism is key for its visualization using viability imaging (Chap. 20).

Conclusion

Cardiomyocyte metabolism is a vast and complicated topic which remains an area of active study. However, FDG-PET can serve as a useful probe to help elucidate the mysteries of the myocardium.

References

1. Régis C, Martineau P, Harel F, Pelletier-Galarneau M. Personalized cardiac imaging with new PET radiotracers. Curr Cardiovasc Imaging Rep. 2020;13(3):11.
2. Tigerstedt R. Die Physiologie des Kreislaufes. Berlin, Germany: Walter de Gruyter; 1921.
3. Randle P. The glucose fatty-acid cycle. Its role in insulin sensitivity and the metabolic disturbances of diabetes mellitus. Lancet. 1963;1:785–9.
4. van der Vusse GJ, Glatz JF, Stam HC, Reneman RS. Fatty acid homeostasis in the normoxic and ischemic heart. Physiol Rev. 1992;72(4):881–940.
5. Luiken JJ, Turcotte LP, Bonen A. Protein-mediated palmitate uptake and expression of fatty acid transport proteins in heart giant vesicles. J Lipid Res. 1999;40(6):1007–16.
6. Schaffer JE, Lodish HF. Expression cloning and characterization of a novel adipocyte long chain fatty acid transport protein. Cell. 1994;79(3):427–36.
7. Gimeno RE, Ortegon AM, Patel S, Punreddy S, Ge P, Sun Y, et al. Characterization of a heart-specific fatty acid transport protein. J Biol Chem. 2003;278(18):16039–44.
8. Luiken JJFP, Koonen DPY, Willems J, Zorzano A, Becker C, Fischer Y, et al. Insulin stimulates long-chain fatty acid utilization by rat cardiac myocytes through cellular redistribution of FAT/CD36. Diabetes. 2002;51(10):3113–9.
9. Fischer Y, Thomas J, Sevilla L, Muñoz P, Becker C, Holman G, et al. Insulin-induced recruitment of glucose transporter 4 (GLUT4) and GLUT1 in isolated rat cardiac myocytes evidence of the existence of different intracellular glut4 vesicle populations. J Biol Chem. 1997;272(11):7085–92.
10. Donthi RV, Huisamen B, Lochner A. Effect of vanadate and insulin on glucose transport in isolated adult rat cardiomyocytes. Cardiovasc Drugs Ther. 2000;14(5):463–70.
11. Tomec RJ, Hoppel CL. Carnitine palmitoyltransferase in bovine fetal heart mitochondria. Arch Biochem Biophys. 1975;170:716–23.
12. Honka H, Solis-Herrera C, Triplitt C, Norton L, Butler J, DeFronzo RA. Therapeutic manipulation of myocardial metabolism: JACC state-of-the-art review. J Am Coll Cardiol. 2021;77(16):2022–39.
13. Goodwin GW, Taegtmeyer H, With the Technical Assistance of Patrick H. Guthrie. Improved energy homeostasis of the heart in the metabolic state of exercise. Am J Physiol-Heart Circ Physiol. 2000;279(4):H1490–501.
14. Bishop SP, Altschuld RA. Increased glycolytic metabolism in cardiac hypertrophy and congestive failure. Am J Physiol-Leg Content. 1970;218(1):153–9.
15. Stanley WC, Recchia FA, Lopaschuk GD. Myocardial substrate metabolism in the normal and failing heart. Physiol Rev. 2005;85(3):1093–129.
16. Manchester J, Kong X, Nerbonne J, Lowry O, Lawrence J Jr. Glucose transport and phosphorylation in single cardiac myocytes: rate-limiting steps in glucose metabolism. Am J Physiol-Endocrinol Metab. 1994;266(3):E326–33.
17. Zorzano A, Sevilla L, Camps M, Becker C, Meyer J, Kammermeier H, et al. Regulation of glucose transport, and glucose transporters expression and trafficking in the heart: studies in cardiac myocytes. Am J Cardiol. 1997;80(3):65A–76A.
18. Kasahara M, Hinkle PC. Reconstitution and purification of the D-glucose transport protein from human erythrocytes. In: Biochemistry of membrane transport. Berlin: Springer; 1977. p. 346–50.
19. Cifuentes M, García MA, Arrabal PM, Martínez F, Yañez MJ, Jara N, et al. Insulin regulates GLUT1-mediated glucose transport in MG-63 human osteosarcoma cells. J Cell Physiol. 2011;226(6):1425–32.
20. Egert S, Nguyen N, Schwaiger M. Myocardial glucose transporter GLUT1: translocation induced by insulin and ischemia. J Mol Cell Cardiol. 1999;31(7):1337–44.
21. Simpson IA, Appel NM, Hokari M, Oki J, Holman GD, Maher F, et al. Blood—brain barrier glucose transporter: effects of hypo-and hyperglycemia revisited. J Neurochem. 1999;72(1):238–47.
22. Boado RJ, Pardridge WM. Glucose deprivation and hypoxia increase the expression of the GLUT1 glucose transporter via a specific mRNA cis-acting regulatory element. J Neurochem. 2002;80(3):552–4.
23. Chen C, Pore N, Behrooz A, Ismail-Beigi F, Maity A. Regulation of glut1 mRNA by hypoxia-inducible factor-1 interaction between H-ras and hypoxia. J Biol Chem. 2001;276(12):9519–25.
24. Young LH, Yin R, Raymond R, Xiaoyue H, Michael C, Jianming R, et al. Low-flow ischemia leads to translocation of canine heart GLUT-4 and GLUT-1 glucose transporters to the sarcolemma in vivo. Circulation. 1997;95(2):415–22.
25. Pessin JE, Bell GI. Mammalian facilitative glucose transporter family: structure and molecular regulation. Annu Rev Physiol. 1992;54(1):911–30.

26. Kraegen EW, Sowden JA, Halstead MB, Clark PW, Rodnick K, Chisholm DJ, et al. Glucose transporters and in vivo glucose uptake in skeletal and cardiac muscle: fasting, insulin stimulation and immunoisolation studies of GLUT1 and GLUT4. Biochem J. 1993;295(1):287–93.

27. Bryant NJ, Govers R, James DE. Regulated transport of the glucose transporter GLUT4. Nat Rev Mol Cell Biol. 2002;3(4):267–77.

28. Shepherd PR, Kahn BB. Glucose transporters and insulin action—implications for insulin resistance and diabetes mellitus. N Engl J Med. 1999;341(4):248–57.

29. Sun D, Nguyen N, DeGrado TR, Schwaiger M, Brosius F 3rd. Ischemia induces translocation of the insulin-responsive glucose transporter GLUT4 to the plasma membrane of cardiac myocytes. Circulation. 1994;89(2):793–8.

30. Rattigan S, Appleby GJ, Clark MG. Insulin-like action of catecholamines and Ca2+ to stimulate glucose transport and GLUT4 translocation in perfused rat heart. Biochim Biophys Acta BBA-Mol Cell Res. 1991;1094(2):217–23.

31. Doenst T, Taegtmeyer H. α-Adrenergic stimulation mediates glucose uptake through phosphatidylinositol 3-kinase in rat heart. Circ Res. 1999;84(4):467–74.

32. Papageorgiou I, Viglino C, Brulhart-Meynet M-C, James RW, Lerch R, Montessuit C. Impaired stimulation of glucose transport in cardiac myocytes exposed to very low-density lipoproteins. Nutr Metab Cardiovasc Dis. 2016;26(7):614–22.

33. Armoni M, Harel C, Bar-Yoseph F, Milo S, Karnieli E. Free fatty acids repress the GLUT4 gene expression in cardiac muscle via novel response elements. J Biol Chem. 2005;280(41):34786–95.

34. Lund S, Holman G, Schmitz O, Pedersen O. Contraction stimulates translocation of glucose transporter GLUT4 in skeletal muscle through a mechanism distinct from that of insulin. Proc Natl Acad Sci. 1995;92(13):5817–21.

35. Grover-McKay M, Walsh SA, Thompson SA. Glucose transporter 3 (GLUT3) protein is present in human myocardium. Biochim Biophys Acta BBA-Biomembr. 1999;1416(1–2):145–54.

36. Aerni-Flessner L, Abi-Jaoude M, Koenig A, Payne M, Hruz PW. GLUT4, GLUT1, and GLUT8 are the dominant GLUT transcripts expressed in the murine left ventricle. Cardiovasc Diabetol. 2012;11(1):1–10.

37. Joost H-G, Bell GI, Best JD, Birnbaum MJ, Charron MJ, Chen Y, et al. Nomenclature of the GLUT/SLC2A family of sugar/polyol transport facilitators. Am J Physiol-Endocrinol Metab. 2002;282(4):E974–6.

38. Cotter DG, Schugar RC, Crawford PA. Ketone body metabolism and cardiovascular disease. Am J Physiol-Heart Circ Physiol. 2013;304(8):H1060–76.

39. Balasse EO, Féry F. Ketone body production and disposal: effects of fasting, diabetes, and exercise. Diabetes Metab Rev. 1989;5(3):247–70.

40. Halestrap AP, Wilson MC. The monocarboxylate transporter family—role and regulation. IUBMB Life. 2012;64(2):109–19.

41. Forsey RG, Reid K, Brosnan JT. Competition between fatty acids and carbohydrate or ketone bodies as metabolic fuels for the isolated perfused heart. Can J Physiol Pharmacol. 1987;65(3):401–6.

42. Crawford PA, Crowley JR, Sambandam N, Muegge BD, Costello EK, Hamady M, et al. Regulation of myocardial ketone body metabolism by the gut microbiota during nutrient deprivation. Proc Natl Acad Sci. 2009;106(27):11276–81.

43. Garland PB, Newsholme EA, Randle PJ. Effect of fatty acids, ketone bodies, diabetes and starvation on pyruvate metabolism in rat heart and diaphragm muscle. Nature. 1962;195(4839):381–3.

44. Abu-Erreish GM, Neely JR, Whitmer JT, Whitman V, Sanadi DR. Fatty acid oxidation by isolated perfused working hearts of aged rats. Am J Physiol-Endocrinol Metab. 1977;232(3):E258.

45. McMillin JB, Taffet GE, Taegtmeyer H, Hudson EK, Tate CA. Mitochondrial metabolism and substrate competition in the aging Fischer rat heart. Cardiovasc Res. 1993;27(12):2222–8.

46. Kates AM, Herrero P, Dence C, Soto P, Srinivasan M, Delano DG, et al. Impact of aging on substrate metabolism by the human heart. J Am Coll Cardiol. 2003;41(2):293–9.

47. Koonen DPY, Febbraio M, Bonnet S, Nagendran J, Young ME, Michelakis ED, et al. CD36 expression contributes to age-induced cardiomyopathy in mice. Circulation. 2007;116(19):2139–47.

48. Wende AR, Abel ED. Lipotoxicity in the heart. Biochim Biophys Acta BBA Mol Cell Biol Lipids. 2010;1801(3):311–9.

49. Van Der Meer RW, Rijzewijk LJ, Diamant M, Hammer S, Schär M, Bax JJ, et al. The ageing male heart: myocardial triglyceride content as independent predictor of diastolic function. Eur Heart J. 2008;29(12):1516–22.

50. Pol CJ, Lieu M, Drosatos K. PPARs: protectors or opponents of myocardial function? PPAR Res. 2015;2015:e835985.

51. Lopaschuk GD, Karwi QG, Tian R, Wende AR, Abel ED. Cardiac energy metabolism in heart failure. Circ Res. 2021;128(10):1487–513.

52. Fillmore N, Levasseur JL, Fukushima A, Wagg CS, Wang W, Dyck JRB, et al. Uncoupling of glycolysis from glucose oxidation accompanies the development of heart failure with preserved ejection fraction. Mol Med. 2018;24(1):3.

53. Kato T, Niizuma S, Inuzuka Y, Kawashima T, Okuda J, Tamaki Y, et al. Analysis of metabolic remodeling in compensated left ventricular hypertrophy and heart failure. Circ Heart Fail. 2010;3(3):420–30.

54. Degens H, de Brouwer KF, Gilde AJ, Lindhout M, Willemsen PH, Janssen BJ, et al. Cardiac fatty acid metabolism is preserved in the compensated hypertrophic rat heart. Basic Res Cardiol. 2006;101(1):17–26.

55. Lei B, Lionetti V, Young ME, Chandler MP, d'Agostino C, Kang E, et al. Paradoxical downregulation of the glucose oxidation pathway despite

enhanced flux in severe heart failure. J Mol Cell Cardiol. 2004;36(4):567–76.

56. Israel O, Weiler-Sagie M, Rispler S, Bar-Shalom R, Frenkel A, Keidar Z, et al. PET/CT quantitation of the effect of patient-related factors on cardiac 18F-FDG uptake. J Nucl Med. 2007;48(2):234–9.

57. Mosterd A, Hoes AW. Clinical epidemiology of heart failure. Heart. 2007;93(9):1137–46.

58. Herrmann G, Decherd JRGM. The chemical nature of heart failure. Ann Intern Med. 1939;12(8):1233–44.

59. Conway MA, Allis J, Ouwerkerk R, Niioka T, Rajagopalan B, Radda GK. Detection of low phosphocreatine to ATP ratio in failing hypertrophied human myocardium by 31P magnetic resonance spectroscopy. Lancet. 1991;338(8773):973–6.

60. Nascimben L, Friedrich J, Liao R, Pauletto P, Pessina AC, Ingwall JS. Enalapril treatment increases cardiac performance and energy reserve via the creatine kinase reaction in myocardium of Syrian myopathic hamsters with advanced heart failure. Circulation. 1995;91(6):1824–33.

61. Tian R, Nascimben L, Kaddurah-Daouk R, Ingwall JS. Depletion of energy reserve via the creatine kinase reaction during the evolution of heart failure in cardiomyopathic hamsters. J Mol Cell Cardiol. 1996;28(4):755–65.

62. Beer M, Seyfarth T, Sandstede J, Landschütz W, Lipke C, Köstler H, et al. Absolute concentrations of high-energy phosphate metabolites in normal, hypertrophied, and failing human myocardium measured noninvasively with 31P-SLOOP magnetic resonance spectroscopy. J Am Coll Cardiol. 2002;40(7):1267–74.

63. Neubauer S, Remkes H, Spindler M, Horn M, Wiesmann F, Prestle J, et al. Downregulation of the Na+−creatine cotransporter in failing human myocardium and in experimental heart failure. Circulation. 1999;100(18):1847–50.

64. Mori J, Alrob OA, Wagg CS, Harris RA, Lopaschuk GD, Oudit GY. ANG II causes insulin resistance and induces cardiac metabolic switch and inefficiency: a critical role of PDK4. Am J Physiol-Heart Circ Physiol. 2013;304(8):H1103–13.

65. Chandler MP, Kerner J, Huang H, Vazquez E, Reszko A, Martini WZ, et al. Moderate severity heart failure does not involve a downregulation of myocardial fatty acid oxidation. Am J Physiol-Heart Circ Physiol. 2004;287(4):H1538–43.

66. Remondino A, Rosenblatt-Velin N, Montessuit C, Tardy I, Papageorgiou I, Dorsaz P-A, et al. Altered expression of proteins of metabolic regulation during remodeling of the left ventricle after myocardial infarction. J Mol Cell Cardiol. 2000;32(11):2025–34.

67. Nascimben L, Ingwall JS, Lorell BH, Pinz I, Schultz V, Tornheim K, et al. Mechanisms for increased glycolysis in the hypertrophied rat heart. Hypertension. 2004;44(5):662–7.

68. Osorio JC, Stanley WC, Linke A, Castellari M, Diep QN, Panchal AR, et al. Impaired myocardial fatty acid oxidation and reduced protein expression of retinoid X receptor-α in pacing-induced heart failure. Circulation. 2002;106(5):606–12.

69. Kalsi K, Smolenski R, Pritchard R, Khaghani A, Seymour A, Yacoub M. Energetics and function of the failing human heart with dilated or hypertrophic cardiomyopathy. Eur J Clin Invest. 1999;29(6):469–77.

70. Razeghi P, Young ME, Alcorn JL, Moravec CS, Frazier O, Taegtmeyer H. Metabolic gene expression in fetal and failing human heart. Circulation. 2001;104(24):2923–31.

71. Taylor M, Wallhaus TR, DeGrado TR, Russell DC, Stanko P, Nickles RJ, et al. An evaluation of myocardial fatty acid and glucose uptake using PET with [18F] fluoro-6-thia-heptadecanoic acid and [18F] FDG in patients with congestive heart failure. J Nucl Med. 2001;42(1):55–62.

72. Lopaschuk GD, Karwi QG, Ho KL, Pherwani S, Ketema EB. Ketone metabolism in the failing heart. Biochim Biophys Acta BBA-Mol Cell Biol Lipids. 2020;1865:158813.

73. Bedi KC Jr, Snyder NW, Brandimarto J, Aziz M, Mesaros C, Worth AJ, et al. Evidence for intramyocardial disruption of lipid metabolism and increased myocardial ketone utilization in advanced human heart failure. Circulation. 2016;133(8):706–16.

74. Aubert G, Martin OJ, Horton JL, Lai L, Vega RB, Leone TC, et al. The failing heart relies on ketone bodies as a fuel. Circulation. 2016;133(8):698–705.

75. Horton JL, Davidson MT, Kurishima C, Vega RB, Powers JC, Matsuura TR, et al. The failing heart utilizes 3-hydroxybutyrate as a metabolic stress defense. JCI Insight. 2019;4(4):e124079.

76. Nielsen R, Jorsal A, Iversen P, Tolbod L, Bouchelouche K, Sørensen J, et al. Heart failure patients with prediabetes and newly diagnosed diabetes display abnormalities in myocardial metabolism. J Nucl Cardiol. 2018;25(1):169–76.

77. WHO. Obesity and overweight fact sheet. Geneva: World Health Organization; 2018.

78. Zheng Y, Ley SH, Hu FB. Global aetiology and epidemiology of type 2 diabetes mellitus and its complications. Nat Rev Endocrinol. 2018;14(2):88–98.

79. Gottdiener JS, Arnold AM, Aurigemma GP, Polak JF, Tracy RP, Kitzman DW, et al. Predictors of congestive heart failure in the elderly: the cardiovascular health study. J Am Coll Cardiol. 2000;35(6):1628–37.

80. Leichman JG, Aguilar D, King TM, Vlada A, Reyes M, Taegtmeyer H. Association of plasma free fatty acids and left ventricular diastolic function in patients with clinically severe obesity. Am J Clin Nutr. 2006;84(2):336–41.

81. Iozzo P. Myocardial, perivascular, and epicardial fat. Diabetes Care. 2011;34(Supplement 2):S371–9.

82. Labbé SM, Grenier-Larouche T, Noll C, Phoenix S, Guérin B, Turcotte EE, et al. Increased myocardial uptake of dietary fatty acids linked to cardiac dysfunction in glucose-intolerant humans. Diabetes. 2012;61(11):2701–10.

83. Eckel J, Reinauer H. Insulin action on glucose transport in isolated cardiac myocytes: signalling pathways and diabetes-induced alterations. Biochem Soc Trans. 1990;18(6):1125–7.

84. Ohtake T, Yokoyama I, Watanabe T, Momose T, Serezawa T, Nishikawa J, et al. Myocardial glucose metabolism in noninsulin-dependent diabetes mellitus patients evaluated by FDG-PET. J Nucl Med. 1995;36(3):456–63.

85. Rijzewijk LJ, van der Meer RW, Lamb HJ, de Jong HWAM, Lubberink M, Romijn JA, et al. Altered myocardial substrate metabolism and decreased diastolic function in nonischemic human diabetic cardiomyopathy. J Am Coll Cardiol. 2009;54(16):1524–32.

86. Ménard SL, Croteau E, Sarrhini O, Gélinas R, Brassard P, Ouellet R, et al. Abnormal in vivo myocardial energy substrate uptake in diet-induced type 2 diabetic cardiomyopathy in rats. Am J Physiol-Endocrinol Metab. 2010;298(5):E1049–57.

87. Dutka DP, Pitt M, Pagano D, Mongillo M, Gathercole D, Bonser RS, et al. Myocardial glucose transport and utilization in patients with type 2 diabetes mellitus, left ventricular dysfunction, and coronary artery disease. J Am Coll Cardiol. 2006;48(11):2225–31.

88. Taegtmeyer H, Roberts AF, Raine AE. Energy metabolism in reperfused heart muscle: metabolic correlates to return of function. J Am Coll Cardiol. 1985;6(4):864–70.

89. Taegtmeyer H, Hems R, Krebs HA. Utilization of energy-providing substrates in the isolated working rat heart. Biochem J. 1980;186(3):701–11.

90. Rosano G, Fini M, Caminiti G, Barbaro G. Cardiac metabolism in myocardial ischemia. Curr Pharm Des. 2008;14(25):2551–62.

91. Braunwald E, Kloner R. The stunned myocardium: prolonged, postischemic ventricular dysfunction. Circulation. 1982;66(6):1146–9.

92. Camici PG, Wijns W, Borgers M, De Silva R, Ferrari R, Knuuti J, et al. Pathophysiological mechanisms of chronic reversible left ventricular dysfunction due to coronary artery disease (hibernating myocardium). Circulation. 1997;96(9):3205–14.

93. Diamond GA, Forrester JS, deLuz PL, Wyatt H, Swan H. Post-extrasystolic potentiation of ischemic myocardium by atrial stimulation. Am Heart J. 1978;95(2):204–9.

94. Fallavollita JA, Malm BJ, Canty JM. Hibernating myocardium retains metabolic and contractile reserve despite regional reductions in flow, function, and oxygen consumption at rest. Circ Res. 2003;92(1):48–55.

95. Depré C, Vanoverschelde J-LJ, Gerber B, Borgers M, Melin JA, Dion R. Correlation of functional recovery with myocardial blood flow, glucose uptake, and morphologic features in patients with chronic left ventricular ischemic dysfunction undergoing coronary artery bypass grafting. J Thorac Cardiovasc Surg. 1997;113(2):371–8.

96. McFalls EO, Hou M, Bache RJ, Best A, Marx D, Sikora J, et al. Activation of p38 MAPK and increased glucose transport in chronic hibernating swine myocardium. Am J Physiol-Heart Circ Physiol. 2004;287(3):H1328–34.

Myocardial Suppression Protocols

4

Michael T. Osborne, Kenechukwu Mezue, and Sanjay Divakaran

Abbreviations

^{18}F-FDG	^{18}F-fluorodeoxyglucose
JSNC	Japanese Society of Nuclear Cardiology
PET	Positron Emission Tomography
SNMMI/ASNC	Society of Nuclear Medicine and Molecular Imaging/ American Society of Nuclear Cardiology

M. T. Osborne (✉) · K. Mezue
Cardiology Division, Department of Medicine,
Massachusetts General Hospital and Harvard Medical
School, Boston, MA, USA

Cardiovascular Imaging Research Center,
Massachusetts General Hospital and Harvard Medical
School, Boston, MA, USA
e-mail: mosborne@mgh.harvard.edu;
kmezue@mgh.harvard.edu

S. Divakaran
Cardiovascular Imaging Program, Departments of
Radiology and Medicine, Brigham and Women's
Hospital and Harvard Medical School,
Boston, MA, USA

Division of Cardiovascular Medicine, Department of
Medicine, Brigham and Women's Hospital and
Harvard Medical School, Boston, MA, USA
e-mail: sdivakaran@bwh.harvard.edu

Introduction

One of the primary challenges in successful ^{18}F-fluorodeoxyglucose positron emission tomography (^{18}F-FDG-PET) imaging of myocardial and intracardiac inflammation is discerning pathologic ^{18}F-FDG uptake from physiologic uptake by background myocardium. Accordingly, patients undergoing cardiovascular ^{18}F-FDG-PET for inflammation must undergo careful preparation prior to imaging to optimize the diagnostic yield of the modality. This chapter will describe the underlying physiology of myocardial and inflammatory cell metabolism, examine the existing evidence for the utility of various preparation techniques, describe current evidence-based consensus recommendations, and identify future directions for further research to optimize inflammatory myocardial ^{18}F-FDG-PET imaging.

Underlying Physiology of Myocardial and Inflammatory Cell Glucose Metabolism

Normal myocytes are able to use both glucose and free fatty acids for metabolism and have variable avidity for glucose under different metabolic conditions. Intake of carbohydrates triggers insulin secretion, which leads to activation of GLUT4 channels in the myocardium to augment glucose uptake. In the absence of insulin, normal myocytes utilize free fatty acids for metabolism [1]. Alternatively, inflammatory cells are only able to utilize glucose for metabolism through uptake via the constitutively expressed GLUT1 and GLUT3 channels [2]. ^{18}F-FDG, a radioactive glucose analog, is phosphorylated upon entry into cells and becomes trapped, allowing an assessment of glucose metabolism using PET imaging. Thus, by manipulating the metabolism of normal myocardium to shift it away from glucose and towards free fatty acids prior to ^{18}F-FDG-PET imaging it is possible to identify pathological inflammation that would otherwise be obscured.

Goals of Preparation for ^{18}F-FDG-PET Imaging

To limit myocyte uptake of glucose and ^{18}F-FDG, the primary goal of patient preparation is to minimize insulin release and glucose availability prior to ^{18}F-FDG-PET imaging of myocardial and intracardiac inflammation. A secondary goal is to augment free fatty acid availability to provide adequate energy for the myocardium in a low insulin state. Ultimately, the sensitivity for detecting highly metabolic inflammatory cells within cardiovascular tissues is optimized by maximally suppressing ^{18}F-FDG uptake by the myocardium. The metabolism of normal myocardium and inflammatory cells and the impact of patient preparation are summarized in Fig. 4.1 [3].

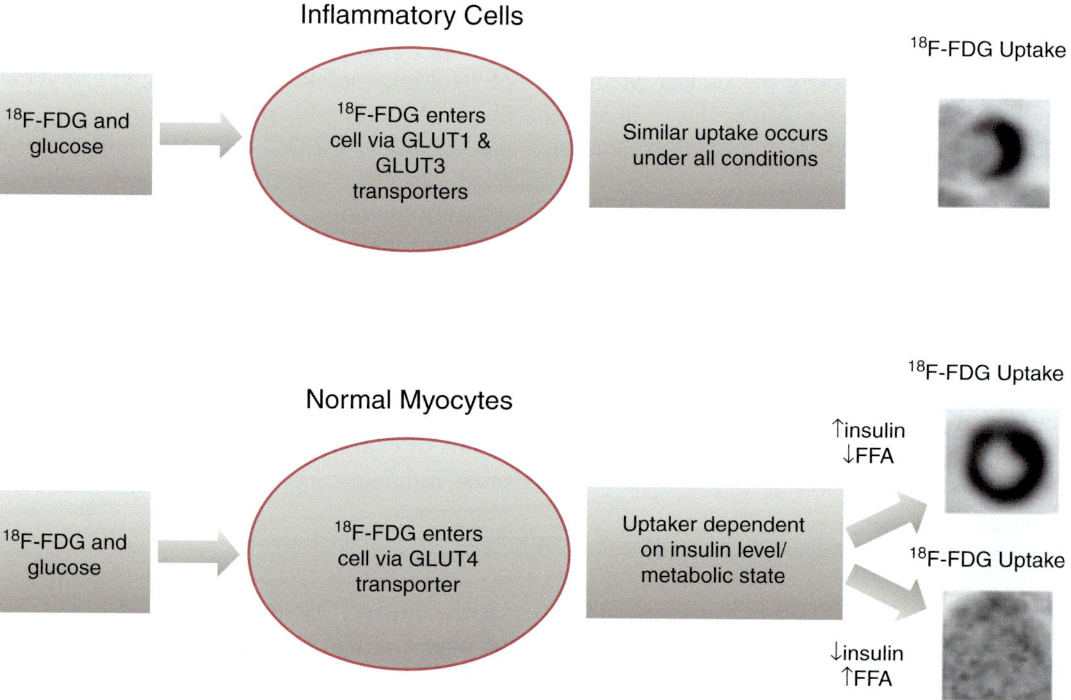

Fig. 4.1 Metabolism of inflammatory cells and normal myocytes under a variety of metabolic conditions and impact of suppressing physiologic myocardial ^{18}F-FDG uptake for inflammatory imaging. *FFA* free fatty acids, *^{18}F-FDG* ^{18}F-fluorodeoxyglucose. (Reprinted with permission [3])

Patterns of Myocardial ¹⁸F-FDG Uptake

The appearance of optimally suppressed ¹⁸F-FDG uptake by normal myocardium leads to a relative paucity of myocardial tracer uptake compared to the blood pool to facilitate identification of areas of abnormal ¹⁸F-FDG uptake. Alternatively, a pattern of intense global myocardial uptake that obscures foci of abnormal ¹⁸F-FDG uptake indicates poor suppression of myocardial uptake. Between these extremes, a finding of focally increased uptake on a background of diffuse ¹⁸F-FDG myocardial uptake can be seen with either poor suppression or with incomplete suppression and superimposed inflammatory pathology. Lastly, focal ¹⁸F-FDG uptake is often seen in the setting of inflammatory pathology; however, focal myocardial ¹⁸F-FDG uptake limited to the lateral wall and basal ring has been reported as normal variants [4]. These patterns can be challenging to distinguish from pathology and the physiology underlying the patterns is not well understood. Images demonstrating these patterns are shown below (Fig. 4.2).

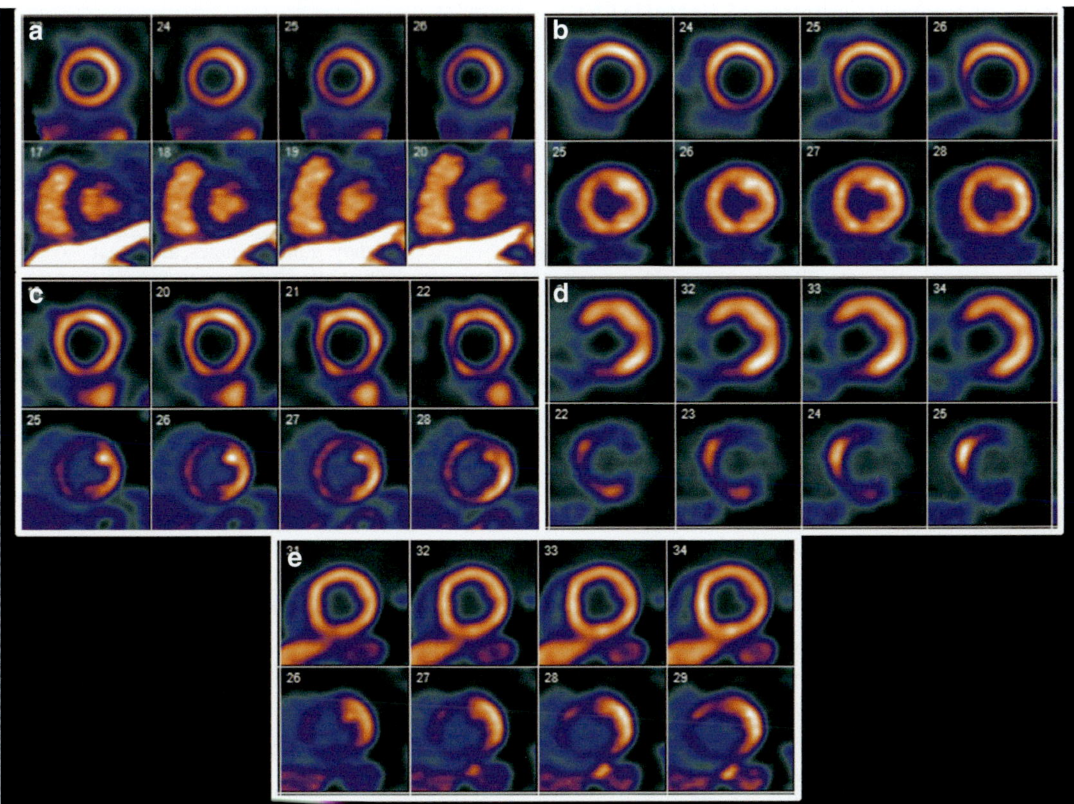

Fig. 4.2 Patterns of myocardial ¹⁸F-FDG uptake following preparation for inflammatory imaging. (**a**) Global suppression. (**b**) Diffuse uptake. (**c**) Focal on diffuse uptake. (**d**) Focal uptake. (**e**) Lateral wall uptake (normal variant). All panels display short axis images with perfusion imaging in the top row and metabolism (¹⁸F-FDG) in the bottom row

Approaches to Suppress Myocardial ^{18}F-FDG Uptake

Dietary Strategies

Prolonged Fasting

Fasting has been widely studied and has become a commonly implemented component of many protocols to suppress myocardial ^{18}F-FDG uptake [3, 5]. The metabolic consequences of fasting include lower insulin release and heightened lipolysis, resulting in a shift towards myocardial utilization of free fatty acids rather than glucose [6]. Although current Society of Nuclear Medicine and Molecular Imaging/American Society of Nuclear Cardiology (SNMMI/ASNC) recommendations support a fast of at least 4–12 h prior to ^{18}F-FDG administration, more recent data suggests that a longer fast of up to 18 h may provide even greater suppression of myocardial ^{18}F-FDG uptake [5, 7, 8]. Fasting for 18 h may also provide the optimal method for myocardial ^{18}F-FDG uptake suppression in isolation for individuals with significant dietary constraints (e.g., vegan and vegetarian diets) [5].

High-Fat Low-Carbohydrate Diet

A high-fat low-carbohydrate diet can be implemented to reduce insulin release and increase available free fatty acids as a method of shifting myocardial metabolism towards free fatty acids rather than glucose. This strategy has been extensively researched, and several studies have shown improved suppression of myocardial ^{18}F-FDG uptake with high-fat low-carbohydrate meals combined with fasting compared to fasting alone [3, 5]. Accordingly, current SNMMI/ASNC recommendations include having at least two meals with >35 g of fat and <3 g carbohydrates on the day prior to the ^{18}F-FDG-PET exam [5]. The Japanese Society of Nuclear Cardiology (JSNC) also recommends a low carbohydrate diet (<5 g) prior to fasting but considers a high-fat diet to be supplemental [8]. Table 4.1 provides a guide of optimal choices for dietary preparation [3].

High-Fat Drink

Multiple studies have evaluated the impact of adding a high-fat drink to a dietary preparation

Table 4.1 Dietary recommendations for optimal suppression of myocardial uptake of ^{18}F-FDG

Consume	Meat fried in oil or butter without breading or broiled (chicken, turkey, bacon, meat-only sausage, hamburgers, steak, fish)
	Eggs (prepared without milk or cheese)
	Oil (an option for patients who are unable to eat and have enteral access or vegan patients) and butter
	Clear liquids (water, tea, coffee, diet sodas, etc.)
Acceptable	Some artificial sweeteners (Sweet'N low, equal, NutraSweet)
	Fast of 18 h or longer if unable to eat with no enteral access or dietary restrictions prevention consumption of advised diet
Avoid	Vegetables, beans, nuts, fruits, and juices
	Bread, grain, rice, pasta, all baked goods
	Sweetened, grilled or cured meats or meat with carbohydrate-containing additives (some sausages, ham, sweetened bacon)
	Dairy products aside from butter (milk, cheese, etc.)
	Candy, gum, lozenges, and sugar
	Alcoholic beverages, soda, and sports drinks
	Mayonnaise, ketchup, tartar sauce, mustard, and other condiments
	Dextrose containing intravenous medications

Reprinted with permission [3]

protocol several hours prior to imaging. This strategy seeks to suppress myocardial ^{18}F-FDG uptake by augmenting free fatty acid availability. While the results of several early studies do not support broad implementation, a recent study describes an effective preparation strategy that includes a high-fat drink as part of a combined approach [3, 5, 9].

Behavioral Strategies

Strenuous exercise triggers augmentation of myocardial glucose uptake and metabolism through activation of catecholaminergic pathways. Accordingly, patients should avoid exercising for 12–24 h before ^{18}F-FDG administration [1].

Pharmacologic Strategies

Heparin

Intravenous heparin increases lipolysis and serum free fatty acids [10]. As such, several institutions administer heparin approximately 15 min prior to ^{18}F-FDG administration as a component of a protocol of myocardial ^{18}F-FDG uptake suppression. The dose given is typically a 50 IU/kg bolus. Nevertheless, the overall body of evidence remains inconclusive and the current SNMMI/ASNC recommendations suggest that heparin administration may be beneficial as an adjunctive component of a preparation strategy while it is not recommended by the JSNC [5, 8].

Calcium Channel Blockers

Intracellular calcium is a known contributor to glucose and ^{18}F-FDG uptake. Although calcium channel blockers reduced myocardial uptake of ^{18}F-FDG in a murine model, they have not been found to be incrementally effective in humans [11].

Communication

It has proven useful to provide careful review of preparation instructions with patients several days in advance of imaging as well as evaluating their adherence to the preparation strategy on the day of imaging prior to radiotracer injection. This allows patients to prepare well in advance of their study as well as to identify patients who are unlikely to have adequate suppression and permit rescheduling without unnecessary radiation exposure [5, 8].

Combination Strategies

Most institutions have preparation protocols that employ more than one of the above approaches in combination to prepare patients for myocardial and intracardiac inflammation imaging with ^{18}F-FDG-PET. The individual component strategies are summarized in Table 4.2.

Table 4.2 Summary of different preparation strategies for myocardial ^{18}F-FDG-PET and their impacts on myocardial metabolism

Strategy grouping	Specific strategies	Impacts on myocardial metabolism
Dietary techniques	Prolonged fasting	Reduced glucose uptake and increased availability of free fatty acids
	High-fat low-carbohydrate diet	Reduced glucose uptake and increased availability of free fatty acids
	High-fat drink	Increased availability of free fatty acids
Behavioral technique	Abstinence from exercise	Reduced glucose uptake
Pharmacologic strategies	Heparin	Increased availability of free fatty acids
	Calcium channel blockers	Reduced glucose uptake
Communication	Review of protocol before preparation and confirmation of adherence prior to imaging	Enhance patient understanding and compliance

Laboratory Values

The relationship between serological measures of glucose and fat metabolism and imaging findings in ^{18}F-FDG-PET imaging of myocardial and intracardiac inflammation has been investigated in several cohorts. The impact of different preparation strategies on serological measures of metabolism has been largely inconsistent to date, although there does appear to be a tendency towards lower blood glucose prior to imaging with a longer duration of fasting [3]. A recent study of serial ^{18}F-FDG-PET imaging showed that the metabolic parameters on serial imaging visits were similar but that these measurements were unrelated to imaging findings [12]. Alternatively, a subsequent single center study that evaluated the effectiveness of a preparation protocol reported that there were significant associations between markers of glucose metabolism and the standardized uptake values of the blood pool and myocardium and established normative ranges of serological measures of metabolic parameters for the study population [9]. Indeed, given the heterogeneity of preparation strategies, it may be that each unique protocol alters metabolism differently, and the establishment of normative values based on a given preparation strategy in a particular population may be necessary to meaningfully assess a particular patient's metabolic state prior to imaging [9, 13].

Patient Populations Requiring Special Considerations

While the above recommendations apply broadly, several patient populations require additional consideration to optimize myocardial suppression of ^{18}F-FDG uptake for inflammation imaging.

Patients with diabetes mellitus create a unique challenge given the need to minimize insulin administration to optimize imaging while balancing patient safety. Current recommendations suggest that patients with diabetes undergo the same preparation strategy as other patients. Those with type I diabetes should receive basal insulin but should minimize short-acting insulin to the extent that it is safe, especially on the day of the study. For those with type 2 diabetes, oral medications and non-insulin injections should be held on the day of the test. Similarly, insulin administration should be minimized to the extent that it is safe [5, 8].

It is important to exclude obstructive coronary disease in patients prior to ^{18}F-FDG-PET imaging if there is clinical suspicion. Ischemic and hibernating myocardium is highly avid for glucose because it lacks the ability to metabolize fatty acids. Accordingly, ischemic territories can exhibit exuberant uptake of ^{18}F-FDG even under fasting conditions, and coronary artery disease should be considered in any patient with ^{18}F-FDG

uptake in a coronary distribution on a study ordered to assess for inflammation [14].

Advanced cardiomyopathy alters myocardial metabolism by increasing glucose metabolism relative to fatty acid metabolism. Although this change in physiology merits consideration, there are presently no recommendations to modify preparation strategies in the setting of cardiomyopathy [15].

Additionally, inpatients who require ^{18}F-FDG-PET myocardial imaging for inflammation also require careful planning. Intravenous medications containing glucose should be avoided. Furthermore, a multidisciplinary approach involving nursing, dieticians, and imaging staff should be employed, in addition to providing the same instructions to the patients that would have been provided in the outpatient setting. As with outpatients, these individuals should be screened carefully for errors in preparation prior to ^{18}F-FDG injection.

Current Recommendations

The most recent SNMMI/ASNC expert consensus document from 2017 provides recommendations to optimize patient preparation based on current evidence. The document supports preparing patients with either: (a) at least two high fat (>35 g) and low carbohydrate (<3 g) meals the day prior to the study followed by a fast ranging from 4 to 12 h or (b) a fast of >18 h. The use of heparin can be considered as an adjunct given its uncertain role in suppressing myocardial glucose utilization. All patients should be contacted with instructions well in advance of the study and should document their meals and preparation for review with lab staff prior to ^{18}F-FDG injection [5]. Since publication of this most recent consensus document, additional support for longer duration fasting has emerged from several centers. Accordingly, if possible, a fast closer to 12 h as part of a combined approach appears to be more favorable [7]. In fact, the JSNC advocates for a longer fasting period of 12–18 h preceded by a low carbohydrate meal in

Table 4.3 SNMMI/ASNC consensus recommendations for myocardial suppression in ^{18}F-FDG-PET Imaging [5]

Beneficial	Maybe beneficial
At least two high-fat (>35 g) low-carbohydrate (<3 g) meals the day prior to imaging followed by a fast of 4–12 h or a fast of >18 h prior to ^{18}F-FDG administration	Use of adjunctive unfractionated heparin as an intravenous bolus (50 IU/kg) 15 min before ^{18}F-FDG administration
Diabetic patients should minimize short-acting insulin and avoid oral agents and non-insulin injections on the day of the study	
The exact preparation strategy should be logged prior to ^{18}F-FDG administration and serial studies should be performed with the same preparation strategy	

its most recent consensus statement [8]. A table of the strategies supported by current SNMMI/ASNC recommendations is provided below (Table 4.3) [5]. Importantly, a recent single center study demonstrated improved efficacy of a protocol based on the SNMMI/ASNC recommendations compared to the previously implemented institutional protocol [7].

Because each institution defines its own strategy for patient preparation for ^{18}F-FDG-PET imaging of myocardial and intracardiac inflammation, it is of paramount importance that all patients adhere to the specified protocol and that the institution performing imaging routinely reviews the quality of imaging results. There should be a goal of >85% successful suppression of myocardial ^{18}F-FDG uptake on these imaging studies.

Future Directions

There remain several key questions that merit ongoing investigation for optimization of ^{18}F-FDG-PET imaging of myocardial and intracardiac inflammation. A multicenter randomized trial comparing preparation strategies to

determine the optimal means of patient preparation should be considered. While serological measures have not yet proven to be useful for the assessment of metabolic status prior to imaging, the identification of an easily measured biomarker that would inform the quality of preparation would be extremely advantageous. Also, the role of machine learning in the interpretation of challenging and heterogeneous images consequent to marginal preparation (e.g., focally increased uptake superimposed on diffuse myocardial uptake) merits additional research. Alternative dietary strategies to reduce myocardial glucose uptake, such as a ketone body infusion, have shown promise in early studies and should be further evaluated [16]. Finally, and importantly, alternative tracers that would not require intensive patient preparation to suppress background myocardial uptake should continue to be investigated. For example, other PET tracers that have already demonstrated potential utility in cardiac sarcoidosis include ^{18}F-fluorothymidine and ^{68}Ga-DOTATATE [17, 18].

References

1. Depre C, Vanoverschelde JL, Taegtmeyer H. Glucose for the heart. Circulation. 1999;99(4):578–88.
2. Mochizuki T, Tsukamoto E, Kuge Y, Kanegae K, Zhao S, Hikosaka K, et al. FDG uptake and glucose transporter subtype expressions in experimental tumor and inflammation models. J Nucl Med. 2001;42(10):1551–5.
3. Osborne MT, Hulten EA, Murthy VL, Skali H, Taqueti VR, Dorbala S, et al. Patient preparation for cardiac fluorine-18 fluorodeoxyglucose positron emission tomography imaging of inflammation. J Nucl Cardiol. 2017;24(1):86–99.
4. Morooka M, Moroi M, Uno K, Ito K, Wu J, Nakagawa T, et al. Long fasting is effective in inhibiting physiological myocardial 18F-FDG uptake and for evaluating active lesions of cardiac sarcoidosis. EJNMMI Res. 2014;4(1):1.
5. Chareonthaitawee P, Beanlands RS, Chen W, Dorbala S, Miller EJ, Murthy VL, et al. Joint SNMMI-ASNC expert consensus document on the role of (18) F-FDG PET/CT in cardiac sarcoid detection and therapy monitoring. J Nucl Cardiol. 2017;24(5):1741–58.
6. Taegtmeyer H. Tracing cardiac metabolism in vivo: one substrate at a time. J Nucl Med. 2010;51(Suppl 1):80S–7S.

7. Christopoulos G, Jouni H, Acharya GA, Blauwet LA, Kapa S, Bois J, et al. Suppressing physiologic 18-fluorodeoxyglucose uptake in patients undergoing positron emission tomography for cardiac sarcoidosis: the effect of a structured patient preparation protocol. J Nucl Cardiol. 2019;28(2):661–71.

8. Kumita S, Yoshinaga K, Miyagawa M, Momose M, Kiso K, Kasai T, et al. Recommendations for (18) F-fluorodeoxyglucose positron emission tomography imaging for diagnosis of cardiac sarcoidosis-2018 update: Japanese Society of Nuclear Cardiology recommendations. J Nucl Cardiol. 2019;26(4):1414–33.

9. Larson SR, Pieper JA, Hulten EA, Ficaro EP, Corbett JR, Murthy VL, et al. Characterization of a highly effective preparation for suppression of myocardial glucose utilization. J Nucl Cardiol. 2019;27(3):849–61.

10. Asmal AC, Leary WP, Thandroyen F, Botha J, Wattrus S. A dose-response study of the anticoagulant and lipolytic activities of heparin in normal subjects. Br J Clin Pharmacol. 1979;7(5):531–3.

11. Demeure F, Hanin FX, Bol A, Vincent MF, Pouleur AC, Gerber B, et al. A randomized trial on the optimization of 18F-FDG myocardial uptake suppression: implications for vulnerable coronary plaque imaging. J Nucl Med. 2014;55(10):1629–35.

12. Alvi RM, Young BD, Shahab Z, Pan H, Winkler J, Herzog E, et al. Repeatability and optimization of FDG positron emission tomography for evaluation of cardiac sarcoidosis. JACC Cardiovasc Imaging. 2019;12(7 Pt 1):1284–7.

13. Osborne MT, Divakaran S. Seeking clarity: insights from a highly effective preparation protocol for suppressing myocardial glucose uptake for PET imaging of cardiac inflammation. J Nucl Cardiol. 2020;27(3):862–4.

14. Schelbert HR, Henze E, Phelps ME, Kuhl DE. Assessment of regional myocardial ischemia by positron-emission computed tomography. Am Heart J. 1982;103(4):588–97.

15. Davila-Roman VG, Vedala G, Herrero P, de las Fuentes L, Rogers JG, Kelly DP, et al. Altered myocardial fatty acid and glucose metabolism in idiopathic dilated cardiomyopathy. J Am Coll Cardiol. 2002;40(2):271–7.

16. Gormsen LC, Svart M, Thomsen HH, Sondergaard E, Vendelbo MH, Christensen N, et al. Ketone body infusion with 3-Hydroxybutyrate reduces myocardial glucose uptake and increases blood flow in humans: a positron emission tomography study. J Am Heart Assoc. 2017;6(3):e005066.

17. Martineau P, Pelletier-Galarneau M, Juneau D, Leung E, Nery PB, de Kemp R, et al. Imaging cardiac sarcoidosis with FLT-PET compared with FDG/perfusion-PET: a prospective pilot study. JACC Cardiovasc Imaging. 2019;12(11 Pt 1):2280–1.

18. Bravo PE, Bajaj N, Padera RF, Morgan V, Hainer J, Bibbo CF, et al. Feasibility of somatostatin receptor-targeted imaging for detection of myocardial inflammation: a pilot study. J Nucl Cardiol. 2019;28(3):1089–99.

Part II

Inflammatory and Malignant Disorders

Patrick Martineau, Matthieu Pelletier Galarneau, and David Birnie

Introduction

Despite having been studied over a century, many aspects of sarcoidosis—including its pathophysiology, diagnosis, and management—continue to confound clinicians and researchers alike. Initially described in 1877 by the English physician Jonathan Hutchinson, this multisystemic condition is characterized by non-caseating granulomas that can involve virtually any organ system. Due to the inter-patient variability in clinical presentation, disease severity, and organs involved, sarcoidosis has historically been referred to by a number of different names and eponyms dependent on the particular constellation of clinical findings, e.g. Lofgren syndrome (lymphadenopathy and skin involvement), Heerfordt syndrome (ocular, salivary gland, and facial nerve involvement), lupus pernio (skin involvement), etc. The introduction of what are essentially subtypes of sarcoidosis obfuscates the situation to a degree as all these conditions reflect a single unifying pathophysiology. Adding to the confusion are the difficulties associated with the diagnosis—sarcoidosis is a diagnosis of exclusion for which no specific tests exist. While serum markers of sarcoidosis are known, these are generally neither sensitive nor specific.

Recently, there has been increased attention on cardiac sarcoidosis (CS) due to the realization that the prevalence of this condition had long been underappreciated (in no small part due to the difficulties inherent in its diagnosis) and of the dire clinical and prognostic implications. Cardiac involvement is the leading cause of death in patients with CS with a 5-year mortality rate estimated to range from 25 to 60% despite treatment [1–3]. As a result, the field has recently seen advances in the development of diagnostic and therapeutic approaches. Fortunately, PET imaging with 2-deoxy-2-[^{18}F]fluoro-D-glucose (FDG) has been shown to be highly sensitive for the detection of inflammatory pathology and has proven itself to be a particularly useful test for the diagnosis and assessment of sarcoidosis, including cardiac involvement.

In this chapter, we review the basics of CS, with particular emphasis on imaging using FDG-PET. We discuss the diagnostic and prognostic significance of FDG-PET findings in patients with CS, as well as compare to other imaging modalities.

P. Martineau (✉)
BC Cancer, Vancouver, BC, Canada
e-mail: patrick.martineau@bccancer.bc.ca

M. P. Galarneau
Montreal Heart Institute, Montréal, QC, Canada
e-mail: Matthieu.pelletier-galarneau@icm-mhi.org

D. Birnie
Arrhythmia Service, Division of Cardiology, Department of Medicine, University of Ottawa Heart Institute, Ottawa, ON, Canada

Histopathology

The etiology of sarcoidosis remains a mystery despite exhaustive attempts to identify a causative agent. To date, the largest study which attempted to shed light on the origins of sarcoidosis was the NIH-funded ACCESS (A Case-Control Etiological Sarcoidosis Study). This study enrolled over 700 subjects, in addition to nearly 30,000 of their first- and second-degree relatives, in an attempt to determine a possible genetic etiology for sarcoidosis but failed to identify either a common agent or genetic locus [4, 5]. Nonetheless, ACCESS was able to confirm familial clustering of sarcoidosis cases, as well as racial variations, supporting a potential genetic component in the pathophysiology of sarcoidosis. Additional support for a genetic component is provided by the observation of a higher incidence rate of sarcoidosis in monozygotic compared to dizygotic twins [6].

Historically, a number of agents have been suggested as possible causative agents of sarcoidosis, including mycobacteria, propionibacteria, mycoplasma, viruses, as well as a variety of inorganic (talc, aluminum, zirconium) and organic (clay, pine tree pollen) substances. Nonetheless, conclusive evidence linking these agents to sarcoidosis has not been forthcoming. Further support for an environmental component of sarcoidosis is an observed variation with geography, seasonal variation, and occupation [7].

Currently, the predominant theory regarding the pathophysiological origins of sarcoidosis is the so-called gene-environment hypothesis—namely that individuals with a genetic predisposition are exposed to a particular environmental trigger, precipitating the disease phenotype [8]. Support for this theory has been garnered by a number of observations including: the above-described genetic component, the particular inflammatory response seen in sarcoidosis patients which is compatible with a Th1-type response triggered by an antigen, as well as an association between the condition and CD4+ T-cells [9]. These elements suggest that sarcoidosis may represent the body's reaction to a poorly degradable antigen resulting in the perpetuation of a chronic inflammatory response.

At the histological level, the hallmark lesions of sarcoidosis consist of granulomas—organized collections of mononuclear phagocytes—which may be associated with additional inflammatory leukocytes [10]. Traditionally, these granulomas are described as non-necrotizing although a degree of central necrosis can be present [10]. An important point to note is that the lesions seen in sarcoidosis are not specific to the condition and can be observed in other granulomatous conditions—as such, sarcoidosis remains a diagnosis of exclusion, and consideration of the clinical presentation, imaging results, as well as pathology results is necessary.

When activated, inflammatory cells overexpress specific glucose transporters—GLUT1, GLUT3, and GLUT4 [11, 12]—leading to an increase in glucose uptake (and, by extension, FDG which acts as a glucose analog) within these cells. It is this uptake which is the key to detecting sarcoidosis lesions on PET imaging.

Epidemiology

The reported incidence of sarcoidosis varies greatly among published studies which may suggest a significant geographical variation (Table 5.1). Sarcoidosis has consistently been reported to be most commonly seen in individuals living in Scandinavian countries, as well as in African Americans, with prevalence rates as high as 215 and 141.4 per 100,000 individuals, in Swedes and African Americans, respectively [13, 14]. However, it is important to note that these results were derived from health care use data which likely underestimates asymptomatic patients or those with limited disease. In addition to race and geography, sarcoidosis incidence has been noted to vary greatly with age and sex. Incidence is noted to peak in middle age, with a slightly greater prevalence in women.

Table 5.1 Reported incidence and prevalence of sarcoidosis

References	Year published	Country	Reported incidence per 100,000	Reported prevalence per 100,000	Age of onset (years)	Female proportion of cases
[13]	2016	Sweden	11.5	160	Male: 45, female: 55	45%
[14]	2016	USA	17.8 (African Americans) 8.1 (Caucasians) 4.3 (Hispanics) 3.2 (Asians)	141.4 (African Americans) 49.8 (Caucasians) 21.7 (Hispanics) 18.9 (Asians)	NR	NR
[108]	2016	USA	11 (overall) 11 (Caucasians) 43 (African Americans) 5 (Hispanics) 6 (others)	100 (overall) 92 (Caucasians) 519 (African Americans) 69 (others)	NR	100%: Only women included in the study
[109]	2017	USA	11.0 (females), 10.5 (males)	NR	Male: 42.8, female: 48.3	50%
[110]	2017	Italy	NR	49	Male: 46.5, female: 53.5	58.3%
[111]	2015	Guadeloupe	2.28	21.09	NR	59%
[112]	2017	France	4.9	30	NR	55%
[113]	2017	Taiwan	NR	2.17	Male: 42, female: 51	63%
[114]	2019	Canada	6.8	143	Male: 45, female: 49	53.1%

NR not reported

Table 5.2 Reported prevalence of cardiac sarcoidosis on imaging studies

References	Year published	Country	N	Prevalence	Modality
[25]	2002	France	31	54.9%	CMR
[23]	2003	France	50	14.0%	CMR
[24]	2005	Holland	82	3.7%	CMR, SPECT
[16]	2008	USA	62	38.7%	CMR, PET
[18]	2009	USA	81	25.9%	CMR
[20]	2011	USA	152	19.0%	CMR
[21]	2013	Germany	155	25.5%	CMR
[17]	2014	Japan	61	31.0%	CMR
[59]	2016	Germany	188	15.4%	CMR
[22]	2016	USA	205	20.0%	CMR

Rates of Cardiac Involvement

The reported prevalence of cardiac involvement varies significantly (Table 5.2). The ACCESS reported a prevalence of CS of only 2.3% [15]; however, it should be noted that studies have consistently revealed that a significant proportion of patients with sarcoidosis without cardiac symptoms have detectable cardiac involvement on imaging, with the proportion ranging from 3.7 to 54.9% [16–25]. Furthermore, comparable results have consistently been seen on autopsy studies. In particular, cardiac sarcoidosis is common among the Japanese population and has been found in up to 58% of sarcoidosis patients [26]. In American populations, autopsy studies have found cardiac involvement in 27–40% of patients [1, 27]. Cardiac involvement has been reported to the predominant cause of death in patients with sarcoidosis, responsible for approximately 50% of sarcoid-related deaths in these patients [28–30], rising to 85% in Japanese patients [26].

Clinical Presentation and Prognosis

The clinical presentation of sarcoidosis is highly variable and dependent on numerous factors, including extent of disease and the organ systems involved. Chronic granulomatous inflammation can result in organ fibrosis and dysfunction. While the clinical significance of this largely depends on the organ or type of tissue affected, such fibrosis in the heart can have significant prognostic implications. In particular, granulomatous infiltration and fibrosis of the heart can precipitate rhythm disturbances, conduction blocks, or even sudden cardiac death when the conduction system is involved (Fig. 5.1) [1, 2, 24, 31–33]. Extensive involvement by cardiac lesions can lead to impaired cardiac function resulting in heart failure [2, 31, 34]. Studies have shown that a large proportion (16–35%) of patients less than 60 years of age presenting with complete heart block, or those with ventricular tachycardia of unknown etiology, have CS [35–38].

Despite this, some patients with cardiac involvement remain asymptomatic—studies have reported that the rate of asymptomatic cardiac involvement in patients with extracardiac disease varies between 3.7% and 54.9% [24, 25].

Cardiac involvement portends a worse prognosis than extracardiac involvement—in particular, CS is reported to be the cause of 85% of sarcoid deaths in Japan [39]—with death being caused by factors such as heart failure and/or arrhythmias.

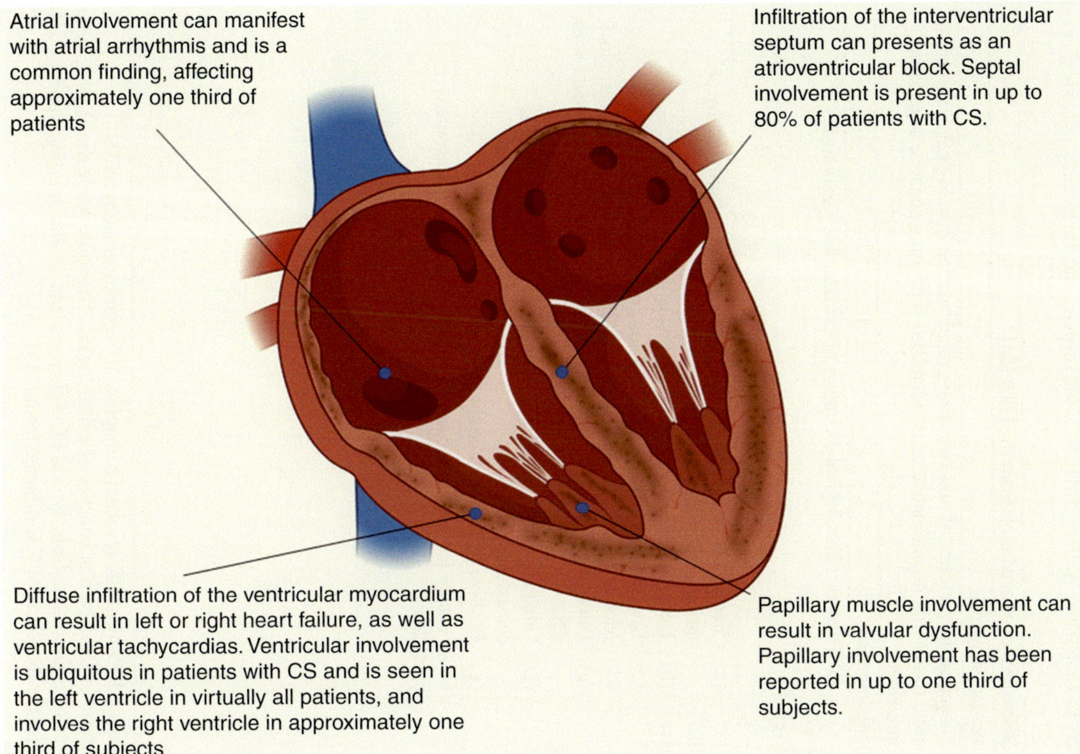

Fig. 5.1 The clinical presentation of cardiac sarcoidosis is variable and is largely dependent on the degree of involvement as well as the location of the lesions

Diagnostic Workup

Due to the lack of a single specific test, the diagnostic workup of patients with CS is comprehensive and takes into account clinical symptoms, serum biomarkers, tissue sampling, and the results of advanced imaging modalities such as PET and MRI.

In order to address this, various diagnostic guidelines have been proposed which incorporate a constellation of clinical symptoms, ECG results, tissue sampling, and imaging findings. There are currently three sets of guidelines used for the diagnosis of CS, all of which propose clinical criteria in order to establish a diagnosis of CS. These are the Japanese Ministry of Health and Welfare (JMHW) criteria, proposed in 1993 [40] and revised in 2007 [41], the World Association for Sarcoidosis and Other Granulomatous Disorders (WASOG) criteria, first published in 1999 [42] and updated in 2014 [43], as well as the more recently published Heart Rhythm Society (HRS) expert consensus statement, also published in 2014 [44]. Most studies examining the use of advanced imaging for the diagnosis of CS use either the JMHW or HRS criteria as gold standard—these criteria are compared in Table 5.3.

A recent study comparing the diagnostic performance of all three sets of criteria compared to an expert, multidisciplinary panel found that a large portion of patients deemed to have CS by the panel failed to satisfy the three diagnostic criteria [45]. Furthermore, the three diagnostic criteria were found to have low concordance; however, it should be noted that the cohort exam-

Table 5.3 Clinical diagnostic criteria for the diagnosis of CS, with the latest Japanese Ministry of Health and Welfare (JMHW) (2006) criteria and the recently published Heart Rhythm Society (HRS) criteria (2014)

2006 modified JMHW guidelines [41]		Expert consensus recommendation from the HRS [44]	
1. Histological diagnosis		1. Histological diagnosis	
CS is confirmed when cardiac biopsy specimens demonstrate non-caseating epithelioid cell granuloma with histological or clinical diagnosis of extracardiac sarcoidosis		CS is diagnosed in the presence of non-caseating granulomas on histological examination of myocardial tissue with no alternative cause identified (including negative organismal stains if applicable)	
2. Clinical diagnosis		2. Clinical diagnosis	
Cardiac sarcoidosis is diagnosed without endomyocardial biopsy or in the absence of typical granulomas on cardiac biopsy when histological or clinical diagnosis of extracardiac sarcoidosis is established and a combination of major or minor diagnostic criteria has been satisfied as follows:		It is probable that there is CS if	(a) There is a histological diagnosis of extracardiac sarcoidosis
≥ 2 of the 4 following major criteria are satisfied:	(a) Advanced atrioventricular block (b) Basal thinning of the ventricular septum (c) Positive cardiac gallium uptake[a] (d) Left ventricular ejection fraction <50%	And one or more of the following is present:	(a) Steroid +/− immunosuppressant responsive cardiomyopathy or atrioventricular block (b) Unexplained reduced LVEF (< 40%) (c) Unexplained sustained (spontaneous or induced) VT (d) Mobitz type II second-degree heart block or third-degree heart block (e) Patchy uptake on dedicated cardiac PET (in a pattern consistent with CS) (f) Late gadolinium enhancement on cardiac MRI (in a pattern consistent with CS) (g) Positive gallium uptake (in a pattern consistent with CS)
Or 1 of the 4 major criteria and ≥2 of the following Minor criteria are satisfied:	(a) Abnormal electrocardiogram findings including ventricular tachycardia, multifocal frequent premature ventricular contractions, complete right bundle branch block, abnormal Q waves, or abnormal axis deviation (b) Abnormal echocardiogram demonstrating regional wall motion abnormalities, ventricular aneurysm, or unexplained increase in wall thickness (c) Perfusion defects detected by myocardial scintigraphy (d) Delayed gadolinium enhancement of the myocardium on cardiac MRI scanning (e) Interstitial fibrosis or monocyte infiltration greater than moderate grade by endomyocardial biopsy	And	Other causes for the cardiac manifestation(s) have been reasonably excluded

CS cardiac sarcoidosis, *LVEF* left ventricular ejection fraction, *PET* positron emission tomography, *MRI* magnetic resonance imaging, *VT* ventricular tachycardia
Note that for both the JMHW and HRS criteria, there are two separate pathways for the diagnosis of CS. The first consists of a histological diagnosis, while the second, more commonly employed, relies on a constellation of findings including pathological diagnosis of extracardiac sarcoidosis, typical ECG changes, and cardiac imaging findings. The JMHW criteria are the first set of diagnostic criteria which explicitly make use of PET results for the diagnosis of CS. Adapted from [115]
[a]FDG-PET is a widely accepted substitute for Ga67 scintigraphy

ined in this study had a high rate of isolated CS which, due to low sensitivity and the difficulties in obtaining a tissue diagnosis of sarcoidosis from endomyocardial biopsy, may partly account for the poor agreement between expert consensus and the various diagnostic criteria.

Serum Biomarkers

Despite the well-known association between sarcoidosis and serum angiotensin converting enzyme (ACE) levels, ACE levels are reported to be elevated in only 60% of patients with sarcoidosis [46]; however, patients treated for hypertension with ACE inhibitors can have suppressed levels of serum ACE—and it should be noted that up to 35% of patients with hypertension in the USA are treated with ACE inhibitors [47]—significantly limiting the utility of this biomarker for the diagnosis of sarcoidosis [48]. A number of additional serum biomarkers have been investigated for the diagnosis and follow-up of sarcoidosis including neopterin, troponin, IL-2, chitotriosidase, lysozyme, serum amyloid A, etc.; however, none of these demonstrates high accuracy for the diagnosis of sarcoidosis [49]. As such, the role of serum biomarkers in the evaluation of sarcoidosis and CS is limited, and serum biomarker results are not included in the diagnostic criteria mentioned above.

Endomyocardial Biopsy

The gold standard for the diagnosis of CS consists of a positive endomyocardial biopsy (EMB). Unfortunately, in part due to the nature of the disease which causes patchy, heterogeneous areas of myocardial infiltration, as well as technical difficulties—sampling being limited to the right-sided heart chambers—the sensitivity of EMB is quite low, reported as 20–30% [39, 50]. Electroanatomical mapping or image-guided biopsy has been reported to improve sensitivity (up to 50%) but most patients with CS are not diagnosed with endomyocardial sampling [51, 52].

ECG Findings

ECG changes frequently serve as a screening test for patients with suspected CS and can demonstrate evidence of structural or functional cardiac abnormalities [16, 53]; however, ECG findings suffer from low sensitivity and specificity for the diagnosis of CS, reported to be 33–58%/22–71%, respectively [31, 54]. Nonetheless, the presence of cardiac symptoms and certain ECG findings, such as bundle branch block, second or third degree atrioventricular block, ventricular arrhythmias, and ST/T changes, can be suggestive of the diagnosis [55–57]. ECG abnormalities in CS patients are common, reported in 12–62% of subjects [2, 24, 58]; however, in patients with clinically silent CS, ECG abnormalities have been reported to be present in only 3.2–8.6% of patients [16–18, 59].

Echocardiography

Echocardiography is often used as the initial cardiac imaging assessment in patients with suspected CS due to it wide availability. While frequently normal in patients with clinically silent CS, symptomatic patients can demonstrate regional wall motion abnormalities, systolic or diastolic dysfunction, basal septal thinning, an increase in left ventricular wall thickness, or a restrictive or dilated cardiomyopathy [16, 60–63]. Occasionally, patients with CS and atrial involvement can demonstrate areas of atrial hypertrophy [64]. None of these findings is specific to CS and patients often require assessment with more advanced imaging modalities. Nonetheless, echocardiography is useful in the initial assessment and follow-up of LV function, an important prognostic indicator.

Cardiac Magnetic Resonance (CMR)

CMR findings are not specific for the diagnosis of CS but typical findings include late gadolinium enhancement (LGE), usually patchy and multifocal. Segments most commonly affected include the basal segments, with LGE usually seen in the midmyocardium and epicardium [20, 65, 66]. CMR enjoys high spatial resolution and allows for accurate assessment of both left and right ventricular function while also assessing for areas of edema and fibrosis. Unfortunately, the use of CMR in patients with suspected CS is often hampered by the presence of cardiac implantable electronic devices (CIED).

FDG-PET Imaging of Patients with CS

Recently, the European Association of Nuclear Medicine (EANM), the European Association of Cardiovascular Imaging (EACVI), the American Society of Nuclear Cardiology (ASNC), and the Society of Nuclear Medicine and Molecular Imaging (SNMMI) have produced multi-society procedural position statements in part to help guide the use of FDG-PET imaging in patients with CS [67, 68].

The EANM, the EACVI, and the ASNC position statement sets forth, among other things, a standardized approach to patient preparation and image acquisition, in addition to a clear set of diagnostic criteria for FDG-PET (in conjunction with perfusion imaging) in patients with suspected CS. These diagnostic criteria support the hypothesis that FDG uptake in cardiac lesions represents sites of active inflammation with the interpretation of these patterns reliant on the distribution of uptake, rather than the degree or intensity of uptake seen. Furthermore, this position statement proposes an imaging approach to the workup of patients with suspected CS (Fig. 5.2) and also highlights the important role that FDG-PET can play in the monitoring of response to immunosuppressive therapy due to the ability of PET to directly visualize inflammatory activity. The views put forth in this position statement largely echo those of the Joint SNMMI–ASNC expert consensus document [68]. Both of these documents make clear the importance of standardized PET acquisition protocols and interpretation criteria. These position statements enumerate multiple clinical scenarios in which PET imaging in patients with known or suspected CS may be helpful.

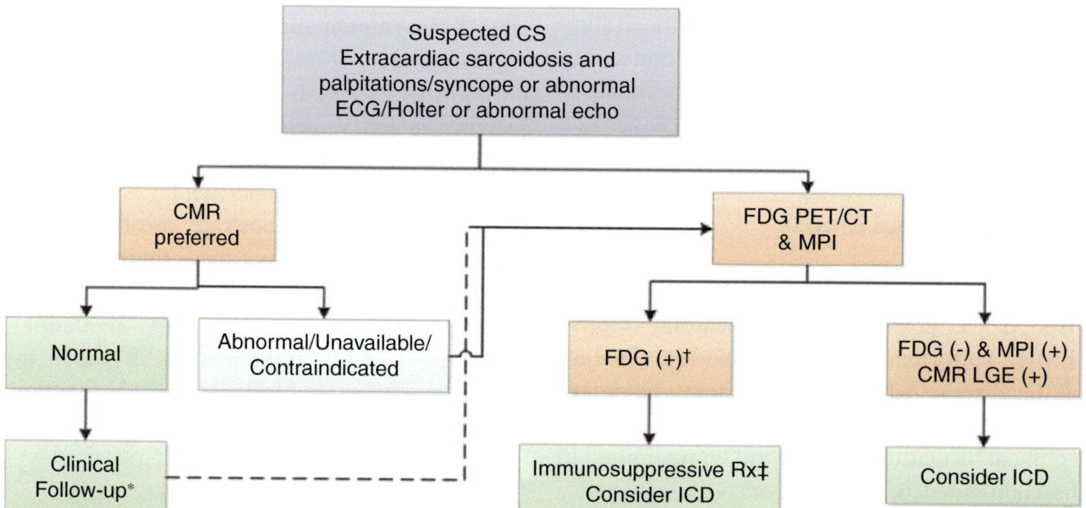

Fig. 5.2 Suggested imaging approach for the assessment of suspected cardiac sarcoidosis suggested by the Cardiovascular and Inflammation and Infection Committees of the European Association of Nuclear Medicine, the European Association of Cardiovascular Imaging, and the American Society of Nuclear Cardiology. *CS* cardiac sarcoidosis, *CMR* cardiovascular magnetic resonance imaging, *ECG* electrocardiogram, *Echo* echocardiogram, *FDG* 18F-fluorodeoxyglucose, *ICD* implantable cardioverter defibrillator, *LGE* late gadolinium enhancement, *MPI* myocardial perfusion imaging, *Rx* therapy. (Reprinted with permission from [67])

Protocols for Cardiac FDG-PET Imaging

Due to the variable nature of physiological cardiac FDG uptake, use of standardized patient preparation protocols is essential when using FDG-PET to assess patients with suspected CS. Further details on the nature of cardiac metabolism and suppression protocols are available in Chaps. 3 and 4. It will be noted that adoption of a structured preparation protocol has been shown to decrease the rate of non-diagnostic studies [69]. Furthermore, Tang et al. performed a systematic review and meta-analysis in order to examine the effects of patient preparation on the diagnostic accuracy of FDG-PET for CS using the JMHW criteria as gold standard [70]. This analysis incorporated 16 studies for a total of 559 patients. The authors found that the diagnostic odds ratio positively correlated with fast duration and heparin use, but not with the use of a high fat low carbohydrate diet.

Interpretation Criteria

Assuming adherence to an appropriate patient preparation protocol, the interpretation of cardiac FDG-PET images is straightforward. As mentioned above, the interpretation of PET cardiac is based on the distribution of uptake and not on the intensity of uptake. Figure 5.3 shows the typical patterns of cardiac FDG uptake encountered in clinical practice. Positive studies for CS should show distinct foci of uptake, or at least heterogeneous uptake, while homogeneous (particularly in the lateral free wall of the left ventricle) or absent uptake should be considered negative for active cardiac sarcoidosis. The distinction of "active" cardiac sarcoidosis is an important one due to the possibility of so-called burnt-out dis-

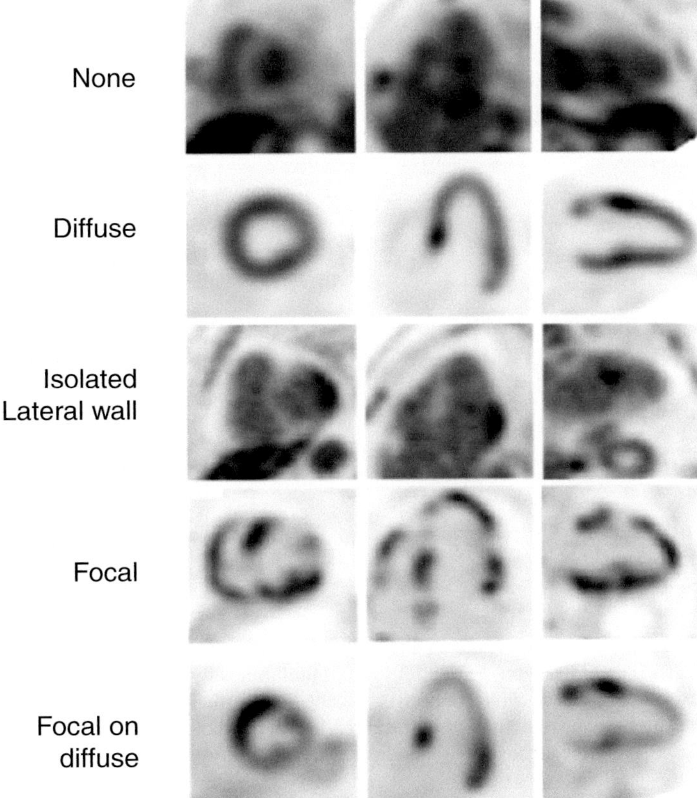

Fig. 5.3 Patterns of cardiac uptake which can be encountered when assessing patients with FDG-PET for suspected CS shown in short, horizontal long, and vertical long axes. The "None," "Diffuse," and "Isolated Lateral wall" patterns are all considered negative for CS. Furthermore, the "Diffuse" pattern should raise the issue of appropriate patient adherence to preparation instructions and such studies may be considered non diagnostic. Positive studies for CS should show focal patterns of activity such as seen in the "Focal" and "Focal on diffuse" patterns. (Reprinted with permission from [115])

ease, i.e. myocardial scarring without evidence of active inflammation. As FDG-PET assesses inflammation, patients with burnt-out disease will not show abnormal findings on this modality; however, cardiac perfusion studies and CMR can show the stigmata of burnt-out CS—namely myocardial scarring—hence the importance of conducting such studies in conjunction with FDG-PET, as recommended by the position statements mentioned above.

One of the important advantages of PET as a whole-body imaging modality is that, in addition to cardiac involvement, extracardiac sarcoidosis can be easily assessed (Fig. 5.4).

Diagnostic Accuracy of FDG-PET for the Assessment of CS

The issue of diagnostic accuracy of FDG-PET for CS is complicated by the lack of a unique reference standard. Furthermore, the results of certain early studies which may not have employed adequate myocardial suppression protocols must be interpreted with caution, as physiological cardiac uptake can be a serious confounder, limiting the effectiveness of FDG-PET. Furthermore, poor correlation between PET results and the JMHW criteria has been reported which brings into question the results of studies reporting the accuracy

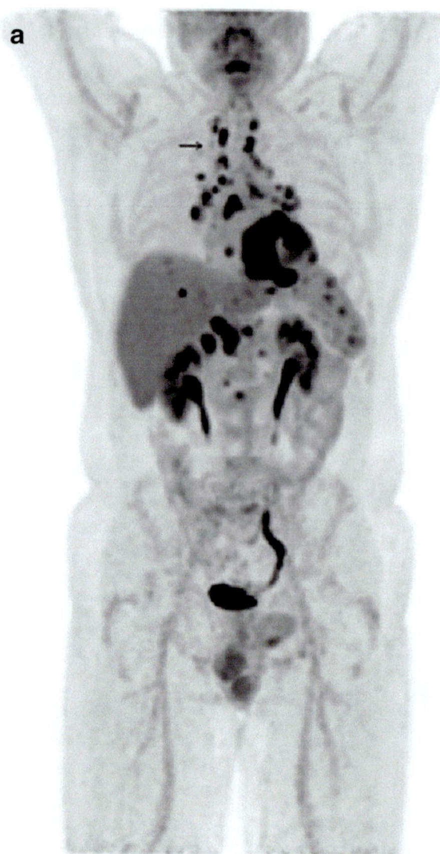

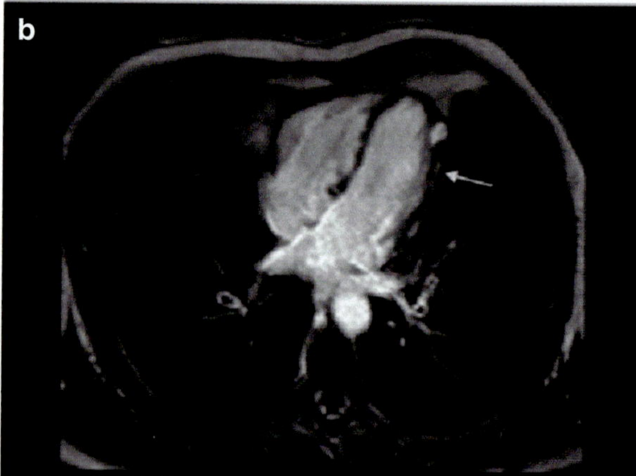

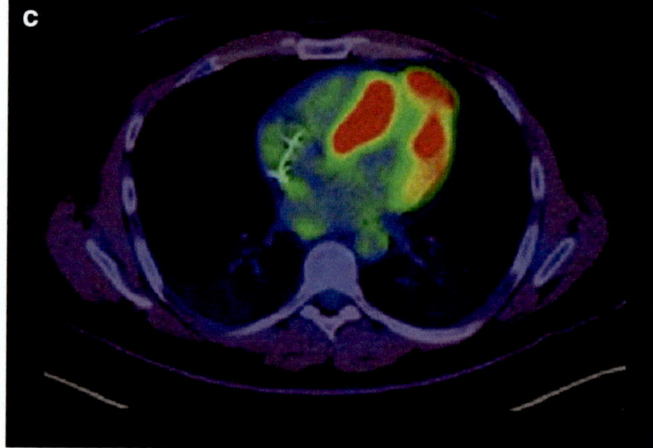

Fig. 5.4 Typical findings in a patient with CS and extracardiac sarcoidosis on FDG-PET. Maximum intensity projection images demonstrate significant myocardial uptake as well as roughly symmetric and bilateral mediastinal/hilar lymphadenopathy (as indicated by the arrow), the typical finding of thoracic sarcoidosis (**a**). In this patient, MRI (**b**) demonstrated patchy myocardial late gadolinium enhancement (as indicated by the arrow), with corresponding activity seen on transaxial FDG-PET/CT images (**c**). (Reprinted with permission from [115])

Table 5.4 Results of studies examining the sensitivity and specificity of FDG-PET for cardiac sarcoidosis

References	Year	N	Preparation	Sensitivity	Specificity	Gold Standard	Country
[116]	2003	17	5 h fast	82%	–	JMHW	Japan
[83]	2004	22	12 h fast	100%	91%	Modified JMHW	Japan
[117]	2005	19	6 h fast, UFH	100%	81%	JMHW	Japan
[72]	2008	21	6 h fast, UFH	88%	38%	JMHW	Japan
[85]	2009	30	18 h fast	85%	90%	JMHW	USA
[84]	2010	24	12 h fast	100%	33%	JMHW	Japan
[73]	2012	24	12 h fast	79%	79%	Modified JMHW	Canada
[118]	2013	43	12 h fast	33%	96%	JMHW	Italy
[96]	2013	58	4 h fast, HFLC diet	50%	95%	JMHW	France
[88]	2014	31	12 h fast, HFLC diet	95%	88%	Modified JMHW	USA
[71]	2014	118	3 h fast, HFLC diet	42%	80%	JMHW	USA
[119]	2014	59	6 h fast, UFH	93%	69%	JMHW	Japan
[120]	2014	19	12 h fast, UFH	75%	73%	JMHW	Japan
[121]	2015	52	12 h fast, UFH	74%	80%	JMHW	Japan
[122]	2015	92	19 h fast, LC diet	97%	83%	Modified JMHW	Japan
[101]	2016	19	15 h fast	33%	88%	JMHW	Denmark
[92]	2017	231	12 h fast, HFLC diet	69%	93%	JMHW	USA
[105]	2017	20	18 h fast	85%	100%	JMHW	Japan

JMHW Japanese Ministry of Health and Welfare Guidelines, *UFH* unfractionated heparin, *HFLC* high fat, low carbohydrate, *LC* low carbohydrate

of PET imaging while using the JMHW criteria as gold standard [71, 72].

Yousef et al., in a meta-analysis of 7 studies including 164 patients, reported a sensitivity and specificity of 89% and 78%, respectively, using the JMHW guidelines as gold standard [73]. A more recent meta-analysis, which updated these results to include 17 studies and 891 subjects, reported a pooled sensitivity and specificity of 0.84 and 0.83, respectively [74] (Table 5.4). The authors suggested that the combination of FDG-PET with perfusion imaging could improve diagnostic accuracy. It should be noted that this meta-analysis only included studies which used the JMHW or modified JMHW criteria as a reference standard and it is unclear how the use of another gold standard (such as the HRS criteria) would impact diagnostic accuracy.

Prognostic Significance

Blankstein et al. examined the relationship between PET abnormalities (perfusion and metabolic) and outcomes in cardiac sarcoidosis patients [71]. Patients were assigned to one of the three categories—normal perfusion and metabolism, abnormal perfusion or metabolism, or abnormal perfusion and metabolism. Primary outcomes considered included all-cause death and documented sustained ventricular tachycardia. This study found that abnormalities in perfusion and metabolism were significantly associated with death and sustained ventricular tachycardia, with the strongest association found in patients with both perfusion defects and metabolic abnormalities. The authors found that focal uptake in the right ventricle was also associated with an increased rate of adverse outcomes which is up to 5 times greater than those without abnormal cardiac perfusion or metabolic findings.

A study comparing the prognostic significance of late gadolinium enhancement (LGE) and myocardial FDG uptake on PET in a group of 56 patients suggested that LGE was predictive of adverse events (defined as sustained ventricular tachycardia, ventricular fibrillation, ICD shock, and all-cause death), while FDG uptake was not [75]. It should be noted that these results differ from those of Blankstein et al. [71].

The prognostic importance of right ventricular involvement was confirmed in a retrospective study by Tuominen et al. involving 137 subjects [76]. This study found that right ventricular involvement, in addition to high total cardiac metabolic activity, was associated with an increased risk of adverse cardiac events (defined as death, reduction in LVEF, or hospitalization due to arrhythmia). The prognostic significance of the extent and severity of FDG-avid cardiac abnormalities in CS was also explored in a retrospective study by Sperry et al. [77]. This study examined the relationship between perfusion PET (using rubidium as a perfusion agent), FDG-PET, and clinical outcomes—in particular, the authors performed survival analysis using a composite endpoint consisting of death, ventricular tachycardia requiring defibrillation, and heart transplantation. Measures of cardiac FDG uptake considered included the summed FDG score, maximum global SUV score, mean global SUV, the standard deviation of global SUV, as well as the coefficient of variation (CoV, defined as the ratio of the standard deviation to the mean) of FDG uptake. Furthermore, the relationship between FDG and perfusion abnormalities was examined. Their results showed that, of the variables examined, the sum rest score (SRS) on perfusion imaging and the CoV on FDG imaging were the best predictors of adverse events.

Subramanian et al. examined the relationship between a novel quantitative measure, the Uptake Index (UI)—defined as the product of the maximum left ventricular SUV and the number of segments with abnormal uptake—and the clinical and echocardiographic response in patients with CS undergoing treatment [78]. This study found that pre-treatment myocardial FDG-PET findings, as assessed by the UI, were an independent predictor of the short-term (4–6 months) clinical and echocardiographic response following the initiation of therapy.

The extent of perfusion abnormalities may have more prognostic significance than the extent of inflammation. A study by Yamamoto et al. [79] examined the prognostic significance of myocardial ischemia—as assessed by ^{123}I-BMIPP SPECT—and myocardial uptake on FDG-PET in 73 subjects with CS and without obstructive coronary artery disease. Patients underwent serial imaging SPECT and PET over a mean follow-up period of 1264 ± 996 days during which time 20 major adverse cardiac events (MACE, defined as all-cause mortality, hospitalization due to heart failure, and sustained ventricular tachycardia/fibrillation) were recorded. Following diagnosis, patients were treated with prednisolone. Those patients with $SUV_{Max} < 4$ on FDG-PET after the introduction of prednisolone for more than 2 years were considered as recurrence-free, while those with $SUV_{Max} > 4$ at least once under treatment were considered to have recurred. The authors found that the higher BMIPP defect scores were predictive of both recurrence and MACE, while FDG findings were not predictive of MACE; however, the metabolic volume (defined as the volume of the left ventricular wall with $SUV \geq 4.0$), total lesion glycolysis (the product of the metabolic volume and mean SUV), and frequency of right ventricular involvement were greater within the recurrence group.

Role in Assessing Response

It is recommended that patients with CS be treated with immunosuppressive drugs when there is evidence of LV dysfunction, ventricular arrhythmias, abnormalities on cardiac imaging (e.g. LGE on CMR, or cardiac uptake on FDG-PET), or when there is RV dysfunction in the absence of pulmonary hypertension [80]. The fact that most of these criteria must be assessed on cross-sectional imaging highlights the important role of advanced imaging modalities for the follow-up of patients with CS undergoing treatment. Furthermore, as neither echocardiography nor CMR is very specific for active cardiac inflammation—which is the aspect of CS most amenable to treatment—FDG-PET may serve as the ideal imaging modality for follow-up in these patients (Fig. 5.5).

One of the advantages of PET imaging is the ease with which quantitative or semi-quantitative assessments of perfusion or metabolic abnormalities can be obtained. Furthermore, many of these quantitative measures have been shown to be associated with high repeatability, an essential

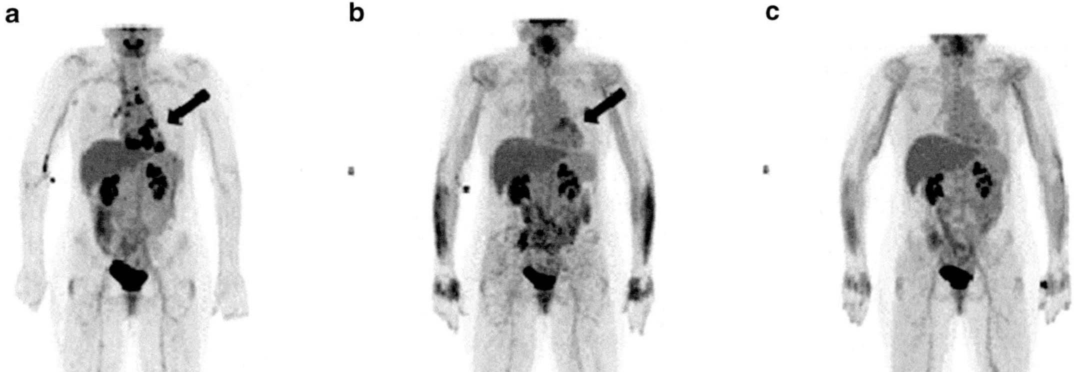

Fig. 5.5 FDG-PET allows for straightforward evaluation of therapeutic response in patients with sarcoidosis. (**a**) shows a baseline FDG-PET of a patient with CS with cardiac (arrow) and mediastinal lymph node involvement. After 3 months of treatment (**b**), the lymphadenopathy has resolved but there is evidence of mild residual inflammation within the heart (arrow). This activity has completely disappeared after an additional 3 months of treatment (**c**)

feature particularly if PET is to be used to measure response to therapy [81, 82]. Measures that have been considered for the assessment of disease activity in CS patients include maximum standardized uptake value (SUV_{Max}), mean segmental SUV, the coefficient of variation (CoV) of myocardial SUVs, the cardiac metabolic activity (CMA), and cardiac metabolic volume (CMV) [71, 83–88]. Some of these measures have been shown to be more revelatory than others. For example, McArdle et al. [86] showed that patients presenting with ventricular tachycardia (VT) had higher values of SUV_{Max} and mean segmental SUV when compared to subjects with atrioventricular block, while Ahmadian et al. [88] have suggested that CMA may be a useful marker for assessing effectiveness of immunosuppressive therapy due to an association with adverse events (including VT and other arrhythmias, congestive heart failure, and heart block).

Several studies have suggested that a decrease in the amount of myocardial inflammation is associated with an improvement in cardiac function and NYHA class [71, 87, 89]. Lee et al. examined the role of FDG-PET/CT for follow-up of 16 patients with CS by comparing various quantitative measures (including maximum (SUV_{Max}), partial-volume corrected mean standardized uptake value (SUV_{Mean}), partial-volume corrected metabolic volume product, and global metabolic volume product) to clinical symptoms, NYHA class, and ECG changes [89]. Results suggested that decreases in both SUV_{Max} and SUV_{Mean} were associated with improvements in clinical measures, while patients with progressive disease failed to show statistically significant decreases in quantitative measures on serial scans; however, one limitation of this study is that the relationship between PET findings and hard cardiac outcomes (e.g. death, arrhythmia, MACE, etc.) was not examined.

Muser et al., in a retrospective study of 20 subjects with a total of 92 PET studies, examined the prognostic significance of SUV_{Max}, partial-volume corrected mean standardized uptake value (SUV_{Mean}), partial-volume corrected volume-intensity product, the volume-intensity product of the entire heart, and the background cardiac metabolic [90]. Over a median follow-up period of 35 months, 18 MACE (including death, heart transplantation, hospitalization for heart failure, and ICD interventions) occurred. It was found that lack of metabolic improvement (as measured by the partial-volume corrected volume-intensity product) was the only predictor of MACE, with a hazard ratio of nearly 19. Furthermore, the authors found a significant inverse relationship between changes in partial-volume corrected volume-intensity product and changes in the LVEF.

A characteristic feature of CS on FDG-PET is heterogeneous myocardial uptake. This heterogeneity is helpful in distinguishing it from other disease processes and has been studied quantitatively through the use of texture analysis. Texture analysis—which consists of a set of computational techniques to study the relationships and inhomogeneity amongst sets of voxels—has been shown to be useful in assessing FDG-PET/CT studies in patients with suspected CS [77, 91–93]. An advantage of texture analysis over other quantitative measures (such as SUV) is that measures of texture can assess the distribution of activity. While much work remains to be done, results to date suggest that texture features could aid in the diagnosis of CS and confer prognostic significance, with many extractable features associated with high inter-operator reproducibility.

Despite these results, the optimal quantitative measure for diagnosis and follow-up has yet to be identified. Furthermore, at least for the purposes of diagnosis, use of these quantitative measures has not been shown to be superior to a visual interpretation by an expert reader. Overall, the use of quantitation of FDG-PET in the assessment of CS continues to be an area of active research.

FDG-PET/MR for the Assessment of CS

Hanneman et al. examined the feasibility of using PET/MR to image cardiac sarcoidosis and myocarditis in 10 subjects with known or suspected cardiac sarcoidosis or myocarditis [94]. They found no significant difference in the number of positive cases between PET/MR and standalone PET/CT or CMR, but they did report a significant decrease in total effective radiation dose between PET/MR and PET/CT.

Wisenberg et al. [95] compared the findings on PET/CT and PET/MR in 10 patients with CS following a single injection of FDG, with patients imaged with both modalities in a single day. They found that the presence of increased uptake, as well as the location of uptake was similar between both modalities. Based on their results, PET/MRI held no clear advantage over PET/CT.

Comparison of FDG-PET/CT to MRI

To date, there has been limited research comparing FDG-PET and CMR in patients with CS. In part, this may be related to the fact that comparing FDG-PET and CMR is inherently limited as both modalities detect different phenomena—FDG-PET is useful for imaging myocardial inflammation but provides essentially no information on the presence or extent of myocardial fibrosis, while CMR is able to detect both inflammation and fibrosis. As such, correlation between FDG-PET and CMR findings has been reported as only mild to moderate [72, 96]. A significant advantage of PET over CMR is the ability to image patients with CIEDs, as well as those with impaired renal function for whom IV contrast may be contraindicated. In addition, PET has the ability to accurately quantify the degree of myocardial inflammation—which is the part of the disease amenable to therapy—and may be better suited for assessing response to treatment on follow-up imaging. Furthermore, PET is highly useful in detecting extracardiac disease, which can be useful in detecting extracardiac sites amenable to biopsy.

A direct comparison between FDG-PET and CMR in 30 untreated patients with CS and conduction system disease (CSD) was provided by Ohira et al. [97]. The modified JMHW 2006 criteria were used as the gold standard for CS. Of the 30 subjects, 20 had abnormalities on both CMR and FDG-PET. After classifying patients into two groups—chronic vs. new-onset CSD—it was found that patients with chronic CSD were more likely to be positive on CMR, while those with new-onset disease were more likely to be positive on FDG-PET. The authors suggested that, despite both CMR and FDG-PET being useful in the assessment of patients with suspected CS, FDG-PET might provide additional information in patients with new-onset CSD.

The respective roles of FDG-PET and CMR in the follow-up of patients with CS were examined in a retrospective study by Coulden et al. [98]. This study examined a total of 31 subjects with biopsy proven extracardiac sarcoidosis and suspected CS, 22 of which received immunosuppressive therapy, all of which underwent repeat CMR and PET after a median 228 days. Treated patients showed a significant decrease in myocardial SUV_{Max} as well as a significant increase in LVEF, with no significant change in volume of LGE post-therapy. The patients not undergoing therapy showed no significant changes in FDG-PET or CMR measures. On the basis of these results, the authors suggested that cardiac FDG-PET findings could serve as a potentially useful surrogate for assessing therapy response.

Future Directions

FDG-PET in the assessment of patients with CS continues to be an area of active research. Outstanding issues include the optimal quantitative measures to use in diagnosis and follow-up as well as the role that PET/MR should play. While FDG-PET has shown itself to be a useful imaging modality in patients with CS, the need for special patient preparation in order to suppress normal myocardial uptake is an important limitation. For this reason, several studies have looked at alternative PET radiotracers—ideally, those without physiological cardiac uptake. To date, numerous other radiotracers have been shown to be able to detect CS on PET including DOTA agents [99–103], fluorothymidine [104, 105], NaF [106], and FMISO [107]. However, compared to FDG, the use of most of these radiotracers is restricted by their limited availability, in addition to reimbursement issues.

Conclusion

The use of FDG-PET for CS is firmly established in clinical practice with this modality offering high diagnostic accuracy, in addition to important diagnostic and prognostic information, distinct from that of other advanced imaging modalities such as CMR. Furthermore, the ability to perform this test in essentially all patients and its straightforward interpretation guarantees it a continued role in the diagnostic armamentarium for CS.

References

1. Roberts WC, McAllister HA Jr, Ferrans VJ. Sarcoidosis of the heart: a clinicopathologic study of 35 necropsy patients (group I) and review of 78 previously described necropsy patients (group II). Am J Med. 1977;63(1):86–108.
2. Yazaki Y, Isobe M, Hiroe M, Morimoto S, Hiramitsu S, Nakano T, et al. Prognostic determinants of long-term survival in Japanese patients with cardiac sarcoidosis treated with prednisone. Am J Cardiol. 2001;88(9):1006–10.
3. Reuhl J, Schneider M, Sievert H, Lutz F-U, Zieger G. Myocardial sarcoidosis as a rare cause of sudden cardiac death. Forensic Sci Int. 1997;89(3):145–53.
4. Baughman R, Bresnitz E, Iannuzzi M, Johns C, Knatterud GL, McLennan G, et al. Design of a Case Control Etiologic Study of sarcoidosis (ACCESS). J Clin Epidemiol. 1999;52(12):1173–86.
5. Rybicki BA, Iannuzzi MC, Frederick MM, Thompson BW, Rossman MD, Bresnitz EA, et al. Familial aggregation of sarcoidosis. Am J Respir Crit Care Med. 2001;164(11):2085–91.
6. Sverrild A, Backer V, Kyvik KO, Kaprio J, Milman N, Svendsen CB, et al. Heredity in sarcoidosis: a registry-based twin study. Thorax. 2008;63(10):894–6.
7. Baughman R, Lower EE, du Bois RM. Sarcoidosis. Lancet. 2003;361:1111–8.
8. Costabel U, Hunninghake GW. ATS/ERS/WASOG statement on sarcoidosis. Sarcoidosis statement committee. American Thoracic Society. European Respiratory Society. World Association for Sarcoidosis and Other Granulomatous Disorders. Eur Respir J. 1999;14(4):735–7.
9. Grunewald J, Kaiser Y, Ostadkarampour M, Rivera NV, Vezzi F, Lötstedt B, et al. T-cell receptor–HLA-DRB1 associations suggest specific antigens in pulmonary sarcoidosis. Eur Respir J. 2016;47(3):898–909.
10. Rosen Y. Pathology of sarcoidosis. In: Respiratory and critical care medicine. New York: Thieme Medical; 2007. p. 036–52.
11. Mochizuki T, Tsukamoto E, Kuge Y, Kanegae K, Zhao S, Hikosaka K, et al. FDG uptake and glucose transporter subtype expressions in experimental tumor and inflammation models. J Nucl Med. 2001;42(10):1551–5.
12. Maratou E, Dimitriadis G, Kollias A, Boutati E, Lambadiari V, Mitrou P, et al. Glucose transporter expression on the plasma membrane of resting and activated white blood cells. Eur J Clin Invest. 2007;37(4):282–90.
13. Arkema EV, Grunewald J, Kullberg S, Eklund A, Askling J. Sarcoidosis incidence and prevalence: a nationwide register-based assessment in Sweden. Eur Respir J. 2016;48(6):1690–9.
14. Baughman RP, Field S, Costabel U, Crystal RG, Culver DA, Drent M, et al. Sarcoidosis in

America analysis based on health care use. ATS. 2016;13(8):1244–52.

15. Baughman RP, Teirstein AS, Judson MA, Rossman MD, Yeager H Jr, Bresnitz EA, et al. Clinical characteristics of patients in a case control study of sarcoidosis. Am J Respir Crit Care Med. 2001;164(10):1885–9.

16. Mehta D, Lubitz SA, Frankel Z, Wisnivesky JP, Einstein AJ, Goldman M, et al. Cardiac involvement in patients with sarcoidosis: diagnostic and prognostic value of outpatient testing. Chest. 2008;133(6):1426–35.

17. Nagai T, Kohsaka S, Okuda S, Anzai T, Asano K, Fukuda K. Incidence and prognostic significance of myocardial late gadolinium enhancement in patients with sarcoidosis without cardiac manifestation. Chest. 2014;146(4):1064–72.

18. Patel MR, Cawley PJ, Heitner JF, Igor K, Parker MA, Jaroudi WA, et al. Detection of myocardial damage in patients with sarcoidosis. Circulation. 2009;120(20):1969–77.

19. Pizarro C, Goebel A, Grohé C, Pabst S, Klein J, Nickenig G, et al. Cardiovascular magnetic resonance-guided diagnosis of cardiac affection in a Caucasian sarcoidosis population. Pneumologie. 2015;69(S1):P299.

20. Patel AR, Klein MR, Chandra S, Spencer KT, DeCara JM, Lang RM, et al. Myocardial damage in patients with sarcoidosis and preserved left ventricular systolic function: an observational study. Eur J Heart Fail. 2011;13(11):1231–7.

21. Greulich S, Deluigi CC, Gloekler S, Wahl A, Zürn C, Kramer U, et al. CMR imaging predicts death and other adverse events in suspected cardiac sarcoidosis. JACC Cardiovasc Imaging. 2013;6(4):501–11.

22. Murtagh G, Laffin LJ, Beshai JF, Maffessanti F, Bonham CA, Patel AV, et al. Prognosis of myocardial damage in sarcoidosis patients with preserved left ventricular ejection fraction. Circ Cardiovasc Imaging. 2016;9(1):e003738. https://doi.org/10.1161/CIRCIMAGING.115.003738.

23. Dhôte R, Vignaux O, Blanche P, Duboc D, Dusser D, Brezin A, et al. Apport de l'IRM dans l'exploration de l'atteinte cardiaque au cours de la sarcoïdose. Rev Med Interne. 2003;24(3):151–7.

24. Smedema J-P, Snoep G, van Kroonenburgh MPG, van Geuns R-J, Dassen WRM, Gorgels AP, et al. Cardiac involvement in patients with pulmonary sarcoidosis assessed at two university medical centers in the Netherlands. Chest. 2005;128(1):30–5.

25. Vignaux O, Dhote R, Duboc D, Blanche P, Devaux J-Y, Weber S, et al. Detection of myocardial involvement in patients with sarcoidosis applying T2-weighted, contrast-enhanced, and cine magnetic resonance imaging: initial results of a prospective study. J Comput Assist Tomogr. 2002;26(5):762–7.

26. Hulten E, Aslam S, Osborne M, Abbasi S, Bittencourt MS, Blankstein R. Cardiac sarcoidosis—state of the art review. Cardiovasc diagn ther. 2016;6(1):50.

27. Silverman KJ, Hutchins GM, Bulkley BH. Cardiac sarcoid: a clinicopathologic study of 84 unselected patients with systemic sarcoidosis. Circulation. 1978;58(6):1204–11.

28. Iwai K, Tachibana T, Takemura T, Matsui Y, Kitalchi M, Kawabata Y. Pathological studies on sarcoidosis autopsy. I. Epidemiological features of 320 cases in Japan. Pathol Int. 1993;43(7–8):372–6.

29. Perry A, Vuitch F. Causes of death in patients with sarcoidosis. A morphologic study of 38 autopsies with clinicopathologic correlations. Arch Pathol Lab Med. 1995;119(2):167–72.

30. Hu X, Carmona EM, Yi ES, Pellikka PA, Ryu J. Causes of death in patients with chronic sarcoidosis. Sarcoidosis Vasc Diffuse Lung Dis. 2016;33(3):275–80.

31. Chapelon-Abric C, de Zuttere D, Duhaut P, Veyssier P, Wechsler B, de Gennes C, et al. Cardiac sarcoidosis: a retrospective study of 41 cases. Medicine. 2004;83(6):315–34.

32. Matsui Y, Iwai K, Tachibana T, Fruie T, Shigematsu N, Izumi T, et al. Clinicopathological study on fatal myocardial sarcoidosis. Ann N Y Acad Sci. 1976;278(1):455–69.

33. Uusimaa P, Ylitalo K, Anttonen O, Kerola T, Virtanen V, Pääkkö E, et al. Ventricular tachyarrhythmia as a primary presentation of sarcoidosis. Europace. 2008;10(6):760–6.

34. Dubrey SW, Falk RH. Diagnosis and management of cardiac sarcoidosis. Prog Cardiovasc Dis. 2010;52(4):336–46.

35. Kandolin R, Lehtonen J, Kupari M. Cardiac sarcoidosis and giant cell myocarditis as causes of atrioventricular block in young and middle-aged adults. Circ Arrhythm Electrophysiol. 2011;4(3):303–9.

36. Nery PB, Beanlands RS, Nair GM, Green M, Yang J, McArdle BA, et al. Atrioventricular block as the initial manifestation of cardiac sarcoidosis in middle-aged adults. J Cardiovasc Electrophysiol. 2014;25(8):875–81.

37. Nery PB, Mc Ardle BA, Redpath CJ, Leung E, Lemery R, Dekemp R, et al. Prevalence of cardiac sarcoidosis in patients presenting with monomorphic ventricular tachycardia. Pacing Clin Electrophysiol. 2014;37(3):364–74.

38. Tung R, Bauer B, Schelbert H, Lynch JP III, Auerbach M, Gupta P, et al. Incidence of abnormal positron emission tomography in patients with unexplained cardiomyopathy and ventricular arrhythmias: the potential role of occult inflammation in arrhythmogenesis. Heart Rhythm. 2015;12(12):2488–98.

39. Sekiguchi M, Numao Y, Imai M, Furuie T, Mikami R. Clinical and histopathological profile of sarcoidosis of the heart and acute idiopathic myocarditis concepts through a study employing endomyocardial biopsy I. sarcoidosis: symposium on secondary myocardial disease. Jpn Circ J. 1980;44(4):249–63.

40. Hiraga H. The guides for the diagnosis of cardiac sarcoidosis: report of the Japanese Research Committee

for Diffuse Lung Disease of Japan Ministry Welfare; 1993. p. 23–4.

41. Hiraga H, Yuwai K, Hiroe M. Diagnostic standard and guidelines for sarcoidosis. Jpn J Sarcoidosis Granulomatous Disord. 2007;27:89–102.

42. Judson M, Baughman R, Teirstein A, Terrin M, Yeager H Jr. Defining organ involvement in sarcoidosis: the ACCESS proposed instrument. ACCESS research group. A case control etiologic study of sarcoidosis. Sarcoidosis Vasc Diffuse Lung Dis. 1999;16(1):75–86.

43. Judson MA, Costabel U, Drent M, Wells A, Maier L, Koth L, et al. The WASOG sarcoidosis organ assessment instrument: an update of a previous clinical tool. Sarcoidosis Vasc Diffuse Lung Dis. 2014;31(1):19–27.

44. Birnie DH, Sauer WH, Bogun F, Cooper JM, Culver DA, Duvernoy CS, et al. HRS expert consensus statement on the diagnosis and management of arrhythmias associated with cardiac sarcoidosis. Heart Rhythm. 2014;11(7):1304–23.

45. Neto MLR, Jellis C, Hachamovitch R, Wimer A, Highland KB, Sahoo D, et al. Performance of diagnostic criteria in patients clinically judged to have cardiac sarcoidosis: is it time to regroup? Am Heart J. 2020;223:106–9.

46. Iannuzzi MC, Rybicki BA, Teirstein AS. Sarcoidosis. N Engl J Med. 2007;357(21):2153–65.

47. Ma J, Lee K-V, Stafford RS. Changes in antihypertensive prescribing during US outpatient visits for uncomplicated hypertension between 1993 and 2004. Hypertension. 2006;48(5):846–52.

48. d'Alessandro M, Bergantini L, Perrone A, Cameli P, Cameli M, Prasse A, et al. Serial investigation of angiotensin-converting enzyme in sarcoidosis patients treated with angiotensin-converting enzyme inhibitor. Eur J Intern Med. 2020;78:58–62.

49. Chopra A, Kalkanis A, Judson MA. Biomarkers in sarcoidosis. Expert Rev Clin Immunol. 2016;12(11):1191–208.

50. Uemura A, Morimoto S, Hiramitsu S, Kato Y, Ito T, Hishida H. Histologic diagnostic rate of cardiac sarcoidosis: evaluation of endomyocardial biopsies. Am Heart J. 1999;138(2):299–302.

51. Kandolin R, Lehtonen J, Graner M, Schildt J, Salmenkivi K, Kivistö S, et al. Diagnosing isolated cardiac sarcoidosis. J Intern Med. 2011;270(5):461–8.

52. Bennett MK, Gilotra NA, Harrington C, Rao S, Dunn JM, Freitag TB, et al. Evaluation of the role of endomyocardial biopsy in 851 patients with unexplained heart failure from 2000–2009. Circ Heart Fail. 2013;6(4):676–84.

53. Hutchinson J. Statement on sarcoidosis. Joint statement of the American Thoracic Society (ATS), the European Respiratory Society (ERS) and the world Association of Sarcoidosis and Other Granulomatous Disorders (WASOG) adopted by the ATS Board of directors and by the ER. Am J Respir Crit Care Med. 1999;160(736):55.

54. Okayama K, Kurata C, Tawarahara K, Wakabayashi Y, Chida K, Sato A. Diagnostic and prognostic value of myocardial scintigraphy with thallium-201 and gallium-67 in cardiac sarcoidosis. Chest. 1995;107(2):330–4.

55. Thunell M, Bjerle P, Stjernberg N. ECG abnormalities in patients with sarcoidosis. Acta Med Scand. 1983;213(2):115–8.

56. Fahy GJ, Marwick T, McCreery CJ, Quigley PJ, Maurer BJ. Doppler echocardiographic detection of left ventricular diastolic dysfunction in patients with pulmonary sarcoidosis. Chest. 1996;109(1):62–6.

57. Gibbons WJ, Levy RD, Nava S, Malcolm I, Marin JM, Tardif C, et al. Subclinical cardiac dysfunction in sarcoidosis. Chest. 1991;100(1):44–50.

58. Kim JS, Judson MA, Donnino R, Gold M, Cooper LT Jr, Prystowsky EN, et al. Cardiac sarcoidosis. Am Heart J. 2009;157(1):9–21.

59. Pizarro C, Goebel A, Dabir D, Hammerstingl C, Pabst S, Grohé C. Cardiovascular magnetic resonance-guided diagnosis of cardiac affection in a Caucasian sarcoidosis population. Sarcoidosis Vasc Diffuse Lung Dis. 2016;32(04):325–35.

60. Ayyala US, Nair AP, Padilla ML. Cardiac sarcoidosis. Clin Chest Med. 2008;29(3):493–508.

61. Agarwal A, Sulemanjee NZ, Cheema O, Downey FX, Tajik AJ. Cardiac sarcoid: a chameleon masquerading as hypertrophic cardiomyopathy and dilated cardiomyopathy in the same patient. Echocardiography. 2014;31(5):E138–41.

62. Sköld C, Larsen F, Rasmussen E, Pehrsson S, Eklund A. Determination of cardiac involvement in sarcoidosis by magnetic resonance imaging and Doppler echocardiography. J Intern Med. 2002;252(5):465–71.

63. Burstow DJ, Tajik AJ, Bailey KR, De Remee RA, Taliercio CP. Two-dimensional echocardiographic findings in systemic sarcoidosis. Am J Cardiol. 1989;63(7):478–82.

64. Hourigan LA, Burstow DJ, Pohlner P, Clarke BE, Donnelly JE. Transesophageal echocardiographic abnormalities in a case of cardiac sarcoidosis. J Am Soc Echocardiogr. 2001;14(5):399–402.

65. Cummings KW, Bhalla S, Javidan-Nejad C, Bierhals AJ, Gutierrez FR, Woodard PK. A pattern-based approach to assessment of delayed enhancement in nonischemic cardiomyopathy at MR imaging. Radiographics. 2009;29(1):89–103.

66. Smedema J-P, Snoep G, van Kroonenburgh MP, van Geuns R-J, Dassen WR, Gorgels AP, et al. Evaluation of the accuracy of gadolinium-enhanced cardiovascular magnetic resonance in the diagnosis of cardiac sarcoidosis. J Am Coll Cardiol. 2005;45(10):1683–90.

67. Slart RH, Glaudemans AW, Lancellotti P, Hyafil F, Blankstein R, Schwartz RG, et al. A joint procedural position statement on imaging in cardiac sarcoidosis: from the cardiovascular and Inflammation & Infection Committees of the European Association of Nuclear Medicine, the European Association of

Cardiovascular Imaging, and the American society of nuclear cardiology. Eur Heart J Cardiovasc Imaging. 2017;18(10):1073–89.

68. Chareonthaitawee P, Beanlands RS, Chen W, Dorbala S, Miller EJ, Murthy VL, et al. Joint SNMMI–ASNC expert consensus document on the role of ^{18}F-FDG PET/CT in cardiac sarcoid detection and therapy monitoring. J Nucl Med. 2017;58(8):1341–53.

69. Christopoulos G, Jouni H, Acharya GA, Blauwet LA, Kapa S, Bois J, et al. Suppressing physiologic 18-fluorodeoxyglucose uptake in patients undergoing positron emission tomography for cardiac sarcoidosis: the effect of a structured patient preparation protocol. J Nucl Cardiol. 2019;28(2):661–71.

70. Tang R, Wang JT-Y, Wang L, Le K, Huang Y, Hickey AJ, et al. Impact of patient preparation on the diagnostic performance of ^{18}F-FDG PET in cardiac sarcoidosis: a systematic review and meta-analysis. Clin Nucl Med. 2016;41(7):e327–39.

71. Blankstein R, Osborne M, Naya M, Waller A, Kim CK, Murthy VL, et al. Cardiac positron emission tomography enhances prognostic assessments of patients with suspected cardiac sarcoidosis. J Am Coll Cardiol. 2014;63(4):329–36.

72. Ohira H, Tsujino I, Ishimaru S, Oyama N, Takei T, Tsukamoto E, et al. Myocardial imaging with 18 F-fluoro-2-deoxyglucose positron emission tomography and magnetic resonance imaging in sarcoidosis. Eur J Nucl Med Mol Imaging. 2008;35(5):933–41.

73. Youssef G, Leung E, Mylonas I, Nery P, Williams K, Wisenberg G, et al. The use of ^{18}F-FDG PET in the diagnosis of cardiac sarcoidosis: a systematic review and metaanalysis including the Ontario experience. J Nucl Med. 2012;53(2):241–8.

74. Kim S-J, Pak K, Kim K. Diagnostic performance of F−18 FDG PET for detection of cardiac sarcoidosis; a systematic review and meta-analysis. J Nucl Cardiol. 2019;27(6):2103–15.

75. Bravo PE, Raghu G, Rosenthal DG, Elman S, Petek BJ, Soine LA, et al. Risk assessment of patients with clinical manifestations of cardiac sarcoidosis with positron emission tomography and magnetic resonance imaging. Int J Cardiol. 2017;241:457–62.

76. Tuominen H, Haarala A, Tikkakoski A, Kähönen M, Nikus K, Sipilä K. FDG-PET in possible cardiac sarcoidosis: right ventricular uptake and high total cardiac metabolic activity predict cardiovascular events. J Nucl Cardiol. 2019;28(1):1–7.

77. Sperry BW, Tamarappoo BK, Oldan JD, Omair J, Culver DA, Richard B, et al. Prognostic impact of extent, severity, and heterogeneity of abnormalities on ^{18}F-FDG PET scans for suspected cardiac sarcoidosis. JACC Cardiovasc Imaging. 2018;11(2_Part_2):336–45.

78. Subramanian M, Swapna N, Ali AZ, Saggu DK, Yalagudri S, Kishore J, et al. Pre-treatment myocardial 18FDG uptake predicts response to immunosuppression in patients with cardiac sarcoidosis. JACC Cardiovasc Imaging. 2021;14(10):2008–16.

79. Yamamoto A, Nagao M, Watanabe E, Imamura Y, Suzuki A, Fukushima K, et al. Prognosis and recurrence in cardiac sarcoidosis: serial assessment of BMIPP SPECT and FDG-PET. J Nucl Cardiol. 2021;28(3):919–29. https://doi.org/10.1007/s12350-021-02567-0.

80. Hamzeh NY, Wamboldt FS, Weinberger HD. Management of cardiac sarcoidosis in the United States: a Delphi study. Chest. 2012;141(1):154–62.

81. Alvi RM, Young BD, Shahab Z, Pan H, Winkler J, Herzog E, et al. Repeatability and optimization of FDG positron emission tomography for evaluation of cardiac sarcoidosis. JACC Cardiovasc Imaging. 2019;12(7 Part 1):1284–7.

82. Miller RJ, Cadet S, Pournazari P, Pope A, Kransdorf E, Hamilton MA, et al. Quantitative assessment of cardiac hypermetabolism and perfusion for diagnosis of cardiac sarcoidosis. J Nucl Cardiol. 2020;29(1):86–96.

83. Okumura W, Iwasaki T, Toyama T, Iso T, Arai M, Oriuchi N, et al. Usefulness of fasting ^{18}F-FDG PET in identification of cardiac sarcoidosis. J Nucl Med. 2004;45(12):1989–98.

84. Tahara N, Tahara A, Nitta Y, Kodama N, Mizoguchi M, Kaida H, et al. Heterogeneous myocardial FDG uptake and the disease activity in cardiac sarcoidosis. JACC Cardiovasc Imaging. 2010;3(12):1219–28.

85. Langah R, Spicer K, Gebregziabher M, Gordon L. Effectiveness of prolonged fasting 18f-FDG PET-CT in the detection of cardiac sarcoidosis. J Nucl Cardiol. 2009;16(5):801–10.

86. Mc Ardle BA, Birnie DH, Klein R, de Kemp RA, Leung E, Renaud J, et al. Is there an association between clinical presentation and the location and extent of myocardial involvement of cardiac sarcoidosis as assessed by ^{18}F-fluorodeoxyglucose positron emission tomography? Circ Cardiovasc Imaging. 2013;6(5):617–26.

87. Osborne MT, Hulten EA, Singh A, Waller AH, Bittencourt MS, Stewart GC, et al. Reduction in ^{18}F-fluorodeoxyglucose uptake on serial cardiac positron emission tomography is associated with improved left ventricular ejection fraction in patients with cardiac sarcoidosis. J Nucl Cardiol. 2014;21(1):166–74.

88. Ahmadian A, Brogan A, Berman J, Sverdlov AL, Mercier G, Mazzini M, et al. Quantitative interpretation of FDG PET/CT with myocardial perfusion imaging increases diagnostic information in the evaluation of cardiac sarcoidosis. J Nucl Cardiol. 2014;21(5):925–39.

89. Lee P-I, Cheng G, Alavi A. The role of serial FDG PET for assessing therapeutic response in patients with cardiac sarcoidosis. J Nucl Cardiol. 2017;24(1):19–28.

90. Muser D, Santangeli P, Castro SA, Liang JJ, Enriquez A, Werner TJ, et al. Prognostic role of serial quantitative evaluation of ^{18}F-fluorodeoxyglucose uptake by PET/CT in patients with cardiac sarcoidosis presenting with

ventricular tachycardia. Eur J Nucl Med Mol Imaging. 2018;45(8):1394–404.

91. Manabe O, Ohira H, Hirata K, Hayashi S, Naya M, Tsujino I, et al. Use of ^{18}F-FDG PET/CT texture analysis to diagnose cardiac sarcoidosis. Eur J Nucl Med Mol Imaging. 2019;46(6):1240–7.

92. Schildt JV, Loimaala AJ, Hippeläinen ET, Ahonen AA. Heterogeneity of myocardial 2-[18F] fluoro-2-deoxy-D-glucose uptake is a typical feature in cardiac sarcoidosis: a study of 231 patients. Eur Heart J Cardiovasc Imaging. 2018;19(3):293–8.

93. Manabe O, Koyanagawa K, Hirata K, Oyama-Manabe N, Ohira H, Aikawa T, et al. Prognostic value of ^{18}F-FDG PET using texture analysis in cardiac sarcoidosis. JACC Cardiovasc Imaging. 2020;13(4):1096–7.

94. Hanneman K, Kadoch M, Guo HH, Jamali M, Quon A, Iagaru A, et al. Initial experience with simultaneous ^{18}F-FDG PET/MRI in the evaluation of cardiac sarcoidosis and myocarditis. Clin Nucl Med. 2017;42(7):e328–34.

95. Wisenberg G, Thiessen J, Pavlovsky W, Butler J, Wilk B, Prato F. Same day comparison of PET/CT and PET/MR in patients with cardiac sarcoidosis. J Nucl Cardiol. 2019;27(6):2118–29.

96. Soussan M, Brillet P-Y, Nunes H, Pop G, Ouvrier M-J, Naggara N, et al. Clinical value of a high-fat and low-carbohydrate diet before FDG-PET/CT for evaluation of patients with suspected cardiac sarcoidosis. J Nucl Cardiol. 2013;20(1):120–7.

97. Ohira H, Birnie DH, Pena E, Bernick J, Mc Ardle B, Leung E, et al. Comparison of ^{18}F-fluorodeoxyglucose positron emission tomography (FDG PET) and cardiac magnetic resonance (CMR) in corticosteroid-naive patients with conduction system disease due to cardiac sarcoidosis. Eur J Nucl Med Mol Imaging. 2016;43(2):259–69.

98. Coulden RA, Sonnex EP, Abele JT, Crean AM. Utility of FDG PET and cardiac MRI in diagnosis and monitoring of immunosuppressive treatment in cardiac sarcoidosis. Radiol Cardiothorac Imaging. 2020;2(4):e190140.

99. Reiter T, Werner RA, Bauer WR, Lapa C. Detection of cardiac sarcoidosis by macrophage-directed somatostatin receptor 2-based positron emission tomography/computed tomography. Eur Heart J. 2015;36(35):2404.

100. Lapa C, Reiter T, Kircher M, Schirbel A, Werner RA, Pelzer T, et al. Somatostatin receptor based PET/CT in patients with the suspicion of cardiac sarcoidosis: an initial comparison to cardiac MRI. Oncotarget. 2016;7(47):77807.

101. Gormsen LC, Haraldsen A, Kramer S, Dias AH, Kim WY, Borghammer P. A dual tracer 68 Ga-DOTANOC PET/CT and ^{18}F-FDG PET/CT pilot study for detection of cardiac sarcoidosis. EJNMMI Res. 2016;6(1):1–12.

102. Pizarro C, Kluenker F, Dabir D, Thomas D, Gaertner FC, Essler M, et al. Cardiovascular magnetic resonance imaging and clinical performance of somatostatin receptor positron emission tomography in cardiac sarcoidosis. ESC heart fail. 2018;5(2):249–61.

103. Slart RH, Koopmans K-P, van Geel PP, Kramer H, Groen HJ, Gan CT-J, et al. Somatostatin receptor based hybrid imaging in sarcoidosis. European j hybrid imaging. 2017;1(1):1–5.

104. Martineau P, Pelletier-Galarneau M, Juneau D, Leung E, Nery PB, de Kemp R, et al. Imaging cardiac sarcoidosis with FLT-PET compared with FDG/perfusion-PET: a prospective pilot study. JACC Cardiovasc Imaging. 2019;12(11 Part 1):2280–1.

105. Norikane T, Yamamoto Y, Maeda Y, Noma T, Dobashi H, Nishiyama Y. Comparative evaluation of ^{18}F-FLT and ^{18}F-FDG for detecting cardiac and extra-cardiac thoracic involvement in patients with newly diagnosed sarcoidosis. EJNMMI Res. 2017;7(1):1–7.

106. Weinberg RL, Morgenstern R, DeLuca A, Chen J, Bokhari S. F-18 sodium fluoride PET/CT does not effectively image myocardial inflammation due to suspected cardiac sarcoidosis. J Nucl Cardiol. 2017;24(6):2015–8.

107. Manabe O, Hirata K, Shozo O, Shiga T, Uchiyama Y, Kobayashi K, et al. 18F-fluoromisonidazole (FMISO) PET may have the potential to detect cardiac sarcoidosis. J Nucl Cardiol. 2017;24(1):329–31.

108. Dumas O, Abramovitz L, Wiley AS, Cozier YC, Camargo CA Jr. Epidemiology of sarcoidosis in a prospective cohort study of US women. Ann Am Thorac Soc. 2016;13(1):67–71.

109. Ungprasert P, Crowson CS, Matteson EL. Influence of gender on epidemiology and clinical manifestations of sarcoidosis: a population-based retrospective cohort study 1976–2013. Lung. 2017;195(1):87–91.

110. Beghè D, Dall' Asta L, Garavelli C, Pastorelli AA, Muscarella M, Saccani G, et al. Sarcoidosis in an Italian province. Prevalence and environmental risk factors. PLoS One. 2017;12(5):e0176859.

111. Coquart N, Cadelis G, Tressières B, Cordel N. Epidemiology of sarcoidosis in Afro-Caribbean people: a 7-year retrospective study in Guadeloupe. Int J Dermatol. 2015;54(2):188–92.

112. Duchemann B, Annesi-Maesano I, de Naurois CJ, Sanyal S, Brillet P-Y, Brauner M, et al. Prevalence and incidence of interstitial lung diseases in a multi-ethnic county of greater Paris. Eur Respir J. 2017;50(2):1602419.

113. Wu C-H, Chung P-I, Wu C-Y, Chen Y-T, Chiu Y-W, Chang Y-T, et al. Comorbid autoimmune diseases in patients with sarcoidosis: a nationwide case–control study in Taiwan. J Dermatol. 2017;44(4):423–30.

114. Fidler LM, Balter M, Fisher JH, To T, Stanbrook MB, Gershon A. Epidemiology and health outcomes of sarcoidosis in a universal healthcare population: a cohort study. Eur Respir J. 2019;54(4):1900444. https://erj.ersjournals.com/content/54/4/1900444.

115. Martineau P, Pelletier-Galarneau M, Juneau D, Leung E, Birnie D, Beanlands RSB. Molecular

imaging of cardiac sarcoidosis. Curr Cardiovasc Imaging Rep. 2018;11(3):6.

116. Yamagishi H, Shirai N, Takagi M, Yoshiyama M, Akioka K, Takeuchi K, et al. Identification of cardiac sarcoidosis with 13N-NH3/^{18}F-FDG PET. J Nucl Med. 2003;44(7):1030–6.

117. Ishimaru S, Tsujino I, Takei T, Tsukamoto E, Sakaue S, Kamigaki M, et al. Focal uptake on ^{18}F-fluoro-2-deoxyglucose positron emission tomography images indicates cardiac involvement of sarcoidosis. Eur Heart J. 2005;26(15):1538–43.

118. Ambrosini V, Zompatori M, Fasano L, Nanni C, Nava S, Rubello D, et al. 18F-FDG PET/CT for the assessment of disease extension and activity in patients with sarcoidosis: results of a preliminary prospective study. Clin Nucl Med. 2013;38(4):e171.

119. Manabe O, Yoshinaga K, Ohira H, Sato T, Tsujino I, Yamada A, et al. Right ventricular ^{18}F-FDG uptake is an important indicator for cardiac involvement in patients with suspected cardiac sarcoidosis. Ann Nucl Med. 2014;28(7):656–63.

120. Ito K, Okazaki O, Morooka M, Kubota K, Minamimoto R, Hiroe M. Visual findings of ^{18}F-Fluorodeoxyglucose positron emission tomography/computed tomography in patients with cardiac sarcoidosis. Intern Med. 2014;53(18):2041–9.

121. Momose M, Fukushima K, Kondo C, Serizawa N, Suzuki A, Abe K, et al. Diagnosis and detection of myocardial injury in active cardiac sarcoidosis—significance of myocardial fatty acid metabolism and myocardial perfusion mismatch. Circ J. 2015;79(12):CJ-15.

122. Yokoyama R, Miyagawa M, Okayama H, Inoue T, Miki H, Ogimoto A, et al. Quantitative analysis of myocardial ^{18}F-fluorodeoxyglucose uptake by PET/CT for detection of cardiac sarcoidosis. Int J Cardiol. 2015;195:180–7.

Myocarditis

Geneviève Giraldeau, Julia Cadrin-Tourigny,
Patrick Martineau, and Matthieu Pelletier-Galarneau

Introduction

Myocarditis is an inflammatory disease of the heart muscle associated with a broad variety of clinical presentations, ranging from chronic, subacute, acute, to fulminant. In myocarditis, inflammation, which may be focal or diffuse, is the primary cause of myocardial dysfunction. Diagnosis requires a high clinical suspicion and exclusion of other causes. Endomyocardial biopsy with histological, immunological, and immunohistochemical analysis represents the gold standard to diagnose myocarditis. Myocarditis can be classified according to the type of inflammatory cells infiltrating the myocardium: lymphocytic, eosinophilic, polymorphic, giant cells, and non-caseous granulomas compatible with cardiac sarcoidosis. The European Society working group on Myocarditis also recommends the inclusion of the following subset: viral myocarditis (PCR proven viral replication), autoimmune myocarditis with or without serum cardiac autoantibodies, and viral and immune myocarditis combining positive viral PCR and positive cardiac antibodies [1]. Myocarditis can lead to entirely reversible injury or can cause myocardial scarring and chronic remodeling with subsequent dilated cardiomyopathy [2]. Prompt diagnosis is therefore important to establish appropriate monitoring and management. Given the importance of early diagnosis and the challenges associated with the non-specific symptoms and variable presentations, better diagnostic tools are needed to improve recognition and follow-up and help identify the etiology of inflammation. In this chapter, the epidemiology, clinical presentation, classification, and treatment options of myocarditis, as well as the current diagnostic strategies and role of cardiac magnetic resonance imaging (CMR) and positron emission tomography (PET) will be reviewed.

Epidemiology

The true incidence of myocarditis is not precisely known partly due to the heterogeneous clinical presentation and because endomyocardial biopsy, which represents the gold standard for the diagnosis of myocarditis, is not always performed [1]. Early clinical recognition is key for appropriate diagnosis and management. A recent study using *International Classification of Diseases* (ninth revision) codes estimated the global prevalence

G. Giraldeau · J. Cadrin-Tourigny
M. Pelletier-Galarneau (✉)
Montreal Heart Institute, Montréal, QC, Canada
e-mail: Matthieu.pelletier-galarneau@icm-mhi.org

P. Martineau
BC Cancer, Vancouver, BC, Canada
e-mail: patrick.martineau@bccancer.bc.ca

of myocarditis to be around 22 per 100,000 person-year [3, 4]. Prevalence of myocarditis on autopsies of young people who succumbed to sudden death is highly variable, ranging from 2 to 42%. In patients with unexplained dilated cardiomyopathy, 9–16% of patients have biopsy proven myocarditis [1]. Thus, although the exact incidence of myocarditis is unknown, it is not a rare entity.

Clinical Presentation

Myocarditis is associated with a broad range of clinical presentations, making its diagnosis challenging. Some patients are completely asymptomatic, while others present with non-specific symptoms including chest pain, shortness of breath, palpitations, and fever. In the most severe cases, patients with myocarditis can initially present with life threatening conditions such as cardiogenic shock and malignant arrhythmias [3]. Interestingly, myocarditis can mimic an acute coronary syndrome, with acute chest pain, with or without EKG changes, ventricular segmental motion abnormalities, and increased troponins (acute or prolonged/sustained). In these patients, coronary angiography will show no significant epicardial stenosis. Myocarditis can also present as new onset or worsening heart failure in the absence of coronary disease. In these cases, symptoms include shortness of breath, fatigue, peripheral edema, and chest pain. It can be accompanied with abnormality of the conduction system (AV block and bundle branch block) or arrhythmias. Finally, it can present with hemodynamic instability due to severe myocardial dysfunction, cardiogenic shock, refractory ventricular arrhythmias, and/or death [1].

Myocarditis Classification

Lymphocytic Viral Myocarditis

Lymphocytic viral myocarditis is, as the name suggests, a viral illness manifesting with lymphocyte infiltration of the myocardium [2].

Frequently, a viral prodrome can be identified preceding the development of cardiac symptoms. Lymphocytic viral myocarditis may be fulminant, acute, subacute, or chronic. Some viruses directly infiltrate myocardial cells, including cardiotropic viruses (adenoviruses, enteroviruses, coxsackieviruses, and echoviruses) and vasculotropic viruses (Parvovirus B19), while others may indirectly infiltrate the heart (Cytomegalovirus, Epstein-Barr virus, Herpes simplex 6). Other viruses such as Influenza, HIV, hepatitis C, and possibly SARS-CoV-2 can cause myocardial inflammation by triggering a cytokine storm or a cellular immune response by molecular mimicry [5]. Fulminant presentation is characterized by critical acute illness but those who survive the acute phase have an excellent long-term prognosis (93% survival without heart transplant). Acute presentation on the other hand despite a less severe initial presentation, is associated with a progressive course associated with greater mortality and more commonly require cardiac transplantation (45% survival without heart transplant) [6]. The use of immunosuppression for lymphocytic viral myocarditis is still controversial. Some studies have shown possible benefits in patient with active lymphocytic myocarditis with positive cardiac autoantibodies and no viral genome in the myocardium [7]. This is hardly applicable in clinical practice as viral PCR is not always routinely performed on endomyocardial biopsies. A case of lymphocytic myocarditis is presented in Figs. 6.1 and 6.2.

Giant Cell Myocarditis

Giant cell myocarditis is considered a rare (about 300 cases described in the literature according to NORD- National Organization for Rare Disorder), fulminant, and rapidly fatal disease. In 20% of cases, it is associated with another autoimmune disease. Inflammation is caused by an inflammatory infiltrate containing giant cells resulting in myocardial destruction. Manifestations include heart failure, ventricular arrhythmias and atrioventricular block, hemodynamic instability, cardiogenic shock, and sudden

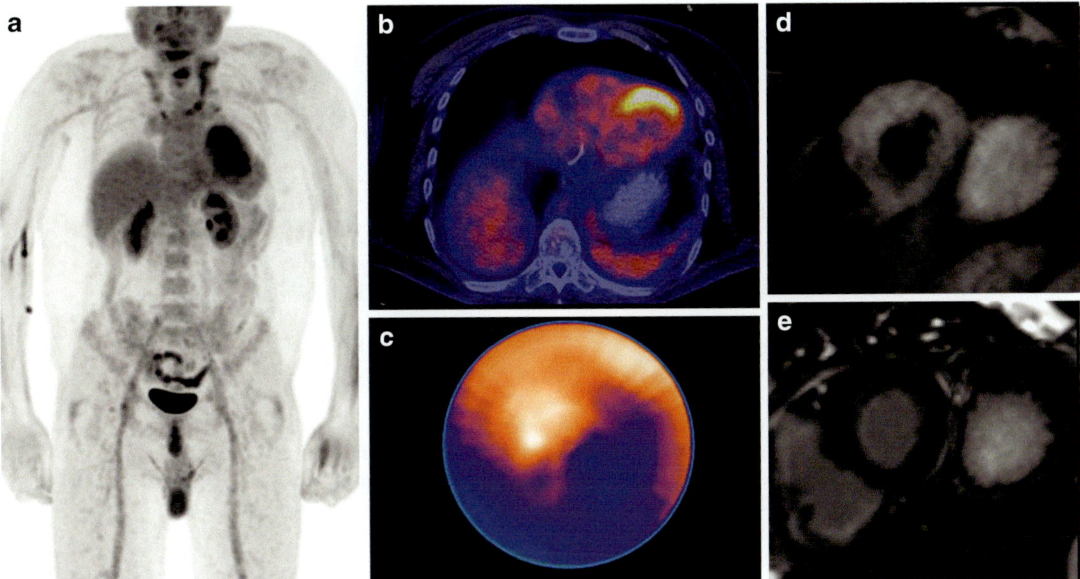

Fig. 6.1 A 41-year-old male with biopsy proven lymphocytic myocarditis. Whole-body FDG-PET maximal intensity projection (MPI) image (**a**), axial FDG-PET/CT image (**b**), and FDG bullseye image (**c**) show relatively extensive increased FDG uptake involving the anteroseptal, anterior, and anterolateral walls, with extension into the lateral basal walls. This uptake distribution does not represent a typical pattern of poor suppression (e.g. isolated lateral wall) and is therefore compatible with inflammation. On CMR, T2-weighted short-tau inversion recovery (STIR) sequences (**d**) show mild edema (ratio heart: muscle 2.1). There was no significant late gadolinium enhancement (**e**)

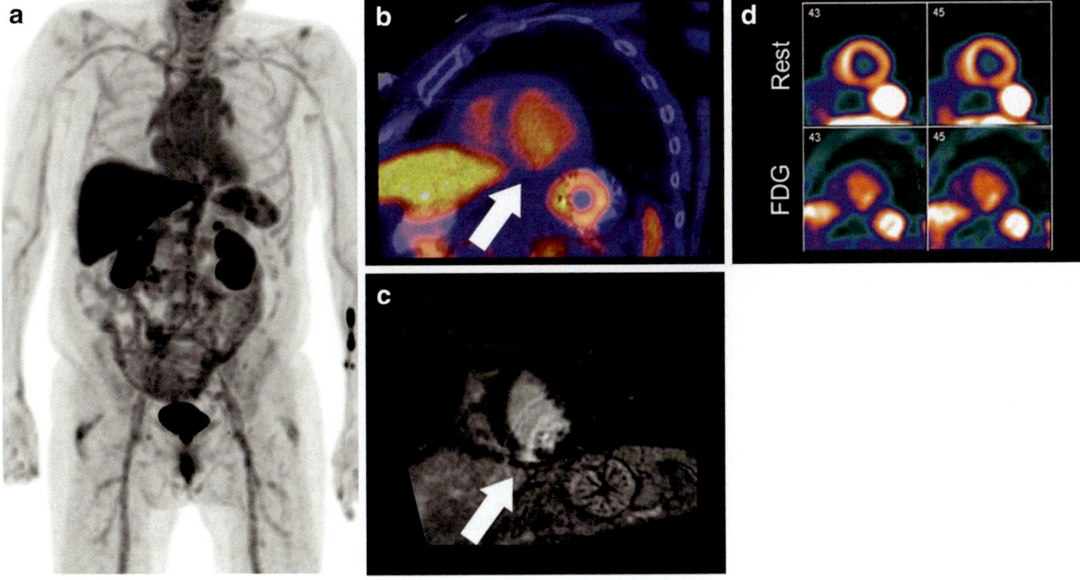

Fig. 6.2 A 60-year-old male referred with myocarditis, non-ischemic cardiomyopathy, and elevated troponins (>10,000). Whole-body FDG-PET maximal intensity projection (MPI) image (**a**) and axial FDG-PET/CT image (**b**) revealed a small area of abnormal FDG uptake (arrow) in the infero-septal wall, corresponding to an area of late gadolinium enhancement on CMR (**c**, arrow). Rubidium rest myocardial perfusion imaging (**d**) demonstrated a corresponding area of focally reduced perfusion

Baseline   Follow up

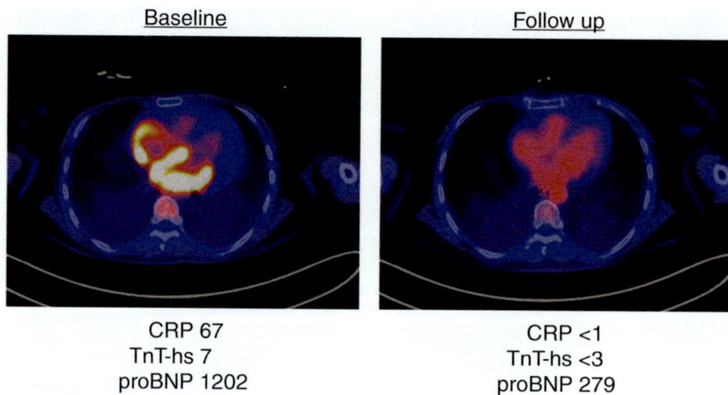

CRP 67
TnT-hs 7
proBNP 1202

CRP <1
TnT-hs <3
proBNP 279

Fig. 6.3 A 60-year-old female who presented with dyspnea. She was found to have thickened atrial walls on echocardiography and atrial late gadolinium enhancement on CMR (not shown). Initial FDG-PET/CT revealed intense (SUV_{max} 15) uptake in both atria with no abnormal uptake in the left or right ventricle. On follow-up study, there is complete resolution of atrial inflammation. A right atrial biopsy confirmed the diagnosis of giant cell myocarditis

death. Without immunosuppression, the rate of death or cardiac transplantation was ~90%, with a median survival of 5.5 months from the onset of symptoms [8]. With immunosuppression, the survival is 65% free of transplantation and 85% with or without transplantation [9]. Giant cell myocarditis is associated with a high risk of sudden death and patients may benefit from a defibrillator [10, 11]. A case of giant cell myocarditis is presented in Fig. 6.3.

Cardiac Sarcoidosis

Sarcoidosis is a multisystemic inflammatory disease causing the formation of non-caseating granulomas. Cardiac involvement is associated with worse prognosis and has been diagnosed in approximately 25% of individuals with systemic sarcoidosis based on autopsy or cardiac imaging studies [12]. The etiology is unknown but it has been hypothesized to be precipitated by exposure to an unknown antigen with subsequent exaggerated immune response in a possibly genetically predisposed individual [12–14]. A frequent initial clinical presentation includes atrioventricular block [15]. Cardiac sarcoidosis is found in as many as 25–35% of patients with AV block under the age of 60–65 [16, 17]. Cardiac sarcoidosis is frequently associated with ventricular arrhythmias and can lead to refractory malignant arrhythmia and ventricular tachycardia (VT) storm and sudden death. It is the underlying diagnosis in 17–18% of patients thought to have idiopathic monomorphic VT [17] and in 10–20% of patient with criteria for arrhythmogenic right ventricular dysplasia (ARVD) [18]. Endomyocardial biopsy is only positive in about 25% of case due to the patchy disease. A common finding on cardiac echocardiography is basal septal thinning and wall motion abnormalities in a noncoronary distribution [19]. CMRI and PET-FDG have been shown useful for the diagnosis of cardiac sarcoidosis and in monitoring response to therapy [19, 20]. Management includes immunosuppression when inflammation is present and early implantation of cardiac defibrillators to prevent sudden death [19, 21]. See Chap. 5 for a more thorough review of cardiac sarcoidosis.

Eosinophilic Cardiomyopathy

Hyper-eosinophilic syndromes (HES) are characterized by persistent marked eosinophilia (>1500 eosinophils/mm^3), absence of a primary cause of eosinophilia (such as parasitic or allergic disease), and evidence of eosinophilic myocardial infiltration. Some other diagnoses involving hypereosinophilia can overlap with cardiac manifestations including Churg-Strauss syndrome, early giant cell myocarditis, hypersensitivity reaction, parasitic infection, Loeffler or tropical endomyocardial fibrosis, and malignancy. The cardiac pathology of HES has traditionally been divided into three stages: (1) acute necrosis, (2) thrombosis, and (3) fibrosis. Clinical manifestations include heart failure, intracardiac thrombus, arrhythmias, and rarely pericarditis. Echocardiographic findings include laminar right and left apical thrombus with possible involvement of posterior mitral leaflets. Management includes normalization of the peripheral eosinophil count, screening for the *FIP1L1-PDGFRA* mutation and treating with imatinib if the mutation is present, and initiating anticoagulant therapy in patients with or at risk for thrombotic complications [22]. Some patients require heart transplantation and more aggressive management of arrhythmias [22, 23].

Diagnosis and Investigation

Clinical history and physical examination may raise the suspicion of myocarditis but presentations are typically non-specific. Non-invasive investigations are useful to improve diagnostic confidence, assess disease severity, and evaluate the need for more invasive investigations. Electrocardiogram (ECG) is easily accessible and routinely performed early in patients with cardiovascular symptoms. ECG of patients with myocarditis is usually abnormal but without any specific or sensitive features. Relatively frequent findings include ST segment abnormalities, atrioventricular block, bundle branch blocks, QRS prolongations, atrial and ventricular arrhythmias, or repolarization abnormalities. Although ECG can neither confirm nor exclude the diagnosis of myocarditis, it should be performed in all patients suspected of myocarditis to exclude other underlying pathology such as acute coronary syndrome. In addition, biomarkers are non-specific for myocarditis [1]; C reactive protein (CRP) is frequently elevated in myocarditis but is not specific and does not confirm diagnosis. Cardiac troponins are frequently elevated, revealing myocardial injury, but are also non-specific and negative troponins do not exclude the diagnosis [24, 25]. Coronary angiography is often performed early to exclude an underlying coronary artery disease that could account for the myocardial dysfunction and cardiac biomarker elevation.

Endomyocardial Biopsy

As stated above, endomyocardial biopsy is the gold standard for the diagnosis of myocarditis. Current guidelines recommend endomyocardial biopsy in the following scenarios, mostly to exclude reversible and treatable cause and establish prognosis [24]:

Class I
1. New onset heart failure of <2 weeks duration associated with a normal-sized or dilated left ventricle and hemodynamic compromise.
2. New onset heart failure of 2 weeks to 3 months duration associated with a dilated left ventricle and new ventricular arrhythmias, second- or third-degree heart block or failure to respond to usual care within 1–2 weeks.

Class IIa
1. Heart failure of >3 months duration associated with a dilated left ventricle and new ventricular arrhythmias, second- or third-degree heart block or failure to respond to usual care within 1–2 weeks.
2. Heart failure associated with a dilated cardiomyopathy of any duration associated with a suspected allergic reaction and/or eosinophilia.
3. Heart failure associated with suspected anthracycline cardiomyopathy.
4. Heart failure associated with unexplained restrictive cardiomyopathy.
5. Suspected cardiac tumors.
6. Unexplained cardiomyopathy in children.

Class IIb
1. New onset heart failure of 2 weeks to 3 months duration associated with a dilated left ventri-

cle without new ventricular arrhythmias or second- or third-degree heart block that responds to usual care within 1–2 weeks.

2. Heart failure of >3 months duration associated with a dilated left ventricle and without new ventricular arrhythmias, second- or third-degree heart block or failure to respond to usual care within 1–2 weeks.

3. Heart failure associated with unexplained hypertrophic cardiomyopathy.

4. Suspected ARVD/C.

5. Unexplained ventricular arrhythmias.

The conventional approach for endomyocardial biopsy consists of acquiring 5–10 samples from the right ventricular septum with access through the right jugular vein or femoral veins. Left ventricular biopsy is feasible and of interest in certain clinical situations and can be combined with right ventricular biopsy to increase the diagnostic yield. Left ventricular biopsy is less frequently performed because of concerns about bleeding, systemic embolization, and possible damage to the aortic valve or mitral subvalvular apparatus. Right ventricular biopsy has a low risk of complications (<2%), which includes arterial puncture, vasovagal reaction, bleeding, arrhythmia, conduction abnormalities, perforation, tamponade, pneumothorax, and death (<0.5%).

The diagnostic yield of a biopsy varies according to underlying disease and timing of the procedure relative to the disease stage. Due to sampling error and evolution of disease over time, a negative biopsy does not entirely rule out myocarditis. For example, sensitivity of biopsy is between 80% and 90% in the very acute (<2 weeks) phase of lymphocytic viral myocarditis and 85% in giant cell myocarditis, while only 20% of right heart biopsies will be positive in cardiac sarcoidosis due to patchy disease involvement [24, 26]. The Dallas criteria, which rely on histological

description of the inflammatory cells, with or without necrosis and/or fibrosis, and immunohistochemistry description, were first introduced in 1986. Although they are often considered the gold standard, they are limited by sampling quality and inter-observer variability in histopathologic interpretation [24].

Echocardiography

Echocardiography is the first line imaging test in patients with suspected myocarditis. In fact, all patients with suspected myocarditis should undergo a transthoracic echocardiography (TTE) and repeated TTE should be performed if there is a clinical or hemodynamical deterioration as myocardial dysfunction can be progressive and evolve rapidly during the acute phase of the disease. ETT findings may include global biventricular dysfunction, regional wall abnormalities, diastolic dysfunction, normal-sized or dilated ventricles, thickened ventricular walls (due to edema), and intraventricular thrombus [1, 27]. Global longitudinal strain is also useful for early diagnosis and follow-up [27].

Cardiac Magnetic Resonance (CMR)

CMR is currently the imaging modality of choice for the diagnosis of myocarditis. In addition to its unrivaled ability to evaluate cardiac function, CMR provides exquisite tissue characterization. The timing of the CMR will depend on hemodynamic stability of the patient and the local availability. Myocarditis is associated with pathophysiological alterations in the myocardium, including hyperemia, increased vascular permeability, edema, necrosis, and fibrosis, all of which can be assessed on CMR (Table 6.1).

Table 6.1 Different CMR findings and their diagnostic accuracy in myocarditis

	Parameter	Prevalence	Sensitivity	Specificity
Edema	T2-ratio	52%	56%	77%
Hyperemia and vascular permeability	EGE	66%	62%	74%
Necrosis	LGE	77%	69%	95%

Adapted from [35]

Presence of edema, or increased water content, will lead to prolonged myocardial T2 relaxation times [28]. A T2 ratio can be calculated by dividing the T2 signal intensity of the myocardium by that of skeletal muscle; a ratio ≥2.0 is indicative of edema [29, 30]. Of note, concurrent skeletal muscle inflammation may lead to a normal T2 ratio despite the presence of myocardial edema. Hyperemia increased vascular permeability, and capillary leak can be assessed on early gadolinium enhancement (EGE) using T1-weighted sequences. Similar to the T2-ratio, a EGE ratio can be calculated by dividing the signal intensity in myocardium to that of skeletal muscle, with ratio ≥4.0 being considered abnormal [31]. Newer sequences aiming at measuring the extracellular space using T1 mapping before and after gadolinium can also be used. Because gadolinium-based contrast agents accumulate in the extracellular space, increased signal is observed after contrast injection. Another hallmark of myocarditis is the presence of necrosis and fibrosis, which can appear as regions of increased signal on T1 images acquired >10 min after administration of gadolinium-based contrast, commonly referred to as late gadolinium enhancement (LGE). Different patterns of delayed contrast enhancement (LGE) have been described and associated with different diagnoses and can provide insight on the etiology of the cardiomyopathy. Lymphocytic myocarditis can cause transmural and/or subepicardial LGE, whereas sarcoidosis can cause patchy, subepicardial, or transmural LGE. Hyper-eosinophilic cardiomyopathy will typically cause subendocardial LGE [32]. Typically, in myocarditis, LGE will follow a non-vascular distribution with subendocardial areas of enhancement, often patchy, and frequently affecting the basal and mid-inferolateral segments. One notable exception is eosinophilic myocarditis which can present as circumferential subendocardial LGE [33]. Finally, other findings on CMR have been associated with the presence of myocarditis, including pericardial effusion, and LV wall motion abnormalities. Interestingly, in the acute phase of myocarditis, the presence of edema without

LGE is associated with better functional recovery and outcomes, while the presence of LGE is associated with adverse outcome, regardless of LVEF [34].

Lake Louise Criteria

On their own, the various diagnostic criteria are neither sensitive nor specific for the diagnosis of myocarditis (Table 6.1). The Lake Louise Criteria (LLC) were developed to address this limitation, by incorporating several criteria to reach a final diagnosis [31]. According to the LLC, CMR findings are compatible with myocardial inflammation in the setting of clinically suspected myocarditis if ≥2 of the following criteria are met: (1) Regional or globally increased T2 signal intensity, (2) increased EGE, and (3) LGE following a non-ischemic pattern. Sensitivity and specificity of the LLC have been reported at 78% and 74%, respectively [35]. In 2018, an updated version of the LLC was presented [30]. The updated LLC, sometimes referred to as the 2018 LLC, stipulate that in patients with a significant pre-test probability of myocarditis, the presence of T2-based markers of edema or T1-based marker of myocardial injury (e.g. EGE, LGE), or both, provides strong evidence of myocardial inflammation [30]. Studies suggest that the 2018 LLC has increased sensitivity compared to the original LLC without any loss in specificity [36], although performance of those new criteria may be affected by the studied population [37].

Positron Emission Tomography

There is a striking paucity of literature on the use of FDG-PET in myocardial inflammation outside of cardiac sarcoidosis. At this time, the literature is limited mainly to small series and case reports, and no prospective study has evaluated the diagnostic performance of FDG-PET/CT in myocarditis. Furthermore, whether FDG-PET has the ability to identify the various types of myocarditis is unknown, and the impact of FDG-PET on the management of patients with suspected myocarditis remains unstudied. Nonetheless, given

Table 6.2 Potential roles of FDG-PET in myocarditis

Initial diagnosis
Distinguish between residual active myocarditis and scarring
Evaluation of prognosis
Assessment of response therapy
Guide biopsy
Assessment of concomitant or precipitating pathology

the central role played by FDG-PET for the initial diagnostic and assessment of therapy response in idiopathic granulomatous myocarditis (cardiac sarcoidosis), it is conceivable that FDG-PET may play a role in the evaluation of patients with suspected myocarditis (Table 6.2). Nonetheless, robust and prospective studies are required.

FDG findings have been described in various types of myocarditis. Abnormal FDG uptake has been reported in myocarditis following viral infection including parvovirus B19 and Epstein-Barr virus [38–42]. Simon et al. reported an interesting case of myocarditis presenting as a manifestation of giant cell arteritis, with intense and diffuse myocardial FDG uptake [43]. In another case report, Gracia et al. showed increased FDG uptake in a patient with eosinophilic myocarditis [44]. Langwieser et al. report a case of relatively intense and focal FDG uptake corresponding to an apical mass in both ventricles in a patient suffering from Loeffler endocarditis, a rare cardiomyopathy caused by eosinophilic infiltration of the endomyocardium [45]. Moriwaki et al. reported a case of eosinophilic myocarditis with intense, predominantly septal uptake after initiation of therapy, which resolved completely following adequate treatment [46].

Kandolin et al. report on 32 subjects with biopsy proven GCM [9]. In their sample, 12 underwent FDG-PET/CT following a cardiac sarcoidosis myocardial suppression protocol in addition to a resting perfusion study. Of those 12 subjects, 10 demonstrated focal uptake, 9 of which had corresponding resting perfusion abnormalities. Two subjects with GCM and without significant FDG uptake had perfusion abnormalities, suggesting a different disease stage and highlighting the importance of acquiring resting perfusion. The authors suggested that guiding biopsy with FDG and CMR findings may improve its yield.

Lamacie et al. reported the case of a patient with GCM who underwent serial FDG-PET/CT scans [47]. On initial FDG-PET, acquired at presentation, there was diffuse and intense FDG uptake in the left and right ventricles, with SUV_{max} of 25. Following 2 weeks of immunosuppressive therapy, uptake reduced significantly with an SUV_{max} of 6.4. After 4 months of therapy, there was no significant residual FDG uptake. Uptake intensity was found to correlate with troponin levels. Similar results were obtained in a patient with fulminant myocarditis, with abnormal FDG uptake resolving after successful therapy [48]. When inflammation subsides, the FDG uptake resolves while LGE typically persists on CMR, allowing to differentiate between active disease and sequelae [20, 49, 50]. This likely explains why the sensitivity of FDG-PET to detect myocarditis related inflammation is highest early after presentation [51]. Using FDG-PET as a biomarker of therapy response may be even more important in eosinophilic myocarditis as serologic markers to monitor cardiac disease are lacking [44, 46].

PET/MR

Given the complementary role of FDG-PET and MR in cardiac sarcoidosis [20] and the critical role of CMR in the evaluation of patients with suspicion of myocarditis, integration of PET and MR into a single study is appealing. This is especially true given that CMR findings do not necessarily correlate with level of myocardial inflammation [29, 52]. Furthermore, there is good but imperfect correlation between CMR and FDG-PET findings. Nensa et al. reported a sensitivity and specificity for FDG-PET of 74% and 97%, respectively, when using CMR (LGE and/or T2) as gold standard [53]. These values of sensitivity and specificity should be interpreted with caution due to the gold standard used. Indeed, FDG-PET and CMR are in fact imaging different aspects of the same pathology. Nonetheless, this highlights the complementary role of the two modalities; a normal CMR does not necessarily exclude the presence of myocardial inflammation, which could be identified on FDG-PET.

Imaging Protocol and Interpretation

PET acquisition should be performed in the same manner as for cardiac sarcoidosis imaging, including use of a myocardial suppression protocol (see Chap. 4). Imaging should be performed relatively early after tracer injection (40–60 min) to avoid creeping myocardial uptake that can be observed on delayed imaging. Resting perfusion images, with SPECT or PET, should also be acquired, especially if CMR LGE sequences are not performed. Increased heterogeneous or focal myocardial uptake should be considered suspicious for myocarditis in the appropriate clinical setting. Image interpretation can be challenging, as contrary to cardiac sarcoidosis, uptake may mimic poorly suppressed myocardium, with either diffuse myocardial uptake or isolated lateral wall uptake [9, 38, 39]. FDG uptake may be very intense and diffuse (Fig. 6.1) or very focal and mild (Fig. 6.2), depending on myocarditis type and timing of imaging (acute inflammation vs.

Table 6.3 Factors to help differentiate between poor myocardial suppression versus diffuse myocardial inflammation as reason for uptake on FDG-PET in patients with suspected myocarditis

Poor suppression more likely	Myocardial inflammation more likely
Suppression protocol not followed	Strict suppression protocol
Normal CRP	Elevated CRP
Normal or low troponins	Elevated troponins
Absence of perfusion defects	Corresponding rest perfusion abnormalities
Diabetic patients	Corresponding MRI abnormalities
Patients receiving high corticosteroid dose	Uptake persists on repeated study
	Very high myocardial uptake with increased marrow and/spleen uptake
	Septal uptake greater than lateral wall uptake
	Atrial uptake

delayed presentation). Table 6.3 presents conditions or circumstances that may help differentiate between poor suppression and diffuse inflammation. When clinical suspicion of poor myocardial suppression is high, PET may be repeated following a 48-h low-carbohydrate-high-fat diet and prolonged fasting. The likelihood of a positive PET study is greater in the presence of resting perfusion and/or CMR abnormalities. It is important to remember that FDG-PET identifies active inflammation and thus, absence of findings on FDG-PET does not exclude remote or quiescent myocarditis, especially when performed >8–10 weeks after onset of symptoms [51] (Fig. 6.4).

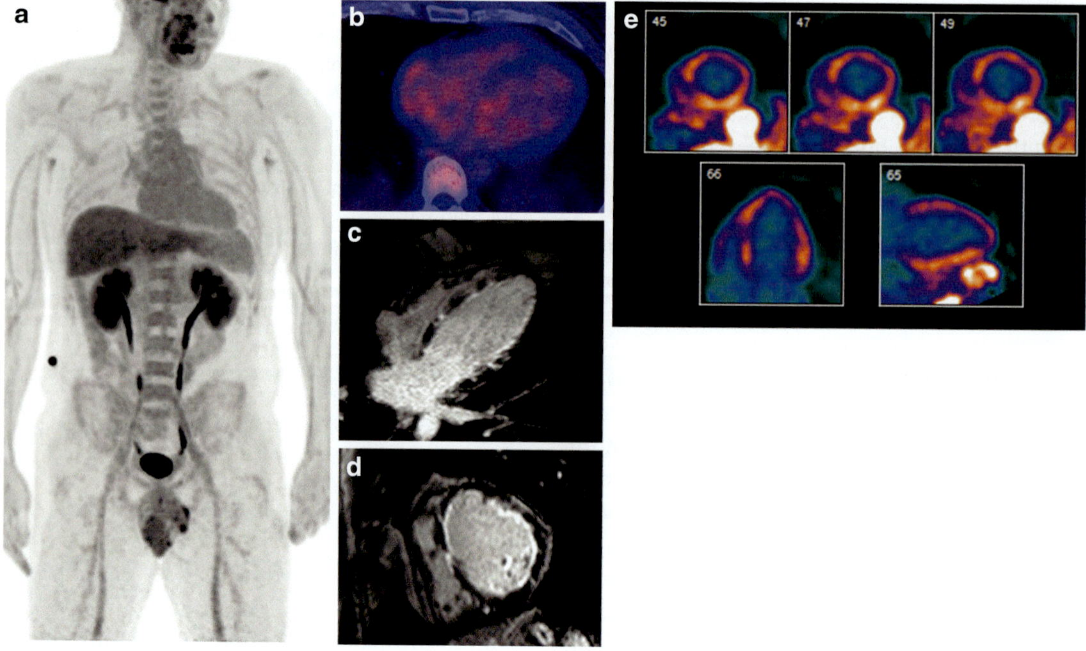

Fig. 6.4 A-29 year-old male with eosinophilic cardiomyopathy. Whole-body FDG-PET maximal intensity projection (MPI) image (**a**) and axial FDG-PET/CT image (**b**) revealed no abnormal myocardial uptake. CMR showed patchy areas of late gadolinium enhancement on 2 chamber (**c**) and short axis (**d**) views. Rubidium rest myocardial perfusion imaging (**e**) demonstrated areas of abnormal perfusion not conforming to coronary anatomy in the mid septal and anterolateral walls

Conclusion

Myocarditis represents a broad range of pathologies characterized by myocardial inflammation. Initial diagnosis of myocarditis can be challenging as clinical presentations are variable and treatment is often limited to supportive therapies. The exact role of FDG-PET in the evaluation of patients with myocarditis remains unclear. The diagnostic performance of FDG-PET depends on the timing of imaging relative to the onset of disease as well as disease subtype. Nonetheless, FDG-PET's unrivaled ability to identify active inflammation may have the potential to help guide therapy. Additional research is needed to better delineate and validate the role of FDG-PET for the evaluation of myocarditis.

References

1. Caforio AL, Pankuweit S, Arbustini E, Basso C, Gimeno-Blanes J, Felix SB, et al. Current state of knowledge on aetiology, diagnosis, management, and therapy of myocarditis: a position statement of the European Society of Cardiology Working Group on myocardial and pericardial diseases. Eur Heart J. 2013;34(33):2636–48, 2648a–2648d.
2. Trachtenberg BH, Hare JM. Inflammatory cardiomyopathic syndromes. Circ Res. 2017;121(7):803–18.
3. Fung E, Fong MW, Correa AJ, Yoon AJ, Grazette LP. Fulminant eosinophilic myocarditis following ICD implantation in a patient with undisclosed nickel allergy. Int J Cardiol. 2015;203:1018–9.
4. Global Burden of Disease Study C. Global, regional, and national incidence, prevalence, and years lived with disability for 301 acute and chronic diseases and injuries in 188 countries, 1990-2013: a systematic analysis for the global burden of disease study 2013. Lancet. 2015;386(9995):743–800.

5. Tschope C, Ammirati E, Bozkurt B, Caforio ALP, Cooper LT, Felix SB, et al. Myocarditis and inflammatory cardiomyopathy: current evidence and future directions. Nat Rev Cardiol. 2021;18(3):169–93.

6. McCarthy RE 3rd, Boehmer JP, Hruban RH, Hutchins GM, Kasper EK, Hare JM, et al. Long-term outcome of fulminant myocarditis as compared with acute (nonfulminant) myocarditis. N Engl J Med. 2000;342(10):690–5.

7. Frustaci A, Chimenti C, Calabrese F, Pieroni M, Thiene G, Maseri A. Immunosuppressive therapy for active lymphocytic myocarditis: virological and immunologic profile of responders versus nonresponders. Circulation. 2003;107(6):857–63.

8. Cooper LT Jr, Berry GJ, Shabetai R. Idiopathic giant-cell myocarditis--natural history and treatment. Multicenter giant cell myocarditis study group investigators. N Engl J Med. 1997;336(26):1860–6.

9. Kandolin R, Lehtonen J, Salmenkivi K, Räisänen-Sokolowski A, Lommi J, Kupari M. Diagnosis, treatment, and outcome of giant-cell myocarditis in the era of combined immunosuppression. Circ Heart Fail. 2013;6(1):15–22.

10. Ekstrom K, Lehtonen J, Kandolin R, Raisanen-Sokolowski A, Salmenkivi K, Kupari M. Incidence, risk factors, and outcome of life-threatening ventricular arrhythmias in giant cell myocarditis. Circ Arrhythm Electrophysiol. 2016;9(12):e004559. https://www.ncbi.nlm.nih.gov/pubmed/27913400.

11. Ekstrom K, Lehtonen J, Kandolin R, Raisanen-Sokolowski A, Salmenkivi K, Kupari M. Long-term outcome and its predictors in giant cell myocarditis. Eur J Heart Fail. 2016;18(12):1452–8.

12. Hulten E, Aslam S, Osborne M, Abbasi S, Bittencourt MS, Blankstein R. Cardiac sarcoidosis-state of the art review. Cardiovasc Diagn Ther. 2016;6(1):50–63.

13. Rybicki BA, Sinha R, Iyengar S, Gray-McGuire C, Elston RC, Iannuzzi MC, et al. Genetic linkage analysis of sarcoidosis phenotypes: the sarcoidosis genetic analysis (SAGA) study. Genes Immun. 2007;8(5):379–86.

14. Spagnolo P, Schwartz DA. Genetic predisposition to sarcoidosis: another brick in the wall. Eur Respir J. 2013;41(4):778–80.

15. Nery PB, Beanlands RS, Nair GM, Green M, Yang J, McArdle BA, et al. Atrioventricular block as the initial manifestation of cardiac sarcoidosis in middle-aged adults. J Cardiovasc Electrophysiol. 2014;25(8):875–81.

16. Kandolin R, Lehtonen J, Kupari M. Cardiac sarcoidosis and giant cell myocarditis as causes of atrioventricular block in young and middle-aged adults. Circ Arrhythm Electrophysiol. 2011;4(3):303–9.

17. Nery PB, Mc Ardle BA, Redpath CJ, Leung E, Lemery R, Dekemp R, et al. Prevalence of cardiac sarcoidosis in patients presenting with monomorphic ventricular tachycardia. Pacing Clin Electrophysiol. 2014;37(3):364–74.

18. Philips B, Madhavan S, James CA, te Riele AS, Murray B, Tichnell C, et al. Arrhythmogenic right ventricular dysplasia/cardiomyopathy and cardiac sarcoidosis: distinguishing features when the diagnosis is unclear. Circ Arrhythm Electrophysiol. 2014;7(2):230–6.

19. Birnie DH, Nery PB, Ha AC, Beanlands RS. Cardiac Sarcoidosis. J Am Coll Cardiol. 2016;68(4):411–21.

20. Martineau P, Pelletier-Galarneau M, Juneau D, Leung E, Birnie D, Beanlands RSB. Molecular imaging of cardiac sarcoidosis. Curr Cardiovasc Imaging Rep. 2018;11(3):6–17.

21. Birnie DH, Sauer WH, Judson MA. Consensus statement on the diagnosis and management of arrhythmias associated with cardiac sarcoidosis. Heart. 2016;102(6):411–4.

22. Ogbogu PU, Rosing DR, Horne MK 3rd. Cardiovascular manifestations of hypereosinophilic syndromes. Immunol Allergy Clin North Am. 2007;27(3):457–75.

23. Antonopoulos AS, Azzu A, Androulakis E, Tanking C, Papagkikas P, Mohiaddin RH. Eosinophilic heart disease: diagnostic and prognostic assessment by cardiac magnetic resonance. Eur Heart J Cardiovasc Imaging. 2021;22(11):1273–84. https://www.ncbi.nlm.nih.gov/pubmed/33432319.

24. Cooper LT, Baughman KL, Feldman AM, Frustaci A, Jessup M, Kuhl U, et al. The role of endomyocardial biopsy in the management of cardiovascular disease: a scientific statement from the American Heart Association, the American College of Cardiology, and the European Society of Cardiology Endorsed by the Heart Failure Society of America and the heart failure Association of the European Society of cardiology. Eur Heart J. 2007;28(24):3076–93.

25. Smith SC, Ladenson JH, Mason JW, Jaffe AS. Elevations of cardiac troponin I associated with myocarditis. experimental and clinical correlates. Circulation. 1997;95(1):163–8.

26. Giraldeau G. The right way to the left ventricle: a better approach to endomyocardial biopsy? Can J Cardiol. 2018;34(10):1247–9.

27. Jeserich M, Konstantinides S, Pavlik G, Bode C, Geibel A. Non-invasive imaging in the diagnosis of acute viral myocarditis. Clin Res Cardiol. 2009;98(12):753–63.

28. Fernández-Jiménez R, Sánchez-González J, Aguero J, Del Trigo M, Galán-Arriola C, Fuster V, et al. Fast T2 gradient-spin-echo (T2-Gra SE) mapping for myocardial edema quantification: first in vivo validation in a porcine model of ischemia/reperfusion. J Cardiovasc Magn Reson. 2015;17:92.

29. Abdel-Aty H, Boyé P, Zagrosek A, Wassmuth R, Kumar A, Messroghli D, et al. Diagnostic performance of cardiovascular magnetic resonance in patients with suspected acute myocarditis: com-

parison of different approaches. J Am Coll Cardiol. 2005;45(11):1815–22.

30. Ferreira VM, Schulz-Menger J, Holmvang G, Kramer CM, Carbone I, Sechtem U, et al. Cardiovascular magnetic resonance in nonischemic myocardial inflammation: expert recommendations. J Am Coll Cardiol. 2018;72(24):3158–76.

31. Friedrich MG, Sechtem U, Schulz-Menger J, Holmvang G, Alakija P, Cooper LT, et al. Cardiovascular magnetic resonance in myocarditis: a JACC white paper. J Am Coll Cardiol. 2009;53(17):1475–87.

32. Cummings KW, Bhalla S, Javidan-Nejad C, Bierhals AJ, Gutierrez FR, Woodard PK. A pattern-based approach to assessment of delayed enhancement in nonischemic cardiomyopathy at MR imaging. Radiographics. 2009;29(1):89–103.

33. Kuchynka P, Palecek T, Masek M, Cerny V, Lambert L, Vitkova I, et al. Current diagnostic and therapeutic aspects of eosinophilic myocarditis. Biomed Res Int. 2016;2016:2829583.

34. Yang F, Wang J, Li W, Xu Y, Wan K, Zeng R, et al. The prognostic value of late gadolinium enhancement in myocarditis and clinically suspected myocarditis: systematic review and meta-analysis. Eur Radiol. 2020;30(5):2616–26.

35. Blissett S, Chocron Y, Kovacina B, Afilalo J. Diagnostic and prognostic value of cardiac magnetic resonance in acute myocarditis: a systematic review and meta-analysis. Int J Cardiovasc Imaging. 2019;35(12):2221–9.

36. Luetkens JA, Faron A, Isaak A, Dabir D, Kuetting D, Feisst A, et al. Comparison of original and 2018 Lake Louise criteria for diagnosis of acute myocarditis: results of a validation cohort. Radiol Cardiothorac Imaging. 2019;1(3):e190010.

37. Gutberlet M, Lücke C. Original versus 2018 Lake Louise criteria for acute myocarditis diagnosis: old versus new. Radiol Cardiothorac Imaging. 2019;1(3):e190150.

38. Nensa F, Poeppel TD, Krings P, Schlosser T. Multiparametric assessment of myocarditis using simultaneous positron emission tomography/magnetic resonance imaging. Eur Heart J. 2014;35(32):2173.

39. Gesa v O, Fabien H, Nicolas L, Karl-Ludwig L, Markus S, Tareq I. Detection of acute inflammatory myocarditis in Epstein Barr virus infection using hybrid ^{18}F-Fluoro-Deoxyglucose–positron emission tomography/magnetic resonance imaging. Circulation. 2014;130(11):925–6.

40. Aleksova N, Juneau D, Dick A, Green M, Birnie D, Beanlands RS, et al. Role of ^{18}F-Fluorodeoxyglucose/positron emission tomography imaging to demonstrate resolution of acute myocarditis. Can J Cardiol. 2017;33(2):293.e3–5.

41. Takano H, Nakagawa K, Ishio N, Daimon M, Daimon M, Kobayashi Y, et al. Active myocarditis in a patient with chronic active Epstein-Barr virus infection. Int J Cardiol. 2008;130(1):e11–3.

42. Abgral R, Dweck MR, Trivieri MG, Robson PM, Karakatsanis N, Mani V, et al. Clinical utility of combined FDG-PET/MR to assess myocardial disease. JACC Cardiovasc Imaging. 2017;10(5):594–7.

43. Simon R, Perel-Winkler A, Bokhari S, Fazlollahi L, Nickerson K. Myocarditis in Giant cell arteritis diagnosed with fluorine 18–labeled Fluorodeoxyglucose positron emission tomography–computed tomography: case report and review of the literature. J Clin Rheumatol. 2020;26(2):e37.

44. Gracia E, Monach P, Shih J. Monitoring of disease activity in eosinophilic myocarditis via pet scans. J Am Coll Cardiol. 2020;75(11 Supplement 1):2559.

45. Langwieser N, von Olshausen G, Rischpler C, Ibrahim T. Confirmation of diagnosis and graduation of inflammatory activity of Loeffler endocarditis by hybrid positron emission tomography/magnetic resonance imaging. Eur Heart J. 2014;35(36):2496.

46. Moriwaki K, Dohi K, Omori T, Tanimura M, Sugiura E, Nakamori S, et al. A survival case of fulminant right-side dominant eosinophilic myocarditis. Int Heart J. 2017;58(3):459–62.

47. Lamacie MM, Aws A, Vidhya N, Ellamae S, David B, Beanlands Rob SB, et al. Serial ^{18}F-Fluorodeoxyglucose positron emission tomography imaging in a patient with Giant cell myocarditis. Circ Cardiovasc Imaging. 2020;13(2):e009940.

48. Tanimura M, Dohi K, Imanaka-Yoshida K, Omori T, Moriwaki K, Nakamori S, et al. Fulminant myocarditis with prolonged active lymphocytic infiltration after hemodynamic recovery. Int Heart J. 2017;58(2):294–7.

49. Palmisano A, Vignale D, Peretto G, Busnardo E, Calcagno C, Campochiaro C, et al. Hybrid FDG-PET/MR or FDG-PET/CT to detect disease activity in patients with persisting arrhythmias after myocarditis. JACC Cardiovasc Imaging. 2020;14(1):288–92.

50. Pelletier-Galarneau M, Ruddy TD. PET/CT for diagnosis and management of large-vessel vasculitis. Curr Cardiol Rep. 2019;21(5):34.

51. Ozawa K, Funabashi N, Daimon M, Takaoka H, Takano H, Uehara M, et al. Determination of optimum periods between onset of suspected acute myocarditis and ^{18}F-fluorodeoxyglucose positron emission tomography in the diagnosis of inflammatory left ventricular myocardium. Int J Cardiol. 2013;169(3):196–200.

52. Chen W, Jeudy J. Assessment of myocarditis: cardiac MR, PET/CT, or PET/MR? Curr Cardiol Rep. 2019;21(8):76.

53. Nensa F, Kloth J, Tezgah E, Poeppel TD, Heusch P, Goebel J, et al. Feasibility of FDG-PET in myocarditis: comparison to CMR using integrated PET/MRI. J Nucl Cardiol. 2018;25(3):785–94.

Pieter H. Nienhuis, Elisabeth Brouwer, and Riemer H. J. A. Slart

Introduction

Large vessel vasculitis (LVV) is a collection of chronic autoimmune conditions characterized by inflammatory lesions in the vessel wall of large- and medium-sized arteries. These vessel wall lesions may result in aneurysm formation, rupture, and dissection in the aorta and stenosis as well as end-organ damage in the medium-sized arteries [1]. There are two major variants of LVV: Takayasu arteritis (TAK) and giant cell arteritis (GCA). TAK is characterized by inflammation of the aorta and its major branches and affects patients under 50 years of age. In GCA, the aorta and its major branches may likewise be affected, but less commonly than in TAK. Instead, the third to fifth-order branches of the aorta such as the temporal and vertebral arteries are affected [2]. Additionally, GCA only presents in patients over 50 years of age, hence age being the main discriminator between the two diseases [3].

Apart from the above-mentioned complications associated with aortic involvement which presents in both TAK and GCA, the frequently affected vessels determine many of the clinical features. In TAK, subclavian artery occlusion leads to limb claudication and pulselessness. Such a clinical course may subsequently be complicated by peripheral ischemia. In GCA, occlusion of cranial arteries leads to headache and jaw claudication. Associated possible complications include vision loss and stroke.

Systemic symptoms such as fever, weight loss, and arthralgia are present in both types of

P. H. Nienhuis
Department of Nuclear Medicine and Molecular Imaging, Medical Imaging Center, University Medical Center Groningen, University of Groningen, Groningen, The Netherlands

Vasculitis Expertise Center Groningen, University Medical Center Groningen, University of Groningen, Groningen, The Netherlands

E. Brouwer
Vasculitis Expertise Center Groningen, University Medical Center Groningen, University of Groningen, Groningen, The Netherlands

Department of Rheumatology and Clinical Immunology, University Medical Center Groningen, University of Groningen, Groningen, The Netherlands

R. H. J. A. Slart (✉)
Department of Nuclear Medicine and Molecular Imaging, Medical Imaging Center, University Medical Center Groningen, University of Groningen, Groningen, The Netherlands

Vasculitis Expertise Center Groningen, University Medical Center Groningen, University of Groningen, Groningen, The Netherlands

Department of Biomedical Photonic Imaging, Faculty of Science and Technology, University of Twente, Enschede, The Netherlands
e-mail: r.h.j.a.slart@umcg.nl

LVV. GCA patients presenting with pain and stiffness of the shoulder or hip girdle are frequently diagnosed with concomitant polymyalgia rheumatica (PMR), belonging to the same disease spectrum as GCA. As many as half of the GCA patients have evidence of PMR [4].

Although both diseases are primarily diagnosed based on clinical suspicion and raised inflammatory markers, various imaging modalities are now frequently used to aid the diagnostic process. In recent recommendations, the early use of imaging in the diagnostic process of GCA has been favored over a temporal artery biopsy, which has historically been considered the diagnostic gold standard [5].

In patients with high clinical suspicion, a positive imaging test may confirm a diagnosis of GCA or TAK. Imaging modalities used to investigate LVV include ultrasonography, magnetic resonance angiography (MRA), computed tomography angiography (CTA), and [^{18}F]-fluorodeoxyglucose positron emission tomography (FDG-PET). Ultrasonography showing a "halo sign" is highly suggestive of GCA. MRA is the primary imaging modality to diagnose TAK by way of showing vessel wall thickening and edema. Additionally, MRA of the cranial arteries may be used to diagnose GCA. CTA may equally be used to detect vessel wall inflammation in the large arteries.

Despite the proven value of the current diagnostic tools, negative results from any diagnostic tool cannot definitively exclude the presence of LVV. For example, a patient may have a negative temporal artery biopsy, ultrasonography without a halo sign, magnetic resonance imaging and computed tomography without wall thickening, but still have LVV as evidenced by a positive FDG-PET/CT.

FDG-PET is a functional imaging technique that is based on detecting enhanced glucose uptake. It is an established tool in the field of oncology, detecting the high glycolytic activity of malignant cells. To anatomically locate FDG uptake, FDG-PET is always used in conjunction with another imaging method, most commonly low-dose CT.

FDG-PET/CT also plays a role in imaging infectious and inflammatory diseases, by detecting the increased glycolytic activity of inflammatory cells such as macrophages [6]. This way, vessel wall inflammation in LVV may be detected on FDG-PET/CT. Given FDG-PET/CT is usually conducted as a whole-body scan, it enables detection of LVV in many regions throughout the body. Using FDG-PET/CT to assess inflammation of the aorta and its first-order branches is already well established in daily clinical practice. Its use to assess vessel wall inflammation in the cranial arteries had always been regarded unfeasible due to the small diameter of these arteries. For example, the superficial branch of the temporal artery has an average diameter of 2 mm, for which PET camera systems did not have sufficient resolution [7]. Additionally, cranial artery uptake was difficult to distinguish from the high physiological FDG uptake of the brain [8]. However, recent studies have shown that procedural adaptions and higher resolution PET camera systems can reveal inflammation in the cranial arteries as well [9–11].

Apart from detecting vessel wall inflammation, FDG-PET/CT may assist the differential diagnosis by enabling the identification of other inflammatory processes that may explain the patient's clinical presentation.

Much remains unknown about how FDG uptake may be interpreted in inflammatory diseases. Increased FDG uptake is mainly noticed in active disease processes with a high rate of metabolism. In LVV, this may be observed in the early phase of the disease process, before anatomic changes in the vessel wall manifest. Therefore, FDG-PET/CT may not show the vessel wall destruction resulting from inflammation and subsequently not capture all clinically significant findings.

In this chapter, the current application of FDG-PET/CT in LVV will be discussed. The technical approach to FDG-PET procedure and image interpretation as well as the role of FDG-PET/CT in the diagnostic workup of LVV forms the backbone of this chapter. Additionally, potential pitfalls of FDG-PET/CT in LVV will be reviewed.

FDG-PET Procedure

The FDG-PET procedure for patients with LVV determines the quality and, therefore, the readability of the FDG-PET images. Important factors in the FDG-PET procedure are patient preparation, image acquisition, and image reconstruction. Standardization of the FDG-PET procedure is paramount to ensure optimal image quality for diagnosis, enable comparison with follow-up imaging, and allow validation of research outcomes [8, 12]. The recommended procedural parameters are summarized in Table 7.1.

Patient Preparation

The main goal of patient preparation is to reduce physiologic tracer uptake in healthy tissues while maintaining or enhancing tracer uptake in inflamed tissues. Because FDG is a glucose analog, glucose may competitively inhibit FDG uptake in tissues. Indeed, serum glucose levels have been found to alter the biodistribution of FDG and lower the diagnostic sensitivity of FDG-PET [13, 14]. Ideally, serum glucose levels do not exceed 7 mmol/L before the FDG

Table 7.1 Summary of recommended patient preparation and image acquisition parameters for FDG-PET/CT in LVV

Parameter	Recommendation
Dietary preparation	Fast for at least 6 h prior to FDG administration Consider a carbohydrate lacking diet for 12–24 h prior to the scan in case of fever of unknown origin or suspected cardiac involvement
Blood glucose levels	Preferably ≤7 mmol/L (126 mg/dL)
Glucocorticoids	Withdraw or delay therapy until after PET, unless there is a risk of ischemic complications
Scan range	Head down to the feet
Incubation time after FDG injection	Standard 60 min

Modified from Slart et al. [8]

administration. For this reason, patients are instructed to fast 6 h before FDG administration. Unlike for certain malignancies, FDG-PET may still enable the detection of inflammatory disorders despite high serum glucose levels [15]. Therefore, hyperglycemia is not considered an absolute contraindication, and patients with (poorly controlled) diabetes may still undergo an FDG-PET [8].

Glucocorticoids form the initial mainstay in the treatment of LVV [16]. Especially when GCA is suspected, glucocorticoid treatment needs to be given without delay to decrease the risk of ischemic complications such as vision loss. For this reason, glucocorticoid treatment may already be started before a diagnosis of LVV can be confirmed by imaging.

However, glucocorticoid treatment may decrease the detectability of LVV on US and FDG-PET imaging [17]. Research revealed that FDG-PET imaging maintains its accuracy for detecting LVV when performed within 3 days of starting glucocorticoid therapy. FDG-PET imaging performed after 10 days of glucocorticoid treatment significantly decreases its diagnostic sensitivity [18]. Glucocorticoids may also increase liver uptake of FDG, resulting in lower diagnostic sensitivity when scoring vascular FDG uptake compared to the liver [19]. Scoring methods will be discussed further below, under "Image Interpretation."

PET Acquisition Procedure

The interval time, defined as the time between FDG injection and acquisition, is one of the main influencing factors of the imaging result. Interval times of approximately 60 min are most frequently used in LVV imaging. Extended interval times of 120 min are more frequently used in atherosclerosis, another type of vessel wall inflammation. In LVV, extended interval times have been shown to decrease FDG uptake in the blood pool, possibly resulting in enhanced detectability of vessel wall uptake due to lower background activity. Interval times of 120 min may identify more patients with clinically active LVV [20]. An important comparative advantage of FDG-PET imaging is its ability to allow assessment of virtually all medium- and large-sized vessels. Imaging from head to knee or from head to feet (whole-body imaging) is, therefore, recommended. Additionally, doubling the imaging time and applying a larger matrix increases the resolution of the images. A higher resolution may be especially beneficial when imaging the arteries of the head and neck due to their smaller size [8].

Image resolution also depends on the chosen image reconstruction settings. Increasing the number of iterations increases the resolution, but also increases image noise. Time-of-flight information must be used during reconstruction and image filtering should be minimized [8].

Interpretation and Reporting of FDG-PET/CT

Arterial FDG uptake may be influenced significantly by several factors. Over the years, several interpretation methods have been proposed for use in clinical practice. The simplest method of FDG-PET interpretation is based on a visual first impression by an experienced reader. This method, also described in literature by the German word "Gestalt," gives fast results, but highly subjective and, subsequently, not standardizable [19]. The interpretation methods are summarized in Table 7.2.

Visual Grading Scales

Visual grading scales may be used to overcome this subjectivity bias, by creating uniform, reproducible, and easy-to-use criteria. Additionally, visual grading scales may also correct for individual differences in systemic FDG uptake by comparing vascular wall uptake to a background organ. To achieve more standardization in clinical practice, 2018 recommendations propose the use of a 0-to-3 visual grading scale that compares

Table 7.2 Summary of FDG-PET/CT interpretation methods for large vessel vasculitis

FDG-PET/CT LVV interpretation methods		
Visual interpretation		
Grading compared to background	Grade 0 (no vascular uptake)	
	Grade 1 (vascular uptake < background)	
	Grade 2 (vascular uptake = background uptake)	
	Grade 3 (vascular uptake > background uptake) Background: Liver Blood pool Lungs Surrounding tissue	
Uptake pattern	Focal (atherosclerosis)	
	Diffuse (vasculitis)	
Semiquantitative interpretation (visual)		
Total vascular score (TVS)	= [Grade Target 1] + [Grade Target 2] + …	
	Vascular targets:	
	Large vessels	Ascending aorta
		Aortic arch
		Descending aorta
		Abdominal aorta
		Pulmonary arteries
		Innominate artery
		Subclavian arteries
		Axillary arteries
		Subclavian arteries
		Iliac arteries
		Femoral arteries
	Cranial vessels	Temporal arteries
		Maxillary arteries
		Vertebral arteries
		Occipital arteries

Table 7.2 (continued)

FDG-PET/CT LVV interpretation methods		
Semiquantitative (SUV)		
Target-to-background ratio (TBR)	= SUV$_{max}$ vascular target/SUV$_{max/mean}$ background	
	Vascular targets:	
	Same as above	
	Background:	
	Blood pool	Superior caval vein
		Inferior caval vein
	Liver	Right lobe

(PET/)CTA/MRA LVV interpretation methods
Regular vascular wall thickness (mm)
Contrast enhancement
Presence of stenosis and/or aneurysm

Modified from Slart et al. [8]

vascular wall uptake to liver [8]. This method is illustrated in Fig. 7.1 and works as follows: grade 0 = no uptake; grade 1 = vascular uptake inferior to liver; grade 2 = vascular uptake equal to liver; grade 3 = vascular uptake superior to liver uptake. Examples of visual grading scores for the large vessels are shown in Fig. 7.1. In active LVV, a smooth linear and segmental pattern of grade 3 visual FDG uptake in the wall of large- and medium-sized arteries is considered a positive FDG-PET. Under immunosuppressive therapy, a grade 2 may be considered positive. In addition to the liver, the blood pool in the vena cava may also be used as background for comparison.

In LVV, all medium- and large-sized vessels may be affected. For FDG-PET interpretation of LVV, it is useful to make a distinction between the large systemic vessels affected in TAK and

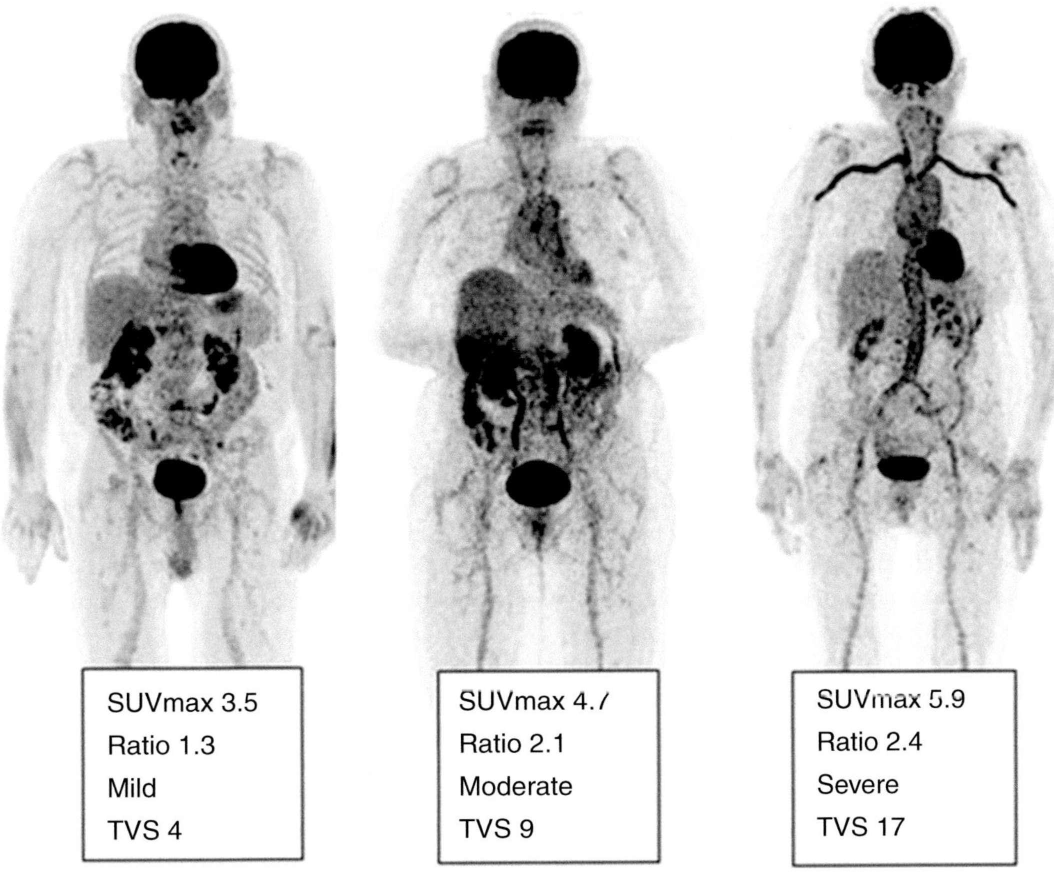

Fig. 7.1 FDG-PET. Mild (grade 1), moderate (grade 2), and severe (grade 3) FDG uptake patterns including SUVmax values of the thoracic aorta in patients with GCA. Ratio is defined as average SUVmax of the thoracic aorta divided by the liver region. The total vascular score (TVS) is the highest for the right-positioned patient. (Modified from Slart et al. [8])

large vessel-GCA (LV-GCA), and between the medium-sized cranial vessels in C-GCA. The initial use of FDG-PET in LVV was based on the assessment of increased tracer uptake in the large systemic vessels [21]. FDG-PET/CT imaging and assessment of the aorta and the common carotid, subclavian, axillary, iliac, and femoral arteries were, increasingly used in the diagnostic workup of GCA and TAK, although to a lesser extent in TAK. Importantly, FDG-PET imaging was not deemed feasible to assess the cranial arteries and, for that reason, not suitable to diagnose C-GCA [22].

Cranial Artery Assessment

Due to procedural adaptions and technical advancements in PET systems in recent years, PET image resolution has increased. The use of digital PET systems and especially systems with time-of-flight capabilities allow for the assessment of extra-cranial artery involvement in GCA. Also, a slight increase in acquisition time of the head/neck area (5 min instead of 2–3 min) improves the visualization of extra-cranial arteries. Diagnosis of C-GCA is possible due to combined assessment of the temporal, maxillary, vertebral, and occipital arteries and may be reported like the visual scoring previously described [9–11] (Fig. 7.2).

Quantification

Until now, only scoring by visual assessment has been discussed. Other types of (semi) quantitative scoring may also be used and may be considered more objective methods of FDG-PET interpretation. Standardized uptake value (SUV) metrics may be calculated by drawing regions of interest (ROI) or volumes of interest (VOI) around the vascular lesions. Additionally, SUV metrics of the target vascular lesion may also be corrected for systemic uptake. By dividing the SUV of the target vascular lesion by the SUV of a background region, a correction can be made for individual differences of tracer uptake depending on weight, injected radiotracer dose, blood glucose levels, and renal clearance.

Frequently used background regions are the liver and the blood pool as measured in the superior or inferior vena cava.

Importantly, semiquantitative measurements using SUV metrics are currently recommended for use in research only [23]. Although studies have shown that SUV metrics can be used for diagnosis, this has not been proven in any large-scale, prospective studies [20, 24, 25]. Moreover, SUV metrics are highly dependent on the FDG-PET imaging procedure, which may make generalization and comparable multicenter diagnostic implementation difficult. Equally, the use of SUV metrics in FDG-PET as a monitoring biomarker or as a predictive tool may provide additional benefit. However, this has not been investigated yet.

Diagnostic Performance

The diagnostic performance of FDG-PET imaging in LVV is good to excellent. The sensitivity of FDG-PET/CT to detect LV-GCA is 80–90% and its specificity is 89–98%, depending on the criteria for reference diagnosis [8, 26]. Diagnostic performance is similar when assessing the cranial arteries in C-GCA, with a sensitivity of 82% and a specificity approaching 100% [9, 10]. In comparison, diagnostic accuracy is lower in TAK patients, a sensitivity of 87% and a specificity of 73%. As stated before, the diagnostic accuracy of FDG-PET in LVV decreases if patients have already been treated with glucocorticoids for more than 3 days [18].

The use of a visual grading scale, as described above, can be extended by calculating a total vascular score (TVS). The TVS is calculated by adding up the visual grading scores of multiple vessels and vascular segments. As expected, a TVS of 4 aortic segments (ascending, arch, descending, and abdominal) and 4 branch arteries (carotid and subclavian) is significantly higher in LVV patients than in controls [27]. It is currently unknown whether TVS also illustrates the disease extent or severity. A recent study concluded that the TVS may be correlated with the global assessment of a physician, but not with patient-reported disease severity [23]. Likewise, it

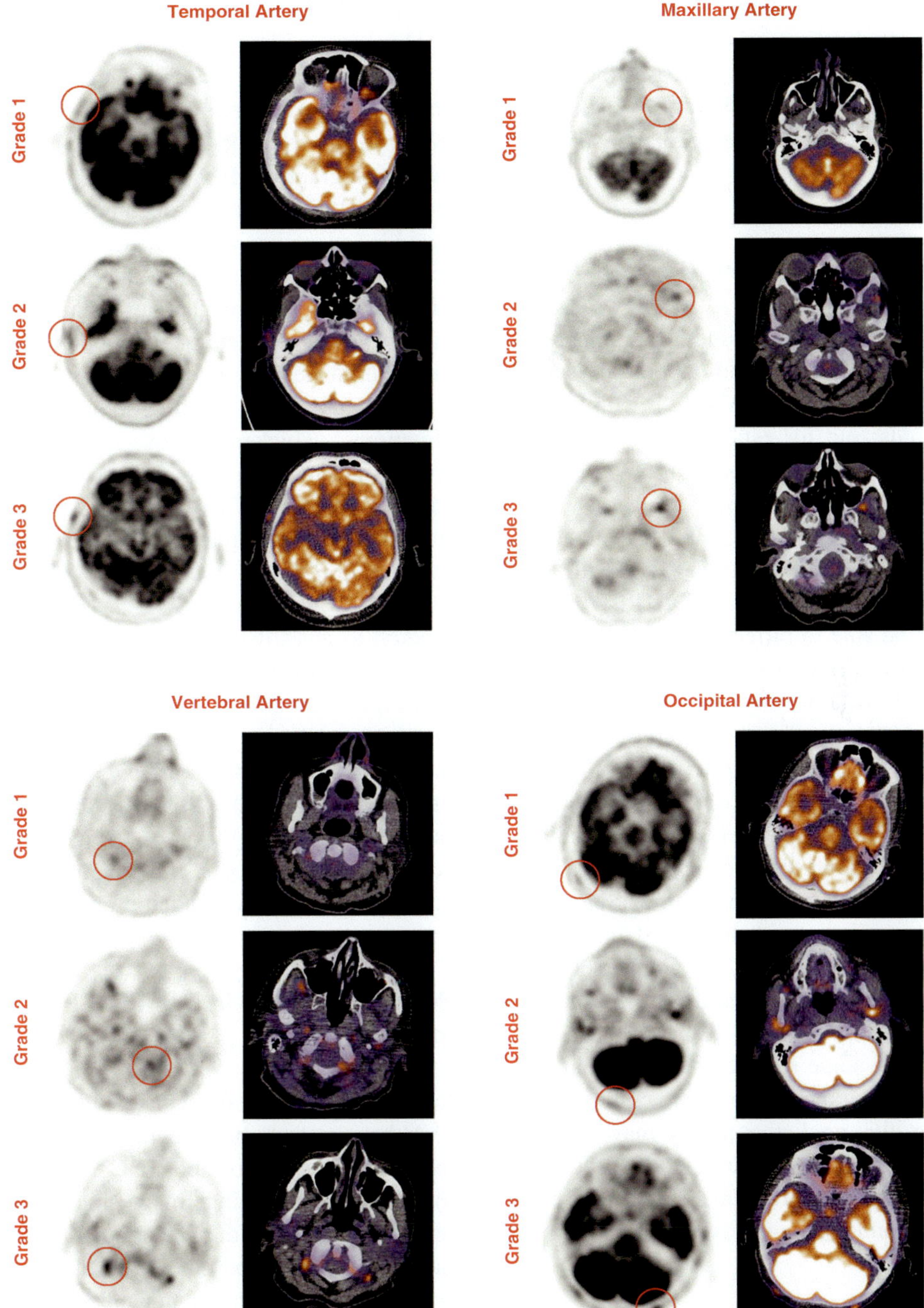

Fig. 7.2 FDG-PET/CT. Mild (grade 1), moderate (grade 2), and severe (grade 3) cranial FDG uptake patterns: temporal artery, maxillary artery, vertebral artery, and occipital artery. The red circle highlights the visually determined area of increased uptake

remains unclear whether including less frequently involved vessels such as the axillary, iliac, and femoral arteries increases the discriminatory value of the TVS. Similarly, including the cranial vessels may increase diagnostic performance [11].

Monitoring and Follow-Up

As described in the introduction, clinical symptoms, physical signs, and laboratory tests are unreliable to diagnose LVV [24]. Similarly, the same holds true for establishing relapsing disease. Over 50% of patients with LVV will experience relapsing disease [16].

The value of serial FDG-PET investigations as an imaging biomarker for LVV is still up for debate [11, 27]. Follow-up FDG-PET/CT imaging may be able to differentiate clinically active and inactive disease by, respectively, higher and lower TVS. Additionally, there may be no correlation between the glucocorticoid dose and TVS, nor between patient-reported assessment and TVS [23]. In studies looking at follow-up FDG-PET scans in LVV patients, FDG uptake was variable in patients with persistent clinical remission, ranging from patients with decreased FDG uptake to patients with increased uptake compared to baseline [25, 28]. Conversely, other studies demonstrated mainly decreased FDG uptake on follow-up scans [29, 30].

Likewise, some research suggests that a high TVS may be predictive for future clinical relapse. However, this predictive ability may depend on the TVS calculation, the number of vascular beds included, the reconstruction techniques used, and the background organ that is used for semiquantitative scoring.

PET Combined with CTA or MRA

Standard FDG-PET/CT imaging in LVV makes use of low-dose CT for attenuation correction and also of anatomic reference for the PET signal. As an imaging tool in LVV, low-dose CT has little added value by itself but can be helpful to distinguish LVV from atherosclerotic activity [31].

Alternatively, PET imaging may be complemented by vascular imaging with angiography, either in the form of CT angiography (CTA) or MR angiography (MRA). When used in conjunction with these imaging techniques, FDG-PET provides visualization of ongoing inflammatory processes, whereas the CTA and MRA can visualize the morphologic changes in the vessel wall, such as wall thickening, aneurysm formation, and arterial stenosis assessment.

Currently, CTA and MRA are used in different situations. Thickening of the vessel wall (>2–3 mm) or aorta dilatation (3–4 cm) on CTA may be indicative of LVV and shows particularly high diagnostic accuracy in TAK [26]. Its use for investigation of the cranial arteries in C-GCA is limited. Conversely, MRA is an established method to investigate mural inflammation in the cranial arteries. By itself, it may also be used to investigate inflammation of the intracerebral arteries, which are precluded from investigation on FDG-PET due to high FDG uptake by the brain. Combined FDG-PET/MRA may synergistically improve diagnosis of C-GCA due to its combined morphologic and functional imaging accompanied by lower radiation burden [32].

Potential Pitfalls in LVV FDG-PET Imaging

Potential pitfalls regarding FDG-PET imaging in LVV have already been mentioned in this chapter. Many aspects of the FDG-PET procedure influence the resulting image, highlighting the importance of procedure standardization. Patient factors, such as blood glucose levels, glucocorticoid use, and body mass, may all influence FDG uptake in the tissues. Other factors, such as renal clearance, metabolic disease, and the use of immunosuppressive drugs may also influence imaging results. Procedural factors such as injected tracer dosage and imaging time delay also influence the FDG-PET image [20].

Image interpretation may also present some challenges. Implementation of the recommended visual scoring methods described above may require additional training. Interpretation of cranial artery uptake may be especially challenging because of the anatomic localization. However, high diagnostic accuracy and reader consensus may be achieved with training [9].

Like LVV, atherosclerosis may show FDG uptake in the arterial wall. Therefore, it may be difficult to distinguish between atherosclerosis and LVV, especially where both diseases may overlap [31]. Hence, one should interpret vascular inflammation in patients with marked calcification on CT with caution. No definitive methods have been devised to differentiate between these types of vascular inflammation, but atherosclerosis seems to present with less intense and patchier FDG uptake compared to LVV, as the latter is a more intense and diffuse pattern [31] (Fig. 7.3).

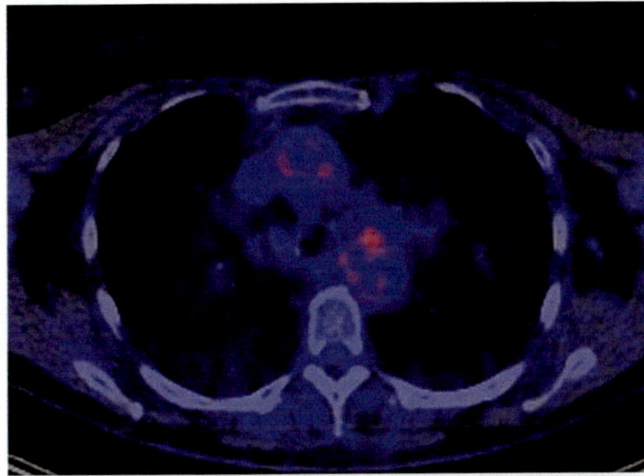
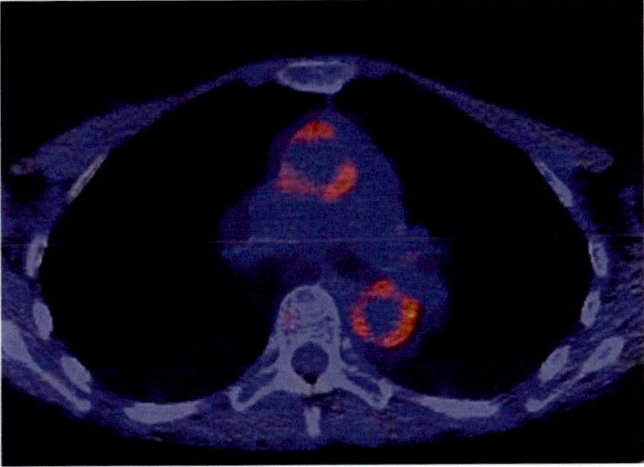

Fig. 7.3 Transverse FDG-PET/CT images of atherosclerotic FDG uptake (above) and vasculitic FDG uptake (below) in the aorta. Vasculitic FDG uptake is characteristically more intense and circumferential compared to atherosclerotic FDG uptake

Perspectives in LVV Imaging

Based on the currently available literature, FDG-PET/CT plays an important role in the diagnosis of LVV, but additional randomized studies are needed to validate the existing evidence. To increase the reproducibility of future research and the generalizability of its results, future studies should take the latest international recommendations on FDG-PET/CT imaging in LVV into account.

Future research should focus on including real-world prospective data and the implementation of FDG-PET/CT with existing diagnostic (imaging) investigations. The development of diagnostic algorithms may further clarify the role of FDG-PET/CT in the diagnostic process and its position within such algorithms. New semiquantitative approaches to FDG-PET/CT interpretation, focusing on SUV metrics, and including TVS, may be of particular benefit in monitoring and prediction of the LVV disease course. An example of a novel semiquantitative metric may be found in the calculation of the total lesion glycolysis (TLG). TLG measurements are already used in oncology and also take the volume of an inflammatory lesion into account, rather than only the intensity of FDG uptake. Although not yet extensively investigated, TLG may prove to be of value in monitoring disease activity [33].

Whole-body PET imaging presents opportunities for truly systemic investigations of LVV, a systemic disease that may present in virtually all large- and medium-sized arteries throughout the body. The availability of the FDG tracer allows for the widespread use and implementation of FDG-PET/CT investigations in LVV. However, FDG remains nonspecific in the investigation of inflammatory processes and cannot provide any information about the nature of inflammation. Additionally, high FDG uptake in the brain precludes FDG-PET from assessing inflammatory processes in the brain, but extra-cranial arteries can be visualized on digital high-resolution PET/CT camera systems.

New PET tracers targeting specific immune cells may open new areas for basic research into LVV as well as more specific characterization and recognition of inflammatory lesions. Macrophage targeting PET tracers, such as ^{18}F-PEG-Folate, and tracers targeting the translocator protein (TSPO) have shown promising results in (auto) inflammatory and vascular diseases [34]. Similarly, tracers targeting the fibroblast activation protein inhibitor (FAPI) are promising, demonstrating low uptake in healthy tissues and showing promise in monitoring disease activity [35, 36].

Importantly, FDG-PET/CT may play an increasing role in clinical practice. Its implementation may be further aided by additional physician training on the interpretation of FDG-PET/CT scans in LVV. Furthermore, the role of FDG-PET/CT in LVV may change in the future, possibly for monitoring and predicting disease course. As the array of investigative (and therapeutic) options increases, and as management will become more personalized, a vasculitis multidisciplinary expert team may ensure optimal use of FDG-PET/CT in LVV. Also training in optimal reading of the FDG-PET/CT for the imager should be supported by the affiliated medical societies.

A patient-centered and multidisciplinary approach has to be accounted for in research too. Therefore, for future research to be built into clinical practice, clinical relevance and patient well-being are essential. This includes minimizing the diagnostic burden where possible and utilizing the strengths of FDG-PET/CT—its high diagnostic performance and whole-body assessment—where necessary.

References

1. Weyand CM, Goronzy JJ. Immune mechanisms in medium and large-vessel vasculitis. Nat Rev Rheumatol. 2013;9:731. http://www.ncbi.nlm.nih.gov/pubmed/24189842.
2. Watanabe R, Berry GJ, Liang DH, Goronzy JJ, Weyand CM. Pathogenesis of Giant cell arteritis and Takayasu arteritis—similarities and differences. Curr Rheumatol Rep. 2020;22(10):68.
3. Jennette J. Overview of the 2012 revised international Chapel Hill consensus conference nomenclature of vasculitides. Clin Exp Nephrol. 2013;17:603–6. http://www.ncbi.nlm.nih.gov/pubmed/24072416.
4. Blockmans D, Stroobants S, Maes A, Mortelmans L. Positron emission tomography in giant cell arteritis and polymyalgia rheumatica: evidence for inflammation of the aortic arch. Am J Med. 2000;108:246–9.
5. Dejaco C, Ramiro S, Duftner C, Besson FL, Bley TA, Blockmans D, et al. EULAR recommendations for the use of imaging in large vessel vasculitis in clinical practice. Ann Rheum Dis. 2018;77:636–43. https://doi.org/10.1136/annrheumdis-2017-212649.
6. Kubota R, Yamada S, Kubota K, Ishiwata K, Tamahashi N, Ido T. Intratumoral distribution of fluorine-18-fluorodeoxyglucose in vivo: high accumulation in macrophages and granulation tissues studied by microautoradiography. J Nucl Med. 1992;33:1972–80. http://www.ncbi.nlm.nih.gov/pubmed/1432158.
7. Marano SR, Fischer DW, Gaines C, VKH S. Anatomical study of the superficial temporal artery. Neurosurgery. 1985;16:786–90. https://academic.oup.com/neurosurgery/article/16/6/786/2752637.
8. Slart RHJA, Glaudemans AWJM, Chareonthaitawee P, Treglia G, Besson FL, Bley TA, et al. FDG-PET/CT (a) imaging in large vessel vasculitis and polymyalgia rheumatica: joint procedural recommendation of the EANM, SNMMI, and the PET interest group (PIG), and endorsed by the ASNC. Eur J Nucl Med Mol Imaging. 2018;45:1250–69.
9. Nielsen BD, Hansen IT, Kramer S, Haraldsen A, Hjorthaug K, Bogsrud TV, et al. Simple dichotomous assessment of cranial artery inflammation by conventional ^{18}F-FDG PET/CT shows high accuracy for the diagnosis of giant cell arteritis: a case-control study. Eur J Nucl Med Mol Imaging. 2019;46:184–93. http://link.springer.com/10.1007/s00259-018-4106-0.
10. Nienhuis PH, Sandovici M, Glaudemans AW, Slart RH, Brouwer E. Visual and semiquantitative assessment of cranial artery inflammation with FDG-PET/CT in giant cell arteritis. Semin Arthritis Rheum. 2020;50:616–23. https://linkinghub.elsevier.com/retrieve/pii/S0049017220300986.
11. Sammel AM, Hsiao E, Schembri G, Bailey E, Nguyen K, Brewer J, et al. Cranial and large vessel activity on positron emission tomography scan at diagnosis and 6 months in giant cell arteritis. Int J Rheum Dis. 2020;23:582–8.
12. Slart RHJA, Glaudemans AWJM, Gheysens O, Lubberink M, Kero T. Procedural recommendations of cardiac PET/CT imaging: and innervation (4Is) -related cardiovascular diseases: a joint collaboration of the EACVI and the EANM. Eur J Nucl Med Mol Imaging. 2020;48(4):1016–39.
13. Bucerius J, Mani V, Moncrieff C, Machac J, Fuster V, Farkouh ME, et al. Optimizing ^{18}F-FDG PET/CT imaging of vessel wall inflammation: the impact of ^{18}F-FDG circulation time, injected dose, uptake parameters, and fasting blood glucose levels. Eur J Nucl Med Mol Imaging. 2014;41:369–83.
14. Wahl L, Henry A, Ethier P. Glucose: effects on tumor and normal in rodents mammary. Radiology. 1992;183:643–7.

15. Rabkin Z, Israel O, Keidar Z. Do hyperglycemia and diabetes affect the incidence of false-negative 18F-FDG PET/CT studies in patients evaluated for infection or inflammation and cancer? A comparative analysis. J Nucl Med. 2010;51:1015–20.

16. Hellmich B, Agueda A, Monti S, Buttgereit F, de Boysson H, Brouwer E, et al. 2018 update of the EULAR recommendations for the management of large vessel vasculitis. Ann Rheum Dis. 2020;79:19–130. https://doi.org/10.1136/annrheumdis-2019-215672.

17. Schmidt WA, Nielsen BD. Imaging in large-vessel vasculitis. Best Pract Res Clin Rheumatol. 2020;34:101589. https://doi.org/10.1016/j.berh.2020.101589.

18. Nielsen BD, Gormsen LC, Hansen IT, Keller KK, Therkildsen P, Hauge EM. Three days of high-dose glucocorticoid treatment attenuates large-vessel 18F-FDG uptake in large-vessel giant cell arteritis but with a limited impact on diagnostic accuracy. Eur J Nucl Med Mol Imaging. 2018;45:1119–28.

19. Stellingwerff MD, Brouwer E, Lensen KJDF, Rutgers A, Arends S, van der Geest KSM, et al. Different scoring methods of FDG PET/CT in giant cell arteritis need for standardization. Medicine (Baltimore). 2015;94:1–9.

20. Quinn KA, Rosenblum JS, Rimland CA, Gribbons KB, Ahlman MA, Grayson PC. Imaging acquisition technique influences interpretation of positron emission tomography vascular activity in large-vessel vasculitis. Semin Arthritis Rheum. 2020;50:71–6. https://doi.org/10.1016/j.semarthrit.2019.07.008.

21. Belhocine T, Blockmans D, Hustinx R, Vandevivere J, Mortelmans L. Imaging of large vessel vasculitis with 18FDG PET: illusion or reality? A critical review of the literature data. Eur J Nucl Med Mol Imaging. 2003;30(9):1305–13.

22. Brodmann M, Lipp RW, Passath A, Seinost G, Pabst E, Pilger E. The role of 2-18F-fluoro-2-deoxy-D-glucose positron emission tomography in the diagnosis of giant cell arteritis of the temporal arteries. Rheumatology. 2004;43:241–2.

23. Rimland CA, Quinn KA, Rosenblum JS, Schwartz MN, Bates Gribbons K, Novakovich E, et al. Outcome measures in large vessel vasculitis: relationship between patient-, physician-, imaging-, and laboratory-based assessments. Arthritis Care Res. 2020;72:1296–304. https://doi.org/10.1002/acr.24117.

24. van der Geest KSM, Sandovici M, Brouwer E, Mackie SL. Diagnostic accuracy of symptoms, physical signs, and laboratory tests for giant cell arteritis: a systematic review and meta-analysis. JAMA Intern Med. 2020;180:1295–304.

25. Walter MA, Melzer RA, Schindler C, Müller-Brand J, Tyndall A, Nitzsche EU. The value of [18F]FDG-PET in the diagnosis of large-vessel vasculitis and the assessment of activity and extent of disease. Eur J Nucl Med Mol Imaging. 2005;32:674–81. https://doi.org/10.1007/s00259-004-1757-9.

26. Duftner C, Dejaco C, Sepriano A, Falzon L, Schmidt WA, Ramiro S. Imaging in diagnosis, outcome prediction and monitoring of large vessel vasculitis: a systematic literature review and meta-analysis informing the EULAR recommendations. RMD Open. 2018;4:101589.

27. Grayson PC, Alehashemi S, Bagheri AA, Civelek AC, Cupps TR, Kaplan MJ, et al. 18F-Fluorodeoxyglucose–positron emission tomography as an imaging biomarker in a prospective, longitudinal cohort of patients with large vessel vasculitis. Arthritis Rheumatol. 2018;70:439–49. https://doi.org/10.1002/art.40379.

28. de Boysson H, Aide N, Liozon E, Lambert M, Parienti JJ, Monteil J, et al. Repetitive 18F-FDG-PET/CT in patients with large-vessel giant-cell arteritis and controlled disease. Eur J Intern Med. 2017;46:66–70.

29. Meller J, Strutz F, Siefker U, Scheel A, Sahlmann CO, Lehmann K, et al. Early diagnosis and follow-up of aortitis with [18F] FDG PET and MRI. Eur J Nucl Med Mol Imaging. 2003;30:730–6. https://doi.org/10.1007/s00259-003-1144-y.

30. Iwabu M, Yamamoto Y, Dobashi H, Kameda T, Kittaka K, Nishiyama Y. F^{-18} FDG PET findings of Takayasu arteritis before and after immunosuppressive therapy. Clin Nucl Med. 2008;33:872–3. https://journals.lww.com/00003072-200812000-00014.

31. Nienhuis PH, van Praagh GD, Glaudemans AWJM, Brouwer E, Slart RHJA. A review on the value of imaging in differentiating between large vessel vasculitis and atherosclerosis. J Pers Med. 2021;11:236. https://www.mdpi.com/2075-4426/11/3/236.

32. Laurent C, Ricard L, Fain O, Buvat I, Adedjouma A, Soussan M, et al. PET/MRI in large-vessel vasculitis: clinical value for diagnosis and assessment of disease activity. Sci Rep. 2019;9:1–7. https://www.nature.com/articles/s41598-019-48709-w.

33. Dellavedova L, Carletto M, Faggioli P, Sciascera A, del Sole A, Mazzone A, et al. The prognostic value of baseline 18F-FDG PET/CT in steroid-naïve large-vessel vasculitis: introduction of volume-based parameters. Eur J Nucl Med Mol Imaging. 2016;43:340–8. https://doi.org/10.1007/s00259-015-3148-9.

34. Jiemy WF, Heeringa P, Kamps JAAM, van der Laken CJ, Slart RHJA, Brouwer E. Positron emission tomography (PET) and single photon emission computed tomography (SPECT) imaging of macrophages in large vessel vasculitis: current status and future prospects. Autoimmun Rev. 2018;17:715–26.

35. Windisch P, Zwahlen DR, Giesel FL, Scholz E, Lugenbiel P, Debus J, et al. Clinical results of fibroblast activation protein (FAP) specific PET for non-malignant indications: systematic review. EJNMMI Res. 2021;11(1):18.

36. Hicks RJ, Roselt PJ, Kallur KG, Tothill RW, Mileshkin L. FAPI PET/CT: will it end the hegemony of 18F-FDG in oncology? J Nucl Med. 2021;62:296–302.

Pericardial Diseases

8

Matthieu Pelletier-Galarneau
and Patrick Martineau

Introduction

The pericardium is composed of two layers: the fibrous layer corresponding to the outer layer and the serous pericardium forming the inner layer, which is attached to the myocardium. It encases the heart and root of the great vessels while providing a physical barrier to external insults such as thoracic infections. In addition, the pericardium contains the pericardial fluid, which reduces friction between the two layers [1].

Pericardial diseases consist of a collection of several diverse pathologies. The symptoms are typically non-specific but can consist of chest pain and/or dyspnea. The severity of the presentation can depend on the underlying etiology and can range from an incidental finding of pericardial effusion in an otherwise asymptomatic patient to life-threatening tamponade. The 2015 European Society of Cardiology (ESC) guidelines for the diagnosis and management of pericardial diseases classify pericardial diseases etiology as infectious vs. non-infectious causes. Non-infectious causes are further divided into autoimmune, neoplastic, metabolic, traumatic, iatrogenic, and drug-related causes (Table 8.1).

Echocardiography should serve as the initial imaging test for the evaluation of suspected pericardial disease. When needed, computed tomography (CT) and cardiac magnetic resonance (CMR) may also be helpful. Fluorodeoxyglucose-positron emission tomography (FDG-PET) is generally reserved for challenging or atypical cases. Nonetheless, FDG-PET may be of value to differentiate between benign and malignant etiologies, as well as to identify extra-cardiac manifestations of systemic conditions that may be responsible for the pericardial disease (Table 8.2). In addition, Gerardin et al. reported that more intense FDG uptake in the pericardial fluid is associated with higher risk of relapse in idiopathic acute pericarditis, highlighting the prognostic value of FDG-PET [2]. FDG-PET, which has an established role in the imaging of both oncological and infectious/inflammatory diseases, and which usually provides whole-body imaging, is ideally suited for these purposes. In this chapter, we review the role and utility of FDG-PET in the assessment of pericardial diseases.

M. Pelletier-Galarneau (✉)
Montreal Heart Institute, Montréal, QC, Canada
e-mail: Matthieu.pelletier-galarneau@icm-mhi.org

P. Martineau
BC Cancer, Vancouver, BC, Canada
e-mail: patrick.martineau@bccancer.bc.ca

Table 8.1 Classification of pericardial diseases etiology

Infectious	Viral	**Most common etiology** *Coxsackievirus, echovirus, Epstein-Barr virus, cytomegalovirus, adenovirus, parvovirus B19, and human herpes virus 6*
	Bacterial	**More frequently in developing countries where tuberculosis is endemic** *Mycobacterium tuberculosis, Coxiella burnetii (Q-Fever), Pneumococcus species, Streptococcus species, Staphylococcus species*
	Fungal	**Rare and typically in immunocompromised patients** *Histoplasma species, Aspergillus, Candida*
	Parasitic	**Very rare** *Echinococcus species, Toxoplasma species*
Non-infectious	Autoimmune	**Connective tissue diseases** Systemic lupus erythematosus, rheumatoid arthritis, Sjögren's syndrome, scleroderma **Others** Sarcoidosis, vasculitis
	Neoplastic	**Primary (very rare)** Pericardial mesothelioma **Secondary (more frequent)** Lung, breast, lymphoma, esophageal, melanoma
	Metabolic	Uremia, myxoedema, anorexia
	Traumatic or iatrogenic	Penetrating thoracic injury, cardiac surgery, post-myocardial infarction, etc.
	Others	Drug-related, amyloidosis, aortic dissection, chronic heart failure

Table 8.2 Potential roles of FDG-PET imaging in the evaluation of patients with pericardial diseases

Potential roles of FDG-PET imaging
Evaluation of patients with probable autoimmune condition to exclude large vessel vasculitis or sarcoidosis
Evaluation of disease activity and extent in patients with suspected TB pericarditis
Evaluation of myocardial inflammation in patients with suspected myopericarditis
Diagnosis and staging of patients with suspected neoplastic pericardial disease
Assessment of relapse risk in idiopathic pericarditis
Assessment of therapy response

Infectious Pericardial Diseases

Pathogens causing infectious pericardial diseases vary based on population, as well as geographical and socio-economical factors. In developed countries, the most common form of pericardial disease is viral pericarditis, with the most frequent virus being coxsackievirus, echovirus, Epstein-Barr virus, cytomegalovirus, adenovirus, parvovirus B19, and human herpes virus 6 [3]. In developing countries where tuberculosis (TB) is endemic, TB is the most frequent causative agent [4]. Patients with tuberculous pericarditis can present with effusive pericarditis, constrictive pericarditis, tamponade, and myopericarditis. *Coxiella burnetii* (Q-fever) pericarditis has also been described, while other bacterial agents less frequently observed. Fungal and parasitic pericarditis is rarely seen [5].

In infectious pericarditis, FDG-PET findings will vary based on the causative agent involved

(Table 8.3). Viral and idiopathic pericarditis typically shows absent to mild, homogeneous pericardial uptake which may be accompanied by a

Table 8.3 Typical FDG distribution of various pericardial disease etiologies

		Uptake distribution	
		Homogeneous	Heterogeneous
Uptake intensity	Mild	Idiopathic Viral Autoimmune Fungal Parasitic Dressler	Fungal Parasitic Neoplastic Iatrogenic Traumatic
	Moderate to intense	Tuberculosis Bacterial	Neoplastic Tuberculosis Traumatic

pericardial effusion (Fig. 8.1) [6, 7]. In tuberculous pericarditis, intense FDG uptake has been described, with SUV values above 5 frequently observed (Fig. 8.2) [7, 8]. In addition, whole-body FDG-PET may allow to detect other areas of infection—this may be helpful in identifying an area more amenable to sampling and may influence differential considerations [9]. In Q-fever, FDG-PET may allow localization of persistent infection foci [10, 11]. In both idiopathic and tuberculous pericarditis, FDG-PET uptake has been shown to predict response to therapy, with responders having higher FDG uptake on the baseline study when compared to non-responders [12].

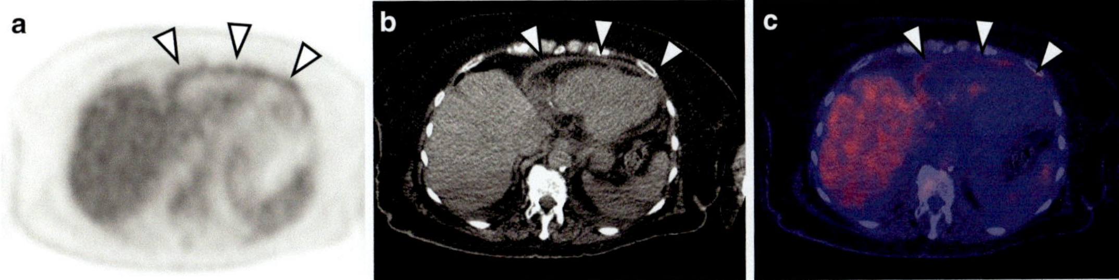

Fig. 8.1 An 89-year-old female referred for weight loss, lower gastrointestinal tract bleed, and pericardial effusion. Axial FDG-PET (**a**), CT (**b**), and fused PET/CT (**c**) images demonstrate mild diffuse pericardial uptake with a small pericardial effusion (arrowheads), attributed to idiopathic pericarditis

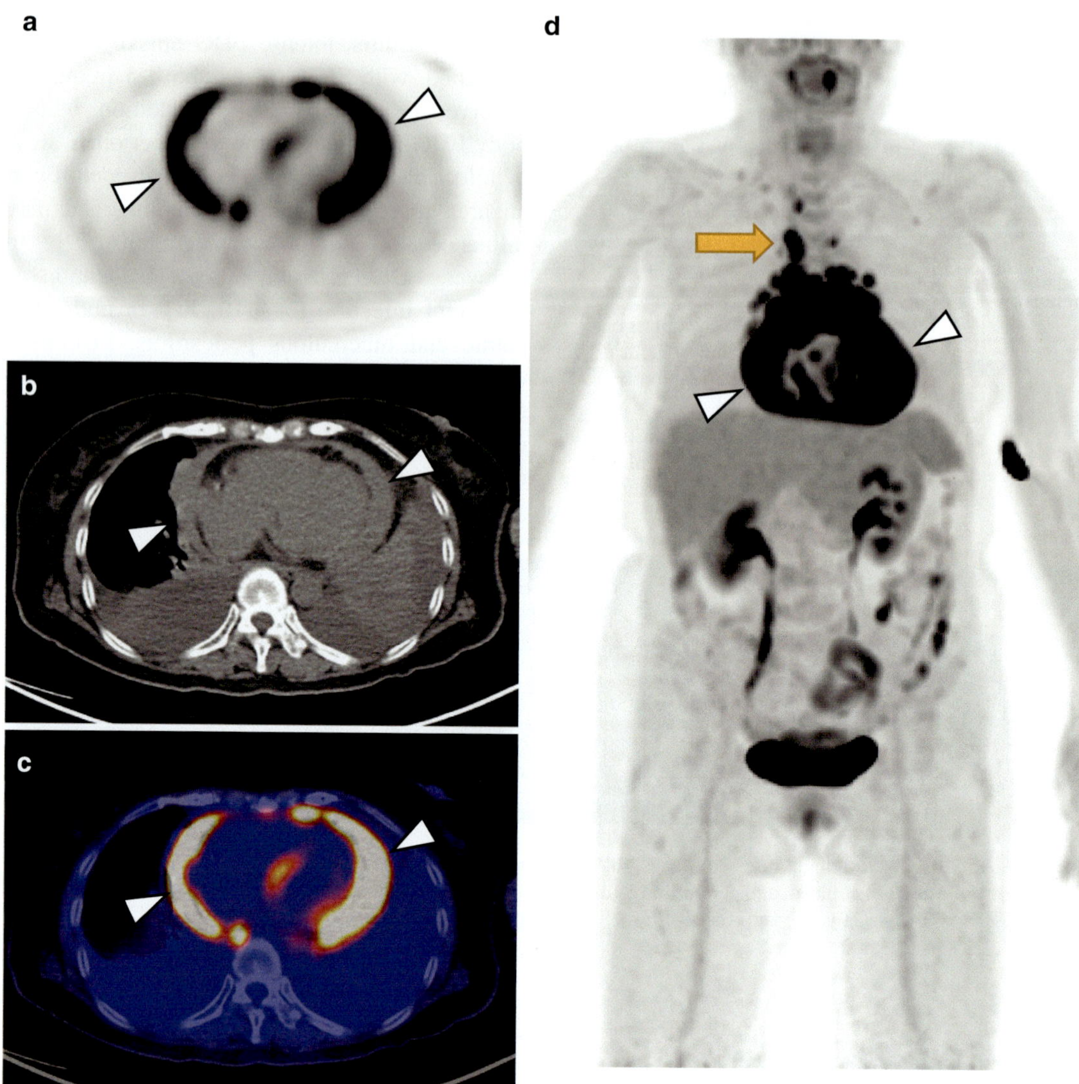

Fig. 8.2 Axial FDG-PET (**a**), CT (**b**), fused PET/CT (**c**), and whole-body MPI (**d**) images of a 73-year-old female referred with an effusive constrictive pericarditis of unknown origin. There is intense (SUV_{max} 14) and somewhat heterogeneous FDG uptake in the pericardial effusion (arrowheads) as well as intense uptake (SUV_{max} 11) in mediastinal lymph nodes (yellow arrow). This pattern of findings is highly suggestive of malignancy or tuberculous pericarditis. The final diagnosis of tuberculous pericarditis was later established on pericardial fluid culture and analysis

Autoimmune Pericardial Diseases

Pericardial diseases may be associated with autoimmune conditions including connective tissue diseases such as systemic lupus erythematosus (SLE), rheumatoid arthritis, and Sjögren's syndrome, as well as sarcoidosis and vasculitis. In these conditions, pericardial diseases typically present as acute or recurrent pericarditis [13]. Pericardial involvement may be caused by the

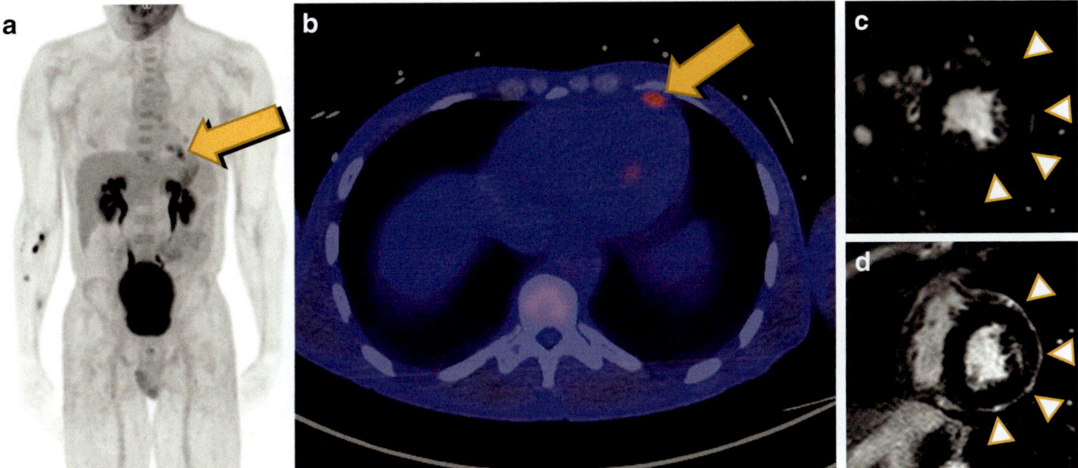

Fig. 8.3 A 53-year-old male referred with a history of Behcet's disease, mouth ulcers, and renal infarctions. Whole-body FDG-PET (**a**) and axial FDG-PET/CT (**b**) images demonstrate mild and focal increased uptake (arrow) in the pericardium. On cardiac magnetic reso- nance, cine short axis images without contrast (**c**) and viability sequences with contrast (**d**) demonstrate enhanc- ing pericardium (arrowheads), compatible with pericardi- tis. The focal uptake is an unusual presentation of pericarditis

systemic inflammatory disease itself or may be precipitated by increased susceptibility to other unrelated illnesses.

FDG-PET can play an important role in the evaluation of patients with suspected autoim- mune causes. In this setting, although PET can detect pericardial inflammation (Fig. 8.3), its strength resides in its ability to assess areas of inflammation on whole-body imaging, which may help reveal the underlying causative pathol ogy and potentially guide biopsy. For example, characteristic FDG-avid mediastinal lymph nodes and lung lesions can point to the diagnosis of sarcoidosis [14], while increased vascular FDG uptake can confirm the presence of large vessel vasculitis [15]. In addition, FDG-PET can readily localize inflammatory arthritis in patients with suspected rheumatoid disease, which is typi- cally symmetrical, FDG-avid, and present in multiple small and large joints and can some- times be accompanied by FDG-avid lymph nodes [16]. In SLE and Sjögren's syndrome, FDG-PET can highlight areas of active inflammation, including in the pericardium, joints, lymph nodes, salivary glands, and lungs [17–19].

Neoplastic Pericardial Diseases

Pericardial diseases associated with malignancy are secondary to metastatic disease in the vast majority of cases, including lung cancer, breast cancer, lymphoma, and melanoma. Primary peri- cardial tumors, most commonly pericardial mesothelioma, are infrequent. Pericardial meso- thelioma is very rare, with an incidence of 0.0022% and represents less than 3% of primary cardiac tumors (see Chap. 10) and may be associ- ated with asbestos exposure [20, 21]. Conversely, secondary pericardial involvement in malignancy is not rare, affecting 1–20% of patients with can- cer based on autopsy studies, but is often under- diagnosed [1, 22, 23]. Neoplastic pericardial diseases may present as acute pericarditis, peri- cardial effusion with or without tamponade, and constrictive pericarditis.

The role of FDG-PET is well established for the diagnosis, staging, and response assessment of neoplastic disease due to the increased FDG uptake seen in most malignancies. Therefore, in cases of suspected neoplastic pericardial disease, FDG-PET with whole-body imaging can be helpful to clarify the etiology of pericardial disease, identify and assess the extent of underlying malignancy, and guide biopsy (Fig. 8.4). Neoplastic pericardial lesions (i.e. metastases) often demonstrate intense and heterogeneous

FDG uptake with corresponding nodularity on CT [24, 25]. In cases of direct spread from an adjacent tumor (typically from a lung primary), an FDG-avid mass involving the pericardium is usually easily identified.

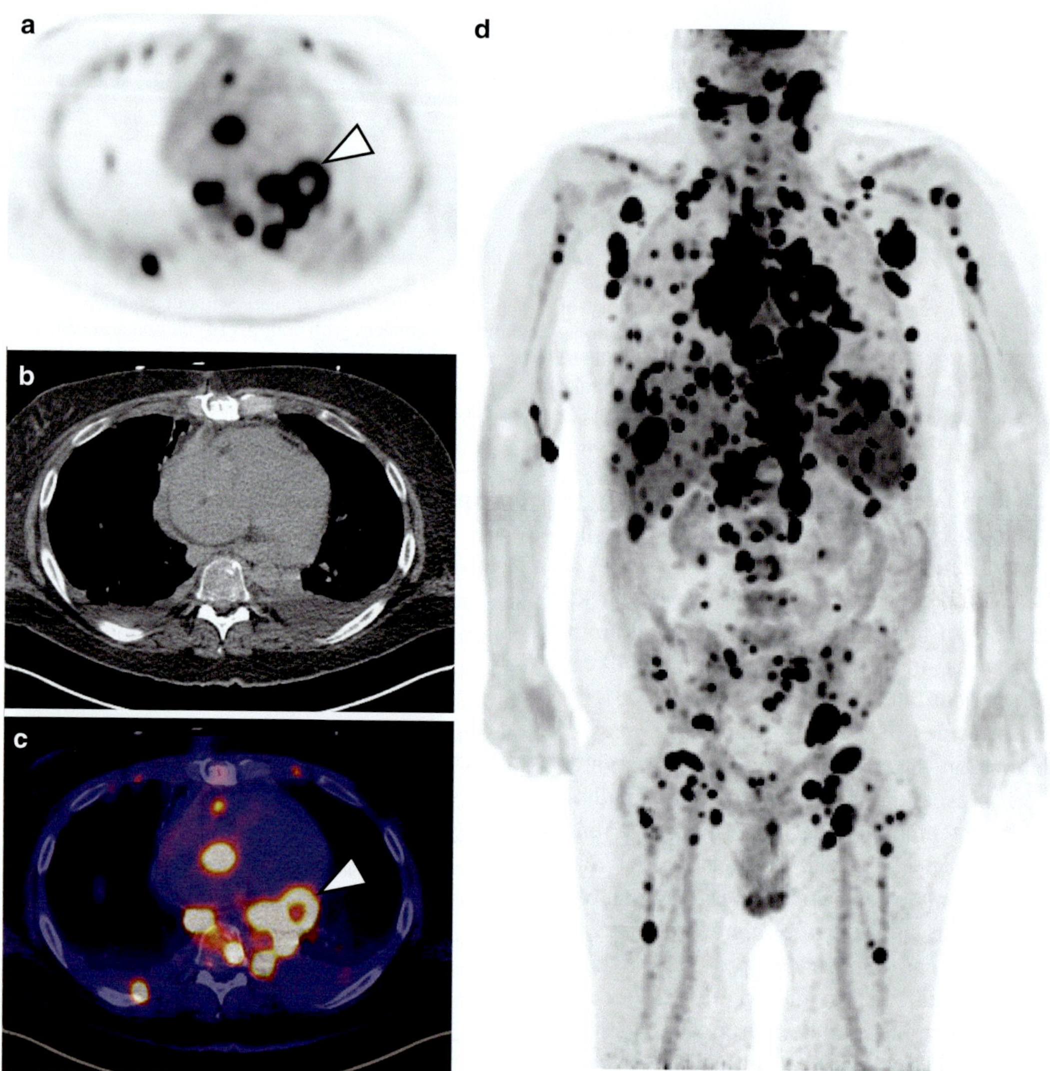

Fig. 8.4 A 43-year-old male with a history of heart transplant presented with sepsis and diarrhea. Axial FDG-PET (**a**), CT (**b**), fused PET/CT (**c**), and whole-body MPI (**d**) demonstrate innumerable foci of intense FDG uptake projecting in lymph nodes as well as within the myocardium, the pericardium (arrowhead), spleen, liver, and bones, compatible with a lymphoproliferative process. The final diagnosis of post-transplant lymphoproliferative disorder (PTLD) was established on biopsy

Other Non-Infectious Pericardial Diseases

Post-cardiac injury syndrome, also called Dressler's syndrome, occurs in the presence of myocardial or pericardial injury, which can be seen following cardiac surgery, myocardial infarction, penetrating injury, pacemaker insertion, etc. It usually occurs within 1–6 weeks following injury [26]. Post-myocardial infarction syndrome became rare following the advent of reperfusion treatments [27]. Nonetheless, in the weeks following a myocardial infarction, especially for patients who did not undergo revascularization or for those with delayed revascularization, symptoms including fever, generalized weakness, and pleuritic chest pain should raise the suspicion of post-myocardial infarction syndrome. On FDG-PET, post-myocardial infarction syndrome is indistinguishable from idiopathic and viral pericarditis and demonstrates mild to moderate, diffusely increased pericardial uptake (Fig. 8.5).

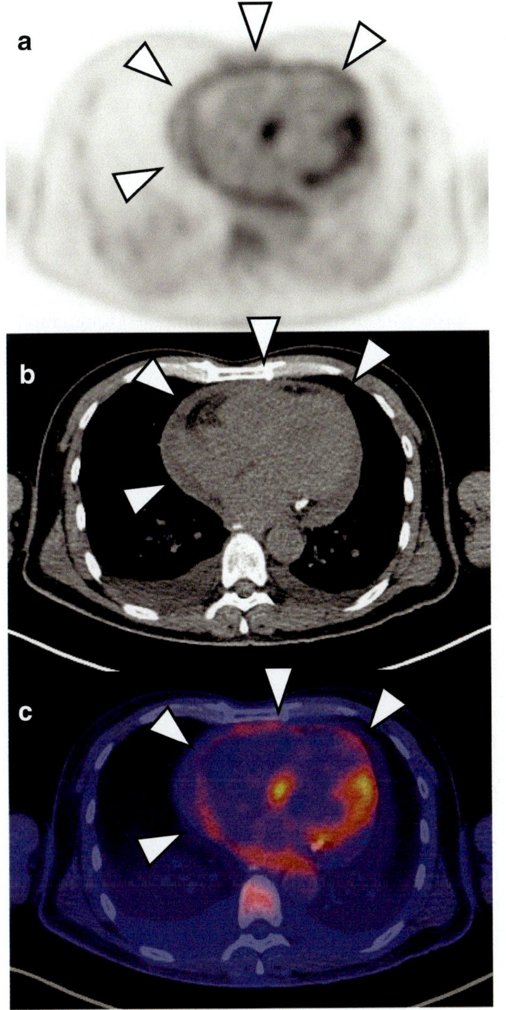

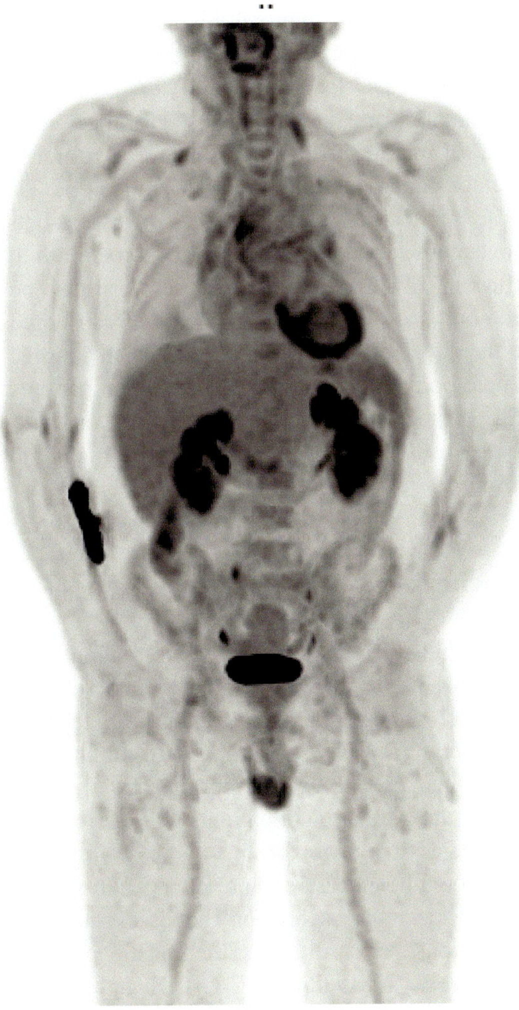

Fig. 8.5 A 57-year-old female referred for fever of unknown origin. The patient had a ST-segment elevation myocardial infarction (STEMI) 2 weeks prior to the study. Axial FDG-PET (**a**), CT (**b**), fused PET/CT (**c**), and whole-body MPI (**d**) images demonstrate mild and diffuse increased uptake within a pericardial effusion, compatible with post-myocardial infarction syndrome (Dressler syndrome)

Post-pericardiotomy syndrome occurs in the weeks following cardiac surgery, with an incidence between 2% and 30% [28]. FDG-PET may reveal diffusely increased pericardial uptake with an associated effusion [29]. Importantly, it may be difficult to differentiate post-operative changes from pericarditis in this context. The distribution of FDG uptake may help distinguish between post-operative changes and post-pericardiotomy syndrome, with the former being more focal and anterior and the latter more diffuse and circumferential.

An unusual cause of non-infectious pericardial disease is IgG4-related disease, which is a rare, multisystemic, immune-mediated, fibro-inflammatory disease often mimicking malignancy [30]. FDG-PET can identify areas of active inflammation and therefore be used for the assessment of organ involvement, therapy response monitoring, and guiding intervention [31]. IgG4-related pericarditis may appear as diffuse or heterogeneous uptake projecting in a pericardial effusion [32]. Coronary involvement can also be seen on occasion, with more focal activity noted at the level of the affected epicardial vessels. Whole-body imaging can be useful in patients with suspected IgG4-related disease in order to assess disease extent as additional, non-cardiac sites of fibrosis and inflammation can be present.

Conclusion

Pericardial diseases are relatively frequent and clarifying the etiology is of paramount importance in order to administer the appropriate therapy and identify potential life-threatening conditions. FDG-PET is emerging as a useful tool for the evaluation of patients with pericardial disease, as it allows for the identification and assessment of disease extent. It has been shown to be especially useful for the assessment of tuberculous pericarditis and neoplastic pericardial lesions. In addition, FDG-PET has shown potential in predicting the response to therapy. Further studies are required to assess the role of FDG-PET, particularly for non-infectious and non-oncological pericardial diseases.

References

1. Adler Y, Charron P, Imazio M, Badano L, Barón-Esquivias G, Bogaert J, et al. 2015 ESC guidelines for the diagnosis and management of pericardial diseases. Eur Heart J. 2015;36(42):2921–64.
2. Gerardin C, Mageau A, Benali K, Jouan F, Ducrocq G, Alexandra J-F, et al. Increased FDG-PET/CT pericardial uptake identifies acute pericarditis patients at high risk for relapse. Int J Cardiol. 2018;271:192–4.
3. Imazio M. Contemporary management of pericardial diseases. Curr Opin Cardiol. 2012;27(3):308–17.
4. Noubiap JJ, Agbor VN, Ndoadoumgue AL, Nkeck JR, Kamguia A, Nyaga UF, et al. Epidemiology of pericardial diseases in Africa: a systematic scoping review. Heart. 2019;105(3):180–8.
5. Melenotte C, Protopopescu C, Million M, Edouard S, Carrieri MP, Eldin C, et al. Clinical features and complications of Coxiella burnetii infections from the French National Reference Center for Q fever. JAMA Netw Open. 2018;1(4):e181580.
6. James OG, Christensen JD, Wong TZ, Borges-Neto S, Koweek LM. Utility of FDG PET/CT in inflammatory cardiovascular disease. Radiogr Rev Publ Radiographics. 2011;31(5):1271–86.
7. Hyeon CW, Yi HK, Kim EK, Park S-J, Lee S-C, Park SW, et al. The role of 18F-fluorodeoxyglucose-positron emission tomography/computed tomography in the differential diagnosis of pericardial disease. Sci Rep. 2020;10(1):21524.
8. Martineau P, Grégoire J, Harel F, Pelletier-Galarneau M. Assessing cardiovascular infection and inflammation with FDG-PET. Am J Nucl Med Mol Imaging. 2021;11(1):46–58.
9. Pelletier-Galarneau M, Martineau P, Zuckier LS, Pham X, Lambert R, Turpin S. 18F-FDG-PET/CT imaging of thoracic and extrathoracic tuberculosis in children. Semin Nucl Med. 2017;47(3):304–18.
10. Eldin C, Melenotte C, Million M, Cammilleri S, Sotto A, Elsendoorn A, et al. 18F-FDG PET/CT as a central tool in the shift from chronic Q fever to Coxiella burnetii persistent focalized infection. Medicine (Baltimore). 2016;95(34):e4287.
11. Barten DG, Delsing CE, Keijmel SP, Sprong T, Timmermans J, Oyen WJ, et al. Localizing chronic Q fever: a challenging query. BMC Infect Dis. 2013;13(1):413.
12. Chang S-A, Choi JY, Kim EK, Hyun SH, Jang SY, Choi J-O, et al. [18F] Fluorodeoxyglucose PET/CT predicts response to steroid therapy in constrictive pericarditis. J Am Coll Cardiol. 2017;69(6):750–2.
13. Knockaert DC. Cardiac involvement in systemic inflammatory diseases. Eur Heart J. 2007;28(15):1797–804.
14. Martineau P, Pelletier-Galarneau M, Juneau D, Leung E, Birnie D, Beanlands RSB. Molecular imaging of cardiac sarcoidosis. Curr Cardiovasc Imaging Rep. 2018;11(3):6–17.

15. Pelletier-Galarneau M, Ruddy TD. PET/CT for diagnosis and management of large-vessel vasculitis. Curr Cardiol Rep. 2019;21(5):34.
16. Hotta M, Minamimoto R, Kaneko H, Yamashita H. Fluorodeoxyglucose PET/CT of arthritis in rheumatic diseases: a pictorial review. Radiographics. 2020;40(1):223–40.
17. Curiel R, Akin EA, Beaulieu G, DePalma L, Hashefi M. PET/CT imaging in systemic lupus erythematosus. Ann N Y Acad Sci. 2011;1228:71–80.
18. Cohen C, Mekinian A, Uzunhan Y, Fauchais A-L, Dhote R, Pop G, et al. 18F-fluorodeoxyglucose positron emission tomography/computer tomography as an objective tool for assessing disease activity in sjögren's syndrome. Autoimmun Rev. 2013;12(11):1109–14.
19. Sharma P, Chatterjee P. 18F-FDG PET/CT in multisystem sjögren syndrome. Clin Nucl Med. 2015;40(5):e293–4.
20. Godar M, Liu J, Zhang P, Xia Y, Yuan Q. Primary pericardial mesothelioma: a rare entity. Case Rep Oncol Med. 2013;2013:283601.
21. Gössinger HD, Siostrzonek P, Zangeneh M, Neuhold A, Herold C, Schmoliner R, et al. Magnetic resonance imaging findings in a patient with pericardial mesothelioma. Am Heart J. 1988;115(6):1321–2.
22. Klatt EC, Heitz DR. Cardiac metastases. Cancer. 1990;65(6):1456–9.
23. Maisch B, Ristic A, Pankuweit S. Evaluation and management of pericardial effusion in patients with neoplastic disease. Prog Cardiovasc Dis. 2010;53(2):157–63.
24. Yi J-E, Yoon HJ, JH O, Youn H-J. Cardiac and pericardial 18F-FDG uptake on oncologic PET/CT: comparison with echocardiographic findings. J Cardiovasc Imaging. 2018;26(2):93–102.
25. Martineau P, Dilsizian V, Pelletier-Galarneau M. Incremental value of FDG-PET in the evaluation of cardiac masses. Curr Cardiol Rep. 2021;23(7):78.
26. Leib AD, Foris LA, Nguyen T, Khaddour K. Dressler Syndrome. In: Stat pearls [internet]. Treasure Island, FL: Stat Pearls; 2021. http://www.ncbi.nlm.nih.gov/books/NBK441988/.
27. Shahar A, Hod H, Barabash GM, Kaplinsky E, Motro M. Disappearance of a syndrome: Dressler's syndrome in the era of thrombolysis. Cardiology. 1994;85(3–4):255–8.
28. Gabaldo K, Sutlić Ž, Mišković D, Knežević Praveček M, Prvulović Đ, Vujeva B, et al. Postpericardiotomy syndrome incidence, diagnostic and treatment strategies: experience AT two collaborative centers. Acta Clin Croat. 2019;58(1):57–62.
29. Salomäki SP, Hohenthal U, Kemppainen J, Pirilä L, Saraste A. Visualization of pericarditis by fluorodeoxyglucose PET. Eur Heart J Cardiovasc Imaging. 2014;15(3):291.
30. Stone JH, Zen Y, Deshpande V. IgG4-related disease. N Engl J Med. 2012;366(6):539–51.
31. Zhang J, Chen H, Ma Y, Xiao Y, Niu N, Lin W, et al. Characterizing IgG4-related disease with 18F-FDG PET/CT: a prospective cohort study. Eur J Nucl Med Mol Imaging. 2014;41(8):1624–34.
32. Matsumiya R, Hosono O, Yoshikawa N, Uehara M, Kobayashi H, Oda A, et al. Elevated serum IgG4 complicated by pericardial involvement with a patchy (18) F-FDG uptake in PET/CT: atypical presentation of IgG4-related disease. Intern Med. 2015;54(18):2337–41.

Daniele Muser, Abass Alavi,
and Pasquale Santangeli

Introduction

Ventricular arrhythmias (VA) include a wide spectrum of clinical entities ranging from idiopathic premature ventricular contractions (PVC) to malignant sustained ventricular tachycardia (VT) or ventricular fibrillation (VF). The mechanisms behind VA are heterogeneous and include triggered activity or exacerbated automaticity in the absence of structural heart disease as well as reentry mechanisms related to the presence of myocardial scar associated with structural heart diseases (SHD) such as ischemic heart disease and non-ischemic cardiomyopathies. Myocardial inflammation may also play a role in the genesis and maintenance of VT in several conditions such as myocarditis, cardiac sarcoidosis (CS), and Chagas cardiomyopathy either by determining cell loss and reparative fibrosis able to sustain reentrant arrhythmias as well as triggered activity and exacerbated automaticity within inflamed areas [1–3]. Recently, a potential role of subclinical myocardial inflammation in patients present-

ing with VA of unexplained origin has been also reported [4]. Cardiac ^{18}F-fluorodeoxyglucose (^{18}F-FDG) positron emission tomography (PET) is the gold standard for evaluation of myocardial inflammation and may be used to improve arrhythmic substrate characterization, risk stratification and identification potential therapeutic targets in patients presenting with VA [5]. In the present chapter, we present the principles and main clinical applications of ^{18}F-FDG PET imaging in the setting of VA.

Mechanistic Bases

Myocardial inflammation contributes to the genesis of VA in several ways [1]. First of all, active inflammation is responsible for direct cell injury leading to myocyte death and consequent replacement fibrosis. The presence of surviving myocardial fibers within fibrous tissue leads to the formation of slow conduction pathways, dispersion of activation and refractoriness which all together create the pathophysiologic basis for reentrant circuits (Fig. 9.1) [6]. Systemic inflammatory response may also promote myocardial electrical instability through cytokine release, electrical remodeling, and sympathetic hyperactivity [7]. Finally, myocardial ischemia as a result of microvascular dysfunction and demand/supply imbalance within the inflamed myocardium can further increase arrhythmogenicity [8].

D. Muser · P. Santangeli (✉)
Cardiac Electrophysiology, Cardiovascular Medicine Division, Hospital of the University of Pennsylvania, Philadelphia, PA, USA
e-mail: pasquale.santangeli@uphs.upenn.edu

A. Alavi
Nuclear Medicine Division, Radiology Department, Hospital of the University of Pennsylvania, Philadelphia, PA, USA

© The Author(s), under exclusive license to Springer Nature Switzerland AG 2022
M. Pelletier-Galarneau, P. Martineau (eds.), *FDG-PET/CT and PET/MR in Cardiovascular Diseases*, https://doi.org/10.1007/978-3-031-09807-9_9

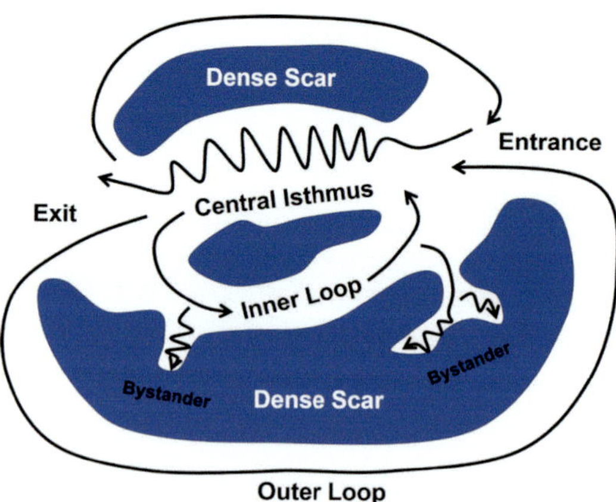

Fig. 9.1 Schematic representation of a reentry circuit as originally described by Stevenson et al. in 1993. In this model, two activation wavefronts propagate around two lines of conduction block sharing a common pathway (central isthmus). Areas of dense scar (blue) cannot be excitable during tachycardia. Bystander pathways can be attached to any point in the circuit and represent areas of tissue activated by the wavefront but not playing an active role in the reentrant circuit

General Principles of ^{18}F-FDG PET/CT Imaging in the Setting of Ventricular Arrhythmias

The possibility to identify myocardial inflammation by the use of ^{18}F-FDG PET relies on the preferential accumulation of ^{18}F-FDG in areas of active inflammation compared to healthy myocardium, thanks to the higher metabolic activity (glucose demand) of inflammatory cells. Considering that in normal circumstances, cardiac metabolism may rely on glucose consumption, physiologic myocardial glucose uptake may represent a major source of false positive results making its suppression of pivotal importance to identify areas of true pathologic involvement [9].

Several strategies have been proposed to achieve adequate suppression of physiologic ^{18}F-FDG uptake including prolonged fasting ($\geq$18 h) preceded by a low-carbohydrate/high-fat content diet to shift cardiac metabolism from a glucose to a free fatty acid one and administration of unfractionated heparin (intravenous bolus of 50 IU/kg 15 min prior to ^{18}F-FDG injection) in order to increase circulating free fatty acid levels [10, 11].

Regrettably, a high variability in myocardial ^{18}F-FDG uptake is still observed even after all the aforementioned precautions, leading to a rate of false positive results of up to 30% [10]. In order to optimize scan reliability, specific criteria have been developed for image interpretation. In particular, diffuse ^{18}F-FDG uptake should always be looked at very suspiciously as a possible result of inadequate suppression, while focal or focal on diffuse uptake patterns are generally regarded as more significant [11]. To further complicate the interpretation of ^{18}F-FDG/PET results, selective uptake of ^{18}F-FDG in the inferolateral wall, even in the presence of a complete suppression of the remaining myocardium, has been reported as a normal physiologic pattern [12, 13]. In this regard, the comparison between ^{18}F-FDG/PET finding and other imaging modalities such CMR with T2-weighted imaging to detect myocardial inflammation and late gadolinium enhancement to detect necrosis/fibrosis may improve its specificity [14]. Other possible sources of false results are represented by misalignment issues due to patient movement or abnormal ^{18}F-FDG uptake surrounding pacemaker (PM) or implantable cardioverter defibrillator (ICD) leads [15, 16]. Recently, the development of new radiotracers which do not physiologically accumulate within healthy myocardium such as Gallium-68 (^{68}Ga) DOTATATE may potentially overcome ^{18}F-FDG limitations. ^{68}Ga-DOTATATE targets somatostatin receptors on activated macrophages which are absent on normal myocardial cells making ^{68}Ga-DOTATATE a selective marker of myocardial inflammation [17].

Cardiac Sarcoidosis

Sarcoidosis is a systemic inflammatory disease characterized by lymphocyte CD4+ mediated formation of non-necrotizing granulomas [18]. Overt cardiac involvement is relatively rare being found in about 5–10% of the patients [19]. Cardiac sarcoidosis is characterized by patchy areas of myocardial inflammation and fibrosis which, depending on the location and severity, may be clinically silent or lead to atrio-ventricular conduction block, supra-ventricular arrhythmias, VA, and progressive heart failure [18]. In the pathophysiologic process of CS there is always a coexistence of lesions at different stages of the disease with areas of active inflammation overlapping areas of dense, metabolically inactive scar (Fig. 9.2) [20, 21]. In patients with CS presenting with recurrent VT, characterization of the arrhythmogenic substrate helps the detection of potential targets for substrate-based ablation but also provides important diagnostic elements and

information to identify patients at high risk of recurrence after catheter ablation (CA) that may benefit from more aggressive medical therapy with immunosuppressive drugs [22]. Interestingly, areas of unipolar voltage abnormality on invasive electroanatomic voltage mapping have been correlated with the presence of active inflammation in areas without a significant amount of scar representing optimal targets for endomyocardial biopsy (EMB), thus improving its sensitivity and specificity which is typically limited by the

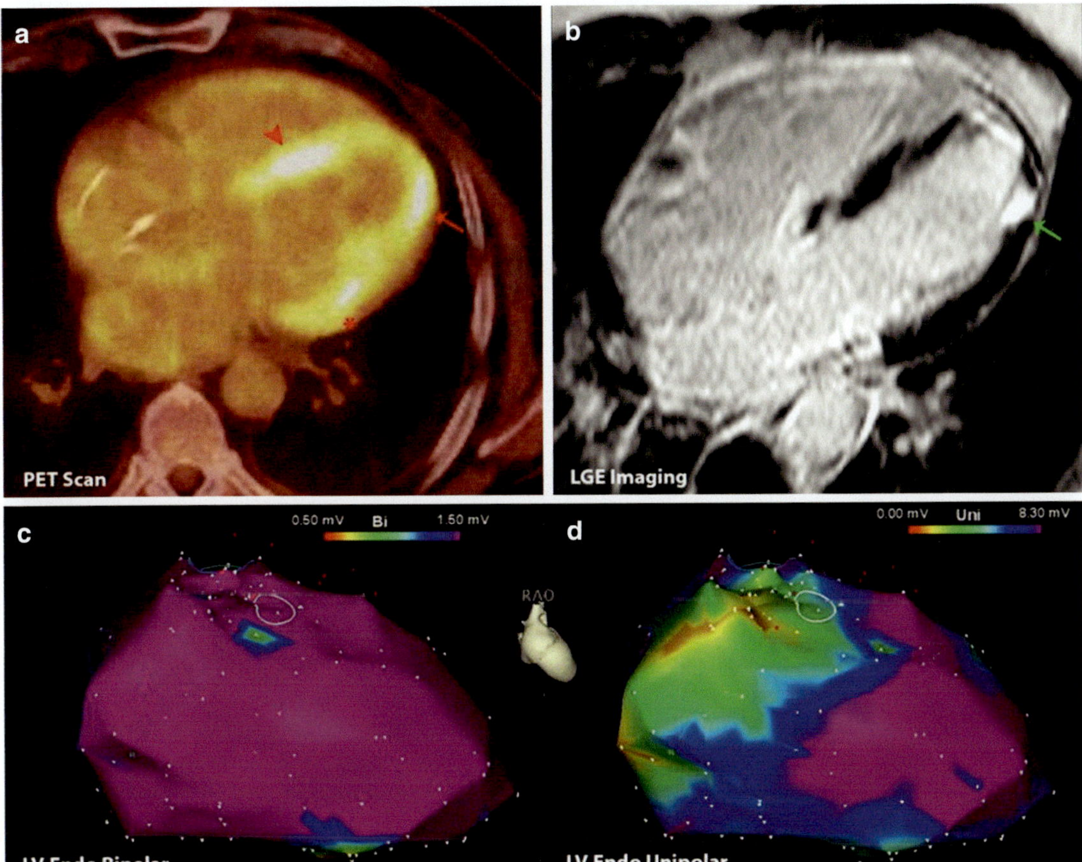

Fig. 9.2 Imaging and electroanatomic findings of a patients with cardiac sarcoidosis and recurrent ventricular tachycardia. Positron emission tomographic (PET) scan (**a–e**) showing active inflammation of the mid-basal inferoseptum (**a**, red arrowhead), basal (**a**, asterix) and apical (**a**, red arrow) anterolateral wall, basal inferior (**e**, red arrow), and anterior (**e**, red arrowhead) walls. Contrast-enhanced magnetic resonance imaging (**b–f**) of the same patient showing diffuse myocardial scar involving the distal anterolateral wall (**b**, green arrow), the anterior wall (**f**, green arrows), and the inferior wall (**f**, green arrowheads). The septum and the basal anterolateral wall do not show scar although they are involved by active inflammation. Left ventricular (LV) endocardial electroanatomic map (EAM; (**c**), (**d**), (**g**), and (**h**)) showing a small area of low bipolar voltage (≤1.5 mV) on the midapical inferior wall (**g**, inferior view) and a more diffuse area of low unipolar voltage (≤8.3) on the basal septum (**d**, right anterior oblique [RAO] view) and inferior wall (**h**, inferior view); unipolar EAM showed areas of abnormal voltage consistent with both scar and inflammation. (Reprinted with permission from Muser et al. [22])

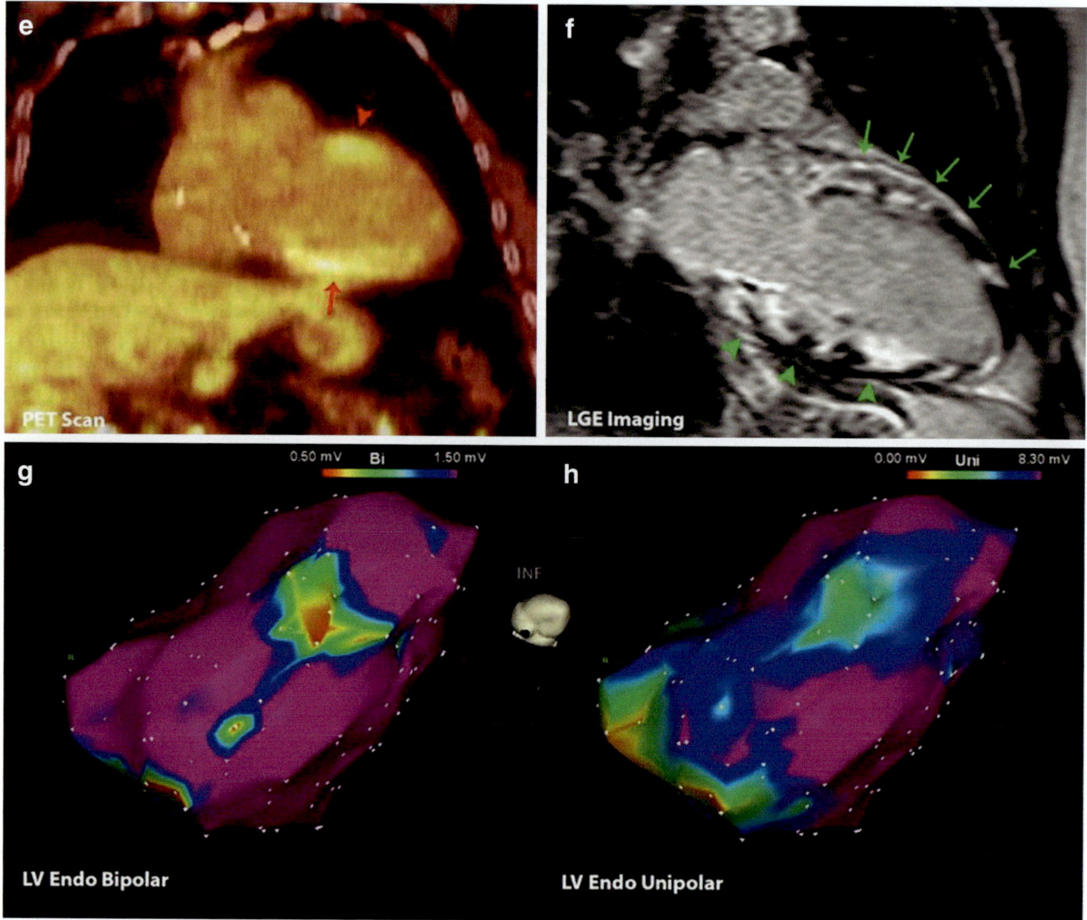

Fig. 9.2 (continued)

patchy distribution of the disease and the presence of areas with dense scar (nonspecific finding on histology) (Fig. 9.3) [5]. The available evidence strongly supports the critical role of scar compared to active inflammation in sustaining VA. In a study including 50 patients with CS, 14% developed VA during follow-up: none among those with LGE-/FDG+, 19% among those with LGE+/FDG+, and 21% among those with LGE+/FDG- [23]. In a series of 42 patients with CS and VT referred for CA who underwent preprocedural ^{18}F-FDG PET and CMR, evidence of active inflammation was found in 48% of the cases, while areas of LGE were almost ubiquitous (90% of the cases) [5]. Interestingly, after quantification of myocardial inflammatory activity in terms of metabolic volume (MV—volume

of the ^{18}F-FDG-avid myocardium) and metabolic activity (MA—product between SUV and MV), myocardial areas showing the presence of abnormal electrograms (representing potential targets for CA) had a higher degree of scar transmurality on CMR and a lower MV and MA compared to those without evidence of abnormal electrograms (Fig. 9.3). Moreover, critical sites for VA determined by electrophysiological mapping appeared more strongly associated with LGE on CMR than with increased ^{18}F-FDG uptake on PET (abnormal electrograms present in 70% of LGE+/PET− myocardial segments vs. 27% of LGE− /PET+ segments) [5]. All the aforementioned data suggest that reentrant VT circuits are strongly associated with presence of scar even in patients with active disease and are located in areas with more

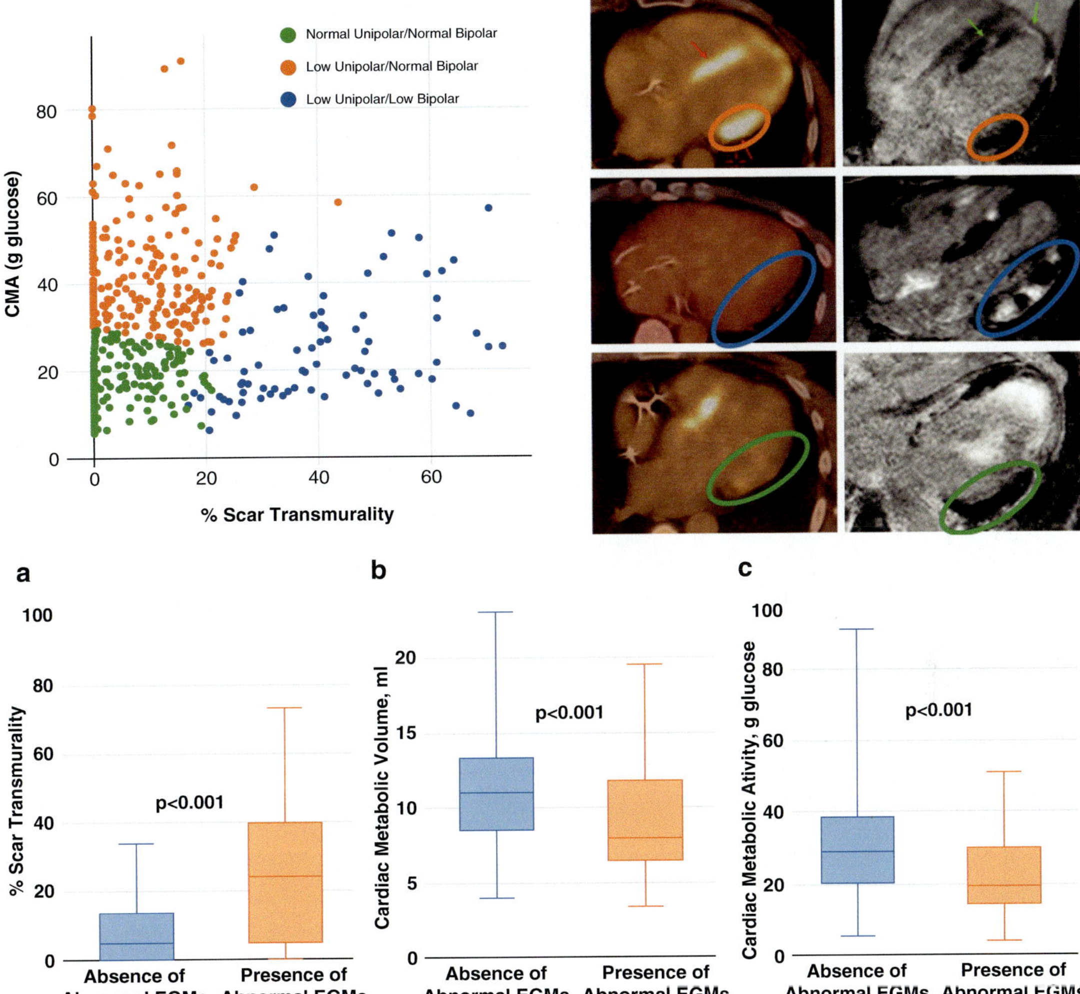

Fig. 9.3 Correlation among presence of scar, inflammation, and electroanatomic findings in patients with cardiac sarcoidosis undergoing ventricular tachycardia ablation Top Panel: Scatter plot representing the distribution of myocardial segments according to imaging and electroanatomic findings. Segments with both normal unipolar and bipolar voltage (green dots) represent the "healthy myocardium" without either scar or inflammation. Segments with low unipolar voltage but normal bipolar voltage (orange dots) represent sites of "active disease" with absence/few scar and presence of active inflammation in which no or only few abnormal electrograms are recorded. Those sites represent potential good targets for endomyocardial biopsy. Segments with both low unipolar and bipolar voltage (blue dots) represent sites of "advanced disease" with high scar transmurality and no/few inflammatory activity. In such sites, abnormal electrograms are frequently recorded representing potential good targets for substrate modification. Bottom Panel: Boxplots demonstrating the higher degree of scar transmurality on CMR (**a**) and the lower degree of inflammation quantified by cardiac metabolic volume (**b**) and cardiac metabolic activity (**c**) within myocardial segments showing the presence of abnormal electrograms (critical sites of VT circuits) compared to those without. (Modified with permission from Muser et al. [5])

extensive fibrous replacement and less inflammation stressing the central role of fibrosis in the genesis of VA. Inflammation still plays an important causative role in VA as the primary source of myocardial damage, cell loss, and fibrotic replacement. To that end, in patients undergoing repeated CA after a first attempt, a significant scar progression has been found only in those with persistent inflammatory activity detected by FDG-PET (Fig. 9.4) [5]. Correspondingly, lack

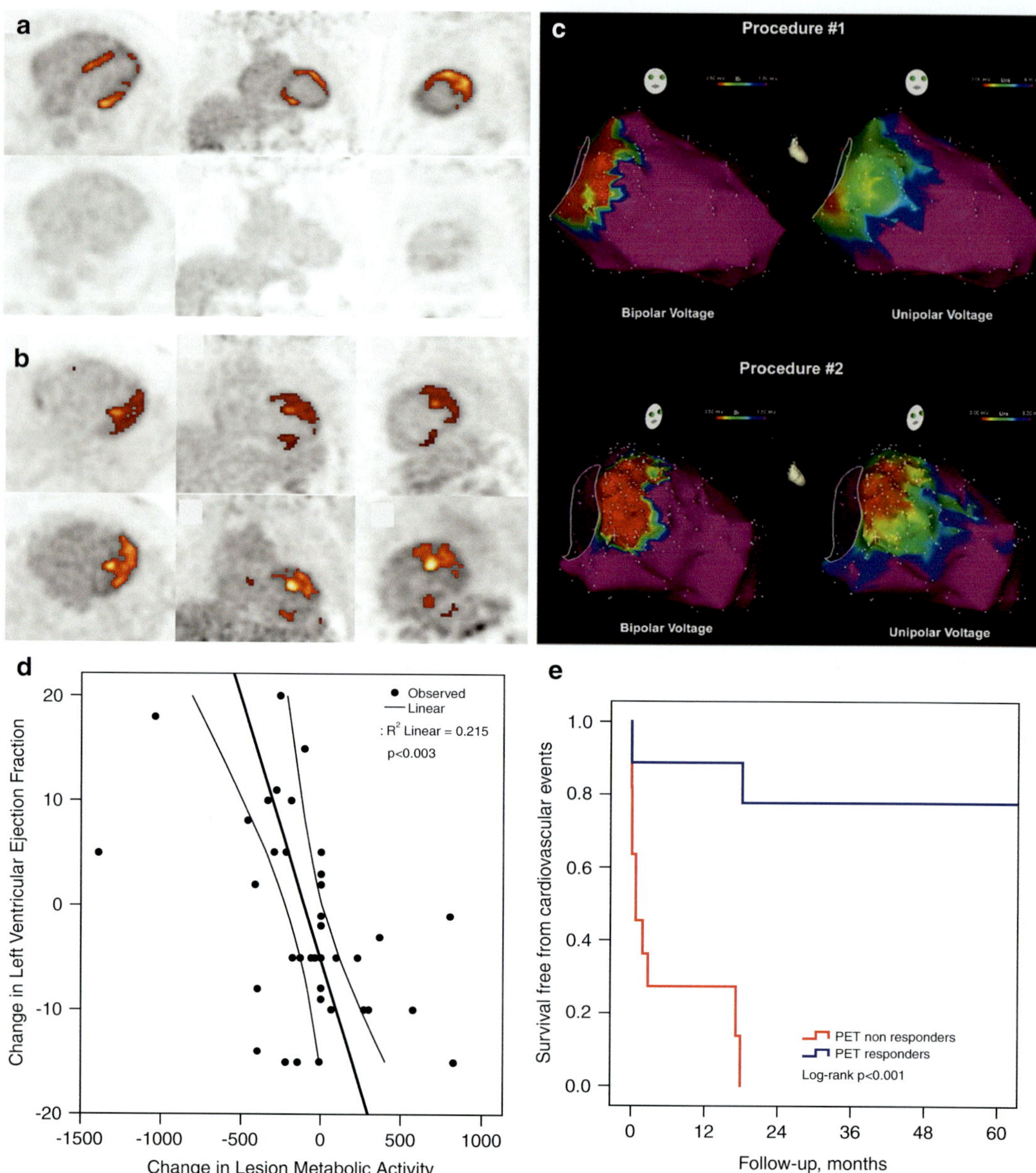

Fig. 9.4 Correlation between [18]FDG-PET evaluation of treatment response, scar progression, and long-term outcomes in patients with cardiac sarcoidosis. (**a**) PET scan in a patient with cardiac sarcoidosis (CS) involving the mid-basal septum, mid-basal anterior, and basal inferior wall of the left ventricle (top row) that demonstrate complete normalization after 6 months of immunosuppressive therapy (bottom row). (**b**) Patient with CS involving the lateral and anterior wall of the left ventricle as well as the anterolateral papillary muscle at baseline (top row) and persistent inflammation despite immunosuppressive treatment (bottom raw). (**c**) Endocardial voltage maps of a patient with persistent myocardial inflammation on FDG-PET and evidence of scar progression between two consecutive ventricular tachycardia ablation procedures performed within 3 months. (**d**) Correlation between changes in lesion metabolic activity and changes in left ventricular ejection fraction in patients undergoing immunosuppressive treatment. (**e**) Kaplan–Meier survival curve showing survival free from cardiovascular events according to metabolic response in patients with CS. (Modified with permission from Muser et al. [5, 24])

of PET improvement after initiation of immuno-suppressive treatment has been associated with worse clinical outcomes at follow-up with a significant inverse relationship between changes in MA and changes in left ventricular ejection fraction (Fig. 9.4) [24, 25]. The presence of abnormal ^{18}F-FDG uptake has also been correlated to long-term risk of recurrence after CA of VT with a fourfold increase risk for those patients with abnormal ^{18}F-FDG uptake at baseline and an adjunctive twofold increase risk for those nonresponders to immunosuppressive therapy [22].

Ventricular Arrhythmias of Unknown Etiology

Subclinical myocardial inflammation may be responsible for VA of otherwise unknown etiology. In a series of 103 patients with non-ischemic heart disease of unknown etiology and VA, evidence of abnormal myocardial ^{18}F-FDG uptake was found in 49% of the cases with signs of extracardiac involvement in 34% of them [4]. Only patients presenting focal or focal on diffuse patterns of myocardial ^{18}F-FDG uptake were considered as PET positive. Among patients who underwent EMB, CS was found in 60% of the cases, non-granulomatous inflammation in 30%, while absence of inflammatory infiltrates was found in the remaining 10%. Among patients treated with CA, a correlation between ^{18}F-FDG PET findings and voltage abnormalities was reported in 79% of the cases. Immunosuppressive treatment was started in 90% of patients with positive ^{18}F-FDG PET showing a trend toward better clinical outcomes. As such these patients may benefit from early detection of underlying inflammation (before irreversible myocardial scarring occurs) and from immunosuppressive medical therapy [4]. Those findings have recently been confirmed by a single center prospective study (Myocarditis And Ventricular Arrhythmia registry—MAVERIC) in which ^{18}F-FDG PET was performed in a series of 107 patients with

frequent (≥5000/24 h) PVC of unexplained etiology [26]. As previously reported, only focal or focal on diffuse myocardial ^{18}F-FDG uptake patterns were considered significant. Patients with positive ^{18}F-FDG PET were treated with immunosuppressive therapy (oral prednisone 40 mg daily tapered 10 mg every 3 weeks for a total of 3 months). In patients who either had a suboptimal or no response at 3 months, a second line immunosuppressive treatment with azathioprine, cyclosporine, mycophenolate, methotrexate, or monoclonal antibodies was considered. ^{18}F-FDG PET scans were repeated every 3 months in order to monitor treatment response and modify therapy accordingly. At baseline 51% of the patients had evidence of abnormal myocardial ^{18}F-FDG uptake and EMB was performed in half of them demonstrating lymphocytic infiltrate in 46% of the cases, CS in 7%, only mild to moderate interstitial fibrosis in 25%, and no pathologic findings in the remaining 25%. Even if EMB did not show the presence of non-caseating granulomas, a diagnosis of CS was made in 24% of the ^{18}F-FDG PET positive patients based upon extracardiac findings, while the remaining 74% of such cases were labeled as idiopathic myocardial inflammation. A total of 46 patients received immunosuppressive treatment with optimal response (≥80% decrease in PVC burden with complete resolution of ^{18}F-FDG uptake on serial PET scans) in 67% of them, suboptimal (<80% decrease in PVC burden with only partial decrease of ^{18}F-FDG uptake) in 15% and no response in the remaining 13% after a mean follow-up of 6 months. Among patients with left ventricular dysfunction, 37% showed an improvement in the mean LVEF. Of note, 54% of the patients did not respond to immunosuppressive treatment with steroids alone and needed a second line treatment [27]. All the above data come from relatively small single center experiences, are burdened by a substantial heterogeneity in treatment strategies -including CA, antiarrhythmic drugs, and type, dose and duration of immunosuppressive therapy - therefore should be considered with caution before being routinely used in clinical practice.

Conclusion

Position emission tomography imaging with ^{18}F-FDG has an increasing role in the field of cardiac electrophysiology helping in diagnosis, risk stratification and management of patients with complex VA by evaluating myocardial inflammation. In the future, the integration of PET imaging with electroanatomic mapping systems could potentially improve VT ablation strategies by identifying critical sites for VT.

Conflict of Interest The authors have no disclosures.

References

1. Lazzerini PE, Capecchi PL, Laghi-Pasini F. Systemic inflammation and arrhythmic risk: lessons from rheumatoid arthritis. Eur Heart J. 2016;38(22):1717–27.
2. Kumar S, Barbhaiya C, Nagashima K, Choi E-K, Epstein LM, John RM, Maytin M, Albert CM, Miller AL, Koplan BA, et al. Ventricular tachycardia in cardiac sarcoidosis characterization of ventricular substrate and outcomes of catheter ablation. Circ Arrhythm Electrophysiol. 2015;8:87–93.
3. Segawa M, Fukuda K, Nakano M, Kondo M, Satake H, Hirano M, Shimokawa H. Time course and factors correlating with ventricular tachyarrhythmias after introduction of steroid therapy in cardiac sarcoidosis. Circ Arrhythm Electrophysiol. 2016;9:e003353.
4. Tung R, Bauer B, Schelbert H, Lynch JP, Auerbach M, Gupta P, Schiepers C, Chan S, Ferris J, Barrio M, Ajijola O, Bradfield J, Shivkumar K. Incidence of abnormal positron emission tomography in patients with unexplained cardiomyopathy and ventricular arrhythmias: the potential role of occult inflammation in arrhythmogenesis. Heart Rhythm. 2015;12:2488–98.
5. Muser D, Santangeli P, Liang JJ, Castro SA, Magnani S, Hayashi T, Garcia FC, Frankel DS, Dixit S, Zado ES, Lin D, Desjardins B, Callans DJ, Alavi A, Marchlinski FE. Characterization of the electroanatomic substrate in cardiac sarcoidosis: correlation with imaging findings of scar and inflammation. JACC Clin Electrophysiol. 2018;4:291–303.
6. Stevenson WG, Khan H, Sager P, Saxon LA, Middlekauff HR, Natterson PD, Wiener I. Identification of reentry circuit sites during catheter mapping and radiofrequency ablation of ventricular tachycardia late after myocardial infarction. Circulation. 1993;88:1647–70.
7. Budzianowski JK, Korybalska K, Bręborowicz A. The role of inflammation in cardiac arrhythmias pathophysiology. J Med Sci. 2016;85:197–204.
8. Klein RM, Vester EG, Brehm MU, Dees H, Picard F, Niederacher D, Beckmann MW, Strauer BE. Inflammation of the myocardium as an arrhythmia trigger. Z Kardiol. 2000;89(Suppl 3):24–35.
9. Camici P, Ferrannini E, Opie LH. Myocardial metabolism in ischemic heart disease: basic principles and application to imaging by positron emission tomography. Prog Cardiovasc Dis. 1989;32:217–38.
10. Manabe O, Yoshinaga K, Ohira H, Masuda A, Sato T, Tsujino I, Yamada A, Oyama-Manabe N, Hirata K, Nishimura M, Tamaki N. The effects of 18-h fasting with low-carbohydrate diet preparation on suppressed physiological myocardial ^{18}F-fluorodeoxyglucose (FDG) uptake and possible minimal effects of unfractionated heparin use in patients with suspected cardiac involvement sarcoidosis. J Nucl Cardiol. 2016;23:244–52.
11. Slart RHJA, Glaudemans AWJM, Gheysens O, Lubberink M, Kero T, Dweck MR, Habib G, Gaemperli O, Saraste A, Gimelli A, Georgoulias P, Verberne HJ, Bucerius J, Rischpler C, Hyafil F, Erba PA. 4Is Cardiovascular Imaging: a joint initiative of the European Association of Cardiovascular Imaging (EACVI) and the European Association of Nuclear Medicine (EANM). Procedural recommendations of cardiac PET/CT imaging: standardization in inflammatory-, infective-, infiltrative-, and innervation- (4Is) related cardiovascular diseases: a joint collaboration of the EACVI and the EANM: summary. Eur Heart J Cardiovasc Imaging. 2020;21:1320–30.
12. Choi Y, Brunken RC, Hawkins RA, Huang SC, Buxton DB, Hoh CK, Phelps ME, Schelbert HR. Factors affecting myocardial 2-[F^{-18}] fluoro-2-deoxy-D-glucose uptake in positron emission tomography studies of normal humans. Eur J Nucl Med. 1993;20:308–18.
13. Iozzo P, Chareonthaitawee P, Di Terlizzi M, Betteridge DJ, Ferrannini E, Camici PG. Regional myocardial blood flow and glucose utilization during fasting and physiological hyperinsulinemia in humans. Am J Physiol Endocrinol Metab. 2002;282:E1163–71.
14. Vita T, Okada DR, Veillet-Chowdhury M, Bravo PE, Mullins E, Hulten E, Agrawal M, Madan R, Taqueti VR, Steigner M, Skali H, Kwong RY, Stewart GC, Dorbala S, Di Carli MF, Blankstein R. Complementary value of cardiac magnetic resonance imaging and positron emission tomography/computed tomography in the assessment of cardiac sarcoidosis. Circ Cardiovasc Imaging. 2018;11:e007030.
15. Dilsizian V, Bacharach SL, Beanlands RS, Bergmann SR, Delbeke D, Dorbala S, Gropler RJ, Knuuti J, Schelbert HR, Travin MI. ASNC imaging guidelines/SNMMI procedure standard for positron emission tomography (PET) nuclear cardiology procedures. J Nucl Cardiol. 2016;23:1187–226.
16. DiFilippo FP, Brunken RC. Do implanted pacemaker leads and ICD leads cause metal-related artifact in cardiac PET/CT? J Nucl Med. 2005;46:436–43.
17. Gormsen LC, Haraldsen A, Kramer S, Dias AH, Kim WY, Borghammer P. A dual tracer (68) Ga-DOTANOC PET/CT and (18) F-FDG PET/

CT pilot study for detection of cardiac sarcoidosis. EJNMMI Res. 2016;6:52.

18. Birnie DH, Nery PB, Ha AC, Beanlands RSB. Cardiac sarcoidosis. J Am Coll Cardiol. 2016;68:411–21.

19. Statement on sarcoidosis. Joint Statement of the American Thoracic Society (ATS), the European Respiratory Society (ERS) and the World Association of Sarcoidosis and other granulomatous disorders (WASOG) adopted by the ATS Board of Directors and by the ERS Executive Committee, February 1999. Am J Respir Crit Care Med. 1999;160:736–55.

20. Patel MR, Cawley PJ, Heitner JF, Klem I, Parker MA, Jaroudi WA, Meine TJ, White JB, Elliott MD, Kim HW, Judd RM, Kim RJ. Detection of myocardial damage in patients with sarcoidosis. Circulation. 2009;120:1969–77.

21. Ohira H, Tsujino I, Ishimaru S, Oyama N, Takei T, Tsukamoto E, Miura M, Sakaue S, Tamaki N, Nishimura M. Myocardial imaging with ^{18}F-fluoro-2-deoxyglucose positron emission tomography and magnetic resonance imaging in sarcoidosis. Eur J Nucl Med Mol Imaging. 2007;35:933–41.

22. Muser D, Santangeli P, Pathak RK, Castro SA, Liang JJ, Magnani S, Hayashi T, Garcia FC, Hutchinson MD, Supple GE, et al. Long-term outcomes of catheter ablation of ventricular tachycardia in patients with cardiac sarcoidosis. Circ Arrhythm Electrophysiol. 2016;9:e004333.

23. Gowani Z, Habibi M, Okada DR, Smith J, Derakhshan A, Zimmerman SL, Misra S, Gilotra NA, Berger RD, Calkins H, Tandri H, Chrispin J. Utility of cardiac magnetic resonance imaging versus cardiac positron emission tomography for risk stratification for ventricular arrhythmias in patients with cardiac sarcoidosis. Am J Cardiol. 2020;134:123–9.

24. Muser D, Santangeli P, Castro SA, Liang JJ, Enriquez A, Werner TJ, Nucifora G, Magnani S, Hayashi T, Zado ES, Garcia FC, Callans DJ, Dixit S, Desjardins B, Marchlinski FE, Alavi A. Prognostic role of serial quantitative evaluation of ^{18}F-fluorodeoxyglucose uptake by PET/CT in patients with cardiac sarcoidosis presenting with ventricular tachycardia. Eur J Nucl Med Mol Imaging. 2018;45(8):1–11.

25. Lee P-I, Cheng G, Alavi A. The role of serial FDG PET for assessing therapeutic response in patients with cardiac sarcoidosis. J Nucl Cardiol. 2017;24:19–28.

26. Lakkireddy D, Turagam MK, Yarlagadda B, Dar T, Hamblin M, Krause M, Parikh V, Bommana S, Atkins D, Di Biase L, Mohanty S, Rosamond T, Carroll H, Nydegger C, Wetzel L, Gopinathannair R, Natale A. Myocarditis causing premature ventricular contractions: insights from the MAVERIC registry. Circ Arrhythm Electrophysiol. 2019;12:e007520.

27. Lakkireddy D, Yarlagadda B, Turagam M, Parikh A, Kola S, Hamblin M, Krause M, Rosamond T, Bommana S, Jaeger M, Carroll H, Nydegger C, Atkins D, Jeffery C, Gopinathannair R. B-LBCT02-02. Myocarditis is an underrecognized etiology of symptomatic premature ventricular contractions—insights from the myocarditis and ventricular arrhythmia (MAVERIC) registry. Heart Rhythm. 2018;15:942–5.

Cardiac Tumors

Patrick Martineau
and Matthieu Pelletier-Galarneau

Introduction

Cardiac masses constitute one of the less well-understood aspects of modern oncology due to a number of reasons. For one, the rarity of primary cardiac tumors is a serious obstacle to conducting studies on the diagnostic approaches and management of these pathologies. Furthermore, while cardiac masses are relatively uncommon findings on imaging, autopsy studies over the course of the last century have repeatedly shown that cardiac involvement in patients with systemic malignancy is relatively prevalent, suggesting that imagers may be systematically understaging the extent of cardiac disease on routine imaging studies. However, with the growing use of FDG-PET for the routine staging and follow-up of patients with systemic malignancy, and the demonstrated utility of this imaging modality in the assessment of cardiac lesions, it may be hoped that this technique could allow for new insights in the evaluation of cardiac tumors.

Cardiac masses include nontumoral lesions in addition to both primary and secondary tumors.

As a rule, primary cardiac tumors are typically rare and benign; however, it is important to note that, due to the dynamic nature of cardiac physiology, even benign pathologies can be associated with high mortality and morbidity with symptom manifestation highly dependent on the location of the mass within the heart and its relation to local structures. Secondary tumors (i.e., metastases) are malignant by definition and constitute the overwhelming majority of cardiac masses.

While most patients with cardiac lesions are asymptomatic [1], clinical manifestations of cardiac masses are myriad and can occur due to pericardial effusion and cardiac tamponade [2, 3], arrhythmia (including atrial fibrillation/flutter, ventricular tachycardia, multifocal atrial tachycardia, and paroxysmal supraventricular tachycardia) [3–6], myocardial infarction (either from tumor embolization into the coronary arteries [7, 8] or from extrinsic compression of the coronary vessels [3, 9, 10]), and tumor embolization [11], with specific symptoms highly dependent on lesion location.

Treatment options depend largely on the tumor type, extent of disease, and the relationship between the tumor and cardiac structures. For example, treatment options in an elderly patient with cardiac involvement from a metastatic lung adenocarcinoma vary drastically from those of a young patient with a primary cardiac rhabdomyoma.

P. Martineau (✉)
BC Cancer, Vancouver, BC, Canada
e-mail: patrick.martineau@bccancer.bc.ca

M. Pelletier-Galarneau
Montreal Heart Institute, Montréal, QC, Canada
e-mail: Matthieu.pelletier-galarneau@icm-mhi.org

Diagnosing cardiac tumors is complicated in part due to the challenges in obtaining a tissue biopsy—as a result, imaging often plays a key role in the diagnosis of these lesions. Several imaging modalities are available for the assessment of cardiac masses and can often provide complimentary information. The most commonly used and widely accessible imaging test is echocardiography—either transthoracic or transesophageal—which provides high-spatial and high-temporal resolution images of lesions, as well as assessment of cardiac function, including the relationship of lesions to valve planes, the presence of pericardial effusions, etc. However, echocardiography can be limited by poor acoustic windows, operator dependency, and poor tissue characterization. Nonetheless, echocardiography typically serves as the initial, and sometimes only, imaging assessment. Contrast-enhanced, cardiac-gated computed tomography (CT) is well-suited for assessing the extent of metastatic disease, provides high spatial resolution imaging, and can be helpful in surgical planning. Cardiac magnetic resonance (CMR) provides superior tissue characterization compared to echocardiography and CT, as well as improved functional assessment compared to CT; however, the technique is limited in patients with impaired renal functions, those with implantable electronic devices, and provides limited information in those patients with secondary cardiac masses. Positron emission tomography (PET) imaging, typically with 2-deoxy-2-[18F]-fluoroglucose, is rarely used in the initial assessment of cardiac masses; however, its role in the assessment of metastatic disease (cardiac or otherwise) is well-established, and studies have shown that it may be particularly well-suited for distinguishing malignant from benign cardiac lesions, as well as assessing for intracardiac tumor recurrence following resection [12]. In addition, in cases of secondary cardiac lesions, PET can be helpful in identifying noncardiac lesions which may be more amenable to tissue sampling than their cardiac counterparts.

Primary Cardiac and Pericardiac Lesions

Epidemiology of Primary Cardiac Lesions

Primary cardiac masses are rare. The prevalence has been reported to vary between 0.0017% and 0.28% with data being derived from autopsy series, which reflects the difficulty of antemortem diagnosis in many cases [13–15]. Furthermore, the great majority of primary cardiac lesions are benign, with myxomas accounting for the bulk of these [14]. Primary malignant cardiac tumors (PMCT) are even more uncommon. A 40-year retrospective review of the SEER program identified their prevalence as 0.008%, with the majority (54.1%) occurring in females with a median age of 50 years [16]. Prognosis is poor with <50% of patients with PMCTs alive 1-year following diagnosis [16].

Types of Primary Cardiac and Pericardiac Masses

A classification of cardiac masses is presented in the fourth edition of the WHO *Classification of Tumours of the Lung, Pleura, Thymus and Heart* [17]. This framework classifies cardiac tumors into one of four separate categories:

1. Benign tumors.
2. Tumors of uncertain biological behavior.
3. Germ cell tumors.
4. Malignant tumors.

As mentioned above, the bulk of primary cardiac tumors are of a benign histology, with only about 10% of these lesions being malignant [18]. Tumors of uncertain biological behavior and germ cell tumors consist of very specific lesion types and are uncommon. Histologically, most primary malignant cardiac tumors in adults belong to the sarcoma (64.8%), lymphoma

Table 10.1 The most common types of cardiac lesions

Primary cardiac lesions			
Malignant		Benign	
Adult	Children	Adult	Children
Angiosarcoma	Rhabdomyosarcoma	Myxoma	Rhabdomyoma
Rhabdomyosarcoma		Lipoma	Teratoma
Mesothelioma		Papillary fibroelastoma	Fibroma
Lymphoma			Myxoma

Common sources of secondary cardiac lesions
Lung
Breast
Esophageal
Melanoma
Sarcoma
Renal cell carcinoma
Lymphoma

Nontumoral lesions
Thrombus
Vegetation

(27.0%), or mesothelioma (8%) types [16]. The specific types of sarcoma vary with age with rhabdomyosarcomas more frequently seen in pediatric patients while angiosarcomas or undifferentiated sarcomas are more common in the adult population. The most frequently seen cardiac lesions are shown in Table 10.1.

Symptoms and Clinical Presentation

The symptomology associated with cardiac lesions is variable and is largely dependent on their location within the heart, pericardium, and great vessels. In general, three broad classes of symptoms are recognized as arising from cardiac lesions. Systemic symptoms can consist of fever, weight loss, arthralgias, and fatigue. In addition, some cardiac lesions present with paraneoplastic symptoms. Cardiac symptoms can consist of cardiac dysfunction (which can occur as a result of lesions filling cardiac chambers or interfering with valve function), arrythmias (typically seen in patients

with lesions present within the myocardium), and cardiac tamponade (secondary to pericardial effusions which are frequently seen in pericardial involvement). Finally, patients with cardiac tumors can develop emboli (pulmonary or systemic) as numerous types of cardiac lesions have embologenic potential. Unfortunately, none of these symptoms are specific for cardiac tumors.

Diagnostic Approach

Cardiac lesions are typically less accessible to tissue sampling than other systemic lesions. As a result, the diagnostic approach in this context relies on the following information:

1. Clinical context/epidemiological likelihood plays a significant role in determining the nature of the lesion.
2. Age is an important diagnostic factor as, for example, certain tumor types are more commonly seen in pediatric patients.

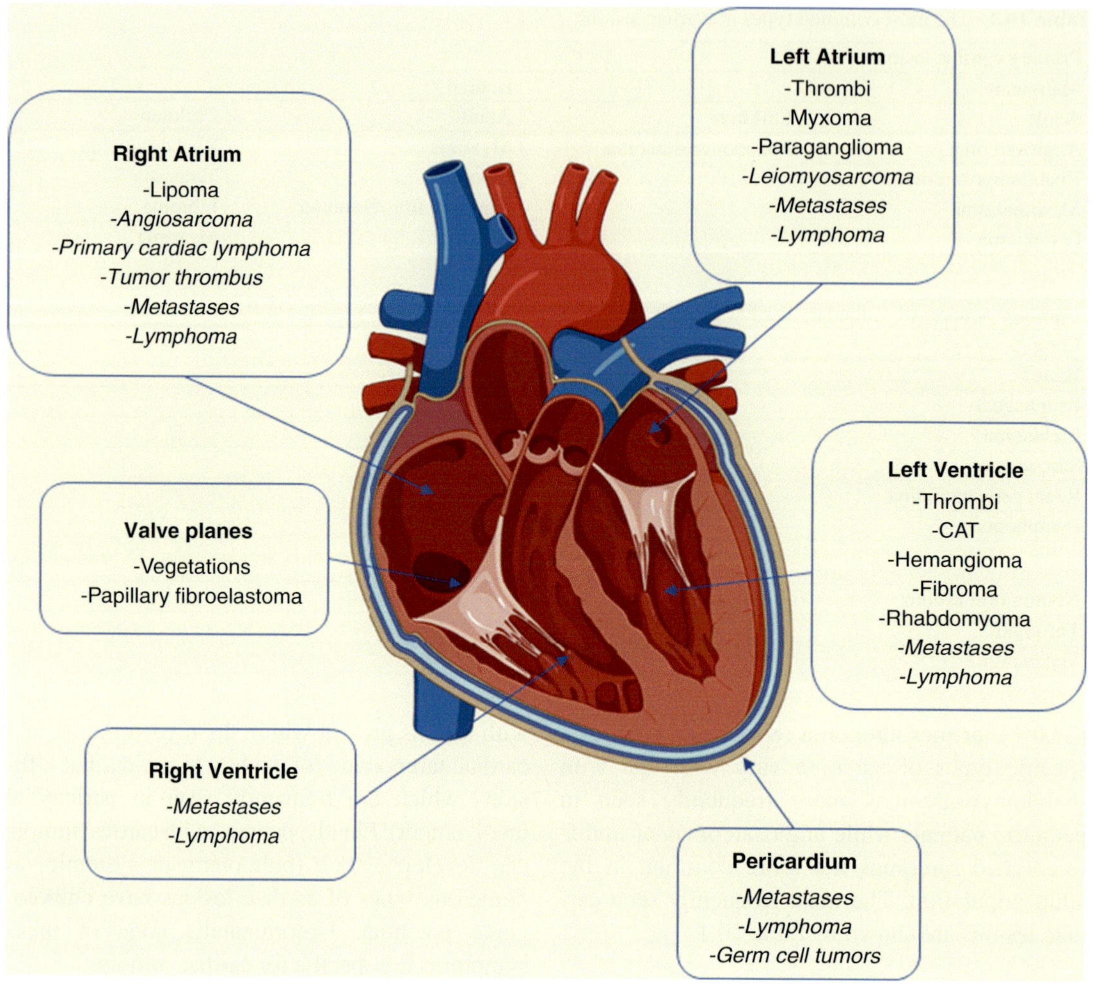

Fig. 10.1 Typical locations of various cardiac lesions. *Malignant lesions.* (Reprinted with permission from [114])

3. Finally, the imaging characteristics (including lesion location, enhancement characteristics, FDG-avidity, sites of additional lesions) are all important factors to consider in the workup of a cardiac mass. The typical locations of various cardiac lesions are shown in Fig. 10.1.

Trans-thoracic echocardiography usually serves as the first-line imaging. If additional imaging is required, trans-esophageal echocardiography, computed tomography (CT), magnetic resonance imaging (MRI), and (increasingly) positron emission tomography (PET) can provide further characterization.

Benign Cardiac Lesions

Intra-Cardiac Thrombi

Thrombi, the most frequently encountered intra-cardiac lesions, are most commonly seen in the left atrium, atrial appendage, and ventricle, but can also be present within the right-sided chambers [19]. Thrombi may be mobile or adherent to the endocardium. Thrombi within the appendages or atria are most commonly seen in patients with arrythmias, atrial enlargement, or mitral valve dysfunction. When seen in the ventricles, these are most commonly associated with apical aneurysms or systolic dysfunction. Thrombi in general are typically seen in patients with hypercoagulability, such as those with malignancy, antiphospholipid syndrome, or in those with intracardiac prosthetic material.

An occasional incidental finding, intracardiac thrombi have been reported on FDG-PET imaging. While FDG uptake is typically low or absent, unusually high uptake has been reported in organizing thrombi [12, 20].

Vegetations

Intra-cardiac vegetations are associated with endocarditis, often appearing as mobile, irregular masses arising along the atrial side of the tricuspid or mitral valves, or along the ventricular side of the pulmonic or aortic valves. Less frequently, vegetations can arise from atrial or ventricular walls [21]. FDG-PET has an established role in the imaging of endocarditis as further discussed in Chaps. 12 and 13.

Patients in hypercoagulable states can also present with noninfective vegetations, termed marantic endocarditis [22]. In this case, the vegetations consist of platelet aggregates and blood interspersed with fibrin. As is in the case of thrombi, FDG accumulation has been described within these lesions [23].

Calcified Amorphous Tumors

Calcified amorphous tumors (CATs) are non-neoplastic lesions of uncertain etiology, characterized by nodular calcifications in a background of amorphous fibrinous material. These lesions are typically pedunculated and can arise in any chamber, but are more common in the left ventricle [24]. Due to the presence of calcifications, the imaging appearance can be suggestive of osteosarcoma, calcified myxoma, or vegetations; however, the histopathological diagnosis of CATs is straightforward. CATs can be encountered in patients with valvular disease (such as mitral annulus complex calcification) and end stage renal disease [25].

Cardiac Myxoma

Atrial myxomas are the most common of the benign cardiac tumors, accounting for approximately two thirds of all primary cardiac masses [26, 27]. Approximately 80% of these lesions arise in the left atrium, and around 80% are attached to the interatrial septum [27]. These rarely arise within the ventricles or from the valves [28]. Ninety percent of patients are diagnosed between the ages of 30 and 60 years [29], and these tumors are 1.5–2 times more common in women [30]. These tumors are rare in children, where they account for about 10% of benign cardiac tumors [31].

Histologically, these tumors consist of multipotent mesenchymal cells. Size, contour, and type of endocardial attachment are variable; however, these are most commonly 3–4 cm in size (but can be much larger [28]), with a lobulated contour, and are often pedunculated. Smaller, pedunculated tumors can be highly mobile and prolapse across the atrioventricular (usually, mitral) valve leading to an element of diastolic filling impairment. Furthermore, myxomas may be covered by a surface thrombus—these are frequently associated with embolization events and present in at least 10–20% of patients [30]. These lesions may calcify (in up to 14% of cases), and occasionally ossify [32].

Diagnosis of cardiac myxomas is usually accomplished by echocardiography, aided by their typical location and appearance. In atypical cases, these can be investigated using advanced imaging. On FDG-PET, most cardiac myxomas demonstrate little to no uptake [33–35].

Therapy consists of surgical excision. Recurrence is rare, except in cases of familial or complex myxomas where recurrence can be seen in 10–20% of cases [36, 37].

The Carney complex is an inherited multiple neuroendocrine neoplasia syndrome. This autosomal dominant condition, associated with mutations of the *PRKAR1A* tumor suppressor gene found on chromosome 17q, is associated with (often multiple) cardiac myxomas, present in the majority of affected individuals.

Papillary Fibroelastoma

These benign endocardial lesions account for the majority (75%) of benign valvular tumors [38]. The most common locations are the downstream side of the aortic valve, followed by the mitral valve, left ventricular endocardium, and the tricuspid valve [39]. At the histopathological level, these tumors are gelatinous and have a frond-like appearance. Like myxomas, these tumors can lead to embolization or impede cardiac function by interfering with valve movement or by obstructing chambers. Surgical resection can be curative. Although experience is limited, these lesions do not appear to be significantly FDG-avid [12].

Lipoma

Cardiac lipomas are most frequently encountered in the right atrium or left ventricle and can be subendocardial (most commonly), subepicardial, or myocardial. These lesions account for approximately 10% of primary benign cardiac lesions [40]. While these lesions can be asymptomatic, the types of symptoms encountered can be related to their location—subendocardial lesions can cause obstructive symptoms while myocardial lesions can lead to arrhythmias. As these are typically encapsulated, embolization is uncommon. Furthermore, the presence of a capsule can help distinguish these lesions from lipomatous hypertrophy of the interatrial septum.

Rhabdomyoma

Rhabdomyomas are the most common primary pediatric cardiac tumors and are most frequently seen in infants and fetuses [41]. Rhabdomyomas are growths consisting of cardiomyocytes and can be considered hamartomas. These are often multiple and located in the interventricular septum or ventricular free wall. Rhabdomyomas can frequently resolve spontaneously [42]. There is an association with tuberous sclerosis with approximately half of infants with tuberous sclerosis found to have rhabdomyomas [43–45].

Fibroma

Cardiac fibromas are the second more commonly encountered primary cardiac tumor in children. Like rhabdomyomas, these are present from birth, but symptoms often present only in the second or third decade of life. These are typically seen in the left ventricular free wall or intraventricular septum [46, 47]. Histologically, they are composed of fibroblasts and collagen fibers along with calcifications [47]. There is an association with familial adenomatous polyposis and Gorlin syndrome [48]. Unlike rhabdomyoma, these tumors do not regress spontaneously, and surgical resection is indicated.

Hemangioma

Hemangiomas and other vascular malformations can be seen in children but are more commonly encountered in adults [49]. In children, these are most commonly present in the right atrium. In adults, these are typically encountered in the left ventricle or associated with cardiac valves. Due to their variable appearance, these are difficult to be distinguished from other lesions and, as they can be infiltrative, can be confused for malignant lesions on imaging.

Tumors of Uncertain Biological Behavior

Cardiac Paraganglioma

Paragangliomas arise from paraganglionic tissue which can be seen at the base of the heart and atrium. These lesions are most commonly seen in the left atrium (55%), interatrial septum (16%), or the anterior wall of the heart (10%) [50]. They are classified as Tumors of Uncertain Biological Behavior but can be aggressive, invading local structures, and should be resected [51]. Like pheochromocytomas, these lesions can be either secretory or nonsecretory. A minority of these tumors can secrete catecholamines which can lead to patients presenting with hypertension, palpitations, headache, and/or diaphoresis. An example is shown in Fig. 10.2.

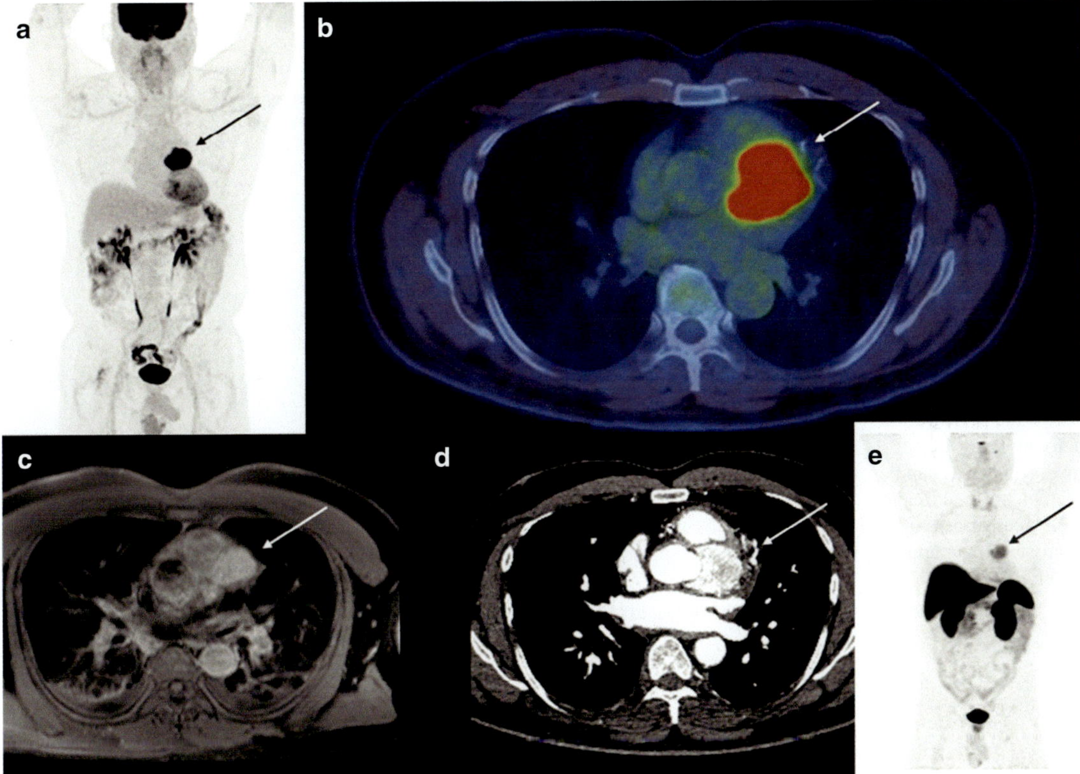

Fig. 10.2 Example of a primary cardiac paraganglioma in a 56-year-old male which demonstrates avid FDG uptake (SUV 27) on maximum intensity projection images (**a**) and trans axial PET/CT (**b**). The lesion is centered between the left atrial appendage and main pulmonary artery and demonstrates homogeneous enhancement on CMR (**c**) and cardiac CT (**d**). In addition, the lesion was noted to be DOTA-avid (**e**)

Germ Cell Tumors

Cardiac germ cell tumors are relatively rare with the majority of cases occurring within the pericardial space [46]. These are usually multilocular and well-defined and often contain fat and/or calcifications [52]. In light of this, MR can be particularly useful in characterizing these lesions. Large pericardial effusions are typically present [53].

Malignant Cardiac Lesions

Given the types of tissue present in the heart, it follows that the bulk of primary malignant cardiac tumors consist of lesions in the sarcoma family. An example is shown in Fig. 10.3. These lesions are usually diagnosed in younger adults, without a clear gender predominance [54]. Clinical presentation is variable and often related

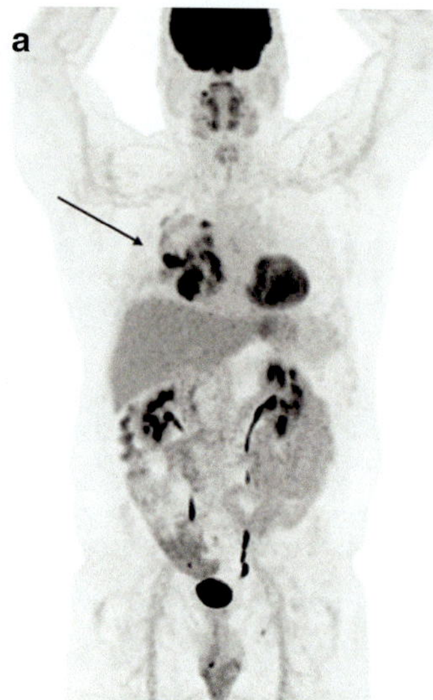
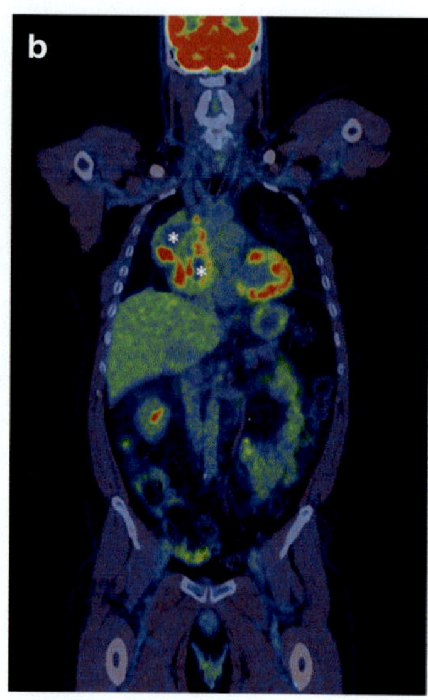

Fig. 10.3 This 49-year-old male was diagnosed with a primary synovial sarcoma of the heart. This large lesion demonstrates significant but heterogeneous FDG uptake (SUV 15) on MIP images (**a**) and was centered at the right atrium, with extension across the pericardium and into the mediastinum as can be seen on coronal images (**b**). Areas of central necrosis (*) are apparent on PET

to the location of the lesion with symptoms comparable to those caused by benign lesions.

Imaging findings suggestive of a malignant lesion include a rapidly growing tumor, necrosis and/or hemorrhage, involvement of multiple chambers, and pericardial effusion; however, none of these features are sensitive or specific [55].

Cardiac Angiosarcoma

This neoplasm of endothelial mesenchymal cells constitutes the most common primary malignant cardiac tumor, accounting for approximately 30–40% of cases [56, 57]. These lesions are more common in males and typically arise in the right atrium (75%) and right atrioventricular groove [15, 58, 59]. Angiosarcomas have a tendency to invade the pericardium, extend into the right ventricle through the tricuspid valve, and involve the right coronary artery. The lesion often appears heterogeneous due to areas of necrosis and hemorrhage. Despite surgery, angiosarcomas have a high rate of recurrence and frequently produce systemic metastases. In fact, metastases can be seen in up to 47–89% of cases, with involvement of the lungs, bone, bowel, and brain reported [60]. Prognosis is poor with survival of a few months without surgery [60].

Leiomyosarcoma

Leiomyosarcomas account for 8–9% of cardiac sarcomas with patients usually presenting in the fourth decade of life [61]. These lesions typically appear as sessile masses arising from the posterior left atrium although involvement of all chambers has been reported [62, 63]. Lesions can be multiple in approximately one third of cases

Rhabdomyosarcoma

Most cases of rhabdomyosarcoma arise in children, with a mean age at presentation of 14 years

[46]. Unlike angiosarcomas and leiomyosarcomas, rhabdomyosarcoma appear to have no clear predilection for any chamber [64]. These primary lesions of striated muscle are the most common pediatric cardiac malignancy [65]. Despite treatment, prognosis is dismal with most patients succumbing in less than 1 year [66].

Primary Cardiac Lymphoma

Primary cardiac lymphoma (PCL) accounts for approximately 27% of primary cardiac malignancies and is the second most common primary cardiac malignancy after sarcomas [67, 68]. Diffuse large B-cell lymphoma (DLBCL) is the most commonly encountered histology (80%), followed by follicular B-cell lymphoma. There is an association with Epstein-Barr virus and AIDS, as well as a prior history of cardiac transplant. In addition, an association with implanted cardiac devices has been reported and thought to be related to a chronic foreign body reaction—this condition has been termed fibrin-associated large B-cell lymphoma [69].

PCL is usually multifocal and most commonly involves the right atrium although any chamber can be involved. Pericardial involvement is reported in one third of cases and superior vena cava involvement in one fourth of cases [70, 71]. Mediastinal lymphadenopathy can be present. Prognosis is poor, and median survival is 12 months [71].

Secondary Cardiac Masses

Epidemiology of Secondary Cardiac Lesions

Secondary (i.e., metastatic) cardiac masses are for more common than primary cardiac tumors. However, the reported prevalence varies greatly, ranging from 2.3% to 18.3% of all patients with malignancy (see Table 10.2)—or roughly 40–50 times more common than primary cardiac masses [72]. All secondary cardiac lesions are consid-

Table 10.2 Results of autopsy studies examining the prevalence of cardiac metastases in patients with malignancy

Reference	Year published	Number of malignancies	Prevalence (%)
Pollia and Gogol [115]	1936	1450	2
Scott and Garvin [116]	1939	1082	10.9
Walther [117]	1948	2027	2.3
Young and Goldman [118]	1954	476	19.1
Gassman et al. [119]	1955	4124	5.0
Hanfling [120]	1960	694	18.3
Berge et al. [121]	1968	2595	4.7
Malaret and Aliaga	1968	250	15.1
Harrer and Lewis [122]	1971	1164	12.6
Kline et al. [79]	1972	716	8.5
Lockwood and Broghamer [123]	1980	1303	14
Mukai et al. [124]	1988	6240	15.0
Karwinski et al. [125]	1989	2564	5.1
Manojlovic [126]	1990	477	8.2
Klatt and Heitz [73]	1990	1095	10.7
MacGee et al. [127]	1991	1311	4.3
Silvestri [128]	1997	1928	8.4
Bussani et al. [74]	2007	7289	9.1

ered malignant, irrespective of histology, due to their potential effect on cardiac function.

Sources of Secondary Cardiac Masses

For males, the most common source of cardiac metastases are lung and esophageal tumors while, in females, most cardiac lesions originate from lung cancer or lymphoma [72]. This is largely due to the prevalence of these malignancies, as well as their proximity to the heart. In particular, lung cancer is associated with a high rate of cardiac disease, with autopsy studies reporting involvement of the heart in approximately one in six cases [73].

Prevalence aside, malignancies with the highest rate of cardiac metastases include melanoma (Fig. 10.4), mesothelioma, and renal cell carcinomas. In particular, melanoma is known to involve the heart in roughly one quarter to one half of patients [73–75], while mesotheliomas affect the heart in nearly one half of cases [74].

Secondary Cardiac Lymphoma

Cardiac involvement is noted in approximately 25% of patients with disseminated lymphoma [76]. Pericardial involvement has been reported to be more frequent in cases of Hodgkin's lymphoma; however, cardiac involvement is more frequently seen in non-Hodgkin's lymphoma [77]. An example is shown in Fig. 10.5.

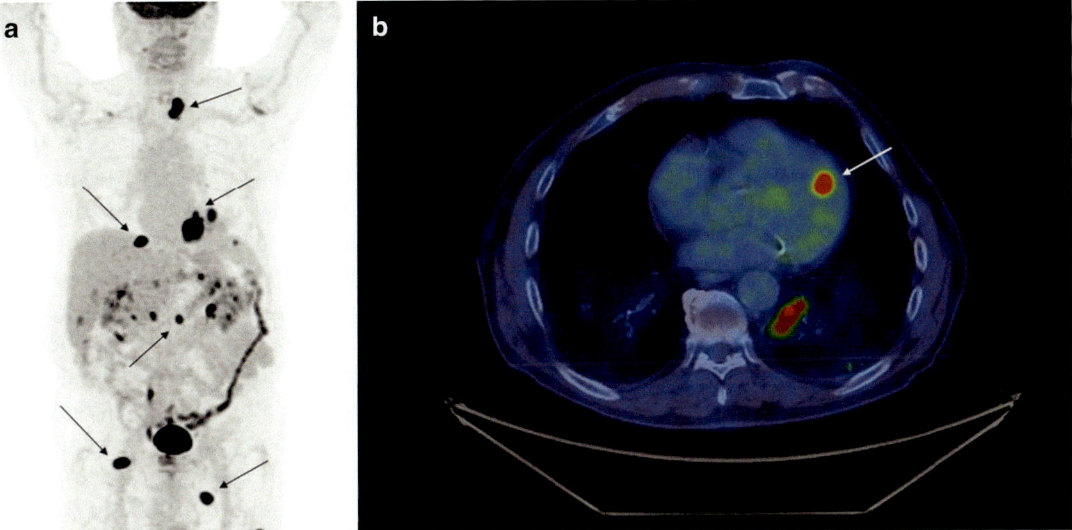

Fig. 10.4 Cardiac metastases from melanoma are well-described in the literature. This 91-year-old man had widespread metastatic melanoma (arrows), best appreci-ated on MIP images (**a**). In addition, there was an obvious lesion in the interventricular septum (**b**, arrow)

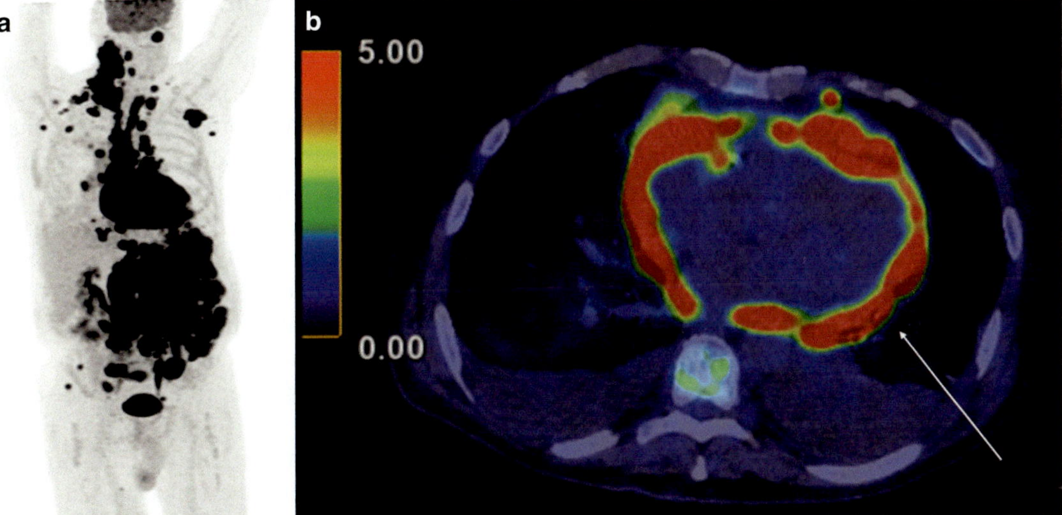

Fig. 10.5 Pericardial or cardiac involvement in lym-phoma is relatively common. This 45-year-old male had extensive diffuse large B-cell lymphoma, best seen on MIP images (**a**). On transaxial PET/CT images (**b**), near-circumferential pericardial disease is visible (arrow)

Miscellaneous Cardiac Lesions

Lipomatous Hypertrophy of the Interatrial Septum

As of the fourth edition of the WHO classification of cardiac tumors, lipomatous hypertrophy of the interatrial septum (LHIS) is no longer considered a distinct cardiac lesion; however, it remains an important diagnostic consideration when evaluating fat-density cardiac tumors. At the histological level, LHIS consists of brown adipocytes and cardiomyocytes. On imaging, LHIS appears as a fat-density lesion within the interatrial septum sparing the fossa ovalis. The presence of brown fat likely explains why LHIS can be distinctly FDG-avid on PET.

Mechanisms of Spread to the Heart and Pericardium

There are four main metastatic pathways to the heart: direct extension, hematogenous dissemination, retrograde lymphatic spread, or by transvenous (tumor thrombus) extension along the superior vena cava (SVC), inferior vena cava (IVC), or pulmonary veins [78]. As is typically seen in oncology, certain tumor types preferentially spread using specific pathways, although dissemination along multiple pathways can also be seen. Studies have suggested that retrograde lymphatic spread may act as the dominant pathway, responsible for the majority of cardiac metastases [3, 79, 80].

The pathway of spread largely determines the location of the resultant cardiac metastases. Metastases spreading through the hematogenous pathway will generally deposit in the endocardium or myocardium due to the nature of coronary circulation. Likewise, metastases spreading through the lymphatics will preferentially accumulate in the sub-epicardium and pericardium where cardiac lymphatic channels are predominantly located. Certain infra-diaphragmatic malignancies such as renal cell carcinoma (RCC) frequently produce tumor thrombi which ascend the IVC into the right atrium, while mediastinal or lung primaries can directly invade the SVC with tumor extending into the right atrium, or by extending along pulmonary veins into the left atrium (Fig. 10.6). Finally, direct invasion can be seen in lung and mediastinal tumors and invariably involves the parietal pericardium before transgressing the visceral pericardium, followed by invasion of the myocardium.

Obstruction of pericardial lymphatics by malignancy can cause impaired pericardial fluid drainage resulting in effusion. Pericardial effusion due to inflammation of the pericardium secondary to tumor infiltration can also occur; however, studies have shown that the majority of patients with malignant pericardial effusions developed cardiac metastases from lymphatic spread [3].

Cardiac Lymphatic Anatomy

The presence of cardiac lymphatics was documented by Rudbeck as early as the seventeenth century; however, the particularities of cardiac and pericardial lymphatic anatomy are often overlooked when compared to other organ systems. For example, in the case of mediastinal lymphatic anatomy, a well-defined classification of nodal stations and their relationship has been proposed and is widely utilized [81].

Studies have revealed that the cardiac lymphatic system is organized into subendocardial, myocardial, and subepicardial plexi [82]. Drainage flows from the subendocardial plexus centrifugally, reaching the subepicardial plexus which resides in the connective tissue between the epicardium and myocardium [83]. From there, drainage proceeds along right and left lymphatic trunks that follow the course of the coronary vessels [84]. Although subject to variation, in the majority of individuals the left efferent trunk merges with the right lower paratracheal lymph node, while the right lymphatic trunk typically joins the left anterior mediastinal lymph node chain [85, 86].

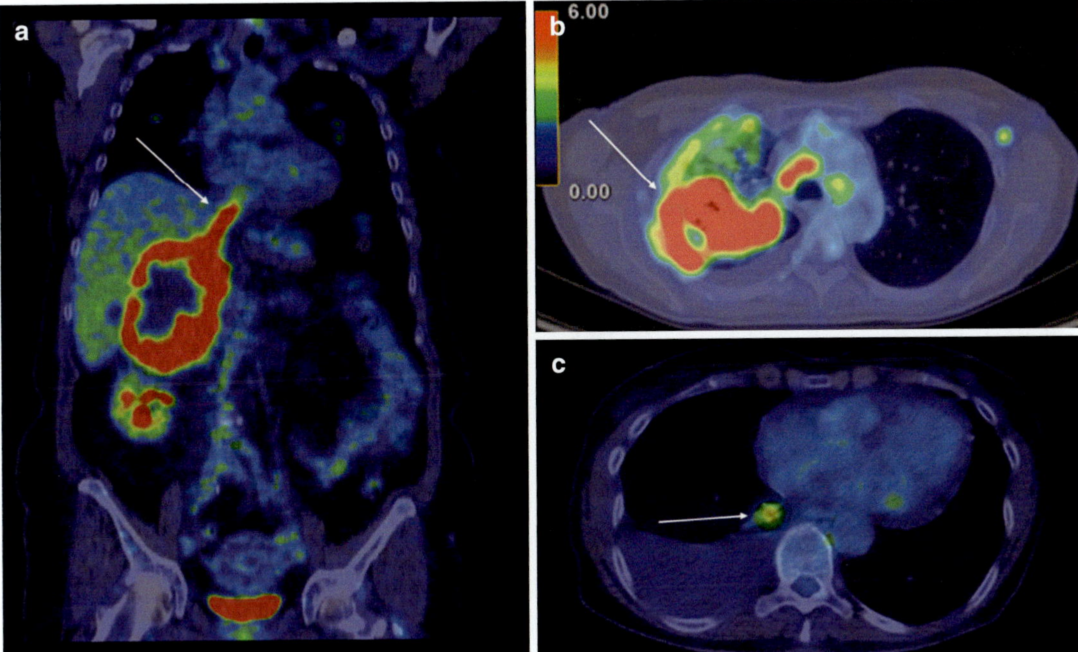

Fig. 10.6 Examples of tumor thrombus. (**a**) This middle-aged woman presented with a right adrenocortical carcinoma which had an associated IVC tumor thrombus extending into the right atrium (arrow). A 52-year-old man had a large adenocarcinoma in the right upper lobe (**b,** arrow) which developed a tumor thrombus within a right-sided pulmonary vein (**c,** arrow)

Lymphatic drainage of the pericardium proceeds by several separate pathways [87]. Drainage of the sternocostal surface of the pericardium proceeds either via efferent pathways laterally toward the phrenic nerves before proceeding caudally to the diaphragm or drains ventrally to prepericardial nodes situated at the anterior junction of the pericardium and diaphragm. The posterior pericardium drains to the upper and lower paratracheal lymph nodes. Drainage from the lateral pericardium is more variable—the more cephalad aspects of the lateral pericardium drain into paratracheal and tracheobronchial nodes, while the more caudal aspects drain into the diaphragm.

Knowledge of cardiac lymphatic anatomy is of practical utility in the assessment of cardiac lesions as lesions at certain locations (i.e., pericardial lymph nodes, lower paratracheal lymph nodes) can help identify those patients at high-risk of cardiac involvement.

Roles of FDG-PET Imaging of Cardiac Masses

Cardiac Metabolism and Patient Preparation for Cardiac FDG-PET

Myocardial metabolism is determined by the Randle cycle which dictates the particular metabolic substrate utilized by cardiomyocytes under varying physiological conditions. These substrates include glucose and free fatty acids (FFAs), with the relative amounts of these nutrients metabolized dictated by availability, endocrine factors, myocardial work, and cardiac perfusion. Prolonged fasting causes upregulation of lipolysis in adipocytes, with an increase in serum FFA levels in addition to a decrease in both circulating glucose and insulin levels. Increased FFAs drives cardiomyocyte metabolism to preferential use of FFAs as metabolic substrate. The ability to use FDG (a glucose analog) to image cardiac pathology is entirely dependent on the ability to distinguish physiological from pathological cardiac uptake. This can best be achieved through the suppression of normal physiological cardiac uptake.

Standard oncology patient preparation protocols (4–6 h of fasting) often result in heterogeneous, diffuse, or focal FDG cardiac uptake in normal patients. As a result, several approaches have been proposed when assessing cardiac pathology including prolonged fasting (5–18 h) [88], a high-fat/low-carbohydrate diet [89], the use of unfractionated heparin infusion, or fasting combined with an unfractionated heparin infusion [90]. However, none of these protocols are universally effective, and approximately 20% of patients will demonstrate unsuppressed benign cardiac FDG uptake [88].

FDG-PET/CT

When investigating cardiac masses with FDG-PET, obtaining cardiac and respiratory gated images is recommended, in order to reduce the effects of motion artifact.

The CT component can provide helpful findings in the characterization of cardiac masses as certain features are more suggestive of benign or malignant lesions [91]. These features are shown in Table 10.3.

A retrospective study by Rahbar et al. examined 24 patients with cardiac masses who underwent FDG-PET/CT. These included seven benign, eight primary, and nine secondary malignant cardiac lesions [92]. PET results were compared to contrast-enhanced CT features. In particular, the features assessed included enhancement, infiltration of surrounding tissues, involvement of the epicardium, irregular tumor margins, presence of necrosis, pericardial effusions, as well as involvement of several cardiac chambers. Malignant lesions were shown to have a standardized uptake value (SUV) significantly greater than those of benign lesions. However, SUV could not be used to distinguish between primary and secondary malignant lesions. Receiver operator characteristic (ROC) analysis showed a sensitivity and specificity of 94% and 100%, respectively, with an optimal cut-off maximum SUV (SUV_{Max}) of 4.2. CT performance was optimal when at least three of the above CT features were present, leading to a sensitivity and specificity of 82% and 86%, respectively.

Similarly, a retrospective study by Qin et al. examined the role of FDG-PET/CT in diagnosis and prognostication of 65 cardiac masses in 64 patients [93]. The studied population included 38 patients with primary and secondary cardiac malignancies, with 27 benign lesions also included in the analysis. Their results showed that numerous PET metrics—including SUV_{Max}, SUV adjusted to lean body mass (SUV_{Lean}), metabolic tumor volume (MTV), and total lesion glycolysis (TLG)—were significantly greater in malignant lesions than benign lesions. Furthermore, SUV_{Max} and SUV_{Lean} were significantly higher in lymphoma than other malignant cardiac lesions. Supplementing the PET findings with CT features—including the infiltration of surrounding tissues, pericardial involvement, the presence of irregular margins, necrosis, pericardial effusion, pleural effusion, and involvement of more than one chamber or vessels—the authors

Table 10.3 CT findings helpful in distinguishing between benign and malignant cardiac masses

CT feature	Benign	Malignant
Size	<5 cm	>5 cm
Number of lesions	Single	Multiple
Location	Intracameral	Intramural
Attachment	Narrow base	Broad base
Margin	Well-defined	Ill-defined
Enhancement	Minimal	Moderate to intense
Invasion	Absent	Can be present
Pericardial effusion	Absent	Can be present

found that the combination of CT features and an $SUV_{Max} > 6.75$ could distinguish between malignant and benign lesions with an accuracy of 92.3%. It was also found that imaging features were useful for prognostication with multivariate Cox regression analysis finding that $SUV_{Max} \geq 6.715$ was an independent prognostic factor while age, gender, and the presence of effusions were not. Similar features were reported in a retrospective study by Meng et al. in 38 patients with cardiac lesions [94]. Shao et al. also showed that SUV could distinguish malignant from benign cardiac lesions in 23 subjects [95].

The increased uptake seen in cardiac lymphoma compared to other cardiac lesions was also reported in a study by Kikuchi et al. [96]. These authors found that the combination of multidetector CT and FDG-PET/CT was able to distinguish DLBCL ($N = 5$) from other cardiac tumors (primary or secondary, $N = 12$) on the basis of significantly greater FDG uptake, in addition to the lesion being located at the right atrioventricular groove, encasement without stenosis of the coronary arteries, and the presence of a large pericardial effusion.

Likewise, the use of contrast-enhanced CT combined with FDG-PET in the evaluation of primary cardiac tumors was examined by Liu et al. [97]. In their retrospective study, 46 primary cardiac tumors were characterized on dual-phase (arterial and venous) contrast-enhanced CT as well as FDG-PET. Seventeen of the 46 lesions had malignant histology. Location in a right-sided chamber, involvement of multiple chambers, involvement of the mediastinum or great vessels, broad base attachment, size (> 5 cm), and at least moderate enhancement were all CT findings compatible with malignancy. Conversely, internal calcification, smooth boundary, and lack of enhancement were findings suggestive of a benign lesion. In terms of PET findings, SUV, SUV adjusted for serum glucose level, as well as tissue to background ratio (TBR) were examined. Among the PET parameters, SUV adjusted for serum glucose level had the highest discriminatory power on ROC analysis. For lesion characterization, contrast-enhanced CT had a diagnostic accuracy of 83%, compared to 85% for FDG-PET. Combining FDG-PET with contrast-enhanced CT significantly improved accuracy to 93%.

D'Angelo et al. retrospectively compared cardiac CT and FDG-PET/CT in 60 subjects [98]. Of these, 40 had malignant masses, including 18 primary cardiac lesions. CT features considered included density, size, calcifications, enhancement, tumor margins, pericardial effusion, invasiveness, and extension of the mass into the adjacent tissues. PET features examined included SUV_{Max}, mean SUV, MTV, and TLG. Of the CT parameters, the presence of irregular margins was the most accurate (91.7%) for differentiating between malignant and benign masses, while intra-tumoral calcifications was the least (31.7%). Of the PET features, TLG had the highest diagnostic accuracy (91.7%) for distinguishing malignant from benign lesions, while SUV_{Max} and MTV both showed good diagnostic performance (accuracies of 89.3% and 86.1%, respectively). SUV_{Max} was found to be an independent prognostic indicator. Based on their findings, the authors also proposed a diagnostic algorithm for the imaging workup of cardiac masses: in the presence of five or more (or two or less) of the CT features, cardiac lesions can accurately be characterized as malignant (or benign); however, PET could be used for further characterization in the remainder of cases, as CT shows insufficient diagnostic accuracy.

Chan et al. compared the results of CMR and FDG-PET for the detectability of cardiac masses in 66 subjects [99]. These authors reported the sensitivity and specificity of FDG-PET to be 70% and 78%, respectively, for cardiac masses (benign or malignant) using CMR as the gold standard. An important limitation of this study is the lack of a dedicated cardiac suppression protocol, or the acquisition of cardiac or respiratory gated images—all factors which could have improved PET performance compared to CMR. They further showed that FDG avidity of cardiac masses (as assessed by SUV) varied with the degree of contrast enhancement on CMR (as measured by signal to noise ratio).

Further comparison of diagnostic modalities was performed by Lemasle et al. who retrospectively studied the roles of various modalities—including TEE, CT, MRI, and PET—for the diagnosis and management of cardiac masses in 119 subjects [100]. Of the various imaging tests, FDG-PET was found to be the most useful modality for distinguishing between benign and malignant lesions.

Despite the observation in the above-mentioned studies that elevated SUVs can be used to identify malignant lesions, it should be noted that several examples of benign cardiac masses with high FDG-avidity have been reported [101–103].

In addition to its utility for lesion characterization, an important use of FDG-PET/CT is for staging—either detection of metastatic disease from primary cardiac malignancies or for identifying cardiac involvement from a systemic malignancy. The use of FDG-PET in this capacity has been described in case reports and one study [93, 104–112]. In the context of cardiac lesions, the detection of metastatic disease can be extremely useful since metastases are likely more amenable to tissue sampling than the cardiac lesion [113]. However, studies to date have not thoroughly examined this.

FDG-PET/MRI

Nensa et al. examined the use of PET/MR for the assessment of cardiac masses [12]. These authors prospectively assessed 16 patients with cardiac masses, in addition to four patients with previously resected cardiac sarcomas. Like the above-described PET/CT studies, these authors found significantly higher SUVs in malignant lesions (primary and secondary) than in benign masses. ROC analysis showed that lesions could be classified as benign or malignant with a sensitivity of 100% and specificity of 92% using an SUV cut-off of 5.2. MR findings including tumor volume, T2 signal characteristics, contrast enhancement, and the presence of pericardial effusion were less useful for lesion characterization. Consent interpretation using all MR features showed an accuracy equal to using SUV. In addition, the combination of con-

sent MR and SUV resulted in a sensitivity and specificity of 100%. In light of the high diagnostic accuracy of both PET and MRI in the assessment of cardiac masses, the authors suggested that this technique should "be reserved for selected cases for which true benefit can be expected."

Conclusion

The role of FDG-PET in the evaluation of patients with cardiac masses continues to be defined and refined. However, the evidence to date lays out a few salient observations. Notably, FDG-PET (combined with either CT or MRI) can distinguish between benign and cardiac masses using measures of FDG-avidity (i.e., SUV, TLG, MTV). In addition, combining PET results with anatomical features can increase the discriminatory power, thus speaking to a synergistic effect of hybrid imaging. Finally, the ability to identify metastatic disease through whole-body imaging is contributory both by helping to characterize the cardiac finding as either a primary or a secondary lesion and in identifying potential biopsy sites.

References

1. Butany J, Nair V, Naseemuddin A, Nair GM, Catton C, Yau T. Cardiac tumours: diagnosis and management. Lancet Oncol. 2005;6(4):219–28.
2. Haskell RJ, French WJ. Cardiac tamponade as the initial presentation of malignancy. Chest. 1985;88(1):70–3.
3. Tamura A, Matsubara O, Yoshimura N, Kasuga T, Akagawa S, Aoki N. Cardiac metastasis of lung cancer. A study of metastatic pathways and clinical manifestations. Cancer. 1992;70(2):437–42.
4. Nakamura A, Suchi T, Mizuno Y. The effect of malignant neoplasms on the heart. A study on the electrocardiographic abnormalities and the anatomical findings in cases with and without cardiac involvement. Jpn Circ J. 1975;39(5):531–42.
5. Yusuf SW, Bathina JD, Qureshi S, Kaynak HE, Banchs J, Trent JC, Ravi V, Daher IN, Swafford J. Cardiac tumors in a tertiary care cancer hospital: clinical features, echocardiographic findings, treatment and outcomes. Heart Int. 2012;7(1):e4. https://doi.org/10.4081/hi.2012.e4.

6. Cates CU, Virmani R, Vaughn WK, Robertson RM. Electrocardiographic markers of cardiac metastasis. Am Heart J. 1986;112(6):1297–303.

7. Virmani R, Khedekar RR, Robinowitz M, McAllister HA. Tumor embolization in coronary artery causing myocardial infarction. Arch Pathol Lab Med. 1983;107(5):243–5.

8. Ackermann DM, Hyma BA, Edwards WD. Malignant neoplastic emboli to the coronary arteries: report of two cases and review of the literature. Hum Pathol. 1987;18(9):955–9.

9. Franciosa JA, Lawrinson W. Coronary artery occlusion due to neoplasm. A rare cause of acute myocardial infarction. Arch Intern Med. 1971;128(5):797–801.

10. Frohlich ED, Shnider BI, Leonard JJ. Antemortem diagnosis of metastatic sarcoma to the heart: a case report. Am Heart J. 1959 Apr;57(4):623–9.

11. Borsaru A, Lau K, Solin P. Cardiac metastasis: a cause of recurrent pulmonary emboli. Br J Radiol. 2007;80(950):e50–3.

12. Nensa F, Tezgah E, Poeppel TD, Jensen CJ, Schelhorn J, Köhler J, et al. Integrated 18F-FDG PET/MR imaging in the assessment of cardiac masses: a pilot study. J Nucl Med. 2015;56(2):255–60.

13. Butany J, Leong SW, Carmichael K, Komeda M. A 30-year analysis of cardiac neoplasms at autopsy. Can J Cardiol. 2005;21(8):675–80.

14. Travis WD. Pathology & genetics tumours of the lung, pleura, thymus and heart. In: World Health Organization classification of tumours; 2004.

15. Reynen K. Frequency of primary tumors of the heart. Am J Cardiol. 1996;77(1):107.

16. Oliveira GH, Al-Kindi SG, Hoimes C, Park SJ. Characteristics and survival of malignant cardiac tumors: a 40-year analysis of >500 patients. Circulation. 2015;132(25):2395–402.

17. Travis WD, Brambilla E, Burke AP, Marx A, Nicholson AG. Introduction to the 2015 World Health Organization classification of tumors of the lung, pleura, thymus, and heart. J Thorac Oncol. 2015;10(9):1240–2.

18. Rahouma M, Arisha MJ, Elmously A, El-Sayed Ahmed MM, Spadaccio C, Mehta K, et al. Cardiac tumors prevalence and mortality: a systematic review and meta-analysis. Int J Surg. 2020;76:178–89.

19. Waller BF, Grider L, Rohr TM, Mclaughlin T, Taliercio CP, Fetters J. Intracardiac thrombi: frequency, location, etiology, and complications: a morphologic review—part I. Clin Cardiol. 1995;18(8):477–9.

20. Chaudhuri KG, Revels JW, Yadwadkar KS, Johnson LS. Intense 18F-FDG uptake in an organizing right atrial thrombus mimicking malignancy. Radiol Case Rep. 2017;12(3):449–54.

21. Chen-Milhone CS, Chakravarthy Potu K, Mungee S. Cardiac Aspergilloma: a rare case of a cardiac mass involving the native tricuspid valve, right atrium, and right ventricle in an immunocompromised patient. Case Rep Cardiol. 2018;2018:6927436.

22. Mazokopakis EE, Syros PK, Starakis IK. Nonbacterial thrombotic endocarditis (marantic endocarditis) in cancer patients. Cardiovasc Hematol Disord Drug Targets. 2010;10(2):84–6.

23. Buteau JP, Morais J, Keu KV. 18F-FDG PET/CT uptake of a nonbacterial thrombotic endocarditis. J Nucl Cardiol. 2016;23(6):1501–3.

24. Reynolds C, Tazelaar HD, Edwards WD. Calcified amorphous tumor of the heart (cardiac CAT). Hum Pathol. 1997;28(5):601–6.

25. de Hemptinne Q, de Cannière D, Vandenbossche J-L, Unger P. Cardiac calcified amorphous tumor: a systematic review of the literature. IJC Heart Vasc. 2015;7:1–5.

26. Prichard RW. Tumors of the heart: review of the subject and report of one hundred and fifty cases. Arch Pathol. 1951;51:98–128.

27. Burke AP, Virmani R. Cardiac myxoma: a clinicopathologic study. Am J Clin Pathol. 1993;100(6):671–80.

28. Reynen K. Cardiac myxomas. N Engl J Med. 1995;333(24):1610–7.

29. Sarjeant JM, Butany J, Cusimano RJ. Cancer of the heart. Am J Cardiovasc Drugs. 2003;3(6):407–21.

30. Pinede L, Duhaut P, Loire R. Clinical presentation of left atrial cardiac myxoma: a series of 112 consecutive cases. Medicine. 2001;80(3):159–72.

31. McAllister HA, Fenoglio JJ. Tumors of the cardiovascular system. Washington, DC: Armed Forces Institute of Pathology; 1978.

32. Grebenc ML, Rosado-de-Christenson ML, Green CE, Burke AP, Galvin JR. From the archives of the AFIP: cardiac myxoma: imaging features in 83 patients. Radiographics. 2002;22(3):673–89.

33. Gheysens O, Cornillie J, Voigt J-U, Bogaert J, Westhovens R. Left atrial myxoma on FDG-PET/CT. Clin Nucl Med. 2013;38(11):e421–2.

34. Okazaki Y, Yamada S, Kitada S, Matsunaga I, Nogami E, Watanabe T, et al. Significance of 18 F-FDG PET and immunohistochemical GLUT-1 expression for cardiac myxoma. Diagn Pathol. 2014;9(1):117.

35. Billet S, Lavie-Badie Y, Hitzel A, Lairez O. What is the role of 18F-FDG uptake intensity in suspected atrial myxoma exploration? J Nucl Cardiol. 2018;25(5):1861–2.

36. Waller DA, Ettles DF, Saunders NR, Williams G. Recurrent cardiac myxoma: the surgical implications of two distinct groups of patients. Thorac Cardiovasc Surg. 1989;37(4):226–30.

37. McCarthy PM, Piehler JM, Schaff HV, Pluth JR, Orszulak TA, Vidaillet HJ, et al. The significance of multiple, recurrent, and "complex" cardiac myxomas. J Thorac Cardiovasc Surg. 1986;91(3):389–96.

38. Mariscalco G, Bruno VD, Borsani P, Dominici C, Sala A. Papillary fibroelastoma: insight to a primary cardiac valve tumor. J Card Surg. 2010;25(2):198–205.

39. Burke A, Jeudy J, Virmani R. Cardiac tumours: an update. Heart. 2008;94(1):117–23.

40. Motwani M, Kidambi A, Herzog BA, Uddin A, Greenwood JP, Plein S. MR imaging of cardiac tumors and masses: a review of methods and clinical applications. Radiology. 2013;268(1):26–43.
41. Freedom R, Lee K-J, MacDonald C, Taylor G. Selected aspects of cardiac tumors in infancy and childhood. Pediatr Cardiol. 2000;21(4):299–316.
42. Günther T, Schreiber C, Noebauer C, Eicken A, Lange R. Treatment strategies for pediatric patients with primary cardiac and pericardial tumors: a 30-year review. Pediatr Cardiol. 2008;29(6):1071–6.
43. Kocabaş A, Ekici F, Cetin II, Emir S, Demir HA, Arı ME, et al. Cardiac rhabdomyomas associated with tuberous sclerosis complex in 11 children: presentation to outcome. Pediatr Hematol Oncol. 2013;30(2):71–9.
44. Harding CO, Pagon RA. Incidence of tuberous sclerosis in patients with cardiac rhabdomyoma. Am J Med Genet. 1990;37(4):443–6.
45. Bosi G, Lintermans J, Pellegrino P, Svaluto-Moreolo G, Vliers A. The natural history of cardiac rhabdomyoma with and without tuberous sclerosis. Acta Paediatr. 1996;85(8):928–31.
46. Burke A, Tavora F. The 2015 WHO classification of tumors of the heart and pericardium. J Thorac Oncol. 2016;11(4):441–52.
47. Burke AP, Rosado-de-Christenson M, Templeton PA, Virmani R. Cardiac fibroma: clinicopathologic correlates and surgical treatment. J Thorac Cardiovasc Surg. 1994;108(5):862–70.
48. Coffin CM. Case 1 congenital cardiac fibroma associated with Gorlin syndrome. Pediatr Pathol. 1992;12(2):255–62.
49. Burke A, Johns JP, Virmani R. Hemangiomas of the heart. A clinicopathologic study of ten cases. Am J Cardiovasc Pathol. 1990;3(4):283–90.
50. Mandak JS, Benoit CH, Starkey RH, Nassef LA Jr. Echocardiography in the evaluation of cardiac pheochromocytoma. Am Heart J. 1996;132(5):1063–6.
51. Huo JL, Choi JC, DeLuna A, Lee D, Fleischmann D, Berry GJ, et al. Cardiac paraganglioma: diagnostic and surgical challenges. J Card Surg. 2012;27(2):178–82.
52. Woodward PJ, Sohaey R, Kennedy A, Koeller KK. From the archives of the AFIP: a comprehensive review of fetal tumors with pathologic correlation. Radiographics. 2005;25(1):215–42.
53. Sklansky M, Greenberg M, Lucas V, Gruslin-Giroux A. Intrapericardial teratoma in a twin fetus: diagnosis and management. Obstet Gynecol. 1997;89(5):807–9.
54. Chen TW-W, Loong HH, Srikanthan A, Zer A, Barua R, Butany J, et al. Primary cardiac sarcomas: a multi-national retrospective review. Cancer Med. 2019;8(1):104–10.
55. Sparrow PJ, Kurian JB, Jones TR, Sivananthan MU. MR imaging of cardiac tumors. Radiographics. 2005;25(5):1255–76.
56. Burke AP, Cowan D, Virmani R. Primary sarcomas of the heart. Cancer. 1992;69(2):387–95.
57. Best AK, Dobson RL, Ahmad AR. Best cases from the AFIP. Radiographics. 2003;23(suppl_1):S141–5.
58. Neragi-Miandoab S, Kim J, Vlahakes GJ. Malignant tumours of the heart: a review of tumour type. Diag Ther Clin Oncol. 2007;19(10):748–56.
59. Burke A. Primary malignant cardiac tumors. Semin Diagn Pathol. 2008;25(1):39–46.
60. Butany J, Yu W. Cardiac angiosarcoma: two cases and a review of the literature. Can J Cardiol. 2000;16(2):197–205.
61. Jellis C, Doyle J, Sutherland T, Gutman J, Mac IA. Cardiac epithelioid leiomyosarcoma and the role of cardiac imaging in the differentiation of intracardiac masses. Clin Cardiol. 2010;33(6):E6–9.
62. Wang J-G, Cui L, Jiang T, Li Y-J, Wei Z-M. Primary cardiac leiomyosarcoma: an analysis of clinical characteristics and outcome patterns. Asian Cardiovasc Thorac Ann. 2015;23(5):623–30.
63. Araoz PA, Eklund HE, Welch TJ, Breen JF. CT and MR imaging of primary cardiac malignancies. Radiographics. 1999;19(6):1421–34.
64. Gilkeson RC, Chiles C. MR evaluation of cardiac and pericardial malignancy. J Magn Reson Imaging. 2003;11(1):173–86.
65. Hwa J, Ward C, Nunn G, Cooper S, Lau K-C, Sholler G. Primary intraventricular cardiac tumors in children: contemporary diagnostic and management options. Pediatr Cardiol. 1994;15(5):233–7.
66. Simsek H, Sahin M, Gumrukcuoglu HA, Tuncer M, Gunes Y. Recurrence of primary cardiac rhabdomyosarcoma without methastasis two years after surgery. Eur J Gen Med. 2012;9(2):146–8.
67. Cresti A, Chiavarelli M, Glauber M, Tanganelli P, Scalese M, Cesareo F, et al. Incidence rate of primary cardiac tumors: a 14-year population study. J Cardiovasc Med. 2016;17(1):37–43.
68. Hudzik B, Miszalski-Jamka K, Glowacki J, Lekston A, Gierlotka M, Zembala M, et al. Malignant tumors of the heart. Cancer Epidemiol. 2015;39(5):665–72.
69. Gruver AM, Huba MA, Dogan A, Hsi ED. Fibrin-associated large B-cell lymphoma: part of the Spectrum of cardiac lymphomas. Am J Surg Pathol. 2012;36(10):1527–37.
70. Travis WD, Brambilla E, Burke AP, Marx A, Nicholson AG. WHO classification of tumours of the lung, pleura, thymus and heart. 4th ed; 2015.
71. Petrich A, Cho SI, Billett H. Primary cardiac lymphoma: an analysis of presentation, treatment, and outcome patterns. Cancer. 2011;117(3):581–9.
72. Lam KY, Dickens P, Chan A. Tumors of the heart. A 20-year experience with a review of 12, 485 consecutive autopsies. Arch Pathol Lab Med. 1993;117(10):1027.
73. Klatt EC, Heitz DR. Cardiac metastases. Cancer. 1990;65(6):1456–9.
74. Bussani R, De-Giorgio F, Abbate A, Silvestri F. Cardiac metastases. J Clin Pathol. 2007;60(1):27–34.

75. Glancy DL, Roberts WC. The heart in malignant melanoma: a study of 70 autopsy cases. Am J Cardiol. 1968;21(4):555–71.

76. Burke A, Tavora F. Hematologic tumors of the heart and pericardium. In: Tumors of the heart and great vessels. Annapolis Junction, MD: American Registry of Pathology; 2015. p. 337–52.

77. Moore JA, DeRan BP, Minor R, Julie A, Fraker TD. Transesophageal echocardiographic evaluation of intracardiac lymphoma. Am Heart J. 1992;124(2):514–6.

78. Goldberg AD, Blankstein R, Padera RF. Tumors metastatic to the heart. Circulation. 2013;128(16):1790–4.

79. Kline IK. Cardiac lymphatic involvement by metastatic tumor. Cancer. 1972;29(3):799–808.

80. Onuigbo WIB. The spread of lung cancer to the heart, pericardium and great vessels. Jpn Heart J. 1974;15(3):234–8.

81. Rusch VW, Asamura H, Watanabe H, Giroux DJ, Rami-Porta R, Goldstraw P. The IASLC lung cancer staging project: a proposal for a new international lymph node map in the forthcoming seventh edition of the TNM classification for lung cancer. J Thorac Oncol. 2009;4(5):568–77.

82. Aagaard CO. Les vaisseaux lymphatiques du cœur chez l'homme et chez quelques mammifières: Illustré par 108 figures originales et 46 autres gravures tous comprises dans le texte. Levin & Munksgaard; French. 1924.

83. Patek PR. The morphology of the lymphactics of the mammalian heart. Am J Anat. 1939;64(2):203–49.

84. Kline I. Lymphatic pathways in the heart. Arch Pathol. 1969;88(6):638–44.

85. Feola M, Merklin R, Cho S, Brockman SK. The terminal pathway of the lymphatic system of the human heart. Ann Thorac Surg. 1977;24(6):531–6.

86. Riquet M, Le Pimpec BF, Souilamas R, Hidden G. Thoracic duct tributaries from intrathoracic organs. Ann Thorac Surg. 2002;73(3):892–8.

87. Eliskova M, Eliska O, Miller AJ. The lymphatic drainage of the parietal pericardium in man. Lymphology. 1995;28(4):208–17.

88. Chareonthaitawee P, Beanlands RS, Chen W, Dorbala S, Miller EJ, Murthy VL, et al. Joint SNMMI–ASNC expert consensus document on the role of 18F-FDG PET/CT in cardiac sarcoid detection and therapy monitoring. J Nucl Med. 2017;58(8):1341–53.

89. Soussan M, Brillet P-Y, Nunes H, Pop G, Ouvrier M-J, Naggara N, et al. Clinical value of a high-fat and low-carbohydrate diet before FDG-PET/CT for evaluation of patients with suspected cardiac sarcoidosis. J Nucl Cardiol. 2013;20(1):120–7.

90. Tang R, Wang JT-Y, Wang L, Le K, Huang Y, Hickey AJ, et al. Impact of patient preparation on the diagnostic performance of 18F-FDG PET in cardiac sarcoidosis: a systematic review and meta-analysis. Clin Nucl Med. 2016;41(7):e327–39.

91. Kassop D, Donovan MS, Cheezum MK, Nguyen BT, Gambill NB, Blankstein R, et al. Cardiac masses on cardiac CT: a review. Curr Cardiovasc Imaging Rep. 2014;7(8):9281.

92. Rahbar K, Seifarth H, Schäfers M, Stegger L, Hoffmeier A, Spieker T, et al. Differentiation of malignant and benign cardiac tumors using 18F-FDG PET/CT. J Nucl Med. 2012;53(6):856–63.

93. Qin C, Shao F, Hu F, Song W, Song Y, Guo J, et al. 18F-FDG PET/CT in diagnostic and prognostic evaluation of patients with cardiac masses: a retrospective study. Eur J Nucl Med Mol Imaging. 2020;47(5):1083–93.

94. Meng J, Zhao H, Liu Y, Chen D, Hacker M, Wei Y, et al. Assessment of cardiac tumors by 18F-FDG PET/CT imaging: histological correlation and clinical outcomes. J Nucl Cardiol. 2020;28(5):2233–43. https://doi.org/10.1007/s12350-019-02022-1.

95. Shao D, Wang S-X, Liang C-H, Gao Q. Differentiation of malignant from benign heart and pericardial lesions using positron emission tomography and computed tomography. J Nucl Cardiol. 2011;18(4):668–77.

96. Kikuchi Y, Oyama-Manabe N, Manabe O, Naya M, Ito YM, Hatanaka KC, et al. Imaging characteristics of cardiac dominant diffuse large B-cell lymphoma demonstrated with MDCT and PET/CT. Eur J Nucl Med Mol Imaging. 2013;40(9):1337–44.

97. Liu E-T, Sun T-T, Dong H-J, Wang S-Y, Chen Z-R, Liu C, et al. Combined PET/CT with thoracic contrast-enhanced CT in assessment of primary cardiac tumors in adult patients. EJNMMI Res. 2020;10(1):1–13.

98. Concetta D'AE, Pasquale P, Giovanni V, Alberto F, Luca B, Ilenia M, et al. Diagnostic accuracy of cardiac computed tomography and 18-F Fluorodeoxyglucose positron emission tomography in cardiac masses. JACC Cardiovasc Imaging. 2020;13(11):2400–11.

99. Chan AT, Josef F, Rocio PJ, Jiwon K, Brouwer LR, John G, et al. Late gadolinium enhancement cardiac magnetic resonance tissue characterization for cancer-associated cardiac masses: metabolic and prognostic manifestations in relation to whole-body positron emission tomography. J Am Heart Assoc. 2019;8(10):e011709.

100. Lemasle M, Badie YL, Cariou E, Fournier P, Porterie J, Rousseau H, et al. Contribution and performance of multimodal imaging in the diagnosis and management of cardiac masses. Int J Cardiovasc Imaging. 2020;36(5):971–81.

101. Zeitouni M, Calais J, Ghodbane W, Ou P, Sannier A, Bouleti C. A cardiac myxoma with intense metabolic activity. Can J Cardiol. 2018;34(1):92.e11–2.

102. Masuda A, Manabe O, Oyama-Manabe N, Naya M, Obara M, Sakakibara M, et al. Cardiac fibroma with high 18F-FDG uptake mimicking malignant tumor. J Nucl Cardiol. 2017;24(1):323–4.

103. Jiang Y, Ma X, Tan Y, Lu Q, Wang Y. Hamartoma of mature cardiac myocytes mimicking malignancy on 18F-FDG PET/CT images. Clin Nucl Med. 2019;44(11):892–4.

104. Bilski M, Kamiński G, Dziuk M. Metabolic activity assessment of cardiac angiosarcoma by 18FDG PET-CT. Nucl Med Rev. 2012;15(1):83–4.

105. Tan H, Jiang L, Gao Y, Zeng Z, Shi H. 18F-FDG PET/CT imaging in primary cardiac angiosarcoma: diagnosis and follow-up. Clin Nucl Med. 2013;38(12):1002–5.

106. Tokmak H, Demir N, Demirkol MO. Cardiac angiosarcoma: utility of [18F] fluorodeoxyglucose positron emission tomography–computed tomography in evaluation of residue, metastases, and treatment response. Vasc Health Risk Manag. 2014;10:399–401.

107. Jain A, Simon S, Elangovan I. 18F-fluorodeoxyglucose positron emission tomography-computed tomography in initial assessment and diagnosis of right atrial angiosarcoma with widespread visceral metastases: a rare case report and review of the literature. Indian J Nucl Med. 2015;30(1):51–4.

108. Liu C, Zhao Y, Yin Z, Hu T, Ren J, Wei J, et al. Right atrial epithelioid angiosarcoma with multiple pulmonary metastasis confirmed by multimodality imaging-guided pulmonary biopsy: a case report and literature review. Medicine (Baltimore). 2018;97(30):e11588.

109. Erdogan EB, Asa S, Aksoy SY, Ozhan M, Halac M. Appearance of recurrent cardiac myxofibrosarcoma on FDG PET/CT. Clin Nucl Med. 2014;39(6):559–60.

110. Taywade SK, Damle NA, Tripathi M, Arun Raj ST, Passah A, Malhi AS, et al. Unusual presentation of rare cardiac tumor: the role of F^{-18}-Fluorodeoxyglucose positron emission tomography/computed tomography. Indian J Nucl Med. 2017;32(2):157–8.

111. Cheng J, Ou X. Prominent bone marrow metastases without concurrent intra-chest metastasis in a case of cardiac Angiosarcoma. Clin Nucl Med. 2020;45(8):638–9.

112. Tripathy S, Tripathi M, Parida GK, Bal C, Shamim SA. Primary cardiac angiosarcoma with extensive visceral metastases: utility of 18F-Fluorodeoxyglucose positron emission tomography-computed tomography in response assessment to Sorafenib. Indian J Nucl Med. 2019;34(3):241–3.

113. Okayama S, Dote Y, Takeda Y, Uemura S, Fujimoto S, Saito Y. Primary cardiac lymphoma: echocardiography and F-18-Fluorodeoxyglucose positron emission tomography in selection of a biopsy site. Echocardiography. 2013;30(1):E13–5.

114. Martineau P, Dilsizian V, Pelletier-Galarneau M. Incremental value of FDG-PET in the evaluation of cardiac masses. Curr Cardiol Rep. 2021;23(7):78.

115. Pollia JA, Gogol LJ. Some notes on malignancies of the heart. Am J Cancer. 1936;27(2):329–33.

116. Scott RW, Garvin CF. Tumors of the heart and pericardium. Am Heart J. 1939;17(4):431–6.

117. Walther H. Krebsmetastasen. Basel: Benno Schwabe; 1948. p. 311.

118. Young J, Goldman IR. Tumor metastasis to the heart. Circulation. 1954;9(2):220–9.

119. Gassman HS, Meadows R, Baker LA. Metastatic tumors of the heart. Am J Med. 1955;19(3):357–65.

120. Hanfling SM. Metastatic cancer to the heart. Circulation. 1960;22(3):474–83.

121. Berge T, Sievers J. Myocardial metastases. A pathological and electrocardiographic study. Br Heart J. 1968;30(3):383.

122. Harrer W. Metastatic tumors involving the heart and pericardium. Pa Med. 1971;74:57–60.

123. Lockwood WB, Broghamer WL. The changing prevalence of secondary cardiac neoplasms as related to cancer therapy. Cancer. 1980;45(10):2659–62.

124. Mukai K, Shinkai T, Tominaga K, Shimosato Y. The incidence of secondary tumors of the heart and pericardium: a 10-year study. Jpn J Clin Oncol. 1988;18(3):195–201.

125. Karwinski B, Svendsen E. Trends in cardiac metastasis. APMIS. 1989;97(7–12):1018–24.

126. Manojlović S. Metastatic carcinomas involving the heart. Review of postmortem examination. Zentralbl Allg Pathol. 1990;136(7–8):657.

127. Mac GW. Metastatic and invasive tumours involving the heart in a geriatric population: a necropsy study. Vichows Archiv A Pathol Anat Histol. 1991;419(3):183–9.

128. Silvestri F, Bussani R, Pavletic N, Mannone T. Metastases of the heart and pericardium. G Ital Cardiol. 1997;27(12):1252.

Matthieu Pelletier-Galarneau, Stephanie Tan, Francois Harel, and Patrick Martineau

Fibrosing Mediastinitis

Fibrosing mediastinitis, also known as sclerosing mediastinitis, is a rare disease characterized by progressive and excessive fibrosis of the mediastinum. Fibrosing mediastinitis typically arises secondary to an infectious or inflammatory pathology. In most cases, fibrosing mediastinitis represents a late complication of an infection by Histoplasma capsulatum, which can be accompanied by an exuberant immune response [1]. Other etiologies of fibrosing mediastinitis have been identified but are thought to be less common with the relative prevalence varying based on geographic location. Infection by Mycobacterium tuberculosis has been identified as a cause of fibrosing mediastinitis and may be more common in areas where tuberculosis is endemic [2]. Noninfectious causes have been reported, including sarcoidosis and mediastinal radiation, and fibrosing mediastinitis has also been associated with immunoglobulin G4-related diseases and vasculitis [2–5]. Clinical presentations are variable and depend on the involved mediastinal structures (Table 11.1). Symptoms, if present, are variable and nonspecific and may include cough, dyspnea, chest pain, face swelling, headaches, dysphagia, odynophagia, etc. The disease typically progresses over the course of several months to years, and symptoms can fluctuate in severity. Treatment typically involves immunosuppressive therapy, and some patients may need surgical intervention to address the complications of the disease.

On CT, fibrosing mediastinitis can have a focal or diffuse appearance [6]. In its more common focal form (82% of cases), fibrosing mediastinitis appears as infiltrative soft tissue limited to a single mediastinal compartment (Fig. 11.1). It is typically found in the middle mediastinal compartment, in the right paratracheal, subcarinal, or hilar region. Stippled or gross calcifications can often be found within these infiltrative areas. In its diffuse form, the soft tissue infiltration

Table 11.1 Sites of fibrosing mediastinitis and associated clinical presentation

Pulmonary vessels	Pulmonary hypertension Pulmonary infarct
Great vessels	Superior vena cava syndrome
Pleura	Constrictive pericarditis Chylothorax
Airways	Pneumonia Atelectasis
Esophagus	Esophageal compression

M. Pelletier-Galarneau (✉) · S. Tan · F. Harel
Montreal Heart Institute, Montréal, QC, Canada
e-mail: Matthieu.pelletier-galarneau@icm-mhi.org

P. Martineau
BC Cancer, Vancouver, BC, Canada
e-mail: patrick.martineau@bccancer.bc.ca

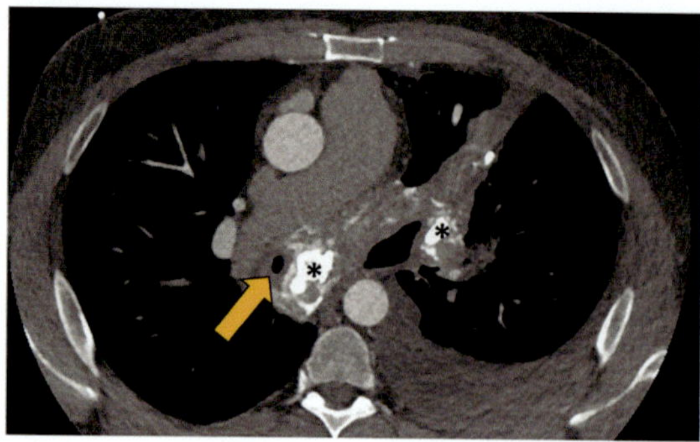 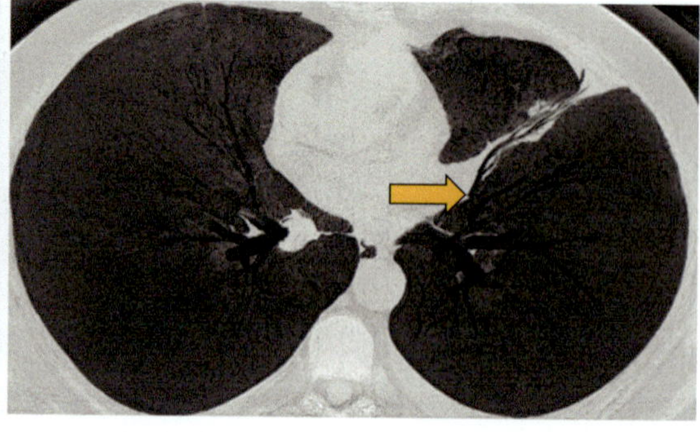

Fig. 11.1 Focal fibrosing mediastinitis. Axial image of a chest CT (left) demonstrates a middle mediastinal tissue infiltrate with calcifications (*). There is encasement of the bronchus intermedius (arrow). Minimal intensity projection (MinIP) axial image (right) shows severe narrowing of the lingular bronchus (arrow) with associated distal atelectasis

involves more than one mediastinal compartment and rarely calcifies.

Fibrosing mediastinitis can encase or invade mediastinal structures. This can cause vessels and airways to narrow [7]. Pulmonary opacities may appear as a result of atelectasis or pneumonia from narrowed airways or pulmonary infarcts from pulmonary vessel occlusion. When fibrosing mediastinitis involves the pericardium, there can be thickening (>4 mm) and calcifications of the pericardium, which can lead to constrictive pericarditis with small cone-shaped ventricles and enlarged atria, as well as septal flattening [8]. Calcified pulmonary, liver or splenic granulomas, or calcified lymph nodes are suggestive of prior histoplasmosis infection and can support the diagnosis of fibrosing mediastinitis [8].

On MRI, soft tissue infiltration related to fibrosing mediastinitis typically shows a signal iso-intense to muscles on T1-weighted images, variable signal on T2-weighted images depending on the degree of fibrosis and inflammation, and heterogeneous enhancement on postcontrast sequences [9]. Calcifications are more difficult to recognize on MRI than on computed tomography because of variable signal intensities and occasionally small size. Usually, calcifications present as hypointense foci on all sequences, but are best confirmed on radiograph or computed tomography [10].

On FDG-PET, fibrosing mediastinitis often represents an incidental finding in the evaluation of patients with suspected neoplasia or other inflammatory or immune pathologies [11].

Fibrosing mediastinitis may present as a hypermetabolic, aggressive-appearing lesion and may be indistinguishable from a neoplastic process (Fig. 11.2). The presence of calcification may suggest a diagnosis of fibrosing mediastinitis in the appropriate clinical setting. Nonetheless, tissue sampling may be required to confirm the diagnosis.

FDG-PET imaging has been proven useful in the assessment of various granulomatous diseases and atypical infections such as sarcoidosis, histoplasmosis, and tuberculosis, by differentiating between active and quiescent disease [12–14]. FDG-PET may play a similar role in the evaluation of patients with fibrosing mediastinitis. However, given the low incidence of the disease, the literature to date is limited to case reports and case series. Ikeda et al. reported the case of a patient with fibrosing mediastinitis causing stricture of the left common carotid artery [15]. On the baseline study, increased FDG uptake was observed in the affected areas while on the follow up scan, following successful immunosuppressive therapy with steroids, the abnormal uptake had resolved completely. Similarly, Takalkar et al. reported a case of a patient with dysphagia, chest pain, and chronic cough, suffering from fibrosing mediastinitis and demonstrating intense FDG uptake in the involved area as confirmed by biopsy [16]. On scans following immunosuppressive therapy, the abnormal uptake resolved significantly. Similar results were reported in a small case series of three patients with fibrosing mediastinitis follow-

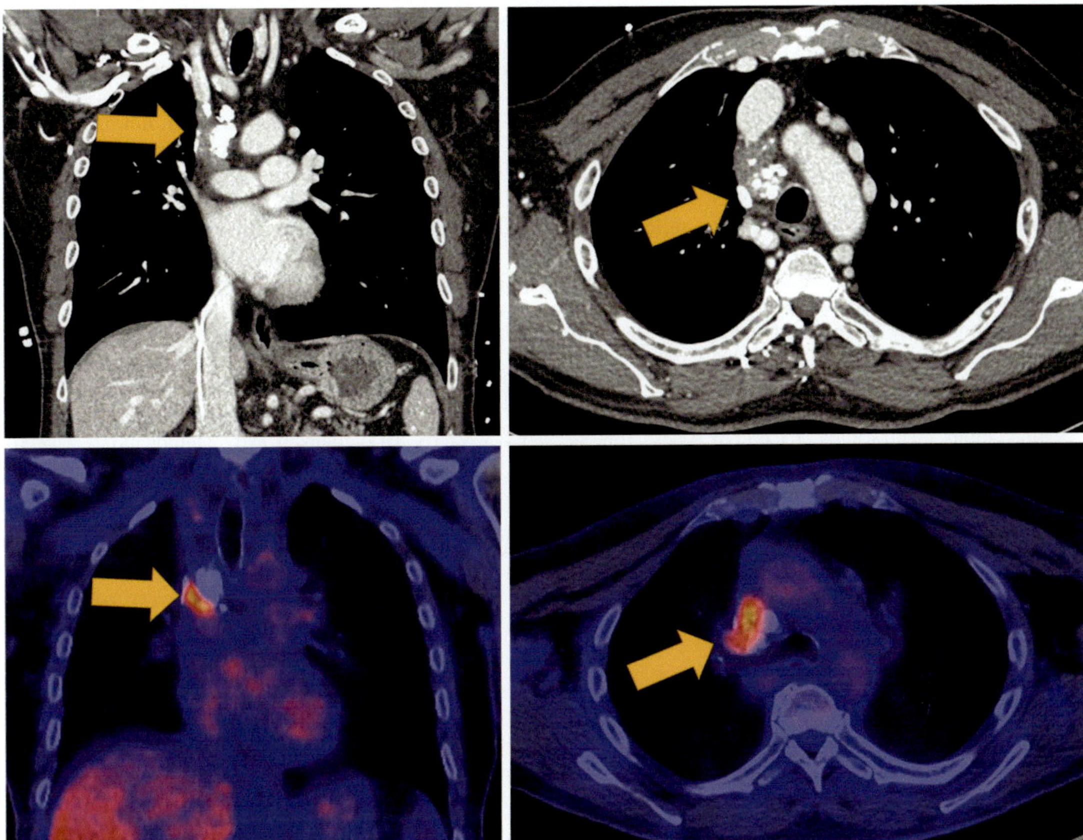

Fig. 11.2 A 71-year-old male with fibrosing mediastinitis. Coronal and axial enhanced CT images (top row) reveal a partially calcified fibrous lesion in the right superior paratracheal region, with obstruction of the superior vena cava (arrow), and extensive collateral venous network (not shown). Corresponding coronal and axial FDG-PET/CT images (bottom rows) reveal moderately increased uptake corresponding to the noncalcified portion of the lesion

ing rituxumab therapy [17]. In another case report, Chong et al. [18] reported a case of quiescent fibrosing mediastinitis which demonstrated no significant FDG uptake. Imran et al. reported the case of a patient with no significant uptake on an initial PET scan, while the disease was quiescent [19]. On a follow-up study, abnormal uptake was seen in a superior mediastinal mass. In that case, uptake intensity appeared to correlate with disease severity. While the evidence supporting the use of FDG-PET in this context remains scant, these reports suggest that there may be a correlation between disease stage and FDG avidity and that FDG could potentially be used to assess response to therapy and progression potential.

References

1. Loyd JE, Tillman BF, Atkinson JB, Des Prez RM. Mediastinal fibrosis complicating histoplasmosis. Medicine (Baltimore). 1988;67(5):295–310.
2. Seferian A, Steriade A, Jaïs X, Planché O, Savale L, Parent F, et al. Pulmonary hypertension complicating fibrosing mediastinitis. Medicine (Baltimore). 2015;94(44):e1800.
3. Rossi GM, Emmi G, Corradi D, Urban ML, Maritati F, Landini F, et al. Idiopathic mediastinal fibrosis: a systemic immune-mediated disorder. A case series and a review of the literature. Clin Rev Allergy Immunol. 2017;52(3):446–59.
4. Morrone N, Gama e Silva Volpe VL, Dourado AM, Mitre F, Coletta EN. Bilateral pleural effusion due to mediastinal fibrosis induced by radiotherapy. Chest. 1993;104(4):1276–8.

5. Hage CA, Azar MM, Bahr N, Loyd J, Wheat LJ. Histoplasmosis: up-to-date evidence-based approach to diagnosis and management. Semin Respir Crit Care Med. 2015;36(5):729–45.
6. Sherrick AD, Brown LR, Harms GF, Myers JL. The radiographic findings of fibrosing mediastinitis. Chest. 1994;106(2):484–9.
7. Weinstein J, Aronberg D, Sagel S. CT of fibrosing mediastinitis: findings and their utility. Am J Roentgenol. 1983;141(2):247–51.
8. Garrana SH, Buckley JR, Rosado-de-Christenson ML, Martínez-Jiménez S, Muñoz P, Borsa JJ. Multimodality imaging of focal and diffuse fibrosing mediastinitis. Radiographics. 2019;39(3):651–67.
9. Kushihashi T, Munechika H, Motoya H, Hamada K, Satoh I, Naitoh H, et al. CT and MR findings in tuberculous mediastinitis. J Comput Assist Tomogr. 1995;19(3):379–82.
10. Akman C, Kantarci F, Cetinkaya S. Imaging in mediastinitis: a systematic review based on aetiology. Clin Radiol. 2004;59(7):573–85.
11. Kan Y, Yuan L, Wang W, Yang J. Unexpected Fibrosing Mediastinitis Shown on FDG PET/CT in a Patient With IgG4-Related Disease. Clin Nucl Med. 2017;42:818–19.
12. Sharma P, Mukherjee A, Karunanithi S, Bal C, Kumar R. Potential role of 18F-FDG PET/CT in patients with fungal infections. Am J Roentgenol. 2014;203(1):180–9.
13. Pelletier-Galarneau M, Martineau P, Zuckier LS, Pham X, Lambert R, Turpin S. 18F-FDG-PET/CT imaging of thoracic and extrathoracic tuberculosis in children. Semin Nucl Med. 2017;47(3):304–18.
14. Martineau P, Pelletier-Galarneau M, Juneau D, Leung E, Birnie D, Beanlands RSB. Molecular imaging of cardiac sarcoidosis. Curr Cardiovasc Imaging Rep. 2018;11(3):6–17.
15. Ikeda K, Nomori H, Mori T, Kobayashi H, Iwatani K, Yoshimoto K, et al. Successful steroid treatment for fibrosing mediastinitis and Sclerosing cervicitis. Ann Thorac Surg. 2007;83(3):1199–201.
16. Takalkar AM, Bruno GL, Makanjoula AJ, El-Haddad G, Lilien DL, Payne DK. A potential role for F-18 FDG PET/CT in evaluation and management of fibrosing mediastinitis. Clin Nucl Med. 2007;32(9):703–6.
17. Westerly BD, Johnson GB, Maldonado F, Utz JP, Specks U, Peikert T. Targeting B lymphocytes in progressive fibrosing mediastinitis. Am J Respir Crit Care Med. 2014;190(9):1069–71.
18. Chong S, Kim TS, Kim B-T, Cho EY. Fibrosing mediastinitis mimicking malignancy at CT: negative FDG uptake in integrated FDG PET/CT imaging. Eur Radiol. 2007;17(6):1644–6.
19. Imran MB, Kubota K, Yoshioka S, Yamada S, Sato T, Fukuda H, et al. Sclerosing mediastinitis: findings on Fluorine-18 Fluorodeoxyglucose positron emission tomography. Clin Nucl Med. 1999;24(5):305–8.

Part III

Cardiovascular Infections

Martina Sollini, Francesco Bartoli, Roberta Zanca, Enrica Esposito, Elena Lazzeri, Riemer H. J. A. Slart, and Paola Anna Erba

Epidemiology, Microbiology, and Pathophysiology of PVE

Cardiovascular infections are a heterogenous group of conditions that can affect various components of the native structure of the heart (pericardium, muscle, endocardium, valves, autonomic nerves, and the vessels) as well as implanted devices such as valve prostheses (all types of prosthetic valves, annuloplasty rings, intracardiac patches, and shunts), cardiovascular implantable electronic devices (CIED), left ventricular assist device catheters, and vascular grafts. The increased use of implantable devices and surgical biomaterials during the last decades have resulted in an increase in related infections as well as associated complications. For example, the expected number of heart valve interventions is estimated to reach more than 800,000 annual procedures worldwide by 2050 [1]. Healthcare-associated infections are the most common non-cardiac complication following cardiac surgery and device implantation affecting about 1.7 million patients each year and associated with nearly 100,000 deaths in the US alone [2, 3].

Infective endocarditis (IE) is a severe disease associated with high morbidity and mortality and whose incidence and severity have remained unchanged or even increased, despite improvements in diagnostic and therapeutic strategies [4, 5]. Recent data such as from the EuroEndo registry, the most comprehensive and far-reaching observational international study involving a cohort of 3116 adult with IE recruited between January 2016 and March 2018 in 40 countries, showed that in-hospital mortality remains very high—around 17.1% of patients—and was more frequent in prosthetic valve endocarditis (PVE). Independent predictors of mortality were the Charlson index, creatinine >2 mg/dL, congestive heart failure, vegetation length >10 mm, cerebral complications, abscess, and failure to undertake surgery when indicated [6].

M. Sollini · R. Zanca
Department of Biomedical Sciences, Humanitas University, Pieve Emanuele (Milan), Italy

F. Bartoli · E. Esposito · E. Lazzeri
Department of Translational Research and Advanced Technologies in Medicine, Regional Center of Nuclear Medicine, University of Pisa, Pisa, Italy

Riemer H. J. A. Slart
University Medical Center Groningen, Medical Imaging Center, University of Groningen, Groningen, The Netherlands

Biomedical Photonic Imaging Group, Faculty of Science and Technology, University of Twente, Enschede, The Netherlands

P. A. Erba (✉)
Department of Translational Research and Advanced Technologies in Medicine, Regional Center of Nuclear Medicine, University of Pisa, Pisa, Italy

University Medical Center Groningen, Medical Imaging Center, University of Groningen, Groningen, The Netherlands
e-mail: p.erba@med.unipi.it

© The Author(s), under exclusive license to Springer Nature Switzerland AG 2022
M. Pelletier-Galarneau, P. Martineau (eds.), *FDG-PET/CT and PET/MR in Cardiovascular Diseases*, https://doi.org/10.1007/978-3-031-09807-9_12

PVE accounts for 20% of all cases of endocarditis and occurs in up to 6% of patients with a prosthetic valve [7]. The frequency of PVE in the EuroEndo registry is also increasing, accounting for 30% of cases [6] as compared to the 26% of cases in the EuroHeart survey [8], 25% in the 2008 French registry [9], and 21% in the International Collaboration on Endocarditis-Prospective Cohort Study reported in 2009 [10].

The epidemiology of aortic PVE is different in patients with surgical aortic valve replacement (SAVR) versus transcatheter aortic valve replacement (TAVR). In SAVR, the incidence of PVE is about 6 per 1000 cases [11] with higher infection rates in cases of bioprosthetic compared to mechanical valves [12]. In TAVR, the incidence rate of PVE is similar to patients with bioprosthetic SAVR [13]. However, TAVR is increasingly being used, and the number of post-TAVR IE is also expected to rise [14]. A major problem with post-TAVR IE is that SAVR is often required to replace the infected valve. However, TAVR patients are often elderly and with more comorbidities, rendering them inoperable or at high risk, thus resulting in a general worst prognosis [15]. In addition, the leaflets of transcatheter valve prostheses contain a greater quantity of metal in the stent frame in contrast to the surgical valves, leading to significant changes in the outcome and management of IE [16].

Early SAVR PVE is typically the result of peri-procedural bacterial contamination of the prosthetic valve, often secondary to seeding from a distant focus of infection such as a catheter or wound infection [17]. In the first days following valve implantation organisms have direct access to the prothesis–annulus interface and the tissue along the sutures in the paravalvular area. They can easily adhere to the fibrinogen and fibronectin in the paravalvular area, resulting in the formation of abscesses. *Staphylococcus aureus*, *Staphylococcus epidermidis*, Gram-negative bacteria, and fungi are the most frequent isolated microorganisms. Staphylococci and streptococci have a penchant for transcatheter valves. Interestingly, in TAVR PVE, enterococci have also been a prominent causative agent in the peri-procedural period [16], likely related to the femoral access in the groin.

Data from the EuroEndo registry confirmed that the microorganisms most often identified were staphylococci (44.1%), oral streptococci (12.3%), enterococci (15.8%), and *Streptococcus gallolyticus* (6.6%). Finally, the number of culture-negative IE observed in the EuroEndo registry (21%) was higher than those previously reported; 14% and 11% observed in the 2002 French survey [9] and 2009 International Collaboration on Endocarditis Prospective Cohort Study [10], respectively.

Late-onset PVE acquired in the community is usually caused by endogenous microbiota organisms also seen in native valve endocarditis, such as streptococci, staphylococci, and enterococci. The prostheses do not allow the organism to adhere to leaflets in the absence of thrombotic material. The sewing ring and sutures become endothelialized a few months after the valve implementation. Alterations in the valve and the paravalvular surface can lead to the formation of microthrombi, to which bacterial organisms can adhere, multiply, and cause an infection [18].

The severity of PVE infection depends upon several factors including the involved microorganism, the maturity of the biofilm developed on the device, the location and type of the biomaterial, and the host defence status [19, 20]. The presence of a biofilm, a community of adherent microorganisms embedded within a self-produced matrix of extracellular polymeric substances, provides a physical barrier leading to antibiotic resistance and host phagocytic defences. Therefore, the only strategy to effectively eradicate the infection is often surgical removal of the infected device.

PVE cannot be diagnosed from a single symptom, sign, or diagnostic test. The heterogeneity of clinical presentations makes a multidisciplinary team approach integrating diagnostic criteria necessary. Microbiology and imaging are currently the benchmarks for a prompt and accurate diagnosis. The standard microbiological investigation includes microorganism identification, and antibiotic susceptibility tests for treatment guidance. Blood culture is the most important initial laboratory test. If antibiotic therapy has been administered prior to the collection of blood cultures, the rate of positive cultures declines, reducing the sensitivity of the diagnostic criteria [21]. Multimodality imaging, including molecular hybrid imaging techniques, is widely used in conjunction with traditional diagnostic criteria.

In this chapter, we will focus on the use of ^{18}F-fluorodeoxyglucose-positron emission tomography/computed tomography (FDG-PET/CT) in PVE. In addition, we will give some insight into recent new developments that might be of particular interest for this field.

Diagnostic Workout

Evidence of valve or intracardiac material involvement on imaging is a major diagnostic criterion of PVE, with echocardiography (ECHO) representing the first-line imaging method. However, it is well known that ECHO has several limitations [22] and other imaging modalities such as CT,

MR, and nuclear imaging have progressively been shown to be useful to demonstrate both valve involvement and the presence of IE-related peripheral complications (metastatic infection and septic embolism), as well as occult predisposing lesions that may be the source of infection. Hybrid imaging combining anatomical imaging and metabolic information as in PET/CT or SPECT/CT has been shown to be particularly useful in the presence of implantable/prosthetic material [23, 24]. Therefore, these techniques have been gradually included in the global assessment of patients with suspected IE, and the 2015 ESC guidelines [25] and the American Heart Association (AHA) 2020 guidelines for the management of patients with valvular heart disease [26] which also recognize the value of the multimodality approach and the importance of team work in the assessment of patients with IE.

Figure 12.1 presents the diagnostic algorithm currently used at our centre. ECHO is the first-

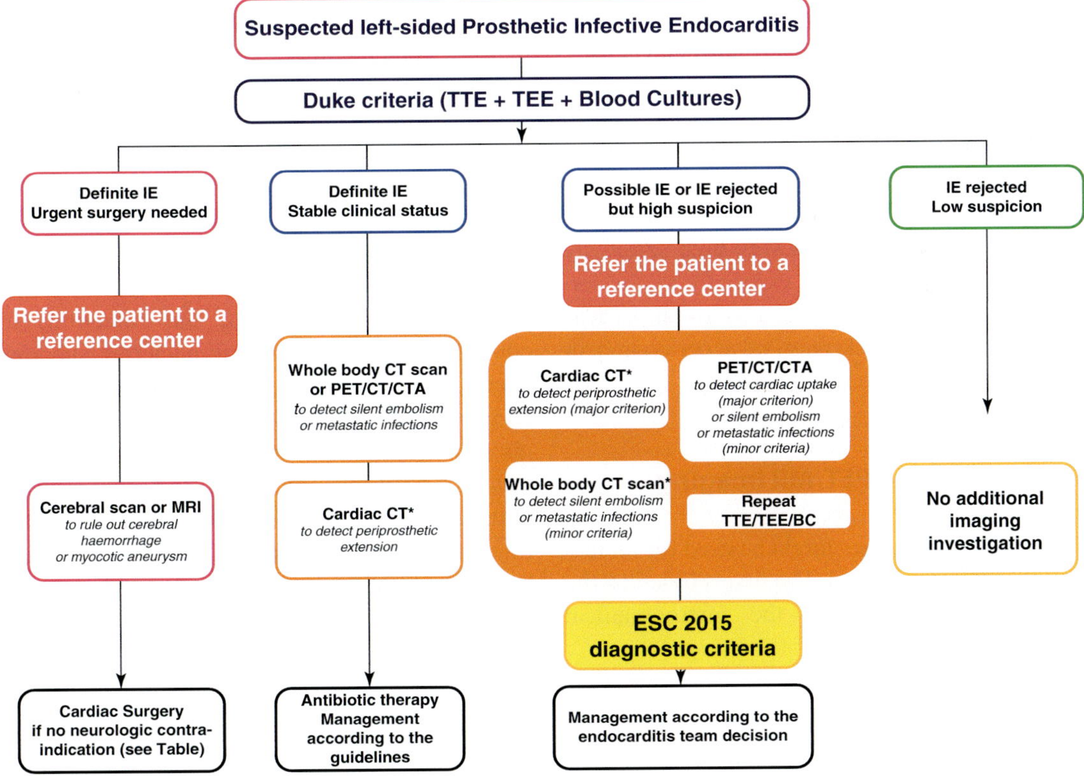

Fig. 12.1 Diagnosis algorithm in suspected prosthetic valve infective endocarditis, reprint with permission from Erba et al. [22]. * If contrast-agent injection is not contra-indicated

line imaging modality performed in suspected IE [22]. Both transthoracic (TTE) and transoesophageal (TEE) echocardiography should be performed [27], with TEE allowing a better evaluation in several situations where TTE has a limited sensitivity [28], such as prosthetic valve IE small vegetations, and in the presence of perivalvular abscess [29]. ECHO is of major importance for the diagnosis of IE, the assessment of the severity of the disease, providing prognostic data including embolic risk, and patient follow-up assessments. The typical ECHO findings in PVE are vegetations and perivalvular complications such as abscess, pseudoaneurysm, new dehiscence of a prosthetic valve, intracardiac fistula, and valve perforation or aneurysm [25]. ECHO is also useful in predicting embolic events, with the size and mobility of vegetations being the stronger predictors of embolic events [30].

In cases of suspected PVE, abnormal uptake at the site of the prosthetic valve on FDG-PET/CT or WBC SPECT/CT is considered a major criterion. Identification on imaging of recent embolic events or infectious aneurysms (silent events) is considered as a minor criterion. The identification of paravalvular lesions by cardiac CT is also a major criterion of the ESC 2015 diagnostic criteria. In fact, ECG-gated cardiac CT (A) enables assessment of both the valve and perivalvular IE lesions with the ability to detect perivalvular lesions (abscesses and pseudoaneurysms) with very high sensitivity and specificity (>95%) [31], especially for the aortic valve [32]. Detection of valvular lesions such as vegetations, leaflet thickening, valve perforation, or valve aneurysm is also feasible [31].

FDG PET/CT and PET/MR Imaging

Two different strategies might be used for molecular imaging of infection. The first is based on the use of agents targeting the microorganism responsible for the infection while the second targets components of the pathophysiological changes of the inflammatory process and/or the host response to the infectious pathogen. FDG is actively incorporated by inflammatory cells (i.e., activated leukocytes, monocyte-macrophages, and CD4+ T-lymphocytes) at the sites of infection due to their overexpression of glucose transporters. FDG-PET/CT in PVE is generally performed using a single acquisition time point (generally at 45–60 min) after the administration of FDG (Fig. 12.2). Advantages of FDG-PET/CT over other nuclear imaging modalities, such as radiolabelled WBC, are the lack of blood handling, a shorter study time that allows the conclusion of the scan within 1–2 h after tracer administration (excluding preparation time), and high target-to-background ratio and higher image resolution.

FDG-PET/CT and PET/MR have an increasingly relevant role in cardiovascular infections and inflammation imaging. They can be used throughout the disease course for different purposes (Fig. 12.3). In the very early phase of the disease, bacteraemia might result in the microorganism adhering to native and/or prosthetic valves. At this stage, the main manifestations of the disease are local as a direct consequence of the vegetation formation. In this phase, ECHO is very useful for identifying valvular abnormalities and early vegetation development. Based on their ability to directly identify the microorganisms sustaining the infection, it could be hypothesized that bacterial specific agents might be the radiopharmaceutical of choice for this early disease phase. At a later phase, once the host immune response to infections has been activated, WBC and other inflammatory cells are recruited at the vegetation site, imaging using radiolabelled WBC and FDG has become effective for detecting local disease extension and/or complication as well as for

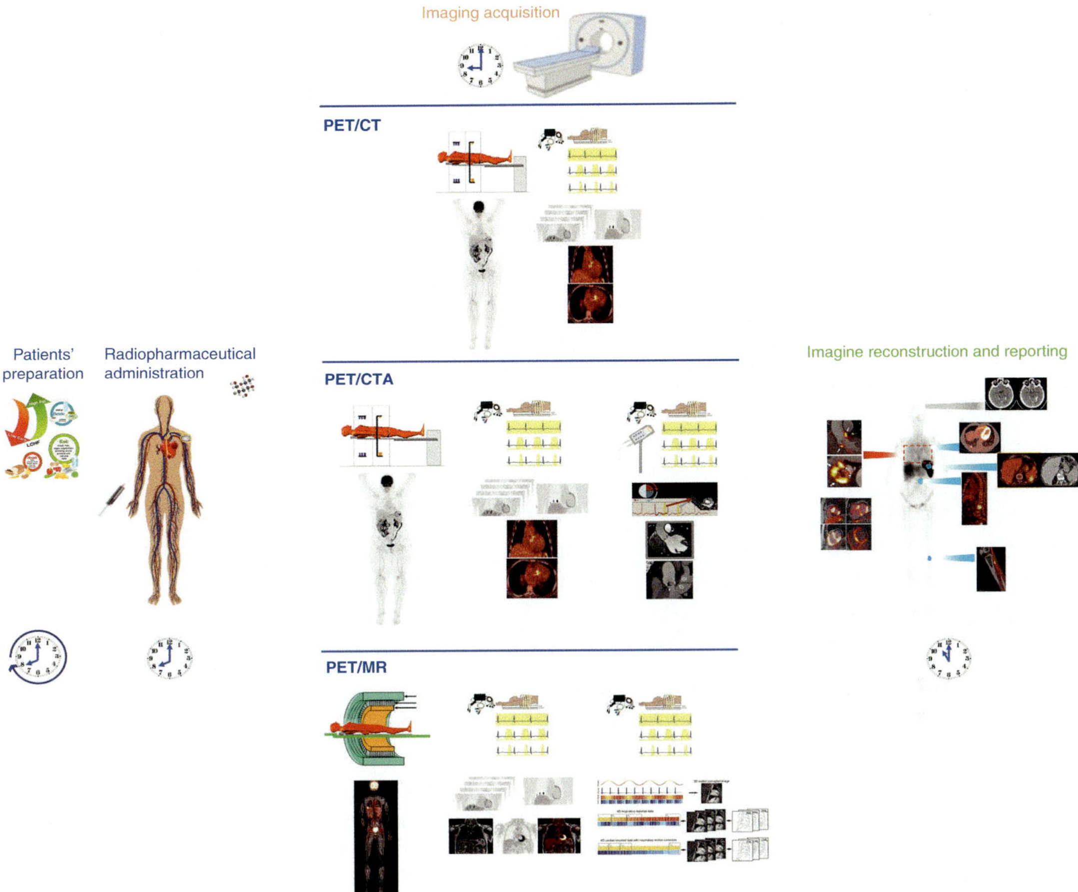

Fig. 12.2 Schematic summary of the use of FDG-PET/CT(A) and PET/MR in the context of cardiovascular infections. First in the right panel, the patient should be properly prepared by at least 24 h of high-fat-low-carb diet followed by 12 h fasting before the radiopharmaceutical administration. After about 1 h, the patient is imaged according to the specific protocol (middle panel, upper row PET/CT, middle row PET/CTA, and lower panel PET/MR). Finally, the images are reconstructed, reoriented, and assessed for the presence of uptake at the valve and extracardiac disease involvement, as in case of septic embolisms, metastatic sites of infection and the portal of entry or alternative source of infections (left panel)

identifying systemic manifestation of the disease caused by embolic detachment from the vegetation/valve. PET/MR, an exciting novel hybrid imaging tool which can assess disease activity together with cardiac anatomy, function, and tissue composition has not been evaluated yet in the context of PVE except in an anecdotal case (Fig. 12.4) [33, 34].

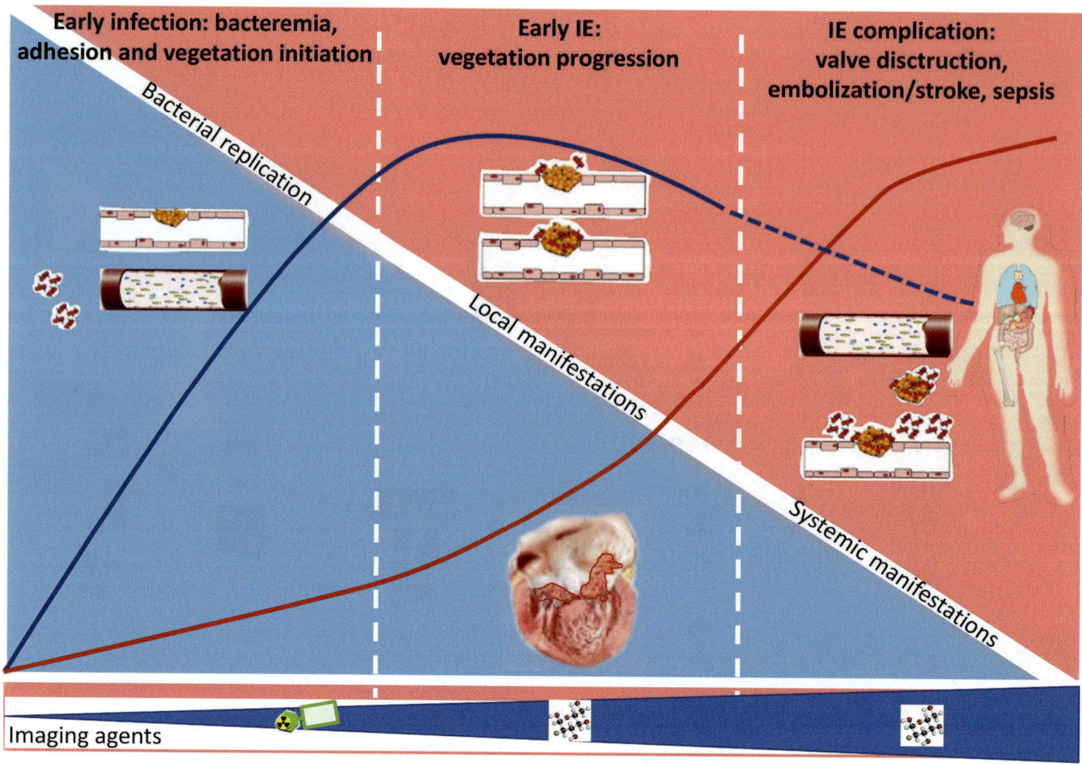

Fig. 12.3 Schematic representation of IE pathogenesis from the microorganism entrance and subsequent heart native valve/prosthetic valve adhesion to local and systemic manifestations of the disease. In the lower panel, the type of radiopharmaceutical agents to be used in relation to the different disease phase: bacterial specific agents potentially leading to early diagnosis or agents identifying the host immune response to infections such as WBC imaging and FDG. The blue curve indicates the intensity of the local infection burden while the red curve the intensity of systemic infection

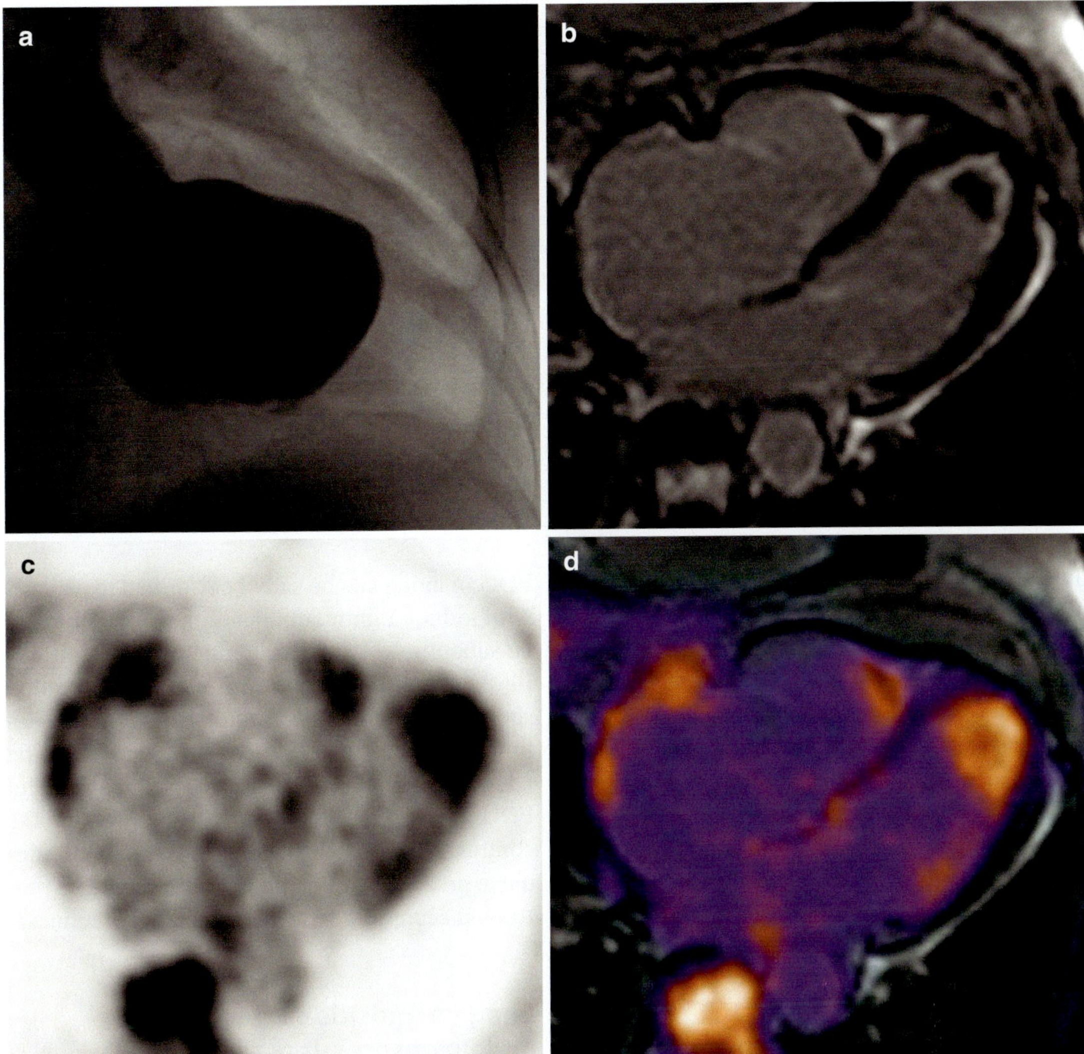

Fig. 12.4 FDG PET/MR images in a case of Loeffler endocarditis. (**a**) Left ventriculography showing thickening of the apical endocardium of the left ventricle. (**b**) Magnetic resonance imaging in four-chamber orientation depicting late gadolinium contrast-enhanced (LGE) lesions restricted circumferentially to the endocardium within the apical region of both ventricles in contrast to an apical mass in the left and right ventricle without LGE. (**c**) FDG-PET in four-chamber orientation demonstrating significant FDG uptake within the whole-apical region of both ventricles. (**d**) Superimposed MRI and FDG-PET in four-chamber orientation, confirming FDG uptake not only in the LGE region but particularly within the apical mass of both ventricles identifying the presence of active inflammatory tissue. (Reprinted from Langwieser et al. [34])

Specific Technical Considerations

For an optimal test, special attention must be paid to the patients' preparation, the imaging protocol, and the study interpretation. An extensive review of the main critical technical issues is provided in the "Recommendation on nuclear and multi-modality imaging in IE and CIED Infections" and in the "EANM Procedural recommendations of cardiac PET/CT imaging standardization in inflammatory-, infective-, infiltrative-, and innervation (4Is)-related cardiovascular diseases: a joint collaboration of the EACVI and the EANM" [35].

Patient Preparation

Patient preparation is very important to reduce the physiological uptake of FDG of the myocardium (see Chap. 4). There is a general agreement to use patient preparation protocols including a high-fat diet lacking carbohydrates for 12–24 h prior to the scan combined with a prolonged fasting period of 12–18 h, with or without the use of intravenous heparin of 50 IU/kg approximately 15 min prior to FDG injection [36–38]. In addition, strenuous exercise should be avoided for at least 12 h prior to the exam. Following FDG injection, and before images are obtained, the patient should continue to fast and should refrain from any physical activity, as both will enhance myocardial glucose uptake. Hyperglycaemia does not represent an absolute contraindication to performing the study [39]. In fact, a study by Rabkin et al. demonstrated that neither diabetes nor hyperglycaemia at the time of the study had a significant effect on the false-negative rate in infection and inflammation imaging [40]. FDG should be injected no sooner than 4 h after subcutaneous injection of rapid-acting insulin or 6 h after subcutaneous injection of short-acting insulin. FDG administration is not recommended on the same day after the injection of intermediate-acting and/or long-acting insulin [41].

Radiopharmaceutical: Administered Activity

The administered activity can vary based on the type of PET scanner used and acquisition duration. The EANM guidelines on FDG-PET imaging in inflammation/infection suggest an administered activity of 2.5–5.0 MBq/kg, which represents 175–350 MBq or 4.7–9.5 mCi for a 70-kg standard adult. In the USA, the recommended FDG administered activity is 370–740 MBq (10–20 mCi) for adults and 3.7–5.2 MBq/kg (0.10–0.14 mCi/kg) for children [39].

Concomitant Treatments

Although antimicrobial treatment for cardiac infection is expected to decrease the intensity of inflammation and therefore FDG accumulation [42], there is currently no evidence to routinely recommend treatment discontinuation before performing PET/CT. The risk of false-negative FDG-PET scans is probably the lowest if the patients are imaged when their CRP is >40 mg/L [43]. This contrasts with inflammatory disorders such as large vessel vasculitis where treatment with steroids can lead to false-negative results [44].

Other Special Considerations

FDG imaging can be safely performed in patients with kidney failure, although image quality may be suboptimal and prone to interpretation pitfalls [45]. Creatinine and/or glomerular filtration should be evaluated, according to national guidelines, if intravenous contrast agents will be administered. If renal function is impaired and FDG-PET/CT examination with intravenous CT contrast agent is deemed necessary, then adequate prevention of nephrotoxicity should be performed according to local or society guidelines.

Image Acquisition Protocol and Postprocessing

Image acquisition generally starts 45–60 min following radiotracer administration, and acquisition duration depends on the sensitivity of the scanner and administered dose. The time interval between FDG injection and scanning is critical if semiquantification using SUV is intended, but less important for visual reading only. Although the recommended interval is 60–90 min for cardiovascular imaging (similar to tumour imaging), 120–180 min is sometimes applied to help assess inflammatory activity in the vascular wall and left ventricle due to lower background activity in the blood pool [39, 46, 47], but these extended time intervals could be less effective in infection detection [48].

A specific acquisition protocol is used for IE imaging. First, a total body acquisition with a field of view extending from skull base to mid thighs is performed. Imaging of the lower limbs and brain can also be considered. Total body FDG-PET imaging is particularly useful in patients with suspected systemic involvement and can identify septic emboli, mycotic aneurysms, and the portal of entry (POE). This first acquisition can be ECG-gated and include a prolonged acquisition of the cardiac region, which can be separately reconstructed to improve evaluation of the heart. A separate and dedicated cardiac bed ECG-gated acquisition may improve image quality, particularly in coronary atherosclerosis assessment and PVE, but supporting literature is scarce [49]. A respiration-averaged low-dose CT can be considered for attenuation correction of the thorax, as this will likely give better alignment between PET and CT over the heart. Otherwise, the recommendations for low-dose CT attenuation correction for tumour imaging with FDG can be followed.

Diagnostic CT angiography (CTA) scan might also be performed, to maximize the diagnostic information provided by the exam. The technical requirements for performing PET/CTA with a hybrid PET/CT scanner are cardiac gating for both techniques and at least a 64-detector row CT. For the evaluation of left-sided PVE, an arterial phase ECG-gated CTA must be performed. When PET/CTA is performed to diagnose device infection, a prospective, ECG-gated, venous phase CTA sequence is recommended to evaluate local soft tissue changes, lead vegetation, and venous thrombosis of the vascular accesses [35]. The routine iodinated contrast injection protocol should be adjusted individually to the patient's body mass index and the scan duration. A typical injection consists of 50–120 mL of isomolar iodinated contrast medium at a flow rate of 4–7 mL/s, followed by a 30–50-mL saline chaser [50]. Optional is the use of diluted contrast which may help define the four heart chambers and make anatomic localization of endocarditis easier (triphasic contrast administration for better delineation of the right and left cardiac chambers).

Medication potentially interacting with intravenous contrast agents (e.g., metformin) and relevant medical history (e.g., compromised renal function) should be taken into consideration. Renal function should generally be assessed in this group of patients before administration of contrast agents because of possible nephrotoxicity. Patients with a higher risk of contrast agent-induced nephrotoxicity include those with an eGFR < 30 mL/min/1.73 m^2 [51]. Furthermore, attention must be paid to patients with a history of previous contrast agent hypersensitivity reactions. Premedication with glucocorticoids and H1- and H2-blockers reduce the risk of an anaphylactic reaction, but unenhanced CT should generally be performed in patients with a known severe contrast reaction.

In cases of IE and CIED infection, combining FDG-PET with CTA is helpful in the identification of a larger number of anatomic lesions and in reducing the number of equivocal scans [52, 53]. CTA can help in the diagnosis of pseudoaneurysm, fistulas, and abscesses associated with infected valves and for the accurate assessment of valve prostheses. CTA is especially useful in patients with aortic grafts, or congenital heart diseases and complex anatomy. Another advantage is that in case of aortic valve IE, CTA can provide useful information about the anatomy of the valve, such as the size or extent of any calcification of the valve and ascending aorta, as it can also differentiate between pannus vs. thrombus/vegetation in case of elevated transvalvular pressure gradients. This information is important for a proper surgical management.

The protocol for cardiac PET/MR in IE requires the acquisition of MR attenuation correction sequences, total body PET, followed by an ECG-gated cardiac PET including the area from the aortic arch to the upper border of the diaphragm (12 cm, with an approximate duration of 30 min). Multiparametric MR sequences are performed simultaneously with PET with different sequences possible such as cine sequences, T1- or T2-weighted turbo spin echo, perfusion, and valvular phase contrast sequences. In case of contrast use, short-axis delayed-enhancement sequences at 10 min following contrast agent injection, with coverage from the base to apex of the heart. Figure 12.2 shows a schematic summary of the FDG-PET/CT, PET/CTA and PET/MR protocol generally used for imaging patients with PVE.

Image Reconstruction

Image reconstruction with and without attenuation correction is recommended to identify potential reconstruction artefacts. Metal artefact reduction techniques are useful to minimize overcorrection. In general, images should be reconstructed according to the guidelines for tumour imaging with FDG-PET/CT [35], using iterative reconstruction with a product of subsets and iterations between 40 and 60. Use of TOF and resolution recovery is recommended as it has been shown to improve disease detectability in cardiac PET [54]. All corrections necessary to obtain quantitative images should be applied during the reconstruction. More advanced image reconstruction methods, such as penalized reconstruction, are possible; however, the use of these methods is rather limited to visual assessment and should not be used interchangeably with regular iterative reconstruction methods [55].

Image Quality Assessment

Image quality should be assessed as suggested in the procedural recommendations of cardiac PET/CT imaging [35] as follows: overall quality (good, average, low), motion artefacts, abnormal biodistribution, quality of FDG suppression in the myocardium (full suppression, partial suppression, unsuppressed). In particular, the proper suppression of FDG signal in the myocardium should be considered before reporting. Physiological myocardial FDG uptake usually occurs in a diffuse intense pattern across the myocardium but can also demonstrate regional variation. In the absence of adequate myocardial suppression, the compliance of the patient to the preparative procedures should be verified, and this information is included in the report. Standard commercial software programs can be applied for reading and quantifying FDG data.

Image Analysis and Interpretation Criteria

FDG-PET/CT images must be visually evaluated. Both CT-attenuation corrected and non-corrected PET images are evaluated in the coronal, transaxial, and sagittal planes, as well as in tridimensional maximum intensity projection (MIP) cine mode. FDG-PET images are visually analysed by assessing increased myocardial FDG uptake, taking into consideration the pattern (focal, focal on diffuse, linear, diffuse), intensity, and relationship to adjacent areas of physiologic distribution (Fig. 12.5). The location, pattern, and intensity of the FDG uptake at the valve should be described and localized as intravalvular (in the leaflets), valvular (following the supporting structure of the valve), or perivalvular (next to the valve). Focal and/or heterogenous perivalvular uptake is the most common finding in case of PVE. In TAVR IE cases, focal or multifocal activity surrounding the prosthetic ring, more intense than the normal pulmonary parenchyma on the non-attenuation-corrected images, is highly suspicious of PVE.

PET information should always be compared with the morphologic information available from the CT, including contrast-enhanced CT scans when available. It must be kept in mind that the sensitivity of FDG for infection and inflammation is not perfect and that even in the absence of significant FDG uptake, a thorough analysis of the CT component is essential.

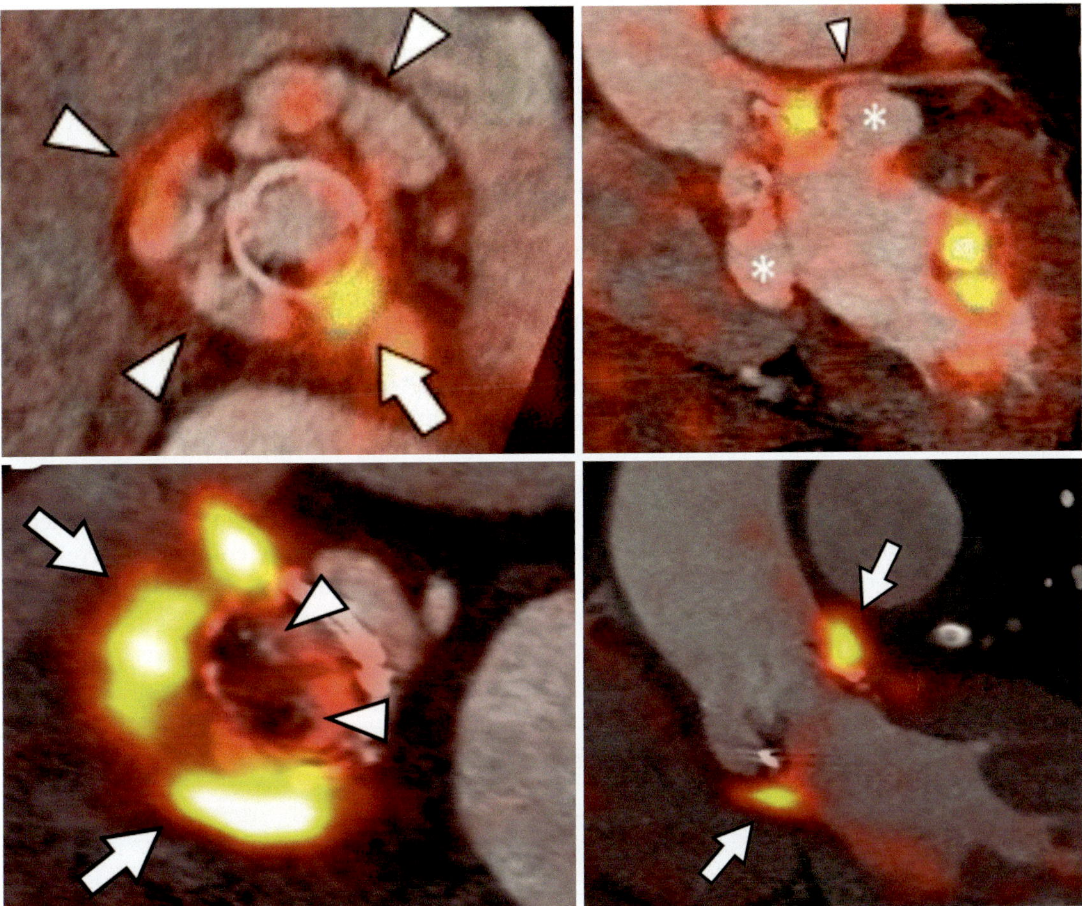

Fig. 12.5 Example of the typical pattern of focal heterogeneous peri-valvular uptake considered a positive finding for FDG-PET/CT in patients with PVE

Semi-quantitative analysis with the standard uptake value (SUV) is possible. However, as opposed to oncology applications, SUV has not been validated in inflammation and infection. If SUV is used, all the factors influencing its quantification should be carefully considered, including those related to patient preparation (glycaemia, concurrent treatment, etc), time of uptake and the use of positive contrast. Although higher SUV may be more suggestive of infection, there is significant overlap with inflammation and uptake distribution must be taken into account in the interpretation.

Several physiological variants and pathological conditions should be recognized to prevent false-positive scan. A physiological variant that might be misinterpreted as PVE is increased activity along the posterior aspect of the heart, which may represent lipomatous hypertrophy of the interatrial septum, presenting as a fat-containing mass with increased FDG uptake [56]. Focally increased FDG uptake might be found in many other conditions such as active thrombi [57], soft atherosclerotic plaques [58], vasculitis [59], primary cardiac tumours [60], cardiac metastases [61], post-surgical inflammation [62], foreign body reactions [63], stitches [64], and Libman-Sacks endocarditis [65]. The use of surgical adhesives (i.e., Bioglue) can result in false-positive scan findings after valve surgery [66]. Post-operative inflammation characterized as diffuse, homogeneous distribution of FDG in the absence of associated anatomic lesions, can also lead to a false-positive scan and can persist for at least 1 year after surgery as suggested by a recent prospective study in patients undergoing FDG-PET/CTA at 1, 6, and 12 months. In fact, the results of this study show that FDG uptake might be present in implanted prosthetic valves from the recent post-operative period, with a typical diffuse and homogenous distribution pattern and mild intensity in relation to post-operative inflammation which can be defined a "normal" FDG morphological and metabolic pattern of non-infected prosthetic valves (Fig. 12.6). Such uptake is very different from the focal/heterogeneous pattern of infected prosthetic valves and remains stable during the first year after surgery [67]. Therefore, based on these results, the 3-month interval recommended in the ESC 2015 guideline [25] seems to lose value, and depending on the level of risk for infection in the presence of noncomplicated valve surgery, scans <3 weeks surgery can be considered [66].

On the other hand, prolonged antimicrobial therapy can reduce FDG intensity despite persistent infections. All these confounder factors should be taken into consideration when interpreting the images. In all cases, correlation with clinical features, ECHO, and CTA findings is necessary. In doubtful cases, white blood cell single-positron emission tomography (WBC-SPECT) can further help define the presence/absence of infection at PVE.

Several semiquantitative parameters have been tested to quantify the FDG uptake in PVE, such as the highest SUV (SUV_{max}) in the valvular region and the prosthetic to background ratio (PBR) which takes into account the variability of the signal related to blood pool activity and image noise, by correcting valve SUV values by background activity in non-affected myocardium. Nonetheless, final interpretation relies on the integration of several parameters

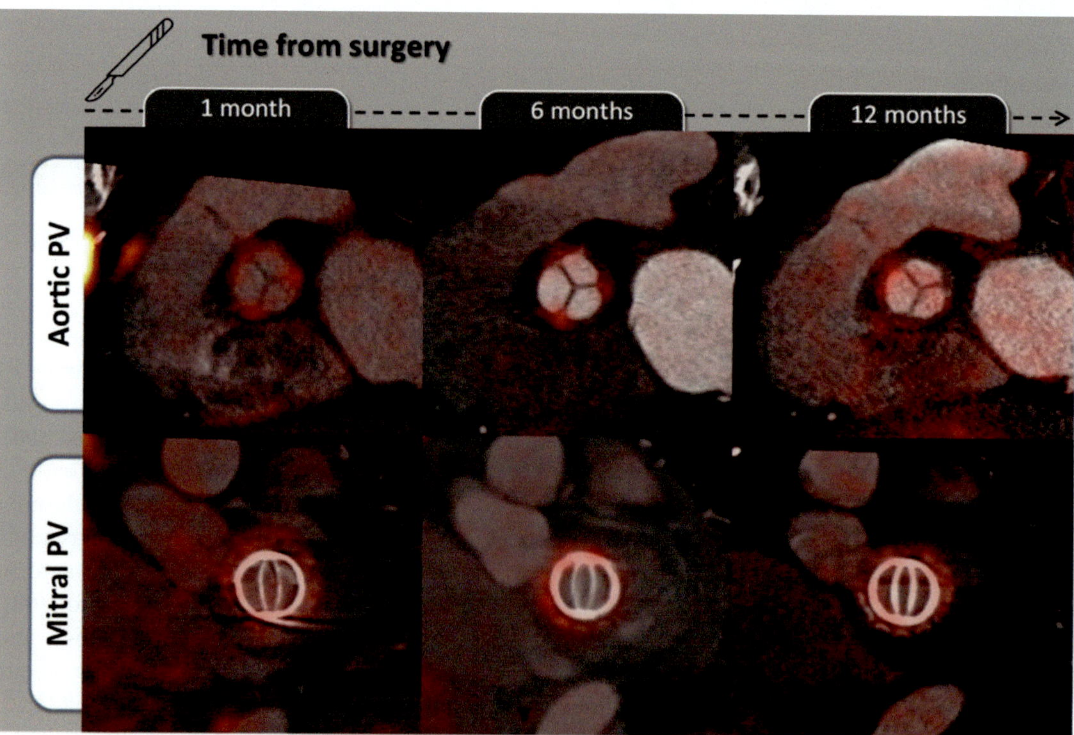

Fig. 12.6 Changes in anatomic and metabolic features over time. Aortic bioprosthesis (upper row) and mitral mechanical prosthesis (lower row) show stable FDG uptake distribution and intensity at 1, 6, and 12 months after surgery. No anatomic lesions appeared at any time point of follow-up. (Reproduced from Roque et al. [67])

including visual analysis and should not rely on a single quantitative index.

Overall Clinical Performance

A recent meta-analysis showed an overall pooled sensitivity and specificity (95% CI, inconsistency I-square statistic) of 0.74 (0.70–0.77, 71.5%) and 0.88 (0.86–0.91, 78.5%) for all cases of endocarditis. For native valve IE, sensitivity was 0.31 (0.21–0.41, 29.4%) and specificity was 0.98 (0.95–0.99, 34.4%). For PVE, sensitivity was 0.86 (0.81–0.89, 60.0%) and specificity was 0.84 (0.79–0.88, 75.2%). Interestingly, the pooled sensitivities and specificities were higher for the 17 most recent studies published after 2015 compared to the nine studies published before 2015, which could be explained by improved imaging techniques and interpretation [68]. The addition of FDG-PET/CT to the modified Duke criteria increased sensitivity for a definite IE from 52–70% to 91–97% [69] by reducing the number of possible PVE cases. This finding has been confirmed in several series [52, 70–76]. The presence of FDG-PET/CT uptake as a major criterion of the ESC 2015 was present in 40.9% of patients without major echo criteria (in this study, ECHO sensitivity was 68.1% [57.5–77.5%] with a specificity of 62.5% [40.6–81.2%] while the sensitivity of FDG-PET/CT was 73.6% [63.3–82.3%] and specificity 75.0% [53.3–90.2%.]). Therefore, by adding FDG-PET/CT in the ESC 2015 classification, the sensitivity of the Duke criteria increased from 57.1% (95% CI: 46.3–67.5%) to 83.5% (95% CI: 74.3–90.5%) (p < 0.001), with a relative decrease in specificity from 95.8% (95% CI: 78.9–99.9%) to 70.8% (95% CI: 48.9–87.4%). However, in cases of high clinical suspicion of IE, the absolute increase in true positive findings was higher than the absolute decrease in the occurrence of

false positive using the ESC 2015 classification instead of the Duke criteria [77]. Indeed, applying the proper interpretation criteria, high sensitivity (87%) and high specificity (92%) have been reported [52, 78], underlying the need to use specific PET/CT criteria (typical findings) in imaging reading and proper discussions of the results within the Endocarditis Team [77].

FDG-PET/CT has been reported to have similar sensitivities for vegetations, perivalvular sequelae, and prosthetic valve dehiscence compared with ECHO [71]. However, the value of FDG-PET/CT is more limited in NVE [79, 80]. The more frequent presence of isolated valve vegetation, rare para-valvular involvement, lower predominance of polymorphonuclear cells, and increased fibrosis in NVE compared with PVE result in reduced inflammatory response and subsequently lower FDG uptake [81]. Notably, the lower sensitivity of FDG-PET/CT is offset by a near perfect specificity for the detection of NVE and an unrivalled ability for identifying septic emboli [79, 82]. Thus, in the case of NVE, the use of FDG-PET/CT is mostly useful for the detection of distant embolic events, a condition currently considered a minor criterion in the 2015 ESC guidelines. The application of gated-PET may further improve it [83].

When FDG-PET/CTA is performed, the sensitivity and specificity increased to 91%, with a positive predictive value of 93% and a negative predictive value of 88% [52, 84]. In association with the Duke criteria, FDG-PET/CTA allowed reclassification of 90% of the cases initially classified as possible IE and provided a more conclusive diagnosis (definite/reject) in 95% of the patients. By adding CTA to PET/CT, it is also possible to assess the entire chest identifying septic pulmonary infarcts and abscesses, evaluate the aorta and the coronary arteries in prevision of surgery. Figures 12.7 and 12.8 present two examples of FDG-PET/CT contribution in patients with suspected PVE.

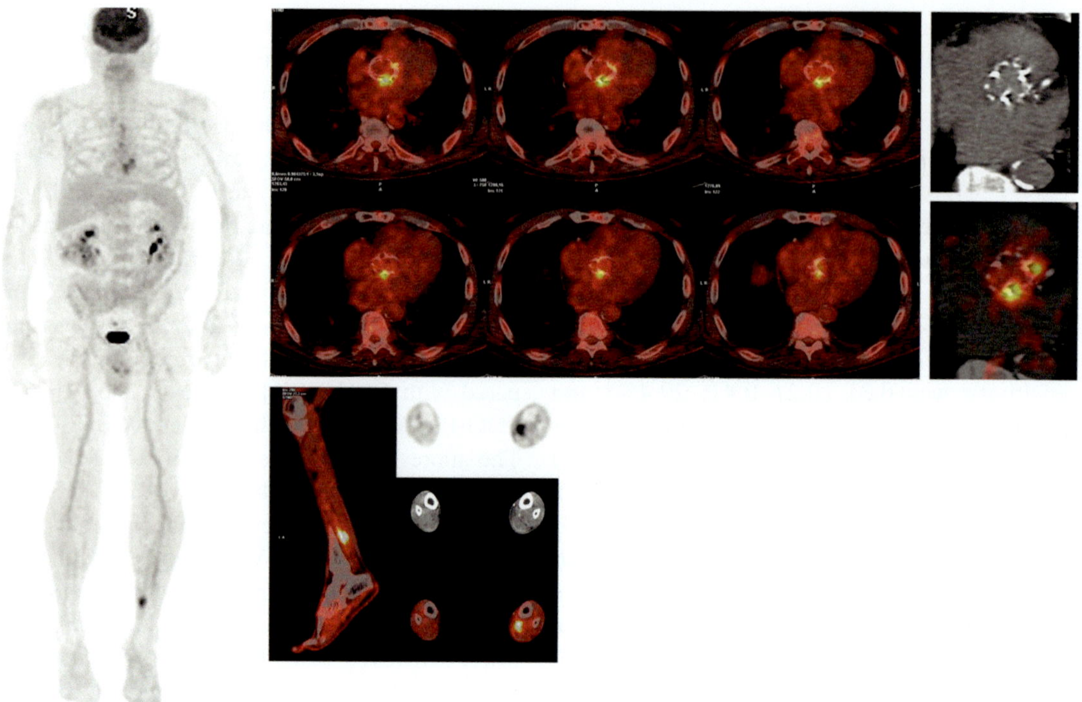

Fig. 12.7 A 73-year-old gentleman with persistent fever. Aortic valve replacement with a biological aortic valve prosthesis was performed in March 2020. TTE and TOE showed a periprosthetic leak. Repeat blood cultures were negative. FDG-PET/CT images (Discovery 710 PET/CT GE Healthcare, from left to right MIP, transaxial superimposed images of the thorax at different levels, and trans- axial CT at upper level and superimposed PET/CT at lower level reconstructed) show a focal area of increased uptake at the perivalvular region, adding a major criterion to the ESC classification, thus resulting in a 'Definite IE'. Furthermore, total body images also show uptake along the tibial artery, consistent of embolic localization as confirmed by follow-up images

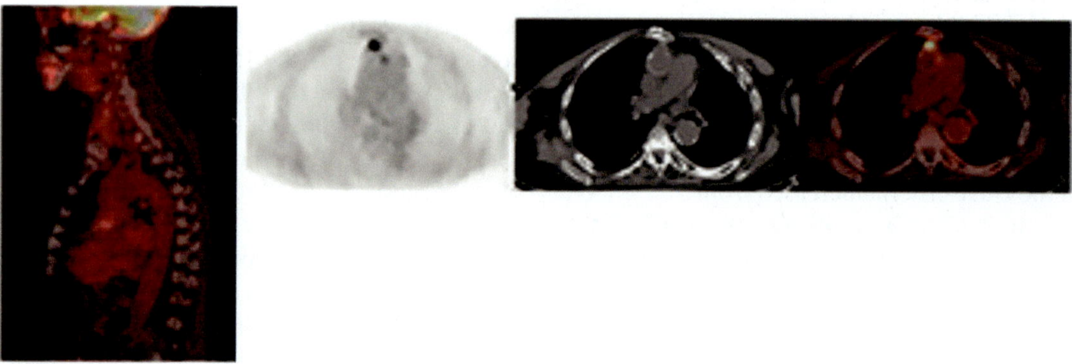

Fig. 12.8 Example of FDG-PET/CT (Discovery 710 PET/CT GE Healthcare) in patients with final diagnosis infection involving the aortic PV as shown by the PET/CT images of the thorax (from left to right, superimposed sag- ittal and transaxial emission, CT and superimposed images valve levels) showing an area of focal radiophar- maceutical uptake limited to the prosthetic aortic valve

Extra-Cardiac Manifestations

Extracardiac manifestations in IE (both NVE and PVE) are reported in 30–80% of patients. Most frequent are embolic stroke or septic embolization to bone, spleen, or kidneys [85]. Importantly, septic emboli are not always associated with symptoms [86–88]. The majority of emboli occur within the first 14 days after treatment initiation [89]. The localization of the emboli and their cerebral/extracerebral proportion vary according to the studies, in particular according to the frequency and modalities of imaging, and the proportion of right-sided and left-sided IE.

Whole-body FDG-PET/CT imaging is particularly useful in patients with suspected or proven PVE to identify septic emboli, mycotic aneurysms, and the POE, with the notable exception of cerebral septic embolism and mycotic aneurysms of intracerebral arteries owing to the high physiological uptake of FDG in the brain (Fig. 12.3). In these cases, CT or MRI is the modality of choice. Typically, septic emboli appear as focal areas of FDG uptake and most often affect the spleen, liver, lungs, and kidneys. Uptake at the intervertebral disks and/or the vertebrae (spondylodiscitis) suggests metastatic infection and can be also observed in muscles and joints (septic arthritis). Embolic events can be clinically silent in 20% of cases, especially those affecting the spleen or brain. On CTA, septic emboli appear as hypodense lesions. FDG-PET is more sensitive and specific than CTA for the detection of septic emboli (Fig. 12.9).

Early detection of septic emboli with FDG-PET/CT has a high sensitivity (87–100%) and specificity (80%) [69], at a reasonable cost-effectiveness, especially in patients with Gram-positive bacteraemia [90]. Extracerebral septic emboli were found in 24–74% of patients with definite IE; most of these peripheral emboli were silent (50–71%) and only revealed by FDG-PET/CT. In a case-control study, FDG-PET/CT detected extra-cardiac lesions in 57.4% of IE patients, representing the only initially positive imaging technique in about half of the patients with embolic events [91]. Detection of metastatic infection by FDG-PET/CT led to change of treatment in up to 35% of patients [92] and a two-fold reduction in the number of relapses [91]. FDG-PET/CT is very accurate in organs with low physiological uptake, but is of limited utility in ruling out the presence of brain emboli [93], where the use of CT/MRI is more appropriate.

The evaluation of disease extent by the identification of extracardiac extension has consequences

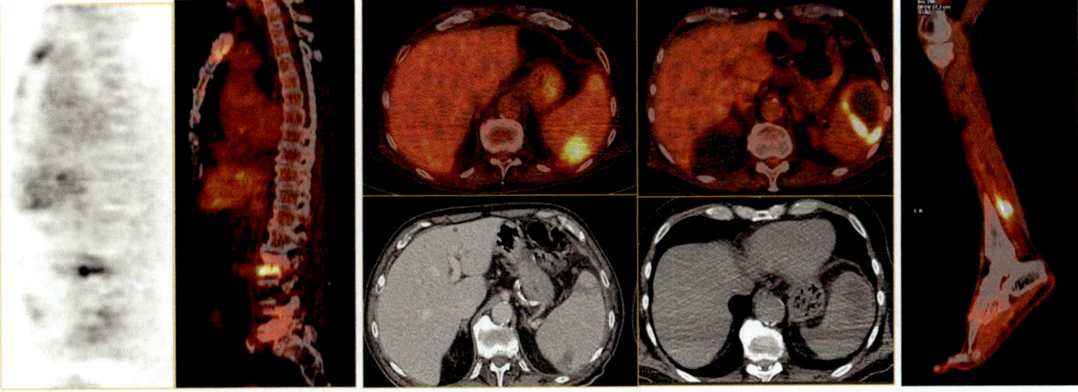

Fig. 12.9 Examples of embolic events detected at FDG-PET/CT (Discovery 710 PET/CT GE Healthcare) in the spine (right panel, sagittal emission, and superimposed images at left panel and corresponding MR images at right panel), spleen emboli (middle, upper panel superimposed PET/CT images, lower panel ceCT images) and in a case of mycotic aneurysm (left panel superimposed PET/CT images). In both cases, increased homogeneous FDG uptake is evident

on therapeutic management of IE, leading to a reduction of the risk of relapse. This has been shown particularly useful in the identification of unexpected infectious foci such as mycotic aneurysms [94], a potential life-threatening complication requiring specific treatment. Indeed, FDG-PET/CT has been demonstrated to lead to a change in therapy in 28% of patients, such as earlier cardiac surgery or initiation of a specific antimicrobial regimen for the treatment of the embolic foci [95]. In addition, in the Kestler case-control study, the systematic use of FDG-PET/CT was associated with a two-fold reduction in the number of IE relapses (9.6 vs. 4.2%) [91].

FDG-PET imaging in IE is also useful to identify the POE. Typical POE that can be identified are dental abscesses, sinusitis, infected central catheters, skin infection, and colonic cancers/polyps [6, 96]. The identification of the infection portal of entry at FDG-PET/CT and subsequent eradication of the sources of infection is particularly important in IE to prevent recurrence, either relapse and/or reinfection, a risk which varies between 2.7% and 22.5% [97–104]. The primary infectious site may be suspected based on the common biotope of the bacteria strain (digestive, skin, catheter). Yet, published research on this topic is very limited. In a recent study, systematic search for the POE identified the site of primary infection in 74% of patients, mainly cutaneous (40%), followed by oral or dental (29%) and gastrointestinal (23%) [105]. FDG-PET/CT has been demonstrated to reveal the source of infection, including cases where the sustaining POE was a neoplasia (colonic cancer) [52]. Once the portal of entry has been identified, risk modification can be attempted.

Multidisciplinary Discussion of Imaging Results

Multidisciplinary discussion of the multimodality imaging and laboratory findings is necessary to enhance their contribution into a clinical planning and decision-making process that delivers quality care in such complex contexts. A multidisciplinary team approach has been recently successfully extended beyond oncology where the work model is successfully established, such as in cases of valvular heart disease (the "Heart Valve Clinic"), particularly in the selection of patients for TAVR procedures, and coronary artery disease for revascularization decisions (Heart Team) [46, 106]. The first example of a multidisciplinary approach in the field of cardiovascular infections is represented by the Endocarditis Team (E-Team), a multidisciplinary "round table" involving specialists involving imaging, cardiologists, cardiac surgeons, infectious disease specialists, microbiologists, and others [25, 107]. This approach has been shown to significantly reduce the in-hospital and 1- and 3-year mortality in France, Italy, and Spain [37, 38]. Putting multimodality imaging in a central position in the diagnostic work-up of patients with suspected cardiovascular infections implies a new professional perspective for the "Clinical Imaging Specialist" who is called to be an active part and contributor within the E-Team. Very recently, this approach has also been recognized by the American Heart Association (AHA) 2020 guidelines for the management of patients with valvular heart disease [26] which now include FDG-PET/CT imaging and a multidisciplinary team approach in the assessment of patients with IE.

Conclusion

The application of multimodality imaging has improved the sensitivity to detect PVE, allowing for the early detection of complications such as septic emboli and metastatic infections even before these become clinically apparent. The role of multimodality imaging in the diagnostic work-up of cardiovascular infections is now well-established and supported by ample evidence. Discussion of the test results in the context of the clinical presentation in the framework of a Multidisciplinary Team Approach is recommended. Novel trends in radiopharmaceuticals developments as well as significant progress in technology, new insights on the various mechanisms that play a role in cardiovascular infections will likely provide in the near future new diagnostic and therapeutic targets for further developments in the field.

References

1. Hoerstrup SP, Weber B. Biological heart valves. Eur Heart J. 2015;36(6):325–6.
2. Kollef MH, Sharpless L, Vlasnik J, Pasque C, Murphy D, Fraser VJ. The impact of nosocomial infections on patient outcomes following cardiac surgery. Chest. 1997;112(3):666–75.
3. Brown PP, Kugelmass AD, Cohen DJ, Reynolds MR, Culler SD, Dee AD, et al. The frequency and cost of complications associated with coronary artery bypass grafting surgery: results from the United States Medicare program. Ann Thorac Surg. 2008;85(6):1980–6.
4. Gabbieri D, Dohmen PM, Linneweber J, Grubitzsch H, von Heymann C, Neumann K, et al. Early outcome after surgery for active native and prosthetic aortic valve endocarditis. J Heart Valve Dis. 2008;17(5):508–24; discussion 25.
5. Dohmen PM, Binner C, Mende M, Daviewala P, Etz CD, Borger MA, et al. Gender-based long-term surgical outcome in patients with active infective aortic valve endocarditis. Med Sci Monit. 2016;22:2520–7.
6. Habib G, Erba PA, Iung B, Donal E, Cosyns B, Laroche C, et al. Clinical presentation, aetiology and outcome of infective endocarditis. Results of the ESC-EORP EURO-ENDO (European infective endocarditis) registry: a prospective cohort study. Eur Heart J. 2019;40(39):3222–32.
7. Wang A, Athan E, Pappas PA, Fowler VG, Olaison L, Paré C, et al. Contemporary clinical profile and outcome of prosthetic valve endocarditis. JAMA. 2007;297(12):1354–61.
8. Tornos P, Iung B, Permanyer-Miralda G, Baron G, Delahaye F, Gohlke-Bärwolf C, et al. Infective endocarditis in Europe: lessons from the Euro heart survey. Heart. 2005;91(5):571–5.
9. Hoen B, Alla F, Selton-Suty C, Béguinot I, Bouvet A, Briançon S, et al. Changing profile of infective endocarditis: results of a 1-year survey in France. JAMA. 2002;288(1):75–81.
10. Murdoch DR, Corey GR, Hoen B, Miró JM, Fowler VG, Bayer AS, et al. Clinical presentation, etiology, and outcome of infective endocarditis in the 21st century: the international collaboration on endocarditis-prospective cohort study. Arch Intern Med. 2009;169(5):463–73.
11. Østergaard L, Valeur N, Ihlemann N, Bundgaard H, Gislason G, Torp-Pedersen C, et al. Incidence of infective endocarditis among patients considered at high risk. Eur Heart J. 2018;39(7):623–9.
12. Glaser N, Jackson V, Holzmann MJ, Franco-Cereceda A, Sartipy U. Aortic valve replacement with mechanical vs. biological prostheses in patients aged 50-69 years. Eur Heart J. 2016;37(34):2658–67.
13. Butt JH, Ihlemann N, De Backer O, Søndergaard L, Havers-Borgersen E, Gislason GH, et al. Long-term risk of infective endocarditis after transcatheter aortic valve replacement. J Am Coll Cardiol. 2019;73(13):1646–55.
14. Ben-Shoshan J, Amit S, Finkelstein A. Transcatheter aortic valve implantation infective endocarditis: current data and implications on prophylaxis and management. Curr Pharm Des. 2016;22(13):1959–64.
15. Martínez-Sellés M, Bouza E, Díez-Villanueva P, Valerio M, Fariñas MC, Muñoz-García AJ, et al. Incidence and clinical impact of infective endocarditis after transcatheter aortic valve implantation. EuroIntervention. 2016;11(10):1180–7.
16. Amat-Santos IJ, Messika-Zeitoun D, Eltchaninoff H, Kapadia S, Lerakis S, Cheema AN, et al. Infective endocarditis after transcatheter aortic valve implantation: results from a large multicenter registry. Circulation. 2015;131(18):1566–74.
17. Pettersson G, Hussain S. Surgical treatment of aortic valve endocarditis. In: Cohn LH, Adams DH, editors. Cardiac surgery in the adult. 5th ed. New York: McGraw Hill Education; 2018. p. 731–41.
18. Mahesh B, Angelini G, Caputo M, Jin XY, Bryan A. Prosthetic valve endocarditis. Ann Thorac Surg. 2005;80(3):1151–8.
19. Donlan RM. Biofilms and device-associated infections. Emerg Infect Dis. 2001;7(2):277–81.
20. Zimmerli W, Sendi P. Pathogenesis of implant-associated infection: the role of the host. Semin Immunopathol. 2011;33(3):295–306.
21. Pazin GJ, Saul S, Thompson ME. Blood culture positivity: suppression by outpatient antibiotic therapy in patients with bacterial endocarditis. Arch Intern Med. 1982;142(2):263–8.
22. Erba PA, Pizzi MN, Roque A, Salaun E, Lancellotti P, Tornos P, et al. Multimodality imaging in infective endocarditis: an imaging team within the endocarditis team. Circulation. 2019;140(21):1753–65.
23. Sollini M, Berchiolli R, Delgado Bolton RC, Rossi A, Kirienko M, Boni R, et al. The "3M" approach to cardiovascular infections: multimodality, multitracers, and multidisciplinary. Semin Nucl Med. 2018;48(3):199–224.
24. Erba PA, Sollini M, Lazzeri E, Mariani G. FDG-PET in cardiac infections. Semin Nucl Med. 2013;43(5):377–95.
25. Habib G, Lancellotti P, Antunes MJ, Bongiorni MG, Casalta JP, Del Zotti F, et al. 2015 ESC guidelines for the management of infective endocarditis: the task force for the Management of Infective Endocarditis of the European Society of Cardiology (ESC). Endorsed by: European Association for Cardio-Thoracic Surgery (EACTS), the European Association of Nuclear Medicine (EANM). Eur Heart J. 2015;36(44):3075–128.
26. Otto CM, Nishimura RA, Bonow RO, Carabello BA, Erwin JP, Gentile F, et al. 2020 ACC/AHA guide-

line for the Management of Patients with Valvular Heart Disease: a report of the American College of Cardiology/American Heart Association joint committee on clinical practice guidelines. Circulation. 2021;143(5):e72–e227.

27. Horstkotte D, Follath F, Gutschik E, Lengyel M, Oto A, Pavie A, et al. Guidelines on prevention, diagnosis and treatment of infective endocarditis executive summary; the task force on infective endocarditis of the European society of cardiology. Eur Heart J. 2004;25(3):267–76.

28. Shively BK, Gurule FT, Roldan CA, Leggett JH, Schiller NB. Diagnostic value of transesophageal compared with transthoracic echocardiography in infective endocarditis. J Am Coll Cardiol. 1991;18(2):391–7.

29. Erbel R, Rohmann S, Drexler M, Mohr-Kahaly S, Gerharz CD, Iversen S, et al. Improved diagnostic value of echocardiography in patients with infective endocarditis by transoesophageal approach. A prospective study. Eur Heart J. 1988;9(1):43–53.

30. Habib G. Embolic risk in subacute bacterial endocarditis: determinants and role of transesophageal echocardiography. Curr Cardiol Rep. 2003;5(2):129–36.

31. Grob A, Thuny F, Villacampa C, Flavian A, Gaubert JY, Raoult D, et al. Cardiac multidetector computed tomography in infective endocarditis: a pictorial essay. Insights Imaging. 2014;5(5):559–70.

32. Feuchtner GM, Stolzmann P, Dichtl W, Schertler T, Bonatti J, Scheffel H, et al. Multislice computed tomography in infective endocarditis: comparison with transesophageal echocardiography and intraoperative findings. J Am Coll Cardiol. 2009;53(5):436–44.

33. Barrio P, López-Melgar B, Fidalgo A, Romero-Castro MJ, Moreno-Arciniegas A, Field C, et al. Additional value of hybrid PET/MR imaging versus MR or PET performed separately to assess cardiovascular disease. Rev Esp Cardiol. 2021;74(4):303–11.

34. Langwieser N, von Olshausen G, Rischpler C, Ibrahim T. Confirmation of diagnosis and graduation of inflammatory activity of Loeffler endocarditis by hybrid positron emission tomography/magnetic resonance imaging. Eur Heart J. 2014;35(36):2496.

35. Slart RHJA, Glaudemans AWJM, Gheysens O, Lubberink M, Kero T, Dweck MR, et al. Procedural recommendations of cardiac PET/CT imaging: standardization in inflammatory-, infective-, infiltrative-, and innervation (4Is)-related cardiovascular diseases: a joint collaboration of the EACVI and the EANM. Eur J Nucl Med Mol Imaging. 2021;48(4):1016–39.

36. Jensen AG, Wachmann CH, Espersen F, Scheibel J, Skinhøj P, Frimodt-Møller N. Treatment and outcome of Staphylococcus aureus bacteremia: a prospective study of 278 cases. Arch Intern Med. 2002;162(1):25–32.

37. Botelho-Nevers E, Thuny F, Casalta JP, Richet H, Gouriet F, Collart F, et al. Dramatic reduction in infective endocarditis-related mortality with a management-based approach. Arch Intern Med. 2009;169(14):1290–8.

38. Chirillo F, Scotton P, Rocco F, Rigoli R, Borsatto F, Pedrocco A, et al. Impact of a multidisciplinary management strategy on the outcome of patients with native valve infective endocarditis. Am J Cardiol. 2013;112(8):1171–6.

39. Jamar F, Buscombe J, Chiti A, Christian PE, Delbeke D, Donohoe KJ, et al. EANM/SNMMI guideline for 18F-FDG use in inflammation and infection. J Nucl Med. 2013;54(4):647–58.

40. Roca M, de Vries EF, Jamar F, Israel O, Signore A. Guidelines for the labelling of leucocytes with (111)in-oxine. Inflammation/infection taskgroup of the European Association of Nuclear Medicine. Eur J Nucl Med Mol Imaging. 2010;37(4):835–41.

41. Boellaard R, Delgado-Bolton R, Oyen WJ, Giammarile F, Tatsch K, Eschner W, et al. FDG PET/CT: EANM procedure guidelines for tumour imaging: version 2.0. Eur J Nucl Med Mol Imaging. 2015;42(2):328–54.

42. de Vries EF, Roca M, Jamar F, Israel O, Signore A. Guidelines for the labelling of leucocytes with (99m)Tc-HMPAO. Inflammation/infection Taskgroup of the European Association of Nuclear Medicine. Eur J Nucl Med Mol Imaging. 2010;37(4):842–8.

43. SNMMI Procedure Standard for ^{99m}Tc Exametazime (HMPAO)-Labeled Leukocyte Scintigraphy for Suspected Infection/Inflammation 3.0. http://www.snmmi.org/ClinicalPractice/content.aspx?ItemNumber=6414#InfecInflamm. Accessed 11 Nov 2021.

44. SNMMI Procedure Standard for 111In-Leukocyte Scintigraphy for Suspected Infection/Inflammation 3.0. http://www.snmmi.org/ClinicalPractice/content.aspx?ItemNumber=6414#InfecInflamm.

45. Erba PA, Conti U, Lazzeri E, Sollini M, Doria R, De Tommasi SM, et al. Added value of 99mTc-HMPAO-labeled leukocyte SPECT/CT in the characterization and management of patients with infectious endocarditis. J Nucl Med. 2012;53(8):1235–43.

46. Vahanian A, Alfieri O, Andreotti F, Antunes MJ, Barón-Esquivias G, Baumgartner H, et al. Guidelines on the management of valvular heart disease (version 2012). Eur Heart J. 2012;33(19):2451–96.

47. Osborne MT, Hulten EA, Murthy VL, Skali H, Taqueti VR, Dorbala S, et al. Patient preparation for cardiac fluorine-18 fluorodeoxyglucose positron emission tomography imaging of inflammation. J Nucl Cardiol. 2017;24(1):86–99.

48. Rabkin Z, Israel O, Keidar Z. Do hyperglycemia and diabetes affect the incidence of false-negative 18F-FDG PET/CT studies in patients evaluated for infection or inflammation and cancer? A comparative analysis. J Nucl Med. 2010;51(7):1015–20.

49. Raplinger K, Chandler K, Hunt C, Johnson G, Peller P. Effect of steroid use during chemotherapy on SUV levels in PET/CT. J Nucl Med. 2012;53(supplement 1):2718.

50. Abbara S, Arbab-Zadeh A, Callister TQ, Desai MY, Mamuya W, Thomson L, et al. SCCT guide-

lines for performance of coronary computed tomographic angiography: a report of the Society of Cardiovascular Computed Tomography Guidelines Committee. J Cardiovasc Comput Tomogr. 2009;3(3):190–204.

51. Nijssen EC, Nelemans PJ, Rennenberg RJ, van der Molen AJ, van Ommen GV, Wildberger JE. Impact on clinical practice of updated guidelines on iodinated contrast material: CINART. Eur Radiol. 2020;30(7):4005–13.

52. Pizzi MN, Roque A, Fernández-Hidalgo N, Cuéllar-Calabria H, Ferreira-González I, Gonzàlez-Alujas MT, et al. Improving the diagnosis of infective endocarditis in prosthetic valves and intracardiac devices with 18F-Fluordeoxyglucose positron emission tomography/computed tomography angiography: initial results at an infective endocarditis referral center. Circulation. 2015;132(12):1113–26.

53. Roque A, Pizzi MN, Cuéllar-Calàbria H, Aguadé-Bruix S. F-FDG-PET/CT angiography for the diagnosis of infective endocarditis. Curr Cardiol Rep. 2017;19(2):15.

54. Schaefferkoetter J, Ouyang J, Rakvongthai Y, Nappi C, El Fakhri G. Effect of time-of-flight and point spread function modeling on detectability of myocardial defects in PET. Med Phys. 2014;41(6):062502.

55. Lindström E, Sundin A, Trampal C, Lindsjö L, Ilan E, Danfors T, et al. Evaluation of penalized-likelihood estimation reconstruction on a digital time-of-flight PET/CT scanner for. J Nucl Med. 2018;59(7):1152–8.

56. Fan CM, Fischman AJ, Kwek BH, Abbara S, Aquino SL. Lipomatous hypertrophy of the interatrial septum: increased uptake on FDG PET. AJR Am J Roentgenol. 2005;184(1):339–42.

57. García JR, Simo M, Huguet M, Ysamat M, Lomeña F. Usefulness of 18-fluorodeoxyglucose positron emission tomography in the evaluation of tumor cardiac thrombus from renal cell carcinoma. Clin Transl Oncol. 2006;8(2):124–8.

58. Williams G, Kolodny GM. Retrospective study of coronary uptake of 18F-fluorodeoxyglucose in association with calcification and coronary artery disease: a preliminary study. Nucl Med Commun. 2009;30(4):287–91.

59. Kobayashi Y, Ishii K, Oda K, Nariai T, Tanaka Y, Ishiwata K, et al. Aortic wall inflammation due to Takayasu arteritis imaged with 18F-FDG PET coregistered with enhanced CT. J Nucl Med. 2005;46(6):917–22.

60. Rahbar K, Seifarth H, Schäfers M, Stegger L, Hoffmeier A, Spieker T, et al. Differentiation of malignant and benign cardiac tumors using 18F-FDG PET/CT. J Nucl Med. 2012;53(6):856–63.

61. Kaderli AA, Baran I, Aydin O, Bicer M, Akpinar T, Ozkalemkas F, et al. Diffuse involvement of the heart and great vessels in primary cardiac lymphoma. Eur J Echocardiogr. 2010;11(1):74–6.

62. Abidov A, D'agnolo A, Hayes SW, Berman DS, Waxman AD. Uptake of FDG in the area of a recently implanted bioprosthetic mitral valve. Clin Nucl Med. 2004;29(12):848.

63. Schouten LR, Verberne HJ, Bouma BJ, van Eck-Smit BL, Mulder BJ. Surgical glue for repair of the aortic root as a possible explanation for increased F-18 FDG uptake. J Nucl Cardiol. 2008;15(1):146–7.

64. Versari A, Casali M. Normal findings with different radiopharmaceuticals, techniques, variants, and pitfalls. In: Lazzeri E, Signore A, Erba PA, Prandini N, Versari A, D' Errico G, et al., editors. Radionuclide imaging of infection and inflammation: a pictorial case-based atlas. Cham: Springer International; 2021. p. 1–27.

65. Dahl A, Schaadt BK, Santoni-Rugiu E, Bruun NE. Molecular imaging in Libman-sacks endocarditis. Infect Dis (Lond). 2015;47(4):263–6.

66. Swart LE, Gomes A, Scholtens AM, Sinha B, Tanis W, Lam MGEH, et al. Improving the diagnostic performance of 18 F-Fluorodeoxyglucose positron-emission tomography/computed tomography in prosthetic heart valve endocarditis. Circulation. 2018;138(14):1412–27.

67. Roque A, Pizzi MN, Fernández-Hidalgo N, Permanyer E, Cuellar-Calabria H, Romero-Farina G, et al. Morpho-metabolic post-surgical patterns of non-infected prosthetic heart valves by [18F]FDG PET/CTA: "normality" is a possible diagnosis. Eur Heart J Cardiovasc Imaging. 2020;21(1):24–33.

68. Wang TKM, Sánchez-Nadales A, Igbinomwanhia E, Cremer P, Griffin B, Xu B. Diagnosis of infective endocarditis by subtype using. Circ Cardiovasc Imaging. 2020;13(6):e010600.

69. Gomes A, Glaudemans AWJM, Touw DJ, van Melle JP, Willems TP, Maass AH, et al. Diagnostic value of imaging in infective endocarditis: a systematic review. Lancet Infect Dis. 2017;17(1):e1–e14.

70. Rouzet F, Chequer R, Benali K, Lepage L, Ghodbane W, Duval X, et al. Respective performance of 18F-FDG PET and radiolabeled leukocyte scintigraphy for the diagnosis of prosthetic valve endocarditis. J Nucl Med. 2014;55(12):1980–5.

71. Saby L, Laas O, Habib G, Cammilleri S, Mancini J, Tessonnier L, et al. Positron emission tomography/computed tomography for diagnosis of prosthetic valve endocarditis: increased valvular 18F-fluorodeoxyglucose uptake as a novel major criterion. J Am Coll Cardiol. 2013;61(23):2374–82.

72. Salomäki SP, Saraste A, Kemppainen J, Bax JJ, Knuuti J, Nuutila P, et al. F-FDG positron emission tomography/computed tomography in infective endocarditis. J Nucl Cardiol. 2017;24(1):195–206.

73. Ricciardi A, Sordillo P, Ceccarelli L, Maffongelli G, Calisti G, Di Pietro B, et al. 18-Fluoro-2-deoxyglucose positron emission tomography-computed tomography: an additional tool in the diagnosis of prosthetic valve endocarditis. Int J Infect Dis. 2014;28:219–24.

74. Bartoletti M, Tumietto F, Fasulo G, Giannella M, Cristini F, Bonfiglioli R, et al. Combined computed tomography and fluorodeoxyglucose positron

emission tomography in the diagnosis of prosthetic valve endocarditis: a case series. BMC Res Notes. 2014;7:32.

75. Fagman E, van Essen M, Fredén Lindqvist J, Snygg-Martin U, Bech-Hanssen O, Svensson G. 18F-FDG PET/CT in the diagnosis of prosthetic valve endocarditis. Int J Cardiovasc Imaging. 2016;32(4):679–86.

76. Duval X, Le Moing V, Tubiana S, Esposito-Farèse M, Ilic-Habensus E, Leclercq F, et al. Impact of systematic whole-body 18F-Fluorodeoxyglucose PET/CT on the Management of Patients Suspected of infective endocarditis: the prospective multicenter TEPvENDO study. Clin Infect Dis. 2021;73(3):393–403.

77. Philip M, Tessonier L, Mancini J, Mainardi JL, Fernandez-Gerlinger MP, Lussato D, et al. Comparison between ESC and Duke criteria for the diagnosis of prosthetic valve infective endocarditis. JACC Cardiovasc Imaging. 2020;13(12):2605–15.

78. Swart LE, Scholtens AM, Tanis W, Nieman K, Bogers AJJC, Verzijlbergen FJ, et al. 18F-fluorodeoxyglucose positron emission/computed tomography and computed tomography angiography in prosthetic heart valve endocarditis: from guidelines to clinical practice. Eur Heart J. 2018;39(41):3739–49.

79. Pelletier-Galarneau M, Abikhzer G, Harel F, Dilsizian V. Detection of native and prosthetic valve endocarditis: incremental attributes of functional FDG PET/CT over morphologic imaging. Curr Cardiol Rep. 2020;22(9):93.

80. Philip M, Delcourt S, Mancini J, Tessonnier L, Cammilleri S, Arregle F, et al. F-fluorodeoxyglucose positron emission tomography/computed tomography for the diagnosis of native valve infective endocarditis: a prospective study. Arch Cardiovasc Dis. 2021;114(3):211–20.

81. de Camargo RA, Sommer Bitencourt M, Meneghetti JC, Soares J, Gonçalves LFT, Buchpiguel CA, et al. The role of 18F-Fluorodeoxyglucose positron emission tomography/computed tomography in the diagnosis of left-sided endocarditis: native vs. prosthetic valves endocarditis. Clin Infect Dis. 2020;70(4):583–94.

82. Primus CP, Clay TA, McCue MS, Wong K, Uppal R, Ambekar S, et al. 18F-FDG PET/CT improves diagnostic certainty in native and prosthetic valve infective endocarditis over the modified Duke criteria. J Nucl Cardiol. 2021. https://doi.org/10.1007/s12350-021-02689-5. Online ahead of print..

83. Boursier C, Duval X, Bourdon A, Imbert L, Mahida B, Chevalier E, et al. ECG-gated cardiac FDG PET acquisitions significantly improve detectability of infective endocarditis. JACC Cardiovasc Imaging. 2020;13(12):2691–3.

84. Pizzi MN, Dos-Subirà L, Roque A, Fernández-Hidalgo N, Cuéllar-Calabria H, Pijuan Domènech A, et al. F-FDG-PET/CT angiography in the diagnosis of infective endocarditis and cardiac device infection in adult patients with congenital heart disease and prosthetic material. Int J Cardiol. 2017;248:396–402.

85. Di Salvo G, Habib G, Pergola V, Avierinos JF, Philip E, Casalta JP, et al. Echocardiography predicts embolic events in infective endocarditis. J Am Coll Cardiol. 2001;37(4):1069–76.

86. Duval X, Delahaye F, Alla F, Tattevin P, Obadia JF, Le Moing V, et al. Temporal trends in infective endocarditis in the context of prophylaxis guideline modifications: three successive population-based surveys. J Am Coll Cardiol. 2012;59(22):1968–76.

87. Selton-Suty C, Célard M, Le Moing V, Doco-Lecompte T, Chirouze C, Iung B, et al. Preeminence of Staphylococcus aureus in infective endocarditis: a 1-year population-based survey. Clin Infect Dis. 2012;54(9):1230–9.

88. Delahaye F, Goulet V, Lacassin F, Ecochard R, Selton-Suty C, Hoen B, et al. Characteristics of infective endocarditis in France in 1991. A 1-year survey. Eur Heart J. 1995;16(3):394–401.

89. Vilacosta I, Graupner C, San Román JA, Sarriá C, Ronderos R, Fernández C, et al. Risk of embolization after institution of antibiotic therapy for infective endocarditis. J Am Coll Cardiol. 2002;39(9):1489–95.

90. Vos FJ, Bleeker-Rovers CP, Sturm PD, Krabbe PF, van Dijk AP, Cuijpers ML, et al. 18F-FDG PET/CT for detection of metastatic infection in gram-positive bacteremia. J Nucl Med. 2010;51(8):1234–40.

91. Kestler M, Muñoz P, Rodríguez-Créixems M, Rotger A, Jimenez-Requena F, Mari A, et al. Role of (18)F-FDG PET in patients with infectious endocarditis. J Nucl Med. 2014;55(7):1093–8.

92. Orvin K, Goldberg E, Bernstine H, Groshar D, Sagie A, Kornowski R, et al. The role of FDG-PET/CT imaging in early detection of extra-cardiac complications of infective endocarditis. Clin Microbiol Infect. 2015;21(1):69–76.

93. Özcan C, Asmar A, Gill S, Thomassen A, Diederichsen AC. The value of FDG-PET/CT in the diagnostic work-up of extra cardiac infectious manifestations in infectious endocarditis. Int J Cardiovasc Imaging. 2013;29(7):1629–37.

94. Mikail N, Benali K, Ou P, Slama J, Hyafil F, Le Guludec D, et al. Detection of mycotic aneurysms of lower limbs by whole-body (18)F-FDG-PET. JACC Cardiovasc Imaging. 2015;8(7):859–62.

95. Van Riet J, Hill EE, Gheysens O, Dymarkowski S, Herregods MC, Herijgers P, et al. (18)F-FDG PET/CT for early detection of embolism and metastatic infection in patients with infective endocarditis. Eur J Nucl Med Mol Imaging. 2010;37(6):1189–97.

96. Erba PA, Lancellotti P, Vilacosta I, Gaemperli O, Rouzet F, Hacker M, et al. Recommendations on nuclear and multimodality imaging in IE and CIED infections. Eur J Nucl Med Mol Imaging. 2018;45(10):1795–815.

97. Heiro M, Helenius H, Hurme S, Savunen T, Metsärinne K, Engblom E, et al. Long-term outcome of infective endocarditis: a study on patients surviving over one year after the initial episode treated in

a Finnish teaching hospital during 25 years. BMC Infect Dis. 2008;8:49.

98. Renzulli A, Carozza A, Romano G, De Feo M, Della Corte A, Gregorio R, et al. Recurrent infective endocarditis: a multivariate analysis of 21 years of experience. Arenzul@tin.It. Ann Thorac Surg. 2001;72(1):39–43.

99. Castillo JC, Anguita MP, Ramírez A, Siles JR, Torres F, Mesa D, et al. Long term outcome of infective endocarditis in patients who were not drug addicts: a 10 year study. Heart. 2000;83(5):525–30.

100. Alexiou C, Langley SM, Stafford H, Lowes JA, Livesey SA, Monro JL. Surgery for active culture-positive endocarditis: determinants of early and late outcome. Ann Thorac Surg. 2000;69(5):1448–54.

101. Kaiser SP, Melby SJ, Zierer A, Schuessler RB, Moon MR, Moazami N, et al. Long-term outcomes in valve replacement surgery for infective endocarditis. Ann Thorac Surg. 2007;83(1):30–5.

102. David TE, Gavra G, Feindel CM, Regesta T, Armstrong S, Maganti MD. Surgical treatment of active infective endocarditis: a continued challenge. J Thorac Cardiovasc Surg. 2007;133(1):144–9.

103. Tornos MP, Permanyer-Miralda G, Olona M, Gil M, Galve E, Almirante B, et al. Long-term complications of native valve infective endocarditis in non-addicts. A 15-year follow-up study. Ann Intern Med. 1992;117(7):567–72.

104. Mansur AJ, Dal Bó CM, Fukushima JT, Issa VS, Grinberg M, Pomerantzeff PM. Relapses, recurrences, valve replacements, and mortality during the long-term follow-up after infective endocarditis. Am Heart J. 2001;141(1):78–86.

105. Delahaye F, M'Hammedi A, Guerpillon B, de Gevigney G, Boibieux A, Dauwalder O, et al. Systematic search for present and potential portals of entry for infective endocarditis. J Am Coll Cardiol. 2016;67(2):151–8.

106. Nishimura RA, Otto CM, Bonow RO, Carabello BA, Erwin JP, Guyton RA, et al. 2014 AHA/ACC guideline for the Management of Patients with Valvular Heart Disease: executive summary: a report of the American College of Cardiology/American Heart Association task force on practice guidelines. Circulation. 2014;129(23):2440–92.

107. Erba PA, Habib G, Glaudemans AWJM, Miro JM, Slart RHJA. The round table approach in infective endocarditis & cardiovascular implantable electronic devices infections: make your e-team come true. Eur J Nucl Med Mol Imaging. 2017;44(7):1107–8.

Gad Abikhzer, Jeremy Y. Levett, Igal A. Sebag,
and Matthieu Pelletier-Galarneau

Acronyms

IE   Infective endocarditis
NVIE   Native-valve infective endocarditis
PVE   Prosthetic valve endocarditis
TEE   Transesophageal echocardiogram
TTE   Transthoracic echocardiogram

Introduction

Although relatively rare, infective endocarditis (IE) is associated with significant morbidity and mortality [1]. The diagnosis of IE is clinically challenging due to diverse and variable clinical presentations, ranging from chronic, to subacute, to rapidly progressive disease. To circumvent these diagnostic difficulties, the Duke criteria were established. The diagnosis of IE mostly relies on a modified version of those criteria (the modified Duke criteria), consisting of major and minor criteria that are composed of clinical and paraclinical findings including blood cultures and echocardiographic findings. Studies have demonstrated that approximately one third of patients investigated for IE are classified as possible IE [2, 3]. In patients categorized as having possible IE by the modified Duke criteria, 24–72% of these patients are subsequently found to have IE following additional investigations, such as repeat TTE or TEE [4, 5]. This ultimately leads to delays in diagnosis and initiation of treatment which is in turn associated with poorer outcomes, including increased rates of irreversible morphologic valvular damage, embolic events, surgery, and death [6, 7]. Advanced multimodality imaging has become increasingly integrated in the diagnosis and evaluation of IE. Although the role of FDG-PET/CT in native valve infective endocarditis (NVIE) is still being defined, there is a growing body of evidence supporting the role for FDG-PET/CT in the diagnosis and staging of this disease.

G. Abikhzer (✉)
Department of Radiology and Nuclear Medicine, Jewish General Hospital, Montreal, QC, Canada

Faculty of Medicine and Health Sciences, McGill University, Montreal, QC, Canada
e-mail: gad.abikhzer@mcgill.ca

J. Y. Levett
Faculty of Medicine and Health Sciences, McGill University, Montreal, QC, Canada

I. A. Sebag
Faculty of Medicine and Health Sciences, McGill University, Montreal, QC, Canada

Division of Cardiology, Jewish General Hospital, Montreal, QC, Canada

M. Pelletier-Galarneau
Montreal Heart Institute, Montréal, QC, Canada
e-mail: Matthieu.pelletier-galarneau@icm-mhi.org

Pathophysiology

The healthy heart is naturally resistant to infection [8]. High pressures, constant hemodynamic

M. Pelletier-Galarneau, P. Martineau (eds.), *FDG-PET/CT and PET/MR in Cardiovascular Diseases*, https://doi.org/10.1007/978-3-031-09807-9_13

flow, and poor adherence to endocardial surfaces prevent infectious organisms from colonizing endocardial structures [8, 9]. A predisposing abnormality of the endocardium, massive bacteremia, or virulent microorganism is therefore usually necessary to cause endocarditis of native valves. The most common predisposing abnormalities of the endocardium are structural in nature, typically involving the heart valves, and include mitral valve prolapse, rheumatic valve disease, calcific or bicuspid aortic valves, congenital heart defects, hypertrophic cardiomyopathy, mural thrombi, ventricular septal defects, or patent ductus arteriosus sites [8, 10–12]. As a result of endothelial damage and activation of the coagulation cascade, the nidus for infection is typically a sterile fibrin-platelet vegetation [8].

Microorganisms colonize and proliferate the endocardium in three stages [13]. First, they begin by circulating in the bloodstream, causing bacteremia. Second, a predisposing abnormality of the endocardium promotes increased adherence and local stasis, enabling the pathogenic agents to adhere to the abnormal or damaged endothelium. Third, the nidus formed by the predisposing abnormality nurtures an environment for microorganism proliferation and inflammation of local structures, leading to the formation of a mature vegetation. As a defensive mechanism from host innate and humoral immunity, as well as from antibiotic penetration, many of the causative endocarditis microorganisms produce a protective matrix of polysaccharide biofilms surrounding the mature vegetation [13].

NVIE is generally classified into two categories: left-sided NVIE (mitral or aortic valve), which represents 80% of infections, or right-sided NVIE (tricuspid or pulmonic valve) [13]. The causative microorganisms vary by sites of infection, etiology of bacteremia, and host risk factors. Staphylococci and streptococci are the most common causative microorganisms, accounting for over 80% of NVIE cases [13]. The consequences of endocarditis can manifest locally and systemically, depending on the progression of disease [13]. Devastating local complications can include valvular, myocardial, or aortic root abscesses with tissue necrosis and conduction

system abnormalities, sudden and severe valvular regurgitation, or aortitis due to adjacent spread of infection [8]. Systemic consequences most commonly manifest as a result of embolization of vegetation material from the heart valve, a devastating complication which can occur in 25–50% of patients [14], or immune-mediated phenomena. Left-sided NVIE lesions can embolize to any tissue, particularly the central nervous system, kidneys, or spleen, whereas right-sided NVIE lesions can be complicated by septic pulmonary embolism, resulting in pulmonary infarction, pneumonia, or empyema [8]. As a result of left-sided NVIE lesions, mycotic aneurysms of major arteries can also form. Furthermore, cutaneous (Osler nodes and Janeway lesions) and retinal emboli are specific features of left-sided NVIE [13].

Epidemiology

While the precise estimate of NVIE incidence is difficult to ascertain due to varying case definitions over time, it is estimated that the crude incidence for the global burden of IE ranges from 1.5 to 11.6 cases per 100,000 person-years [15]. NVIE is a fatal disease unless treated appropriately, with a mortality rate of approximately 25% despite standard of care therapy [1]. Early diagnosis and management is essential to preventing significant morbidity and mortality. In high-income countries, the mean age of patients with NVIE has significantly increased over the past century [1]. This is primarily attributable to the changing etiology and predisposing cardiac risk factors of patients with NVIE. Rheumatic heart disease, primarily affecting the mitral valve, has historically been the most frequent underlying etiology of NVIE. However, in the past two decades, its proportion has decreased to ≤5% in developed countries [1]. Other risk factors including increasing age [16] structural heart disease [11], poor dentition or dental infection [17], injection drug use [18], and healthcare-associated NVIE [19] have become prevalent in high-income countries and have changed the distribution of etiologies. At the time that endocarditis develops, approximately 75% of patients have a preexisting structural cardiac abnormality [11]. In developing countries, rheumatic heart disease remains the most common underlying heart condition [20].

Clinical Presentation and Diagnosis

Historically, the diagnosis of NVIE was made on the clinical diagnosis of active valvulitis (such as a cardiac murmur or chest pain), embolic sequela, and immunological vascular phenomena in concurrence with positive blood cultures [13]. However, the latest advancements in developed countries have resulted in a shift toward earlier clinical presentations due to healthcare-associated NVIE with *Staphylococcus aureus* infection. Accordingly, many of the classic pathognomonic signs and symptoms associated with NVIE do not manifest, with most patients (approximately 90% of cases) presenting with fever of unknown origin (FUO) [1, 21]. The diverse and nonspecific nature of symptoms, as well as the clinical variability in presentations, complicates early diagnosis and identification of patients who would be optimal candidates for early effective antibiotic therapy or surgical inter-vention. Therefore, the ability to accurately diagnose or exclude NVIE in a timely manner is of utmost clinical importance in reducing morbidity and mortality.

Currently, the diagnosis of NVIE requires a combination of clinical manifestations, microbiological analysis, and imaging results. The modified Duke clinical diagnostic criteria integrate these three spheres, weighing findings as either major or minor criteria, and allowing clinicians and investigators to reach a definite, possible, or rejected diagnosis of IE (Table 13.1) [22]. The definite diagnosis of IE is established in the presence of pathologic criteria, two major clinical criteria, one major clinical criterion, and three minor clinical criteria, or five minor clinical criteria (definite IE). In the presence of one major criterion and one minor clinical criterion, three minor criteria, IE is considered possible (possible IE). IE is rejected if a firm alternate diagnosis is made, clinical manifestations resolve with antibiotic therapy for less than or equal to 4 days, there is no pathologic evidence of IE at surgery or autopsy with antibiotic therapy for less than or equal to 4 days, or clinical criteria for a definite or possible diagnosis are not met (rejected IE). While the modified Duke criteria remain the gold standard for the diagnosis of IE, they are limited

Table 13.1 Modified Duke criteria for the diagnosis of IE

Definite IE
Pathological criteria
Pathologic lesions—Vegetation or intracardiac abscess demonstrating active endocarditis on histology, OR
Microorganisms—Demonstrated by culture or histology of a vegetation or intracardiac abscess
Clinical criteria
Using specific definitions listed below:
2 major clinical criteria, OR
1 major and 3 minor clinical criteria, OR
5 minor clinical criteria
Possible IE
Presence of 1 major and 1 minor clinical criteria OR presence of 3 minor clinical criteria
Rejected IE
A firm alternate diagnosis is made
Resolution of clinical manifestations with antibiotic therapy for ≤4 days
No pathologic evidence of IE is found at surgery or autopsy with antibiotic therapy for ≤4 days
Clinical criteria for definite or possible IE not met

(continued)

Table 13.1 (continued)

Major clinical criteria

Blood culture positivity for either of the following:

1. Typical microorganism (viridans group streptococci, *Streptococcus gallolyticus*, HACEK organisms, *Staphylococcus aureus*, and community-acquired enterococci in the absence of a primary focus) from two separate blood cultures.
2. Persistent bacteremia (two positive cultures >12 h apart, three positive cultures or a majority of four or more culture-positive results >1 h apart).

Evidence of endocardial involvement from either of the following:

1. Echocardiographic findings of mobile mass attached to a valve or a valve apparatus, abscess, or new partial dehiscence of a prosthetic valve.
2. New valvular regurgitation.

Serology:

Single positive blood culture for *Coxiella burnetii* or an antiphase 1 IgG antibody titer of $\geq 1/800$

Minor clinical criteria

Predisposing condition:

Intravenous drug use

Predisposing cardiac condition

Vascular phenomena:

Arterial embolism

Septic pulmonary embolism

Mycotic aneurysm

Intracranial hemorrhage

Conjunctival hemorrhage

Janeway lesions

Description: Adapted from Li et al. Proposed modifications to the Duke criteria for the diagnosis of infective endocarditis. Clin. Infect. Dis., 2000, 30, 4, 633–638 [22]

HACEK Haemophilus spp., *Aggregatibacter* spp., *Cardiobacterium hominis*, *Eikenella corrodens*, or *Kingella* spp.; *IE* infective endocarditis, *NVIE* native-valve infective endocarditis

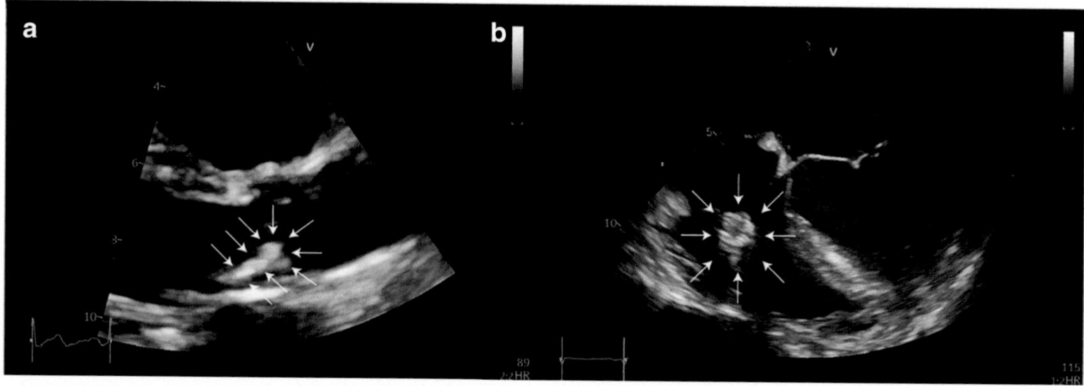

Fig. 13.1 Representative echocardiographic findings of NVIE. Description: (**a**) Transthoracic echocardiogram still image of a large, pedunculated, and prolapsing vegetation on the atrial surface of the noncoronary cusp of the aortic valve. (**b**) Transesophageal echocardiogram still image of a rounded, large, echo density on the atrial surface of the tricuspid valve leaflet

by their reliance on the presence of positive microbiological criteria and typical echocardiographic findings (Fig. 13.1), which remain the cornerstone of an IE diagnosis.

Transthoracic echocardiography (TTE) is only moderately sensitive (75%) for the detection of a vegetation in native valves [23], and blood cultures can be negative in up to 10% of cases [6]. Although the minority of cases (20%), the sensitivity of TTE is highest in right-sided IE due to the tricuspid and pulmonic valves' proximity to the chest wall [13]. In patients with clinically suspected IE but equivocal or negative TTE, transesophageal echocardiography (TEE) is the gold standard and improves sensitivity and specificity to more than 90% with better detection of the main cardiac complications (vegetation, abscess, leaflet perforation, and pseudoaneurysm) [6, 23]. However, its invasiveness and feasibility are important considerations, with major complication rates ranging between 0.2% and 0.5% [24–26]. Furthermore, false positives can occur with thrombi, fibrous strands on the aortic valve, and cardiac tumors. The sequential and indeterminate diagnostic evaluations can ultimately lead to delays in diagnosis and initiation of treatment, which are in turn related to a poorer outcome with increased rates of progressive and potentially irreparable structural damage, embolic events, surgery, and death [6, 7].

Management

The management of IE requires a multidisciplinary approach, including input from cardiologists, infectious disease specialists, and cardiovascular surgeons [7]. The standard of care is for all patients to receive antimicrobial therapy, and a subset of patients may benefit from cardiovascular surgical intervention [7, 13]. Antibiotics can be started on an empirical basis as soon as three blood cultures have been collected from separate venipuncture sites [7, 13]. The empirical antibiotic regimens for native valve endocarditis are based on guidelines [27], although they can be modified with the assistance of an infectious disease consultant, according to blood culture results, resistance patterns, and the clinical severity of infection [7]. In light of the primary purpose of antimicrobial therapy to completely eradicate infection within cardiac vegetations, an extended course of intravenous therapy is generally required (extending up to 6 weeks in severe cases) [13]. In addition to antimicrobial therapy, surgical intervention is required in approximately 50% of cases [28]. In the only randomized trial published to date on the effect of early surgical intervention versus conventional treatment for NVIE, early surgical intervention was found to

significantly reduce the primary composite endpoint of in-hospital mortality and embolic events by 90% [29]. The three most common indications for surgery are heart failure caused by valvular regurgitation or obstruction, uncontrolled or complex infection involving valve leaflet and paravalvular tissue destruction, and prevention of embolism [6, 7, 13].

FDG-PET/CT Imaging

Fluorodeoxyglucose-positron emission tomography/computed tomography (FDG-PET/CT) has become extremely useful for infectious disease imaging such as FUO [30], sternal wound infections [31], vascular graft infections [32], spondylodiscitis [33], cardiovascular implantable electronic device (CIED) infections [34, 35], and prosthetic valve IE (PVE) [36, 37]. Activated granulocytes involved in the infectious and inflammatory response have a high expression of glucose transporters (GLUT1 and GLUT3) and increased hexokinase activity [38]. Use of FDG-PET/CT for infection imaging compared to SPECT radiotracers yields several advantages including excellent image resolution, lack of blood manipulation, lower radiation exposure, and a shorter procedure for both the patient and technical staff, allowing results to be available in less than 2 h after injection. FDG-PET/CT is especially useful in patients with renal failure or those who are allergic to contrast media. FDG has, however, several limitations in the evaluation of cardiovascular infection. Physiological myocardial uptake can mask or limit the distinction between physiological uptake at the base of the myocardium and pathological valvular activity. Cardiac suppression protocols consisting of fasting (12-18 h), high-fat-low-carbohydrate diet, and in some centers IV heparin are recommended prior to imaging (see Chap. 4) [39–41]. This preparation delays the scheduling of an FDG-PET/CT by 20 h, as well as being inconvenient for the patient. Despite optimal preparation, partial or complete failure of suppression of physiological myocardial activity may be present in 5–15% of scans

[42]. Additionally, FDG is not an infection-specific radiotracer with uptake in inflammation and malignancy. The ongoing development of novel infection-specific PET radiotracers yield promise to further improve on IE diagnosis, although none are yet clinically available [43]. In the context of PVE, specificity of FDG may be affected by uptake in post-operative inflammation and foreign body inflammation surrounding prosthetic material or surgical adhesives [44]; in the setting of suspected NVIE, these confounders are not present which explains the near perfect specificity of abnormal valvular uptake in NVIE. Given the absence of physiological valvular activity in native valves, any focal valvular activity above background or blood pool, after excluding papillary muscle activity or residual physiological myocardial activity at the base of the myocardium, is considered positive for NVIE on FDG-PET/CT (Fig. 13.2). The added value of standardized uptake values (SUV) in this context has not yet been demonstrated [45]. In heavily calcified native valves, very mild activity can rarely be present, and it is also important to verify non-attenuation corrected images to ensure over-correction artifacts.

The role of FDG-PET/CT in suspected PVE has been well studied and introduced as a major criterion for the diagnosis of PVE in the 2015 European Society of Cardiology (*ESC*) guidelines [36]. The role of FDG-PET/CT for NVIE is less well defined and studied than for PVE, mainly because of its higher false-negative rate and the excellent diagnostic performance of TEE in NVIE yielding less diagnostic dilemmas. Initial PET/CT studies included small subgroups of NVIE patients within larger subgroups of PVE patients and resulted in very poor sensitivity [46, 47]. In a dedicated retrospective study of 88 patients with suspected NVIE, 20 patients had NVIE according to multidisciplinary consensus. Of these 20 patients, nine (45%) had abnormal valvular FDG uptake [36]; however, septic emboli were detected in 48 (55%) cases [48]. A

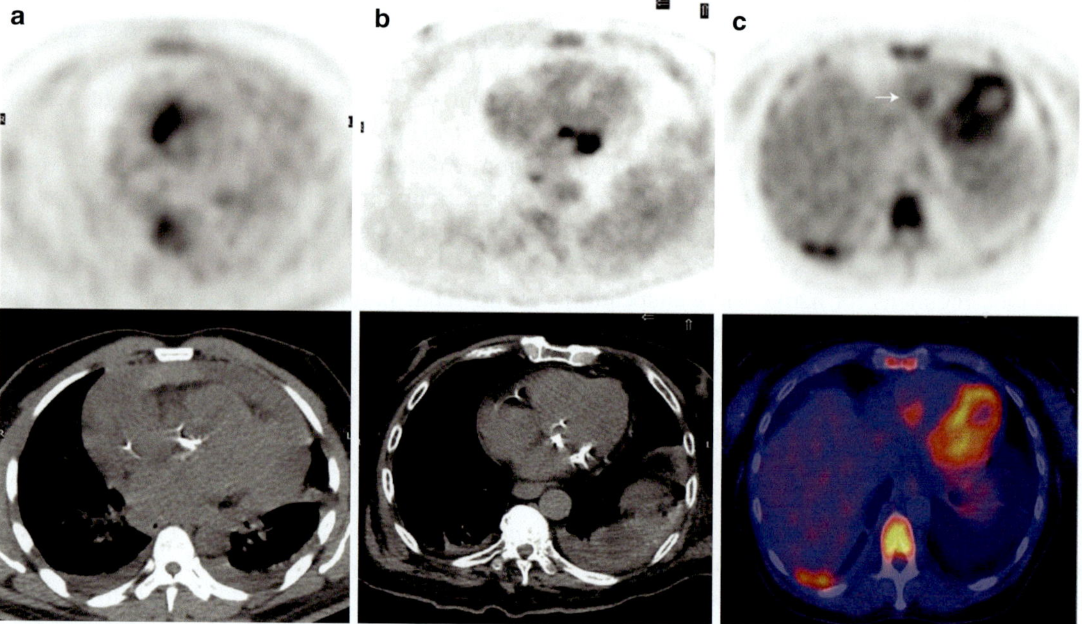

Fig. 13.2 Representative examples of abnormal native valve uptake in patients with IE. Description: (**a**) Aortic valve endocarditis complicate by para-valvular abscess and hemorrhagic pericardial effusion on CT. (**b**) Mitral valve endocarditis with intense multifocal uptake in a mitral valve with annular calcifications, which can be a predisposing factor for IE. (**c**) Tricuspid valve endocarditis with abnormal mild, focal uptake above background (red arrow). Septic lung emboli are also present. *FDG PET/CT* fluorodeoxyglucose (18F)-positron emission tomography/computed tomography

dedicated retrospective study of 75 patients with NVIE who underwent FDG-PET/CT demonstrated a sensitivity of 17.5% and specificity of 100%. Integration of PET/CT to the ESC in this context increased sensitivity to 69.8% from 63.5% without affecting specificity [49]. In an observational prospective study of patients referred for suspicion of left-sided NVIE and PVE, only 10/46 subjects with final diagnosis of NVIE had abnormal FDG uptake on consensus interpretation, yielding a sensitivity of 22%, while none of the 69 subjects without NVIE had a positive FDG-PET/CT study [50]. The largest contribution of FDG-PET/CT in this patient population was the appropriate reclassification of 11/26 (42%) patients from *Possible IE* to *Definite IE*. Of note, imaging in this study was performed with an older generation analog PET system. In the European Infective Endocarditis Registry (EURO-ENDO), a prospective observational cohort including 156 centers from 40 countries, a low sensitivity of 28% was observed. Further, they reported that FDG-PET/CT is performed in less than 10% of suspected NVIE cases [51]. In the French registry study, although only 24% of NVIE patients had abnormal valvular uptake, 51% had extracardiac findings such as septic emboli or identification of portal of entry. FDG-PET/CT in this patient population changed management in 31% through modification of the length of antibiotic therapy or surgery. PET/CT modified classification or management mainly in patients with non-contributory echocardiogram or *Possible IE* [52]. These registry studies only reported pooled sensitivity encompassing numerous centers using a variety of PET/CT scanners with different technology. Poor reported sensitivity for NVIE can be improved through use of more recent PET/CT devices. In a retrospective study dedicated to NVIE using the best available analog PET/CT, abnormal FDG uptake was identified in 21 of the 31 subjects with NVIE, yielding a sensitivity of 67.7% [5]. However, when excluding subjects with suboptimal myocardial suppression interfering with study interpretation, the sensitivity rose to 77%. Incorporating FDG-PET/CT uptake as a new major criterion, eight of 18 subjects (44.4%) with *Possible IE* and a final

diagnosis of IE were appropriately reclassified as *Definite IE*. A meta-analysis, with only four studies in the NVIE category, demonstrates a near perfect specificity of FDG-PET/CT for NVIE at 98%, but low pooled sensitivity at 31%. However, their results suggest that technological advances have contributed to higher accuracy for all subtypes of IE, where pooled sensitivity and specificity were higher in studies published since 2015 than those between 2009 and 2014 [40]. In another meta-analysis including seven NVIE studies, pooled sensitivity was 36.3%, with pooled specificity of 99.1%. Pooled positive likelihood ratio, negative likelihood ratio, and diagnostic odds ratio were 8.3, 0.6, and 15.3, respectively [45].

The relatively low sensitivities of FDG-PET/CT for NVIE can at least partly be accounted for by physiological and technical factors. The more frequent presence of isolated valve vegetations, rare para-valvular involvement, lower predominance of polymorphonuclear cells, and increased fibrosis in NVIE compared to PVE, result in reduced inflammatory response and subsequently lower FDG uptake [50]. False-negative studies have been associated with antibiotic use in some studies, although duration of antibiotic therapy before uptake normalization is unknown and other studies show no diagnostic effect from the use of antibiotics on FDG-PET/CT [45]. Poor myocardial suppression is associated with a 4.8 odds ratio of having a false-negative study when inadequate myocardial suppression is present [5]. Most importantly, the low reported sensitivity for NVIE can be partly explained by the technical properties of the PET systems used in these studies, with lower sensitivity and inferior spatial resolution, limiting their ability to detect small foci of uptake. Technological advances in PET/CT camera design have considerably enhanced resolution and contrast, with the possibility of significantly improving the detection of NVIE. The development of digital PET/CT systems with silicon photodiodes, replacing photomultiplier tubes used in the analog PET devices promises to further improve small lesion detection, as is present in NVIE, through improved sensitivity, contrast, and resolution of these devices [53]. Vegetation size on echocardiography is on average smaller in false-negative PET cases compared to true-positive cases (9.6 ± 5.9 mm vs. 14.4 ± 6.1, p = 0.049) [5], but within the resolution of digital PET/CT devices. Additionally, new scanner technology allows gated acquisition to account for both respiratory and cardiac motions. Hence, the blurring of FDG uptake related to the motion of the vegetations on the valves, which limits the sensitivity of the test, could be improved with ECG-gated and respiratory-gated acquisitions which "freezes" motion and subsequent blurring of uptake in the infected valves [54]. The use of dual time point imaging in patients with equivocal valvular activity can increase sensitivity by increased target to background ratio on delayed images through decreased blood pool activity or through the reproduction of equivocal foci of valvular uptake on two distinct acquisitions which raises the suspicion of true focal valvular uptake rather than statistical noise or reconstruction artifacts [5].

The most useful role for FDG-PET/CT in the evaluation of patients with suspected NVIE given its limited sensitivity but near-perfect specificity and the excellent performance of TEE appears to be as additional major or minor criteria to the modified Duke criteria which may help to decrease the number of patients in the subgroup classified as *possible IE*. This indication of FDG-PET/CT for *possible IE* cases is in addition to its role in the evaluation for septic emboli in cases with *definite IE* as recommended by the ESC guidelines [45, 55]. The ACC/AHA 2020 guidelines state that FDG-PET/CT is reasonable as adjunct diagnostic imaging in some patients with possible IE [7]. FDG-PET/CT may be particularly useful in patients with suspicion of IE who cannot undergo the more invasive TEE.

Extracardiac Manifestations of Infective Endocarditis

There has been a paradigm shift in the evaluation of IE, with increased awareness of the systemic nature of the disease. Identification of extracardiac manifestations in patients with IE is critical as they can significantly impact patient management decisions and outcome. Extracardiac infectious findings are present in 25–50% of patients [14] and can include cerebral emboli, spondylodiscitis, septic arthritis, pneumonia, abscesses, and mycotic aneurysm (Figs. 13.3 and 13.4). Infectious manifestations can represent septic emboli or an initial site of infection which seeded the heart valve causing the IE. Gastrointestinal polyps and cancers as well as various other malignancies, which may represent the etiology of IE in several cases, are detected by FDG-PET/CT in approximately 10% of patients investigated for IE [56]. Extracardiac manifestations identified on FDG-PET/CT are unknown or unsuspected in the majority of cases and may lead to change in management in about 10% of patients [56].

In addition to infection and cancers, other reactive changes can be observed on whole-body FDG-PET/CT such as increased bone marrow and splenic activity. In IE, increased marrow and splenic activity, defined as uptake greater than liver, has been attributed to hematological diffusion of bacteria and/or cytokines, indicating a systemic inflammatory response to the disease. Increased marrow and splenic uptake is considered an indirect sign of IE and is correlated with C-reactive protein levels as well as the major criterion of positive blood cultures [57]. Specifically, in NVIE, diffuse splenic uptake is present in 58.7% of NVIE cases and has been proposed as

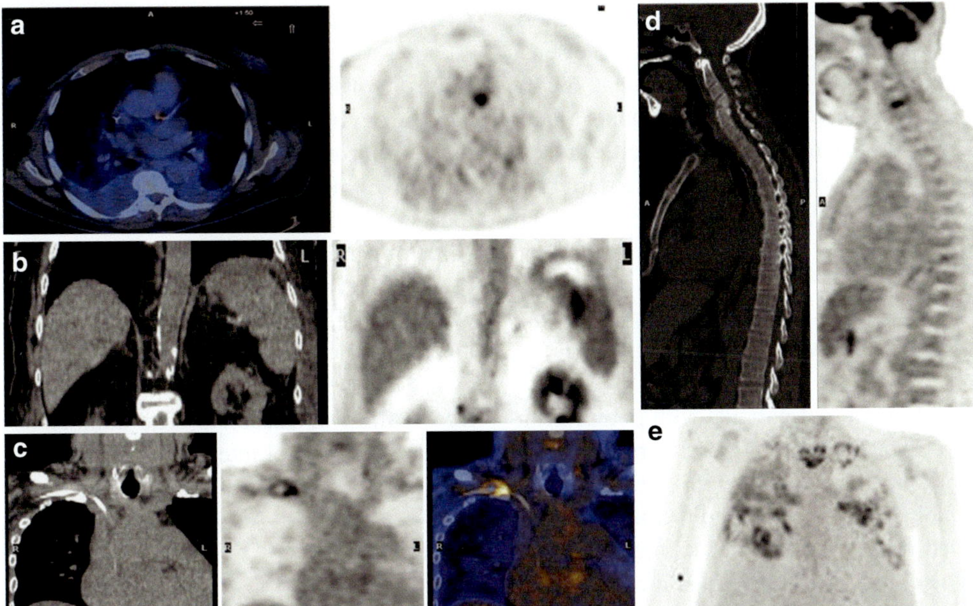

Fig. 13.3 Examples of septic embolic disease in various patients with IE. Description: (**a**) Left main coronary septic arteritis. (**b**) Septic splenic infarct. (**c**) Infected PICC line. (**d**) Cervical spondylodiscitis. (**e**) Extensive septic lung disease in a patient with tricuspid NVIE. *FDG-PET/CT* fluorodeoxyglucose (18F)-positron emission tomography/computed tomography, *PICC* = peripherally inserted intravenous catheter

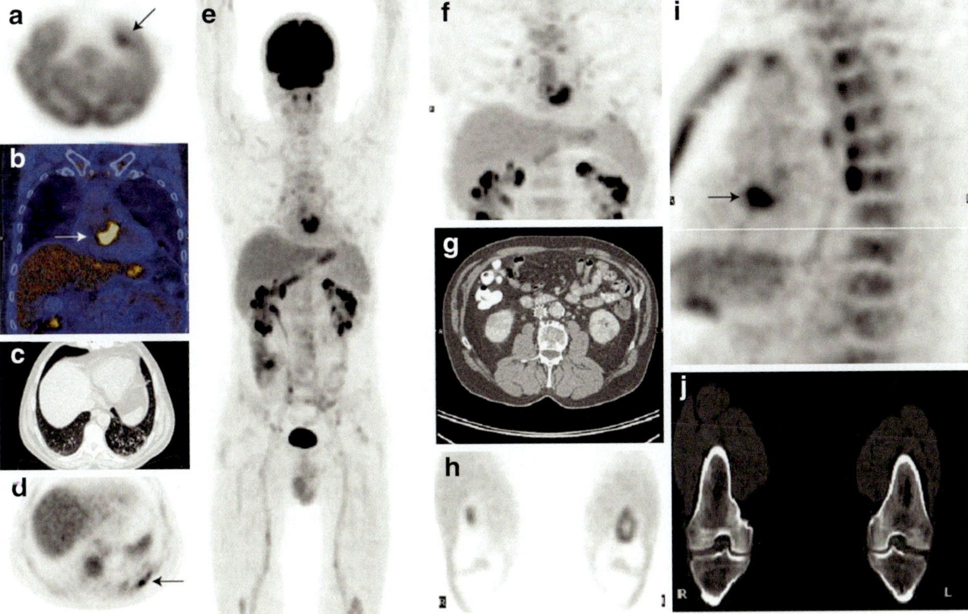

Fig. 13.4 FDG-PET/CT images of a patient referred for suspected lymphoma with night sweats and fever, diagnosed on FDG-PET/CT with native valve endocarditis and extensive embolic disease. Description: Intense uptake is present in the aortic valve (**b**, **j**). There is evidence of embolic disease to the brain (**a**, arrow), lungs (**c**, **d**-arrow), kidneys (**f**, **g**), prevertebral soft tissues (**i**) and bone (**j**). *FDG-PET/CT* fluorodeoxyglucose (18F)-positron emission tomography/computed tomography

an additional minor criterion over ESC criteria already including PET, to further increase sensitivity to 74.6% of the ESC criteria at 69.8%, compared to 63.5% for modified Duke criteria [49]. However, this finding is nonspecific and can be medication related or present in a variety of other inflammatory, infectious, or malignant conditions.

Prognostic Value

Early identification of patients with poorer prognosis is critical as more aggressive management may improve their outcome [58, 59]. Several well-established patient-related factors have been associated with worse prognosis, including older age, diabetes mellitus, and heart failure. Other histopathological and echocardiographic features, including *staphylococcus aureus* as causative organism, vegetation size, peri-annular complications, and severe valve regurgitation have also been associated with worse prognosis [36, 60]. In a prospective study of 47 patients with IE who underwent FDG-PET/CT imaging, the infectious complications and relapse rate were significantly lower when compared to a matched control group of 94 patients with IE who did not undergo FDG-PET/CT imaging [61] In a multivariate model, applying the best predictive model for major adverse cardiac events, the four leading predictors of additional independent prognostic value were as follows: C-reactive protein >100 mg/L, severe mitral regurgitation, positive FDG-PET/CT scan, and FDG-PET/CT scan with moderate-to-intense metabolic uptake. Unlike the PVE subgroup in this study, FDG-PET/CT was not predictive of a major adverse cardiac event in the NVIE subgroup, but moderate-to-intense FDG uptake was associated with a hazard ratio of 8.8 to predict new embolic events [62]. These data suggest that FDG-PET/CT provides independent prognostic information.

Conclusion

The role of FDG-PET/CT in NVIE is currently evolving with technological advances promising to improve sensitivity for abnormal uptake on native valves, while maintaining near-perfect specificity. Clinically, the greatest added value of FDG-PET/CT appears to be in patients classified as *Possible IE,* as well as in patients with *definite IE* for the systemic staging of the disease with potential prognostic significance.

Declaration of Interests The authors have no relevant conflicts of interest to disclose.

References

1. Murdoch DR, Corey GR, Hoen B, Miro JM, Fowler VG Jr, Bayer AS, et al. Clinical presentation, etiology, and outcome of infective endocarditis in the 21st century: the International Collaboration on Endocarditis-Prospective Cohort Study. Arch Intern Med. 2009;169(5):463–73.
2. Baddour LM, Wilson WR, Bayer AS, Fowler VG Jr, Tleyjeh IM, Rybak MJ, et al. Infective endocarditis in adults: diagnosis, antimicrobial therapy, and management of complications: a Scientific Statement for Healthcare Professionals From the American Heart Association. Circulation. 2015;132(15):1435–86.
3. Topan A, Carstina D, Slavcovici A, Rancea R, Capalneanu R, Lupse M. Assessment of the Duke criteria for the diagnosis of infective endocarditis after twenty-years. An analysis of 241 cases. Clujul Med. 2015;88(3):321–6.
4. Habib G, Derumeaux G, Avierinos JF, Casalta JP, Jamal F, Volot F, et al. Value and limitations of the Duke criteria for the diagnosis of infective endocarditis. J Am Coll Cardiol. 1999;33(7):2023–9.
5. Abikhzer G, Martineau P, Gregoire J, Finnerty V, Harel F, Pelletier-Galarneau M. [(18)F]FDG-PET CT for the evaluation of native valve endocarditis. J Nucl Cardiol. 2020;29(1):158–65.
6. Cahill TJ, Prendergast BD. Infective endocarditis. Lancet. 2016;387(10021):882–93.
7. Otto CM, Nishimura RA, Bonow RO, Carabello BA, Erwin JP 3rd, Gentile F, et al. 2020 ACC/AHA Guideline for the management of patients with valvular heart disease: executive summary: a Report of the American College of Cardiology/American Heart

Association Joint Committee on Clinical Practice Guidelines. J Am Coll Cardiol. 2021;77(4):450–500.

8. Thiene G, Basso C. Pathology and pathogenesis of infective endocarditis in native heart valves. Cardiovasc Pathol. 2006;15(5):256–63.

9. Lepeschkin E. On the relation between the site of valvular involvement in endocarditis and the blood pressure resting on the valve. Am J Med Sci. 1952;224(3):318–9.

10. Michel PL, Acar J. Native cardiac disease predisposing to infective endocarditis. Eur Heart J. 1995;16(Suppl B):2–6.

11. Griffin MR, Wilson WR, Edwards WD, O'Fallon WM, Kurland LT. Infective endocarditis. Olmsted County, Minnesota, 1950 through 1981. JAMA. 1985;254(9):1199–202.

12. van der Meer JT, Thompson J, Valkenburg HA, Michel MF. Epidemiology of bacterial endocarditis in The Netherlands I. Patient characteristics. Arch Intern Med. 1992;152(9):1863–8.

13. Holland TL, Baddour LM, Bayer AS, Hoen B, Miro JM, Fowler VG Jr. Infective endocarditis. Nat Rev Dis Primers. 2016;2:16059.

14. Thuny F, Di Salvo G, Belliard O, Avierinos JF, Pergola V, Rosenberg V, et al. Risk of embolism and death in infective endocarditis: prognostic value of echocardiography: a prospective multicenter study. Circulation. 2005;112(1):69–75.

15. Bin Abdulhak AA, Baddour LM, Erwin PJ, Hoen B, Chu VH, Mensah GA, et al. Global and regional burden of infective endocarditis, 1990-2010: a systematic review of the literature. Glob Heart. 2014;9(1):131–43.

16. Hill EE, Herijgers P, Claus P, Vanderschueren S, Herregods MC, Peetermans WE. Infective endocarditis: changing epidemiology and predictors of 6-month mortality: a prospective cohort study. Eur Heart J. 2007;28(2):196–203.

17. Lockhart PB, Brennan MT, Thornhill M, Michalowicz BS, Noll J, Bahrani-Mougeot FK, et al. Poor oral hygiene as a risk factor for infective endocarditis-related bacteremia. J Am Dent Assoc. 2009;140(10):1238–44.

18. Pericàs JM, Llopis J, Athan E, Hernández-Meneses M, Hannan MM, Murdoch DR, et al. Prospective Cohort Study of Infective Endocarditis in People Who Inject Drugs. J Am Coll Cardiol. 2021;77(5):544–55.

19. Fowler VG Jr, Miro JM, Hoen B, Cabell CH, Abrutyn E, Rubinstein E, et al. Staphylococcus aureus endocarditis: a consequence of medical progress. JAMA. 2005;293(24):3012–21.

20. Watt G, Lacroix A, Pachirat O, Baggett HC, Raoult D, Fournier PE, et al. Prospective comparison of infective endocarditis in Khon Kaen, Thailand and Rennes, France. Am J Trop Med Hyg. 2015;92(4):871–4.

21. Silverman ME, Upshaw CB Jr. Extracardiac manifestations of infective endocarditis and their historical descriptions. Am J Cardiol. 2007;100(12):1802–7.

22. Li JS, Sexton DJ, Mick N, Nettles R, Fowler VG Jr, Ryan T, et al. Proposed modifications to the Duke criteria for the diagnosis of infective endocarditis. Clin Infect Dis. 2000;30(4):633–8.

23. Habib G, Badano L, Tribouilloy C, Vilacosta I, Zamorano JL, Galderisi M, et al. Recommendations for the practice of echocardiography in infective endocarditis. Eur J Echocardiogr. 2010;11(2):202–19.

24. Daniel WG, Erbel R, Kasper W, Visser CA, Engberding R, Sutherland GR, et al. Safety of transesophageal echocardiography. A multicenter survey of 10,419 examinations. Circulation. 1991;83(3):817–21.

25. Hilberath JN, Oakes DA, Shernan SK, Bulwer BE, D'Ambra MN, Eltzschig HK. Safety of transesophageal echocardiography. J Am Soc Echocardiogr. 2010;23(11):1115–27; quiz 220-1.

26. Seward JB, Khandheria BK, Oh JK, Freeman WK, Tajik AJ. Critical appraisal of transesophageal echocardiography: limitations, pitfalls, and complications. J Am Soc Echocardiogr. 1992;5(3):288–305.

27. Gould FK, Denning DW, Elliott TS, Foweraker J, Perry JD, Prendergast BD, et al. Guidelines for the diagnosis and antibiotic treatment of endocarditis in adults: a report of the Working Party of the British Society for Antimicrobial Chemotherapy. J Antimicrob Chemother. 2012;67(2):269–89.

28. Prendergast BD, Tornos P. Surgery for infective endocarditis: who and when? Circulation. 2010;121(9):1141–52.

29. Kang DH, Kim YJ, Kim SH, Sun BJ, Kim DH, Yun SC, et al. Early surgery versus conventional treatment for infective endocarditis. N Engl J Med. 2012;366(26):2466–73.

30. Kouijzer IJE, van der Meer JWM, Oyen WJG, Bleeker-Rovers CP. Diagnostic yield of FDG-PET/CT in fever of unknown origin: a systematic review, meta-analysis, and Delphi exercise. Clin Radiol. 2018;73(6):588–9.

31. Hariri H, Tan S, Martineau P, Lamarche Y, Carrier M, Finnerty V, et al. Utility of FDG-PET/CT for the detection and characterization of sternal wound infection following sternotomy. Nucl Med Mol Imaging. 2019;53(4):253–62.

32. Rojoa D, Kontopodis N, Antoniou SA, Ioannou CV, Antoniou GA. 18F-FDG PET in the diagnosis of vascular prosthetic graft infection: a diagnostic test accuracy meta-analysis. Eur J Vasc Endovasc Surg. 2019;57(2):292–301.

33. Glaudemans AW, de Vries EF, Galli F, Dierckx RA, Slart RH, Signore A. The use of (18)F-FDG-PET/CT for diagnosis and treatment monitoring of inflam-

matory and infectious diseases. Clin Dev Immunol. 2013;2013:623036.

34. Sarrazin JF, Philippon F, Tessier M, Guimond J, Molin F, Champagne J, et al. Usefulness of fluorine-18 positron emission tomography/computed tomography for identification of cardiovascular implantable electronic device infections. J Am Coll Cardiol. 2012;59(18):1616–25.

35. Abikhzer G, Turpin S, Bigras JL. Infected pacemaker causing septic lung emboli detected on FDG PET/CT. J Nucl Cardiol. 2010;17(3):514–5.

36. Habib G, Lancellotti P, Antunes MJ, Bongiorni MG, Casalta JP, Del Zotti F, et al. 2015 ESC Guidelines for the management of infective endocarditis: The Task Force for the Management of Infective Endocarditis of the European Society of Cardiology (ESC). Endorsed by: European Association for Cardio-Thoracic Surgery (EACTS), the European Association of Nuclear Medicine (EANM). Eur Heart J. 2015;36(44):3075–128.

37. Pizzi MN, Roque A, Fernandez-Hidalgo N, Cuellar-Calabria H, Ferreira-Gonzalez I, Gonzalez-Alujas MT, et al. Improving the diagnosis of infective endocarditis in prosthetic valves and intracardiac devices with 18f-fluordeoxyglucose positron emission tomography/computed tomography angiography: initial results at an Infective Endocarditis Referral Center. Circulation. 2015;132(12):1113–26.

38. Vaidyanathan S, Patel CN, Scarsbrook AF, Chowdhury FU. FDG PET/CT in infection and inflammation— current and emerging clinical applications. Clin Radiol. 2015;70(7):787–800.

39. Manabe O, Yoshinaga K, Ohira H, Masuda A, Sato T, Tsujino I, et al. The effects of 18-h fasting with low-carbohydrate diet preparation on suppressed physiological myocardial (18)F-fluorodeoxyglucose (FDG) uptake and possible minimal effects of unfractionated heparin use in patients with suspected cardiac involvement sarcoidosis. J Nucl Cardiol. 2016;23(2):244–52.

40. Soussan M, Brillet PY, Nunes H, Pop G, Ouvrier MJ, Naggara N, et al. Clinical value of a high-fat and low-carbohydrate diet before FDG-PET/CT for evaluation of patients with suspected cardiac sarcoidosis. J Nucl Cardiol. 2013;20(1):120–7.

41. Slart R, Glaudemans A, Gheysens O, Lubberink M, Kero T, Dweck MR, et al. Procedural recommendations of cardiac PET/CT imaging: standardization in inflammatory-, infective-, infiltrative-, and innervation- (4Is) related cardiovascular diseases: a joint collaboration of the EACVI and the EANM: summary. Eur Heart J Cardiovasc Imaging. 2020;21(12):1320–30.

42. Martineau PP-GM, Juneau D, Leung E, Birnie D, Beanlands RSB. Molecular imaging of cardiac sarcoidosis. Curr Cardiovasc Imaging Rep. 2018;11(6):6–17.

43. Chen W, Dilsizian V. Molecular imaging of cardiovascular device infection: targeting the bacteria or the host-pathogen immune response? J Nucl Med. 2020;61(3):319–26.

44. Juneau D, Pelletier-Galarneau M. Revisiting the relevance of the 3-month safety period in the evaluation of prosthetic valve endocarditis with FDG-PET/CT. J Nucl Cardiol. 2020;28(5):2269–71.

45. Kamani CH, Allenbach G, Jreige M, Pavon AG, Meyer M, Testart N, et al. Diagnostic performance of (18)F-FDG PET/CT in native valve endocarditis: systematic review and bivariate meta-analysis. Diagnostics. 2020;10(10):754.

46. Salomaki SP, Saraste A, Kemppainen J, Bax JJ, Knuuti J, Nuutila P, et al. (18)F-FDG positron emission tomography/computed tomography in infective endocarditis. J Nucl Cardiol. 2017;24(1):195–206.

47. Granados U, Fuster D, Pericas JM, Llopis JL, Ninot S, Quintana E, et al. Diagnostic accuracy of 18F-FDG PET/CT in infective endocarditis and implantable cardiac electronic device infection: a cross-sectional study. J Nucl Med. 2016;57(11):1726–32.

48. Kouijzer IJE, Berrevoets MAH, Aarntzen E, de Vries J, van Dijk APJ, Oyen WJG, et al. 18F-fluorodeoxyglucose positron-emission tomography combined with computed tomography as a diagnostic tool in native valve endocarditis. Nucl Med Commun. 2018;39(8):747–52.

49. Philip M, Delcourt S, Mancini J, Tessonnier L, Cammilleri S, Arregle F, et al. (18) F-fluorodeoxyglucose positron emission tomography/computed tomography for the diagnosis of native valve infective endocarditis: a prospective study. Arch Cardiovasc Dis. 2021;114(3):211–20.

50. de Camargo RA, Sommer Bitencourt M, Meneghetti JC, Soares J, Goncalves LFT, Buchpiguel CA, et al. The role of 18F-Fluorodeoxyglucose positron emission tomography/computed tomography in the diagnosis of left-sided endocarditis: native vs. prosthetic valves endocarditis. Clin Infect Dis. 2020;70(4):583–94.

51. Habib G, Erba PA, Iung B, Donal E, Cosyns B, Laroche C, et al. Clinical presentation, aetiology and outcome of infective endocarditis. Results of the ESC-EORP EURO-ENDO (European infective endocarditis) registry: a prospective cohort study. Eur Heart J. 2019;40(39):3222–32.

52. Duval X, Le Moing V, Tubiana S, Esposito-Farese M, Ilic-Habensus E, Leclercq F, et al. Impact of systematic whole-body 18F-fluorodeoxyglucose PET/CT on the management of patients suspected of infective endocarditis: the prospective multicenter TEPvENDO study. Clin Infect Dis. 2020;73(3):393–403.

53. Hsu DFC, Ilan E, Peterson WT, Uribe J, Lubberink M, Levin CS. Studies of a next-generation silicon-photomultiplier-based time-of-flight PET/CT system. J Nucl Med. 2017;58(9):1511–8.

54. Boursier C, Duval X, Bourdon A, Imbert L, Mahida B, Chevalier E, et al. ECG-gated cardiac FDG PET acquisitions significantly improve detectability of infective endocarditis. JACC Cardiovasc Imaging. 2020;13(12):2691–3.

55. Wang TKM, Sanchez-Nadales A, Igbinomwanhia E, Cremer P, Griffin B, Xu B. Diagnosis of infective endo-

carditis by subtype using (18)F-Fluorodeoxyglucose positron emission tomography/computed tomography: a contemporary meta-analysis. Circ Cardiovasc Imaging. 2020;13(6):e010600.

56. Holle SLK, Andersen MH, Klein CF, Bruun NE, Tonder N, Haarmark C, et al. Clinical usefulness of FDG-PET/CT for identification of abnormal extra-cardiac foci in patients with infective endocarditis. Int J Cardiovasc Imaging. 2020;36(5): 939–46.

57. Boursier C, Duval X, Mahida B, Hoen B, Goehringer F, Selton-Suty C, et al. Hypermetabolism of the spleen or bone marrow is an additional albeit indirect sign of infective endocarditis at FDG-PET. J Nucl Cardiol. 2020;28(6):2533–42.

58. Thuny F, Beurtheret S, Mancini J, Gariboldi V, Casalta JP, Riberi A, et al. The timing of surgery influences mortality and morbidity in adults with severe complicated infective endocarditis: a propensity analysis. Eur Heart J. 2011;32(16):2027–33.

59. Chen W, Dilsizian V. FDG PET/CT for the diagnosis and management of infective endocarditis: expert consensus vs. evidence-based practice. J Nucl Cardiol. 2019;26(1):313–5.

60. Otto CM, Nishimura RA, Bonow RO, Carabello BA, Erwin JP 3rd, Gentile F, et al. 2020 ACC/AHA guideline for the management of patients with valvular heart disease: a report of the American College of Cardiology/American Heart Association Joint Committee on Clinical Practice Guidelines. Circulation. 2021;143(5):e72–e227.

61. Kestler M, Munoz P, Rodriguez-Creixems M, Rotger A, Jimenez-Requena F, Mari A, et al. Role of (18) F-FDG PET in patients with infectious endocarditis. J Nucl Med. 2014;55(7):1093–8.

62. San S, Ravis E, Tessonier L, Philip M, Cammilleri S, Lavagna F, et al. Prognostic value of (18) F-fluorodeoxyglucose positron emission tomography/ computed tomography in infective endocarditis. J Am Coll Cardiol. 2019;74(8):1031–40.

Cardiovascular Implantable Electronic Device Infection

Besma Mahida, Jérémie Calais, and François Rouzet

Introduction

Cardiac Implantable Electronic Device (CIED) Infections

Cardiac implantable electronic device (CIED) implantations, such as pacemakers, cardiac resynchronization therapy devices, and implantable cardiac defibrillators, have significantly increased in number in the past decades [1] as the indications are continuously expanding and because of the aging of the population. Despite improvements of CIED designs and preventive measures, CIED infection incidence, morbidity, mortality [2] are still increasing and represent an economic burden [3].

CIED infection mainly results from generator pocket contamination during implantation [4] with a risk of spread to the leads resulting in cardiac device-related infective endocarditis (CDRIE) [2, 5]. Less frequently, CIED infection results from hematogenous contamination from a distant focal infection [4]. Since CIED infection involves most frequently the generator pocket, the main infectious agents responsible for CIED infections are Gram-positive organisms, predominantly staphylococcal species. The virulence factors of the infectious agents are their ability to initiate microbial adhesion to the device surface and to produce a thick multilayered biofilm concurring to resistance to antibiotic therapy [6].

The most frequent clinical signs of CIED infection are the consequence of local reaction to generator pocket infection that include erythema, pain, swelling, tenderness, discharge, or ulceration [7]. However, these local signs can be missing and CIED systemic infection or CDRIE might have misleading presentation with nonspecific symptoms such as fever, chills, night sweats, or distant septic embolic events (pulmonary, spondylodiscitis) [8, 9]. The diagnostic work-up of CIED infection and/or CDRIE is based on the modified Duke-Li criteria that combine clinical findings, laboratory tests, bacterial cultures (blood and extracted device), and evidence of vegetation on lead or valve by transesophageal echocardiography (TEE) or other imaging modalities [2]. However, the final diagnosis may be challenging, given the variety of clinical presentations and the artifacts of echocardiography due to prosthetic materials [10]. Because therapeutic management of CIED infection/CDRIE often results in complete system removal and/or prolonged anti-

B. Mahida · F. Rouzet (✉)
APHP, Service de Médecine Nucléaire, Hôpital Bichat, Paris, France

Université Paris Cité, Paris, France

Inserm U1148, Paris, France
e-mail: francois.rouzet@aphp.fr

J. Calais
Ahmanson Translational Theranostics Division, Department of Molecular and Medical Pharmacology, David Geffen School of Medicine, UCLA, Los Angeles, CA, USA

biotic therapy [2, 11], an accurate diagnosis is necessary. Recently, the European Societies [2] included as a class 1 recommendation nuclear imaging with both ^{18}F-flurodeoxyglucose (FDG) positron emission tomography/computed tomography (PET/CT) and radiolabeled white blood cell (WBC) single-photon emission computed tomography/computed tomography (SPECT)/CT in the diagnostic criteria.

For inflammatory and infectious diseases indications, FDG PET/CT signal relies on metabolic activity at sites with high concentrations of activated neutrophils and monocyte/macrophages with increased glucose transporters (GLUT) and hexokinase (HK) expression [12].

Left Ventricular Assist Device (LVAD) Infection

Left ventricular assist device (LVAD) is s a life-saving therapy for patients with advanced chronic heart failure, as a bridge to heart transplant or as destination therapy. As LVAD implantations are increasing due to a shortage in organ donations, LVAD infections are rising [13]. LVAD infection is associated with higher risk of pump thrombosis, longer hospital stay duration, requirement for LVAD replacement, and failure to transplant [14].

LVAD infection was described by the International Society for Heart and Lung Transplantation (ISHLT) and classified into (1) "VAD-specific infections," referring to the infection of the hardware components or the body surfaces containing them (including infections of the pump, cannula, anastomoses, the pocket infections, and the percutaneous driveline or tunnel); (2) "VAD-related infections," referring to IE, bloodstream infection and mediastinitis with high infection mortality rating at 70% in VAD-related IE and mediastinitis; and (3) "non-VAD infections," referring to septic events that are not directly related to the presence of the LVAD hardware [15].

The most frequent type of LVAD infection occurs on the driveline, commonly from pathogens of the skin microbiome, including *S. aureus*, coagulase negative staphylococci and *Corynebacterium* spp., while *Candida* is less frequently found [16].

Currently, there are no standard guidelines for LVAD infection diagnosis management; therefore, the impact of nuclear medicine imaging is not yet well established in LVAD infections. However, recent studies reported on the usefulness of FDG PET/CT and/or comparison with WBC SPECT/CT in localizing and assessing the site of LVAD infection [17–21].

Diagnostic Work-Up of CIED and LVAD Infections

Clinical Signs

Due to the variety and absence of specificity of symptoms, the diagnosis of CIED infection is challenging. Infections involve most frequently the generator pocket. Localized generator pocket infection signs range from pocket wound inflammation to external purulent drainage of the device [22].

In the presence of exposed generator or proximal leads, the CIED should be considered infected regardless of microbiology results. Therefore, assessing the potential extension of CIED infection is important for therapy management. Superficial infection of the pocket wound does not require total hardware extraction as it concerns the cutaneous and subcutaneous tissues, allowing a conservative treatment while generator pocket infection, which can be associated with lead infection, CIED systemic sepsis, and/or CDRIE [23], requires a more invasive strategy.

In the absence of visible signs of local infection, CIED systemic infection and CDRIE diagnosis are more challenging with predominantly nonspecific symptoms such as distant septic emboli, mainly pulmonary [24], or vertebral osteomyelitis and discitis [9]. Similarly, the diagnosis of LVAD infection is challenging because clinical presentation may range from nonspecific symptoms such as erythema, warmth, to purulent drainage around the driveline exit site and the difficulty to localize the infection source, involving either superficial or deep components of the device [25].

Microbiology

Most pathogens responsible for CIED and LVAD infections are cutaneous organisms considering that infections most frequently originate from the generator pocket or the percutaneous driveline. However, cultures sampled from blood and from any suspected infected site(s) should be systematically performed before antibiotics initiation in patients with CIED who develop fever without typical signs of local infection.

Imaging

The 2019 European Society of Cardiology (ESC) recommendations for CIED infection diagnosis management [2] rely on multimodality imaging that includes FDG PET/CT and WBC SPECT/CT along with echography and CT.

Echocardiography

Transthoracic echocardiography (TTE) and transesophageal echocardiography (TEE) are recommended for the assessment of lead vegetation and/or valvular involvement in suspected CIED infections with a clear superiority of TEE for vegetation detection and size measurement [2, 26]. Echocardiography remains the first-line diagnostic tool in the assessment of patients with CIED infection or CDRIE suspicion. However, limitations and inconclusive cases impair the Duke-Li classification sensitivity [10].

Cardiac CT

Cardiac contrast-enhanced (CE) computed tomography (CT) provides anatomical information to detect the presence of vegetations and local complications such as abscesses, pseudoaneurysms, fistulas, or septic embolization [27]. The 2015 ESC modified criteria for the diagnosis of IE included cardiac CT in the assessment of paravalvular lesions as a major criterion for IE diagnosis, which might allow the diagnosis of CDRIE. However, CE-CT can be limited by iodinated contrast agent contraindication and the presence of metallic artifacts generated by the CIED or LVAD hardware.

Endocarditis Team

The recent 2019 ESC consensus on CIED infection highlighted the role of a multidisciplinary approach that includes cardiologists, cardiovascular surgeons, infectious diseases specialists, clinical microbiologists, echocardiographers, radiologists, and nuclear medicine physicians. A multidisciplinary approach can significantly reduce the 1-year mortality of IE [28].

Prognosis

The prognosis of patients with infected CIED is poor, with a mortality rate of 5%–8% at 30-day and 20% at 1 year due to cardiac and extracardiac complications [29, 30]. Patients with comorbidities have a higher mortality rate. CIED infection remains a serious, life-threatening condition that requires usually the complete removal of the hardware, as a delay in device removal might worsen prognosis [31].

FDG PET/CT

Basic Principles

FDG PET/CT is a nuclear imaging modality often used for assessing infectious and inflammatory diseases. Fluorine-18 (18F) is a cyclotron-produced radioisotope with a half-life of 109.7 min that decays by emitting positrons, which can be detected with a PET scanner. 18F-FDG is a glucose analogue, which enters cells via glucose transporter (GLUT), and then undergoes phosphorylation by hexokinase (HK). However, phosphorylated 18F-FDG is a metabolic dead end, which accumulates within cells during the 1-h delay separating injection from acquisition resulting in major signal amplification.

Inflammatory cells (activated neutrophils, macrophages, monocytes, and lymphocytes) express high levels of glucose transporters, especially GLUT1 and GLUT3, and have hexokinase activity, which translate into an increased FDG uptake [32]. The European Association of Nuclear Medicine and the Society of Nuclear Medicine issued guidelines for performing FDG PET/CT in patients with suspected infection [33].

Patient Preparation

The main goal is to inhibit physiological myocardial FDG uptake to enable the visualization of increased FDG signal foci. This can be achieved by combining a no-carbohydrate high-fat meal >12 h before the scan and a fasting period of >12 h [34]. As usual with FDG PET, pregnancy, diabetes, and serum glucose level should be checked before FDG injection [33].

Tracer Administration

In Europe the recommended administered activity of FDG ranges between 2.5 and 5.0 MBq/kg. In the United States, it ranges between 370 and 740 MBq. Administered activity should be adapted for infants and children according to pediatric dosage. In case of suspected CIED infection, radiopharmaceuticals should be administrated in the contralateral arm to avoid the potential pitfall of accumulated FDG along the leads mimicking septic locations [33].

Imaging Procedure

The image acquisition should be performed 60 min after FDG administration, from vertex to toes (total-body acquisition) for the detection of distant septic emboli, in whole-body mode, using steps of 1.5–3 min per bed position. CT acquisition parameters can be used as detailed in the EANM tumor imaging guidelines [35] and always adapted to the CT scanner performance and to the specific radiologic society guidelines. PET images should be reconstructed using cor-rections for attenuation, dead time, random events, and scatter, according to the PET/CT scanner performance. Whenever possible, ECG-gated acquisitions in the thorax should be performed as it improves EI detection and might be helpful with CDRIE diagnosis [36].

Interpretation Criteria

The analysis of the FDG PET/CT images relies on visual criteria. Both attenuation-corrected (AC) and non-attenuation-corrected (NAC) images centered on the CIED should be analyzed carefully by scrolling through each of the axial, coronal, and sagittal views of the PET only, CT only, fused PET/CT images. The local analysis should focus on the signal around the generator-pocket site, along the leads and in the valves. Increased FDG uptake above the background around CIED generator-pocket and leads (extravascular, intravascular, or intracardiac) should be considered suspicious. The 3D MIP images and the whole-body FDG PET/CT images should be carefully analyzed for the detection of other foci of infection which could represent the primary site of infection or distant secondary septic locations (lungs, spleen, spine, mycotic aneurysms).

The main cause of false-positive FDG-PET is inflammation (acute, sub-acute, chronic) caused by the surgery or the presence of foreign body. Therefore, the time from CIED implantation to imaging is crucial information that must be collected and incorporated in the overall interpretation of the study.

The final FDG PET/CT diagnosis of CIED infection relies on the combination of multiple features. Visual analysis is the method of reference. The semi-quantitative parameters do not allow the differentiation of infection vs. inflammation (range values overlap) and should be used only as a complement to the visual analysis.

Signs in favor of infection include high-intensity uptake, uptake visible on both AC and NAC images, focal uptake on the leads, heterogeneous and intense signal around the generator, continuity of the FDG PET signal to the surrounding tissues (muscle, skin), presence of distant septic locations (especially in the lungs), and time from CIED implantation to imaging of >2 months. Signs that do not suggest infection include uptake visible only on the AC or the NAC, diffuse and homogeneous moderate uptake, presence of metallic artifacts, and time from CIED implantation to imaging of <2 months.

Factors that decrease the intensity of the signal and thus the sensitivity of the scan include exposure to antibiotic therapy, metallic artifacts, partial volume effect, and motion artifacts. Whenever possible, the scan should be performed as early as possible in the course of the disease before treatment initiation and include ECG-gated acquisitions centered on the thorax. The use of CT contrast may enhance the visualization of the anatomic structures and thus be helpful in some cases.

Although FDG PET/CT offers the possibility of semi-quantitative analysis, current available studies describing the use of values such as a maximum standardized uptake value (SUV_{max}) or a semi-quantitative ratio (SQR) to assess areas of FDG uptake did not report a significant improvement in discriminating infected from non-infected devices [37]. The visual analysis is the method of reference, especially for CDRIE detection.

CIED Infections

Recently, the use of nuclear medicine imaging in suspected CIED infection and CDRIE has increased, especially in cases of suspected CIED infections with no local signs of infection at generator pocket and non-conclusive echocardiography. In these challenging situations, the 2019 ESC guidelines recommend [2] total-body FDG PET/CT to assess the extent of disease, with distant septic emboli being considered as a minor criterion for CIED infection diagnosis, and to localize the portal of entry.

Two recent meta-analyses by Juneau et al. [38] and Mahmood et al. [37] reported high sensitivity and specificity of FDG PET/CT for the diagnosis of CIED infection: pooled sensitivity of 87% (95% CI, 82–91%) and 83% (95% CI 78–86%), and pooled specificity of 94% (95% CI, 88–98%) and 89 (95% CI 84–94%), respectively. Mahmood et al. estimated a higher sensitivity of 96% (95% CI 86–99%) and specificity of 97% (95% CI 86–99%) for pocket infection diagnosis. Although generator pocket infection is mainly a clinical diagnosis, FDG PET/CT can be useful in situations with uncertain diagnosis [39]. The diagnostic accuracy for the detection of lead infections or CDRIE is lower with a reported sensitivity and specificity of 76% (95% CI 65–85%) and 83% (95% CI 72–90%), respectively [37]. The main technical limitations are the partial volume effect and cardiac motion artifact.

Extracardiac complications occur in 30–80% of patients [40, 41] and are known to increase mortality and worsen prognosis [42]. The ability of FDG PET/CT to detect distant extracardiac complications such as septic emboli and metastatic infection provides incremental diagnostic and prognostic information for CIED infection and CDRIE [2, 43]. Septic pulmonary emboli and spondylodiscitis are the most frequent distant infectious sites [9]. Septic pulmonary emboli are a common finding in CIED lead infection and CDRIE involving tricuspid valve infection. The presence of multiple and bilateral foci of FDG uptake, often associated with matching parenchymal opacities on CT, is highly suggestive of septic emboli and accordingly of infection of the device [44]. In a prospective study, Amraoui et al. evaluated 35 patients with a definite diagnosis of CDRIE by Duke-Li criteria, and spondylodiscitis was identified on FDG PET/CT in 20% of patients, some being completely asymptomatic [45]. Vascular septic emboli and mycotic aneurysms are usually asymptomatic but might lead to vascular rupture, a life-threatening complication (Fig. 14.1). The most common localization is in the brain and can be detected by MRI; however, it might occur anywhere else [46–48] (Fig. 14.2). The other frequent sites of septic emboli are the same as encountered in IE and include the spleen and bone marrow. Boursier et al. demonstrated, in a cohort of 129 patients including 88 subjects with a definite diagnosis of IE, that diffuse high FDG uptake in the spleen and/or bone marrow (defined as superior to liver uptake) can be an indirect sign of IE [49].

Although FDG PET/CT has an added value to the modified Duke-Li criteria for the diagnosis of

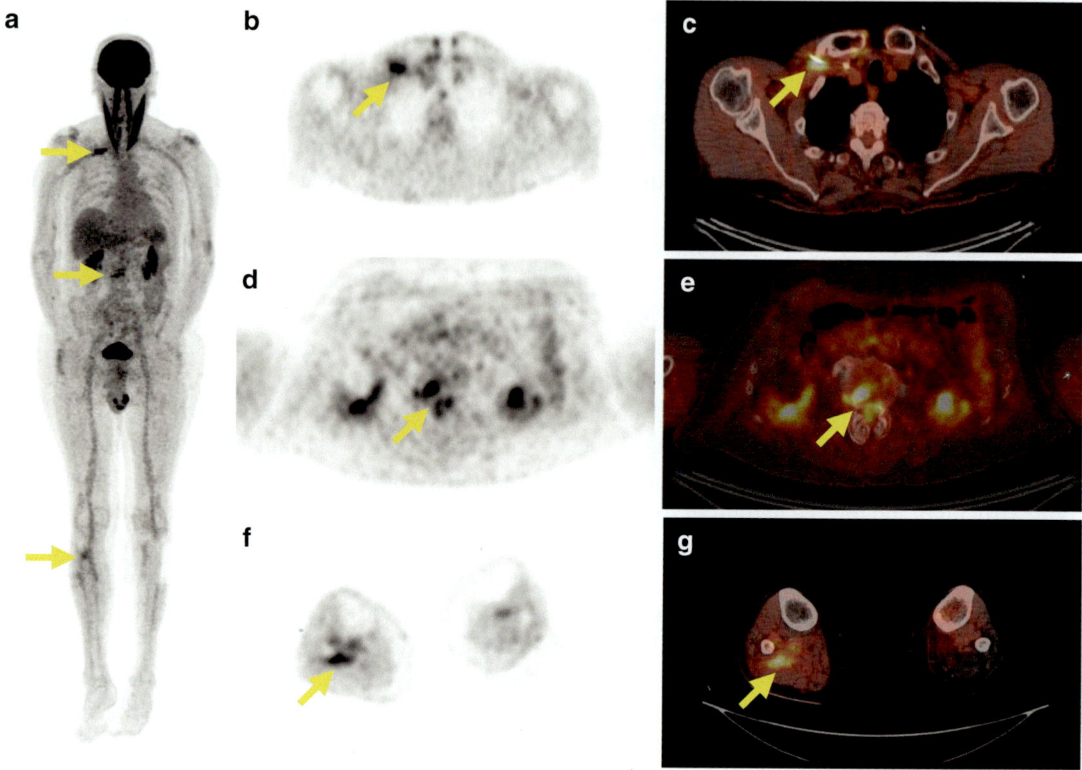

Fig. 14.1 An 83-year-old male who underwent cardiac electronic device (CIED) implantation 5 years prior. The patient had native mitral endocarditis. EI diagnosis was based on the visualization of a vegetation on echocardiography and positive *E. faecalis* blood cultures. 18F-flurodeoxyglucose (FDG) positron emission tomography/computed tomography (PET/CT) scan did not show significant uptake on the native mitral valve. However, it showed intense FDG uptake (yellow arrows) on distant sites along the PM lead, L2-L3 vertebrae, and the tibial fibular arterial trunk ((**a**) whole body FDG PET maximum intensity projection images). (**b**) Axial FDG PET. (**c**) Fused axial PET/CT chest images showed intense uptake along the PM lead. Extraction of the device confirmed the lead infection. (**d**) Axial FDG PET. (**e**) Fused axial PET/ CT spine images showed intense FDG uptake on L2-L3 suspicious for spondylodiscitis that was confirmed on MRI—the patient was asymptomatic. (**f**) Axial FDG PET. (**g**) Fused axial PET/CT of the lower limbs showed focal uptake on the tibial fibular arterial trunk suggesting mycotic aneurysm

CIED infections [44, 50], it is important to point out the limitations of the technique. The main limitation is the lack of specificity of FDG uptake for infection as FDG also accumulates at sites of aseptic inflammation. This can lead to false-positive cases, especially in the immediate period after device implantation, or in patients with intense inflammatory reaction to foreign body. Another important factor to consider is the delay between antibiotics initiation and the scan: sensitivity decreases with duration of the antimicrobial therapy [44, 51]. FDG PET/CT should be performed as early as possible when CIED infection is suspected.

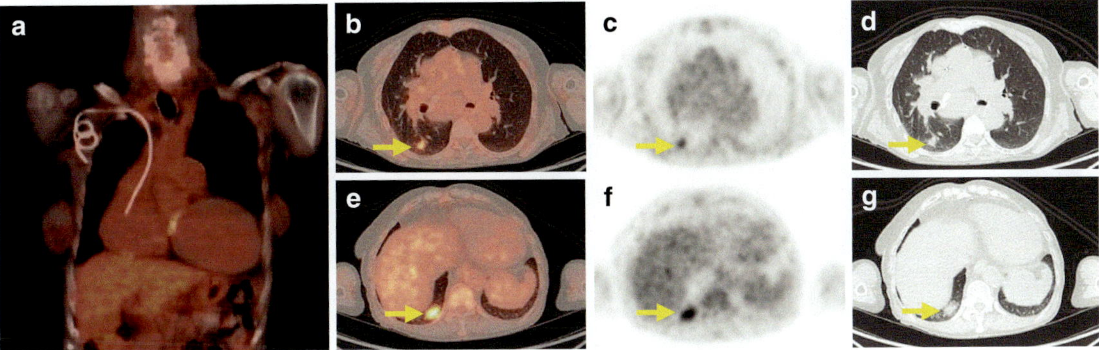

Fig. 14.2 A 75-year-old female with a prior history of CIED infection 2 years earlier. The patient underwent generator removal but only partial leads extraction. The patient had persistent episodes of fever and positive MRSA blood cultures. Echocardiography was inconclusive. The FDG PET/CT scan showed no abnormal uptake on the remaining lead ((**a**) fused coronal PET/CT) but significant intense focal uptake in the right lung (yellow arrows) (PET axial images (**c** and **f**)) corresponding to a lung parenchymal opacity on fused axial PET/CT images (**b** and **e**) and axial CT images (**d** and **g**). FDG PET/CT images of septic lung emboli helped to diagnose the CIED infection. The patient was treated with suppressive antibiotic therapy

LVAD Infections

In their case series, systematic review, and meta-analysis, Tam et al. analyzed the diagnostic accuracy of FDG PET/CT in suspected LVAD infections [20]. Despite limited data, they reported a high sensitivity of 92% (95%CI: 82–97%) and a more variable specificity of 83% (95% CI: 24–99%). The limitations that impair FDG PET/CT specificity for the diagnostic of CIED infection also apply with LVAD. Kim et al. evaluated the impact of FDG PET/CT on patient management and outcome in LVAD infections [18]. FDG PET/ CT localized infection among 28 of the 35 patients analyzed. According to FDG PET/CT findings, patients were considered as noninfected, infected with peripheral infection limited to the exit wound site and/or driveline, or infected with central infection extending to components of the LVAD (cannula and/or pump pocket). During the follow-up, the majority of deaths occurred in patients with central versus peripheral infection groups, and none of the noninfected patients died. FDG PET/ CT should be performed in early stages of suspected LVAD infection to obtain the best impact on the patient management (Fig. 14.3).

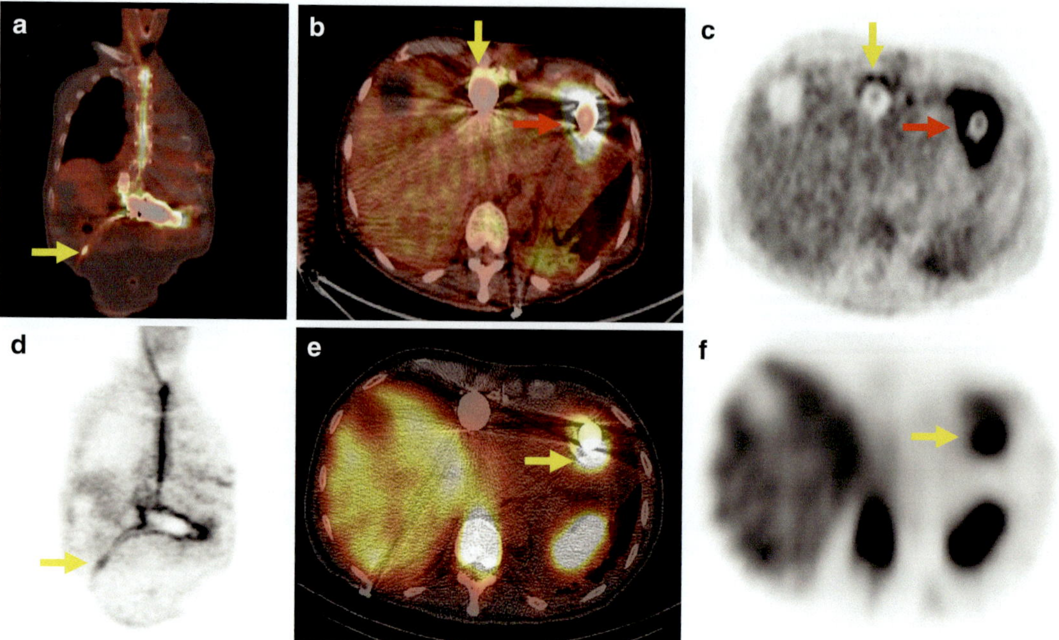

Fig. 14.3 A 72-year-old male referred for suspected left ventricular assist device (LVAD) infection, 2 months after device implantation with fever and *Klebsiella pneumonia*-positive blood culture. The patient underwent FDG PET/CT and WBC SPECT/CT 2 weeks later: (**a**) fused coronal PET/CT images and (**d**) FDG PET maximum intensity projection images showed multifocal device-related infection on all components, including a focal intense FDG uptake along the driveline (yellow arrows) corresponding to a percutaneous exit infection that was proven after sur-gery. (**b**) Fused axial PET/CT and (**c**) axial FDG PET showed intense FDG uptake on the inflow cannula (red arrows) concordant with WBC SPECT/CT images (**e**) and (**f**) (yellow arrows) consistent with infection. FDG uptake along the LVAD pump (yellow arrows) was not associated with corresponding increased uptake on WBC SPECT/CT images obtained 24 h after tracer injection. The device was not removed, and the patient was treated with suppressive antibiotic therapy

Comparison with WBC SPECT/CT

WBC SPECT/CT is the current benchmark radionuclide technique for infection imaging in soft tissues [52]. Although there are limited data on the role of WBC SPECT/CT in CIED infection, the available results show excellent specificity and significant sensitivity [44, 53, 54].

FDG PET/CT has a higher sensitivity for the detection of CIED infection/CDRIE than WBC SPECT/CT because of its greater spatial resolution and contrast. Total-body FDG PET/CT also has the advantage of detecting distant infection sites and portal of entry. However, WBC SPECT/CT has a higher specificity than FDG PET/CT. In their retrospective study, Calais et al. evaluated 48 consecutive patients with clinically suspected CIED infection who had both FDG PET/CT and WBC SPECT/CT, reporting a sensitivity of 100% for FDG PET/CT and a specificity of 100% for WBC SPECT/CT. Prolonged antibiotherapy before imaging had the same consequence on both modalities by decreasing their sensitivity which emphasizes the importance of performing nuclear medicine imaging before or shortly after initiating treatment. In this study, more than half of patients that were initially considered with possible CIED infection based on the modified Duke-Li score at admission and were correctly reclassified as rejected or definite infection based on the results FDG PET/CT or WBC SPECT/CT scan. Hence, in the presence of a suspected CIED infection, FDG PET/CT should be performed as first-line nuclear imaging technique and can be followed by WBC SPECT/CT imaging in case of an inconclusive result (Fig. 14.4).

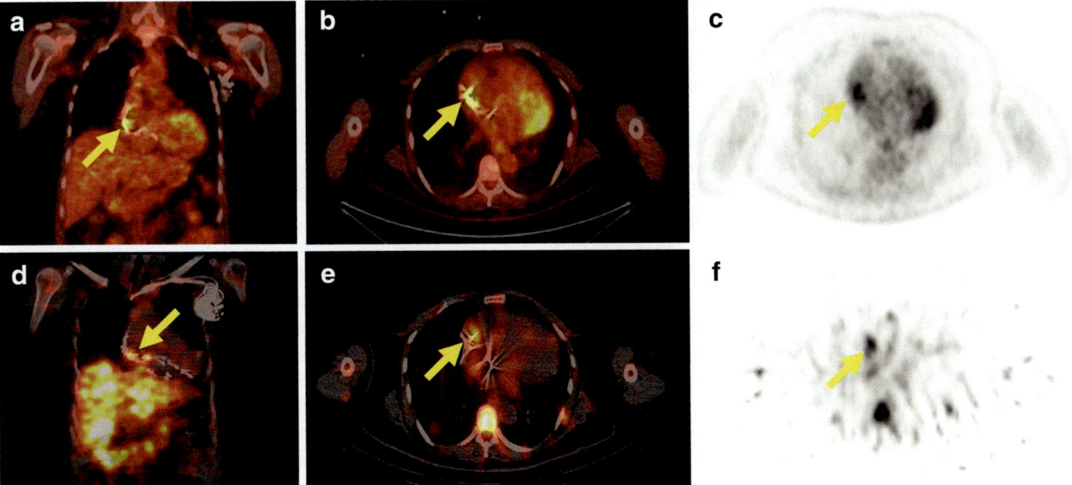

Fig. 14.4 Concordant true-positive 18F-flurodeoxyglucose (FDG) positron emission tomography/computed tomography (PET/CT) and radiolabeled white blood cell (WBC) single photon emission computed tomography/computed tomography (SPECT/CT) in a 63-year-old male who underwent cardiac electronic device (CIED) implantation 4 months before FDG PET/CT images. The patient was referred for fever, non-conclusive echocardiography and negative blood cultures. As per the Duke-Li criteria, CIED infection was initially graded as possible. FDG PET/CT showed intense 18FDG uptake along the leads in the superior vena cava and right atrium suspicious of lead infection (yellow arrows). The extraction of the device confirmed the lead infection: (**a**) FDG PET fused coronal images; (**b**) fused axial PET/CT images; (**c**) axial PET images; (**d**) fused coronal WBC SPECT/CT images obtained 24 h after tracer injection; (**e**) fused axial WBC SPECT/CT images; (**f**) axial WBC SPECT images

Perspectives

FDG PET/CT and WBC SPECT/CT are included as complementary tools in the Novel 2019 International CIED Infection Criteria [2]. However, FDG PET/CT lacks specificity, and WBC SPECT/CT requires dedicated equipment, direct handling of blood products, is time consuming and has limited capacity for total body scanning. Ideally, the key strengths of both techniques should be combined. The development of new radiopharmaceuticals and the technological advancements of detection systems may improve further the performances of nuclear imaging of infection.

tion and no specific signs of hardware involvement. Whole-body FDG PET/CT influences the therapeutic decisions and outcomes by improving the diagnosis performance of the Duke-Li score, by enabling assessment of the extracardiac components of the device, and by identifying the portal of entry or septic emboli. FDG PET/CT's lack of specificity may be overcome by associating WBC SPECT/CT as a second-line imaging technique when needed. FDG PET/CT and WBC SPECT/CT should be performed in early stage of suspected infection to avoid sensitivity loss following antibiotics initiation.

Conclusions

FDG PET/CT is a highly sensitive imaging technique now established in the management of patients with CIED and LVAD infections, particularly in patients with suspected bloodstream infec-

References

1. Mond HG, Proclemer A. The 11th world survey of cardiac pacing and implantable cardioverter-defibrillators: calendar year 2009: a world Society of Arrhythmia's project. Pacing Clin Electrophysiol. 2011;34(8):1013–27.
2. Blomström-Lundqvist C, Traykov V, Erba PA, Burri H, Nielsen JC, Bongiorni MG, et al. European heart

rhythm association (EHRA) international consensus document on how to prevent, diagnose, and treat cardiac implantable electronic device infections-endorsed by the Heart Rhythm Society (HRS), the Asia Pacific Heart Rhythm Society (APHRS), the Latin American Heart Rhythm Society (LAHRS), International Society for Cardiovascular Infectious Diseases (ISCVID) and the European Society of Clinical Microbiology and Infectious Diseases (ESCMID) in collaboration with the European Association for Cardio-Thoracic Surgery (EACTS). Europace. 2020;22(4):515–49.

3. Gitenay E, Molin F, Blais S, Tremblay V, Gervais P, Plourde B, et al. Cardiac implantable electronic device infection: detailed analysis of cost implications. Can J Cardiol. 2018;34(8):1026–32.

4. Nagpal A, Baddour LM, Sohail MR. Microbiology and pathogenesis of cardiovascular implantable electronic device infections. Circ Arrhythm Electrophysiol. 2012;5(2):433–41.

5. Krahn AD, Longtin Y, Philippon F, Birnie DH, Manlucu J, Angaran P, et al. Prevention of arrhythmia device infection trial: the PADIT trial. J Am Coll Cardiol. 2018;72(24):3098–109.

6. Patel R. Biofilms and antimicrobial resistance. Clin Orthop Relat Res. 2005;437:41–7.

7. Bongiorni MG, Burri H, Deharo JC, Starck C, Kennergren C, Saghy L, et al. 2018 EHRA expert consensus statement on lead extraction: recommendations on definitions, endpoints, research trial design, and data collection requirements for clinical scientific studies and registries: endorsed by APHRS/HRS/LAHRS. Europace. 2018;20(7):1217.

8. Athan E, Chu VH, Tattevin P, Selton-Suty C, Jones P, Naber C, et al. Clinical characteristics and outcome of infective endocarditis involving implantable cardiac devices. JAMA. 2012;307(16):1727–35.

9. Rodriguez Y, Greenspon AJ, Sohail MR, Carrillo RG. Cardiac device-related endocarditis complicated by spinal abscess. Pacing Clin Electrophysiol. 2012;35(3):269–74.

10. Dundar C, Tigen K, Tanalp C, Izgi A, Karaahmet T, Cevik C, et al. The prevalence of echocardiographic accretions on the leads of patients with permanent pacemakers. J Am Soc Echocardiogr. 2011;24(7):803–7.

11. Rickard J, Tarakji K, Cheng A, Spragg D, Cantillon DJ, Martin DO, et al. Survival of patients with biventricular devices after device infection, extraction, and reimplantation. JACC Heart Fail. 2013;1(6):508–13.

12. Mochizuki T, Tsukamoto E, Kuge Y, Kanegae K, Zhao S, Hikosaka K, et al. FDG uptake and glucose transporter subtype expressions in experimental tumor and inflammation models. J Nucl Med. 2001;42(10):1551–5.

13. Daneshmand MA, Rajagopal K, Lima B, Khorram N, Blue LJ, Lodge AJ, et al. Left ventricular assist device destination therapy versus extended criteria cardiac transplant. Ann Thorac Surg. 2010;89(4):1205–9; discussion 1210.

14. Kilic A, Acker MA, Atluri P. Dealing with surgical left ventricular assist device complications. J Thorac Dis. 2015;7(12):2158–64.

15. Hannan MM, Husain S, Mattner F, Danziger-Isakov L, Drew RJ, Corey GR, et al. Working formulation for the standardization of definitions of infections in patients using ventricular assist devices. J Heart Lung Transplant. 2011;30(4):375–84.

16. Nienaber JJC, Kusne S, Riaz T, Walker RC, Baddour LM, Wright AJ, et al. Clinical manifestations and management of left ventricular assist device-associated infections. Clin Infect Dis. 2013;57(10):1438–48.

17. Litzler P-Y, Manrique A, Etienne M, Salles A, Edet-Sanson A, Vera P, et al. Leukocyte SPECT/CT for detecting infection of left-ventricular-assist devices: preliminary results. J Nucl Med. 2010;51(7):1044–8.

18. Kim J, Feller ED, Chen W, Liang Y, Dilsizian V. FDG PET/CT for early detection and localization of left ventricular assist device infection: impact on patient management and outcome. JACC Cardiovasc Imaging. 2019;12(4):722–9.

19. de Vaugelade C, Mesguich C, Nubret K, Camou F, Greib C, Dournes G, et al. Infections in patients using ventricular-assist devices: comparison of the diagnostic performance of 18F-FDG PET/CT scan and leucocyte-labeled scintigraphy. J Nucl Cardiol. 2019;26(1):42–55.

20. Tam MC, Patel VN, Weinberg RL, Hulten EA, Aaronson KD, Pagani FD, et al. Diagnostic accuracy of FDG PET/CT in suspected LVAD infections: a case series, systematic review, and meta-analysis. JACC Cardiovasc Imaging. 2020;13(5):1191–202.

21. Ten Hove D, Treglia G, Slart RHJA, Damman K, Wouthuyzen-Bakker M, Postma DF, et al. The value of 18F-FDG PET/CT for the diagnosis of device-related infections in patients with a left ventricular assist device: a systematic review and meta-analysis. Eur J Nucl Med Mol Imaging. 2021;48(1):241–53.

22. Uslan DZ, Sohail MR, St Sauver JL, Friedman PA, Hayes DL, Stoner SM, et al. Permanent pacemaker and implantable cardioverter defibrillator infection: a population-based study. Arch Intern Med. 2007;167(7):669–75.

23. Knigina L, Kühn C, Kutschka I, Oswald H, Klein G, Haverich A, et al. Treatment of patients with recurrent or persistent infection of cardiac implantable electronic devices. Europace. 2010;12(9):1275–81.

24. Klug D, Lacroix D, Savoye C, Goullard L, Grandmougin D, Hennequin JL, et al. Systemic infection related to endocarditis on pacemaker leads: clinical presentation and management. Circulation. 1997;95(8):2098–107.

25. Leuck A-M. Left ventricular assist device driveline infections: recent advances and future goals. J Thorac Dis. 2015;7(12):2151–7.

26. Flachskampf FA, Wouters PF, Edvardsen T, Evangelista A, Habib G, Hoffman P, et al. Recommendations for transoesophageal echocardiography: EACVI update 2014. Eur Heart J Cardiovasc Imaging. 2014;15(4):353–65.

27. Habib G, Lancellotti P, Antunes MJ, Bongiorni MG, Casalta J-P, Del Zotti F, et al. 2015 ESC guidelines for the management of infective endocarditis: the task force for the Management of Infective Endocarditis of the European Society of Cardiology (ESC). Endorsed by: European Association for Cardio-Thoracic Surgery (EACTS), the European Association of Nuclear Medicine (EANM). Eur Heart J. 2015;36(44):3075–128.

28. Botelho-Nevers E, Thuny F, Casalta JP, Richet H, Gouriet F, Collart F, et al. Dramatic reduction in infective endocarditis-related mortality with a management-based approach. Arch Intern Med. 2009;169(14):1290–8.

29. Boersma LV, Barr CS, Burke MC, Leon AR, Theuns DA, Herre JM, et al. Performance of the subcutaneous implantable cardioverter-defibrillator in patients with a primary prevention indication with and without a reduced ejection fraction versus patients with a secondary prevention indication. Heart Rhythm. 2017;14(3):367–75.

30. Bannay A, Hoen B, Duval X, Obadia J-F, Selton-Suty C, Le Moing V, et al. The impact of valve surgery on short- and long-term mortality in left-sided infective endocarditis: do differences in methodological approaches explain previous conflicting results? Eur Heart J. 2011;32(16):2003–15.

31. Viganego F, O'Donoghue S, Eldadah Z, Shah MH, Rastogi M, Mazel JA, et al. Effect of early diagnosis and treatment with percutaneous lead extraction on survival in patients with cardiac device infections. Am J Cardiol. 2012;109(10):1466–71.

32. Love C, Tomas MB, Tronco GG, Palestro CJ. FDG PET of infection and inflammation. Radiographics. 2005;25(5):1357–68.

33. Jamar F, Buscombe J, Chiti A, Christian PE, Delbeke D, Donohoe KJ, et al. EANM/SNMMI guideline for 18F-FDG use in inflammation and infection. J Nucl Med. 2013;54(4):647–58.

34. Morooka M, Moroi M, Uno K, Ito K, Wu J, Nakagawa T, et al. Long fasting is effective in inhibiting physiological myocardial 18F-FDG uptake and for evaluating active lesions of cardiac sarcoidosis. EJNMMI Res. 2014;4:1.

35. Boellaard R, Delgado-Bolton R, Oyen WJG, Giammarile F, Tatsch K, Eschner W, et al. FDG PET/CT: EANM procedure guidelines for tumour imaging: version 2.0. Eur J Nucl Med Mol Imaging. 2015;42(2):328–54.

36. Boursier C, Duval X, Bourdon A, Imbert L, Mahida B, Chevalier E, et al. ECG-gated cardiac FDG PET acquisitions significantly improve detectability of infective endocarditis. JACC Cardiovasc Imaging. 2020;13(12):2691–3.

37. Mahmood M, Kendi AT, Farid S, Ajmal S, Johnson GB, Baddour LM, et al. Role of 18F-FDG PET/CT in the diagnosis of cardiovascular implantable electronic device infections: a meta-analysis. J Nucl Cardiol. 2019;26(3):958–70.

38. Juneau D, Golfam M, Hazra S, Zuckier LS, Garas S, Redpath C, et al. Positron emission tomography and single-photon emission computed tomography imaging in the diagnosis of cardiac implantable electronic device infection: a systematic review and meta-analysis. Circ Cardiovasc Imaging. 2017;10(4):e005772.

39. JAT S, Barlow G, Chambers JB, Gammage M, Guleri A, Howard P, et al. Guidelines for the diagnosis, prevention and management of implantable cardiac electronic device infection. Report of a joint working party project on behalf of the British Society for Antimicrobial Chemotherapy (BSAC, host organization), British Heart Rhythm Society (BHRS), British cardiovascular society (BCS), British heart valve society (BHVS) and British Society for Echocardiography (BSE). J Antimicrob Chemother. 2015;70(2):325–59.

40. Duval X, Le Moing V, Tubiana S, Esposito-Farèse M, Ilic-Habensus E, Leclercq F, et al. Impact of systematic whole-body 18F-Fluorodeoxyglucose PET/CT on the management of patients suspected of infective endocarditis: the prospective multicenter TEPvENDO study. Clin Infect Dis. 2020;73(3):393–403. https://doi.org/10.1093/cid/ciaa666/5850646.

41. Murdoch DR, Corey GR, Hoen B, Miró JM, Fowler VG, Bayer AS, et al. Clinical presentation, etiology, and outcome of infective endocarditis in the 21st century: the international collaboration on endocarditis-prospective cohort study. Arch Intern Med. 2009;169(5):463–73.

42. Hill EE, Herijgers P, Claus P, Vanderschueren S, Herregods M-C, Peetermans WE. Infective endocarditis: changing epidemiology and predictors of 6-month mortality: a prospective cohort study. Eur Heart J. 2007;28(2):196–203.

43. Habib G, Erba PA, Iung B, Donal E, Cosyns B, Laroche C, et al. Clinical presentation, aetiology and outcome of infective endocarditis. Results of the ESC-EORP EURO-ENDO (European infective endocarditis) registry: a prospective cohort study. Eur Heart J. 2019;40(39):3222–32.

44. Calais J, Touati A, Grall N, Laouénan C, Benali K, Mahida B, et al. Diagnostic impact of 18F-Fluorodeoxyglucose positron emission tomography/computed tomography and white blood cell SPECT/computed tomography in patients with suspected cardiac implantable electronic device chronic infection. Circ Cardiovasc Imaging. 2019;12(7):e007188.

45. Amraoui S, Tlili G, Sohal M, Berte B, Hindié E, Ritter P, et al. Contribution of PET imaging to the diagnosis of septic embolism in patients with pacing lead endocarditis. JACC Cardiovasc Imaging. 2016;9(3):283–90.

46. Mikail N, Benali K, Ou P, Slama J, Hyafil F, Le Guludec D, et al. Detection of mycotic aneurysms of lower limbs by whole-body (18)F-FDG-PET. JACC Cardiovasc Imaging. 2015;8(7):859–62.

47. Mikail N, Benali K, Mahida B, Vigne J, Hyafil F, Rouzet F, et al. 18F-FDG-PET/CT imaging to diag-

nose septic emboli and mycotic aneurysms in patients with endocarditis and cardiac device infections. Curr Cardiol Rep. 2018;20(3):14.

48. Calais J, Pasi N, Nguyen V, Hyafil F. Mycotic aneurysm in a pulmonary artery detected with 18F-fluorodeoxyglucose positron emission tomography/computed tomography imaging. Eur Heart J. 2017;38(46):3474.

49. Boursier C, Duval X, Mahida B, Hoen B, Goehringer F, Selton-Suty C, et al. Hypermetabolism of the spleen or bone marrow is an additional albeit indirect sign of infective endocarditis at FDG-PET. J Nucl Cardiol. 2020;28(6):2533–42. https://doi.org/10.1007/s12350-020-02050-2.

50. Jerónimo A, Olmos C, Vilacosta I, Ortega-Candil A, Rodríguez-Rey C, Pérez-Castejón MJ, et al. Accuracy of 18F-FDG PET/CT in patients with the suspicion of cardiac implantable electronic device infections. J Nucl Cardiol. 2020;29(2):594–608.

51. Diemberger I, Bonfiglioli R, Martignani C, Graziosi M, Biffi M, Lorenzetti S, et al. Contribution of PET imaging to mortality risk stratification in candidates to lead extraction for pacemaker or defibrillator infection: a prospective single center study. Eur J Nucl Med Mol Imaging. 2019;46(1):194–205.

52. Signore A, Jamar F, Israel O, Buscombe J, Martin-Comin J, Lazzeri E. Clinical indications, image acquisition and data interpretation for white blood cells and anti-granulocyte monoclonal antibody scintigraphy: an EANM procedural guideline. Eur J Nucl Med Mol Imaging. 2018;45(10):1816–31.

53. Erba PA, Sollini M, Conti U, Bandera F, Tascini C, De Tommasi SM, et al. Radiolabeled WBC scintigraphy in the diagnostic workup of patients with suspected device-related infections. JACC Cardiovasc Imaging. 2013;6(10):1075–86.

54. Holcman K, Małecka B, Rubiś P, Ząbek A, Szot W, Boczar K, et al. The role of 99mTc-HMPAO-labelled white blood cell scintigraphy in the diagnosis of cardiac device-related infective endocarditis. Eur Heart J Cardiovasc Imaging. 2020;21(9):1022–30.

Vascular Graft Infection

Elite Arnon-Sheleg and Zohar Keidar

Introduction

Vascular grafts or prostheses are used for the treatment of occlusive vascular disease, life-threatening aortic aneurysms, and aortic dissection. Autologous vascular grafts are made with the patient's vessels (commonly the long saphenous vein). Biological grafts can also be created from human donor vessels (allografts) or bovine vessels (xenografts). Synthetic grafts can be made from polyethylene-terephthalate (commercially known as Dacron) or polytetrafluoroethylene (PTFE, commercially known as Gore-Tex). Grafts are divided into extracavitary grafts, located in the groin (80% of cases) and lower limbs or intracavitary grafts, located in the abdomen (70% of cases) and thorax [1]. Grafts may be implanted surgically or as endografts.

Endografts are frequently used for intracavitary locations. In the last two decades, thoracic endovascular aortic repair (TEVAR) has been gradually replacing open intervention with surgical replacement of the aorta with a synthetic graft. Currently, TEVAR is accepted as the treatment of choice for most cases of thoracic aortic disease that have anatomic feasibility [2]. Major complications related to vascular grafts include occlusion (due to thrombosis or intimal hyperplasia), distal emboli, periprosthetic seroma (fluid collection), pseudoaneurysm, structural degeneration, erosion into adjacent structures, and infection [3].

Vascular graft infections (VGI) are considered to be one of the most severe and life-threatening complications of vascular graft insertion, are a major cause of morbidity and mortality, and are associated with a high economic cost. The treatment of an infected graft is based on its surgical removal, revascularization, and adjunctive antimicrobial therapy. The removal of an infected graft is associated with a mortality rate of 18–30%, while leaving the infected graft "in situ" can lead to a mortality rate approaching 100% despite prolonged antimicrobial treatment [4, 5]. Early diagnosis can lead to early treatment and improve patient outcome, but the diagnosis of VGI is highly complex, as the clinical manifestations are nonspecific, and there is no "gold standard" diagnostic test.

E. Arnon-Sheleg (✉)
Department of Nuclear Medicine, Galilee Medical Center, Naharia, Israel

Department of Diagnostic Radiology, Galilee Medical Center, Naharia, Israel

Azrieli Faculty of Medicine, Bar-Ilan University, Safed, Israel
e-mail: elitea@gmc.gov.il

Z. Keidar
Department of Nuclear Medicine, Faculty of Medicine, Technion—The Israeli institute of Technology, Haifa, Israel
e-mail: Z_keidar@rambam.health.gov.il

Frequency, Pathogenesis, and Clinical Presentation

The incidence of VGI ranges between 0.5% and 6% and differs according to the graft's location. Intracavitary grafts are less likely to be infected, with infection occurring in up to 1% of abdominal aortic grafts and in 1.5–2% of aorto-femoral grafts. The incidence of infection in extracavitary grafts is higher and reaches 6% for grafts located in the groin [6].

The most common cause of graft infection is intraoperative bacterial contamination, followed by direct spread of infection from a contiguous site such as a surgical wound infection or erosion of a vascular graft into adjacent bowel wall. Bacteremia is an infrequent cause for VGI, with the highest risk for hematogenous infection during the early postoperative period (<2 months) [4]. The pathogenesis of graft infection differs according to the graft's location. Infection of extracavitary grafts usually occurs due to surgical wound infection or intraoperative contamination, while intracavitary graft infections occur due to mechanical erosion, bacteremia, or contiguous infection from an adjacent site such as spondylodiscitis [7].

The common microorganisms involved in VGI have changed over the years. Early published studies found *Staphylococcus aureus* as the most common causative pathogen. Later studies show a more diverse microbiological spectrum of infection, with coagulase-negative staphylococci found to be the most common causative microorganism. In addition, multidrug-resistant strains, polymicrobial and fungal infections are becoming more frequent. These changes can be explained by the use of prophylactic anti-staphylococcal antibiotics, improvement in surgical techniques, the growing tendency to perform surgery on patients with multiple underlying comorbidities and the evolution of hospital flora [1, 4].

The graft material can potentially influence its susceptibility to infection. Autologous grafts are generally less susceptible to infection due to their microcirculation. Dacron grafts were found in in-vitro studies to be more likely to harbor bacteria that can adhere to its surface and are therefore coated with collagen and antibiotics to prevent infections [1, 8]. In-vivo studies have not found actual differences in prevalence of VGI among the different graft materials [9].

The clinical manifestations of VGI are highly variable and change according to the graft location, the causative microorganism, and the duration of time since surgery.

Early VGI occur within the first 4 months after surgery, involve virulent organisms introduced at the time of surgery (such as *S. aureus*), and are usually easier to diagnose since the signs and symptoms of infection and inflammation are more apparent. The patient may present with systemic signs of infection as well as local signs of infection, including erythema and tenderness of the skin overlying the graft, sinus tract drainage, abscess, and limb ischemia. Late VGI occur after 4 months, are usually indolent, and can present with no evidence of systemic sepsis [1]. Intracavitary VGI may have no obvious physical findings. Intra-abdominal VGI may present with abdominal pain and signs of sepsis. Aortic grafts can erode into the third or fourth portion of the duodenum, resulting in intermittent, polymicrobial bacteremia of fecal flora or occasionally gastrointestinal tract bleeding (Fig. 15.1). Intrathoracic VGI that involves the aortic root can present with signs and symptoms similar to those of infective endocarditis, including fever, chills, heart failure, and disruption of the anastomotic suture line of the aortic root, which can result in sudden massive hemorrhage. Septic emboli can occur in the central nervous system or peripherally [4]. While all vascular graft infections are associated with high morbidity and mortality, those involving the thoracic aorta are the most catastrophic, with reported mortality rates ranging from 25% to 75% [10] (Fig. 15.2).

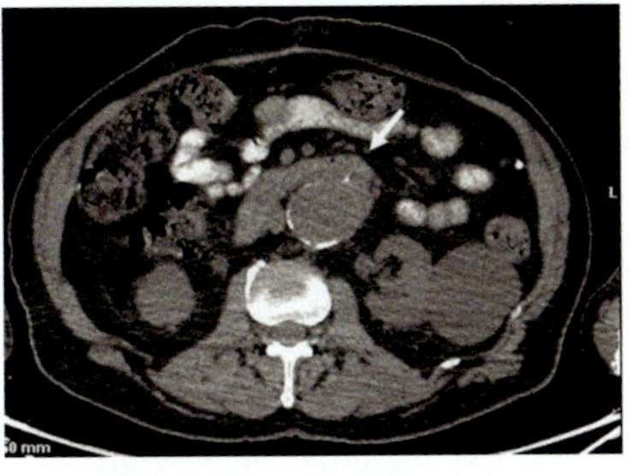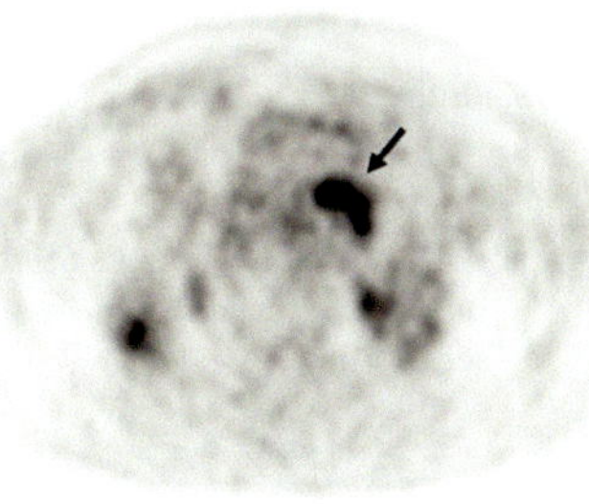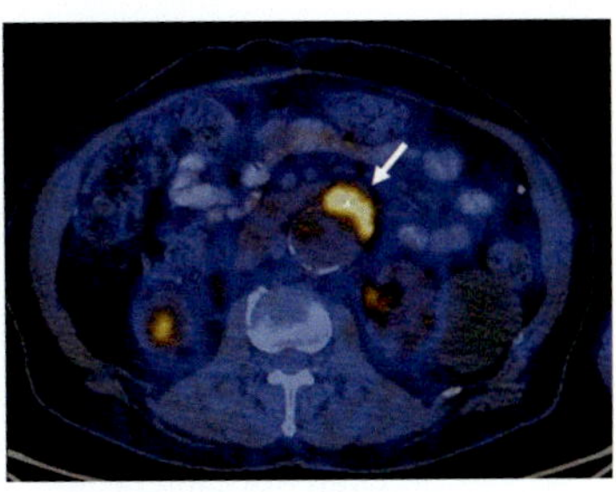

Fig. 15.1 Graft infection with suspected erosion of bowel wall. A 71-year-old man with an aorto-bi-femoral graft implanted 20 years ago sent for investigation of a new aneurism found at the proximal graft anastomosis. Transaxial CT (left), PET (middle), and fused PET/CT slice (right) show increased FDG uptake in the anterior part of a vascular graft in the abdominal aorta and posterior part of the distal duodenum (arrows), suspicious for graft infection with an erosion to adjacent bowel

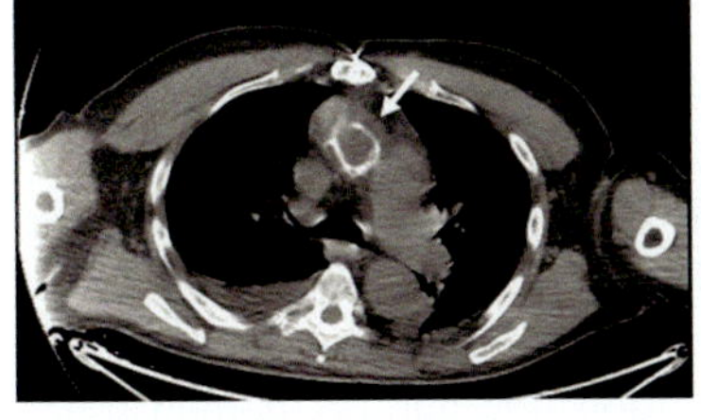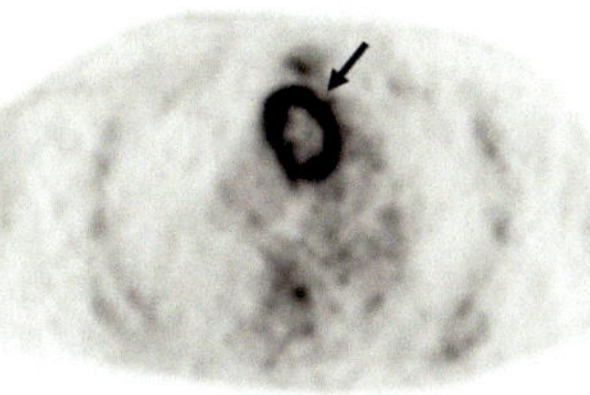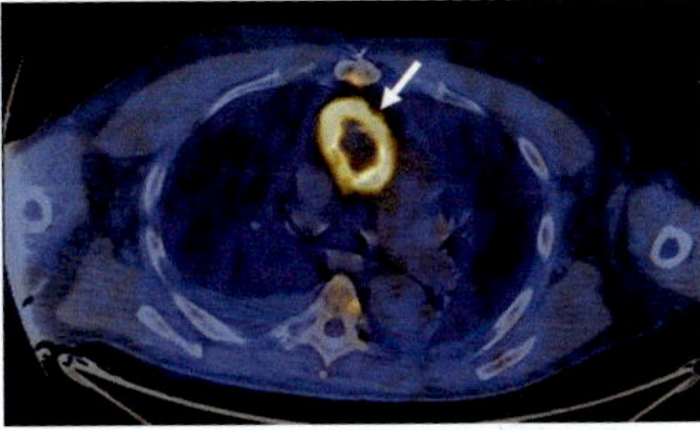

Fig. 15.2 Infected graft in the ascending aorta A 70-year-old man, 5 years after aortic valve and ascending aorta replacement presented with fever and *S. aureus* bacteremia. Transaxial CT (left), PET (middle), and fused PET/CT slice (right) show increased FDG uptake in the circumference of a vascular graft in the ascending aorta, consistent with graft infection

Diagnosis of VGI

The gold standard for the diagnosis of VGI is a positive bacterial culture obtained from the infected graft. Appropriate specimens for bacterial cultures include surgically explanted prosthetic materials, intra-operatively obtained tissue from the infected area, or at least three samples from a perigraft fluid collection. Fluid collections can be aspirated percutaneously directed by ultrasound or CT [9]. In 2016, the Management of Aortic Graft Infection (MAGIC) group of experts introduced criteria for the diagnosis of aortic graft infection, which included minor and major criteria divided into three categories: clinical/surgical, radiology, and laboratory. According to the MAGIC criteria, VGI is suspected in a patient with any isolated major criterion or minor criteria from two of the three categories and is diagnosed in the presence of a single major criterion along with any other criterion (major or minor) from another category (Table 15.1) [5].

Imaging is essential in diagnosing VGI and its accompanying complications, including discontinuation of its structural integrity, perigraft gas or fluid collections, anastomotic leak, pseudoaneurysms, and graft-enteric erosion or fistula. Imaging also contributes to guiding perigraft fluid aspiration and to optimal surgical treatment planning [7]. The MAGIC classification includes major and minor radiological criteria. Major criteria for the diagnosis of VGI are considered to be perigraft fluid more than 3 months after insertion, perigraft gas more than 7 weeks after insertion, and increase in perigraft gas volume in serial imaging tests. Minor radiological criteria include suspicious perigraft gas/fluid, aneurysm expansion, pseudoaneurysm formation and signs of infection spreading to adjacent structures such as focal bowel wall thickening and discitis/osteo-

Table 15.1 The magic criteria for the diagnosis of VGI [5]

	Clinical/surgical	Radiology	Laboratory
Major criteria	– Pus around graft – Open wound with exposed graft or communicating sinus – Fistula formation (aorto-enteric or aorto-bronchial) – Graft insertion in an infected site, mycotic aneurysm or pseudoaneurysm	– Perigraft fluid on CT >3 months after insertion – Perigraft gas >7 weeks after insertion – Increase in perigraft gas volume on serial imaging	– Organisms recovered from an explanted graft – Organisms recovered from an intra-operative specimen – Organisms recovered from a percutaneous aspirate of perigraft fluid
Minor criteria	– Localized clinical features of VGI (erythema, warmth, purulent discharge) – Fever ≥38°C with VGI as the most likely cause	– Suspicious perigraft gas/fluid/soft tissue; aneurysm expansion; pseudoaneurysm formation; focal bowel thickening; discitis/osteomyelitis – Suspicious metabolic activity on FDG PET/CT; uptake in radiolabeled WBC scan	– Positive blood culture with no other apparent source – Abnormally elevated inflammatory markers

myelitis [5]. Imaging methods include radiological and nuclear medicine modalities.

Ultrasonography (US)

US is a noninvasive method with several advantages including repeatability, availability, cost-effectiveness, and a high safety-profile, but is also operator-dependent and can be hampered by the patient's body habitus. US is considered more useful in extra-cavitary graft assessment and can help in the evaluation of perigraft fluid collections, distinguish a fluid collection from a hematoma or pseudoaneurysm, and can be used for US-guided aspiration of a collection [7, 9].

Computed Tomography Angiography (CTA)

CTA is considered as the first-choice imaging modality and was the reference imaging standard for diagnosis of VGI for many years, particularly for intra-cavitary grafts. CTA can demonstrate perigraft fluid, gas or inflammatory tissue, pseudoaneurysm, signs of inflammation or infection in adjacent structures and fistula formation. Although CTA's diagnostic performance is better than that of US, its sensitivity and specificity are moderate [9]. Reinders-Folmer's meta-analyses published in 2018 showed an overall pooled sensitivity of 67% and specificity of 63% for detecting VGI. In addition, the authors demonstrated that isolated CTA usually does not provide enough information for establishing the diagnosis of VGI [11]. CTA has higher false-negative rates and a sensitivity of only 55.5% in low-grade or early VGI, as the findings are difficult to differentiate from postoperative changes. It is more accurate, with a sensitivity and specificity of about 85–94%, in late VGI or infections accompanied by complications such as abscesses in adjacent structures or fistula. Radiological follow-up with serial CTA can increase diagnostic accuracy by showing persistent or worsening findings. Like US, CT can be used for guided aspiration of perigraft fluid [7].

Magnetic Resonance Angiography (MRA)

MRA has several advantages over CTA including the absence of radiation exposure, the use of non-iodinated contrast material, and the possible application of advanced imaging techniques such as functional or dynamic imaging. However, this modality has a longer acquisition time, lower availability and tolerability, and higher costs.

Metallic stents can cause ferromagnetic artifacts and may in some cases be MR-incompatible. MRA can demonstrate small perigraft fluid collections with a greater resolution than CT but, like CT, cannot distinguish a postoperational collection from an infected collection. MRA is more accurate than CT in differentiating perigraft fluid from inflammation or fibrosis [7].

Radiolabeled White Blood Cell (WBC) Scintigraphy

Labeled WBC scintigraphy is a gamma-camera-based nuclear medicine study that is considered the imaging modality of choice for the diagnosis of several infective diseases [12]. Leukocytes, specifically granulocytes, can be labeled with ^{111}In or [99m]Tc. The latter has been more commonly used in recent years due to preferable physical characteristics and less radiation exposure to the patient. The labeled granulocytes migrate to the infection site and accumulate there over time [7]. The European Society of Nuclear Medicine (EANM) guidelines published in 2018 recommend several (at least dual) time point image acquisitions of the investigated regions, with times corrected for isotope decay. Early post injection images (30 min to 1 h) and delayed images (2–4 h) may be sufficient for the diagnosis of VGI, but the addition of late images (20–24 h) is strongly recommended in equivocal cases, low grade or chronic infections, and in follow-up studies. The use of single-photon emission computed tomography (SPECT/CT) increases the diagnostic accuracy and helps in evaluating the infection's extent and location [11, 12]. Interpretation is derived by comparing the uptake intensity in the suspected site of infection between the early and late images. Infection is characterized by increased intensity of uptake over time, while in a sterile inflammation site the labeled WBC uptake will decrease or be stable over time. A study by Puges et al. published in 2019 found WBC scintigraphy as the most accurate method of diagnosing VGI, with sensitivity and specificity of 89.5% and 90.9%, respectively, and a negative predictive value of 97.2% [13]. A meta-analysis published in 2018 comprising 14 studies supported this conclusion with WBC scintigraphy having the highest diagnostic performance in the diagnoses of VGI [11]. Despite the accuracy of this method, the recently published European Society for Vascular Surgery 2020 Clinical Practice Guidelines on the Management of Vascular Graft and Endograft Infections does not recommend labeled WBC scintigraphy as the first-choice nuclear medicine imaging method due to several limitations [9]. The WBC labeling procedure is a time-consuming process, requires highly trained personal, may expose the staff to infected blood products, and has prolonged acquisition times. The method's accuracy is reduced in intracavitary grafts as the tracer is eliminated via the intestinal tract and physiologically taken up in the bone marrow, leading to a difficult interpretation of the aorta [9].

FDG PET/CT in VGI

FDG PET/CT has emerged in the last decades as a useful imaging method for infectious and inflammatory diseases. ^{18}F-FDG, a glucose analog, accumulates in activated inflammatory cells, especially neutrophils and monocytes/macrophages, and in microorganisms such as bacteria or fungi [14]. PET with co-registered CT allows a precise localization of FDG uptake with higher quality images than gamma camera-produced images, and the total procedure time is considerably shorter than labeled WBC scintigraphy (2–3 h vs. 20–24 h). FDG PET/CT can contribute to the early diagnosis of VGI, before clinical, biological, or radiological criteria are evident. In a study by Puges et al., three patients who were negative for VGI according to clinical criteria were correctly diagnosed with infection using FDG PET/CT [13]. Like labeled WBC scintigraphy, FDG PET/CT has the ability to demonstrate additional foci of infection other than the infected graft, and aid in the assessment of the extent of disease [13]. Several studies that aimed to investigate the role of FDG PET/CT in the diagnosis of VGI have been published since 2005, with evidence supporting its accuracy. Earlier studies conducted with FDG PET (without CT) showed high sensitivity but lower specificity. The addition of a co-registered CT leads to an increase in diagnostic accuracy, especially the specificity [11, 15]. This can be explained by the additional information provided by the CT images which aids in accurate localization of the FDG uptake and distinguishing between VGI and infection in a perigraft collection, and provides information on the morphological appearance of the graft's boundaries (Fig. 15.3). Recent meta-analyses showed that FDG PET/CT had pooled sensitivity and specificity ranging between 94–96% and 74–80%, respectively, in the diagnosis of VGI [11, 16, 17].

Scarce information is available concerning the accuracy and performance of FDG PET/CT in intra-thoracic VGI, but several studies have shown this to be an accurate and effective method which can be used to clarify the precise extent and location of an infected graft and guide further

therapy [18–20]. A study by Guether et al. published in 2015 included 26 patients after cardiac and proximal aortic surgery (including aortic valve replacement, aortic root reconstruction or replacement, and ascending aortic and arch replacement) who underwent FDG PET/CT imaging for suspected graft infection. Conventional CT was positive for infection in 13 cases (50%) compared to 22 cases (85%) on PET/CT. In almost 30% of the cases, FDG PET/CT provided substantial additional diagnostic information in comparison with CT alone. Maximum sensitivity (89%) and specificity (100%) in prediction of infection was found when using a cutoff for maximum standardized uptake value (SUV_{max}) of 7.25 (see further explanation in "interpretation criteria/methods") [18]. A study by Dong et al. published in 2019 included 16 infected and eight uninfected thoracic aorta grafts. Using a visual grade score, sensitivity, specificity, and accuracy of 94%, 50%, and 79%, respectively, were found ($P < 0.05$). Focal FDG

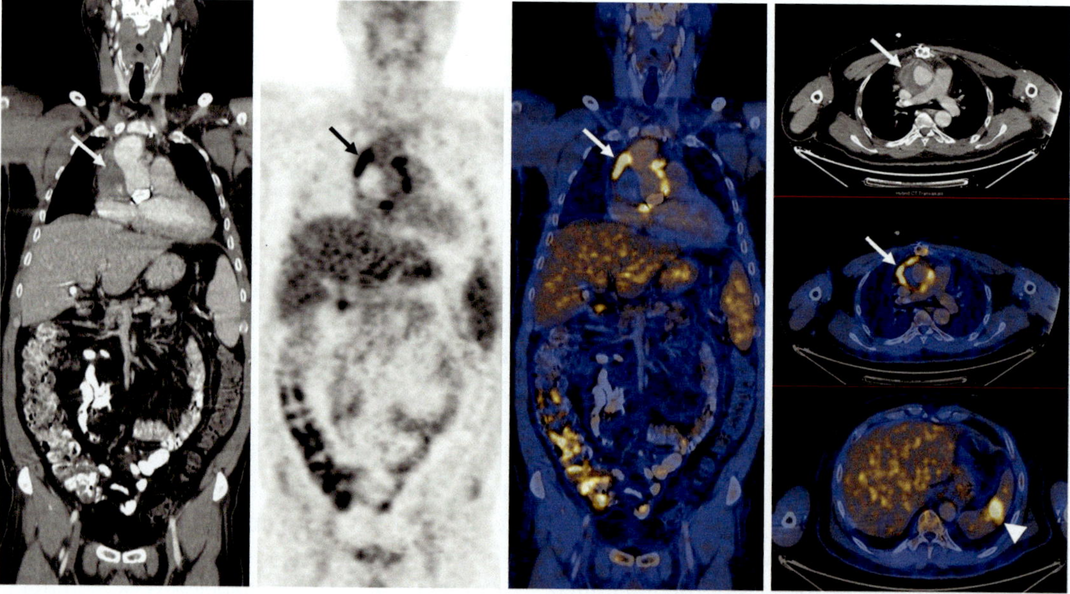

Fig. 15.3 Infected graft in the ascending aorta accompanied by a collection. A 48-year-old man with a history of rheumatic heart disease, 25 years after aortic valve, and ascending aorta replacement with a homograft (biologic prosthesis). Hospitalized with fever and bacteremia. CT, PET, and fused PET/CT slices show increased uptake in the circumference of a fluid collection surrounding the graft in the ascending aorta (arrows), consistent with infected graft. Increased uptake is also seen in a hypodense lesion in the spleen, consistent with an infected embolus (arrowhead)

uptake was noted in 25% of the uninfected and 81% of the infected grafts ($P < 0.05$). Delayed imaging did not differentiate between infected and uninfected grafts but improved the PET image quality [19]. A recent study published in 2020 by Lucinian et al. included 39 subjects following aortic root replacement surgery, 14 with confirmed infection, and 25 without infection according to gold standard criteria. FDG PET/CT studies performed after a myocardial suppression protocol (24 h high-fat, low-carbohydrate diet, 12 h fasting, and intravenous heparin) were retrospectively reviewed. Homogeneous uptake patterns were observed more frequently in noninfected subjects compared with infected subjects ($p = 0.0001$). The presence of heterogeneous uptake (focal or soft tissue extension) at the prosthetic valve, aortic root, or ascending aorta was observed more frequently in infected subjects (85.7% vs. 20.0%; $p = 0.0001$) and was a significant predictor of infection (odds ratio: 24.0; 95% confidence interval: 4.0–143.6; $p = 0.0005$). Tissue-to-background ratio (TBR) was significantly higher in infected subjects compared with noninfected subjects. Furthermore, the presence of heterogeneous uptake combined with a TBR >2.0 was observed more frequently in the infected group than in the noninfected group (85.7% vs. 12.0%; $p < 0.0001$) [20].

PET/CT Acquisition Protocol

The EANM/SNMMI Guideline for FDG Use in Inflammation and Infection details the recommended acquisition parameters for performing a PET/CT study [21]. Other than the usual 4 h fast, no specific patient preparation is needed before the scan is performed. Suppression of the physiological FDG uptake in the myocardium with a lipid-rich diet or other means is not necessary unless aortic grafts involving the aortic root/valve are being investigated. A low-dose CT can be performed for attenuation correction and anatomic localization, but in our experience a diagnostic CT with injection of iodinated contrast material (unless contraindicated) is preferable for localization and interpretation of the findings.

Interpretation Criteria/Methods

Several interpretation criteria for FDG PET/CT in the investigation of VGI have been proposed, including visual assessment of the pattern of uptake (homogenous vs. focal/heterogeneous), tissue-to-background ratio (TBR), calculated maximum standardized uptake value (SUV_{max}), and a visual grading scale (VGS) using a 5-point scale comparing uptake-to-background tissue and urine [7]. The 5-point VGS is graded as follows: grade 0, FDG uptake similar to that in the background; grade I, low FDG uptake, comparable with inactive muscles and fat; grade II, moderate FDG uptake, clearly visible, and higher than uptake by inactive muscles and fat; grade III, strong FDG uptake, but distinctly less than the physiologic urine bladder activity; and grade IV, very strong FDG uptake, comparable with the physiologic urinary activity of the bladder [22] (Fig. 15.4). Currently, there is no consensus regarding the SUV_{max} threshold for diagnosis of VGI with values ranging from 3.5 to 8.0 in the different studies employing this method [15].

A meta-analysis by Rojoa et al. published in 2019 comprising 12 studies with 433 grafts (202 proven as infected) found a pooled sensitivity and specificity of 89% and 61%, respectively, for the VGS method, 93% and 78% for a focal pattern of uptake, 98% and 80% for SUV_{max}, and 57% and 76% for TBR. Dual time point PET imaging (DTPI) was also investigated but only by a single study included in the meta-analysis that found a sensitivity and specificity of 100% and 88%, respectively [15]. A meta-analysis published in 2020 by Reinders-Folmer et al. comprising 13 studies found a pooled sensitivity and specificity of 90% and 59%, respectively, for FDG uptake intensity (assessed with a VGS), 94% and 81% for uptake pattern (focal vs. homogeneous), and 95% and 77% for using SUV_{max} measurements [23]. All of the methods showed a pooled sensitivity of 90% or higher but demonstrated variable specificities. The uptake pattern interpretation method demonstrated the best diagnostic accuracy and the authors suggested it should be implemented as an interpretation crite-

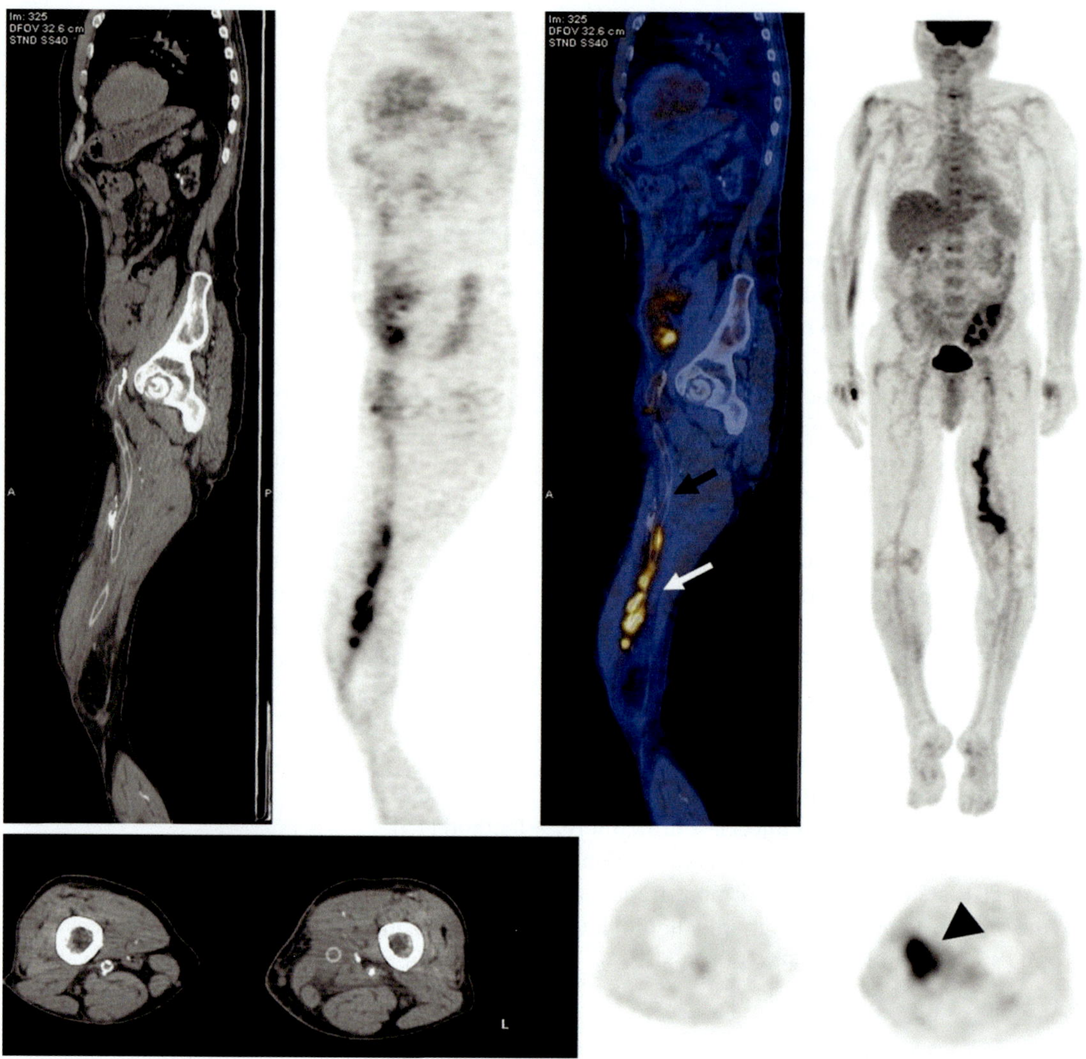

Fig. 15.4 Infection in the distal part of a femoral-popliteal graft. A 75-year-old man with kidney transplant and a femoral-popliteal synthetic bypass implanted 2 years ago. Presented with new onset of pain and swelling in the distal thigh. Sagittal CT, PET, and fused PET/CT slice (upper row) and MIP image (upper row right) and transaxial CT and PET (lower row) show increased uptake in the distal part of the vascular graft (white arrow and black arrowhead). According to the visual grading scale (VGS) analysis method, the uptake is graded as level IV (stronger than the uptake in the bladder) and is consistent with graft infection. No uptake is seen in the proximal part of the graft (black arrow)

rion in future guidelines on FDG PET/CT assessment of VGI [23].

Another tool suggested by Saleem et al. for quantifying the distribution of FDG in the evaluation of vascular graft is termed textural features analysis. This method is based on assessing the spatial arrangement of voxels in a predefined volume of interest. Spatial heterogeneity is indicative of VGI. Using this method, the authors found a sensitivity of 80% and a specificity of 100% [24]. A recent study by Einspieler et al. including 50 suspected aortic VGI demonstrated a diagnostic accuracy of 90% utilizing SUV_{max} as a quantitative measure and a modified 5-point VGS as qualitative measure (taking into account both ^{18}F-FDG uptake pattern around the graft and the ^{18}F-FDG uptake in the liver as reference). The authors suggested that a multiparametric assessment could overcome the limitations of single-mode evaluation [25]. Further prospective, multicenter studies are necessary for the validation of these methods.

Limitations and Pitfalls

There are several causes for false-negative and false-positive results of FDG PET/CT in the investigation of suspected VGI. Increased FDG uptake can be seen in inflammatory changes around the vascular graft during the immediate postoperative period. FDG uptake reaches its peak in the first few weeks after surgery and tends to return to normal values after 4 weeks. Performing the study soon after surgery may result in a false-positive result [15]. FDG uptake in an infection localized in the vicinity of a vascular graft, such as an infected hematoma or lymphocele, may also cause false-positive results [26, 27]. A pattern of linear low-grade FDG uptake can be seen in both native and synthetic grafts. A study by Keidar et al. demonstrated diffuse FDG uptake in most of the noninfected grafts included in their study (92%). The uptake pattern differed according to the graft material. Dacron grafts were characterized by inhomogeneous uptake and Gore-Tex grafts by diffuse homogeneous patterns of uptake. Native vein grafts showed a significant decrease in uptake over time, whereas synthetic grafts showed no change in intensity in a follow-up of up to 16 years [28]. This phenomenon can be explained by a chronic aseptic inflammatory reaction to the foreign material in the synthetic grafts, mediated by macrophages, fibroblasts, and foreign body giant cells [29]. False-positive results can also result from an inhomogeneous/patchy FDG uptake pattern observed in cases where surgical adhesives (such as Bioglue) were applied during the graft placement. In a study by Bowles et al. of 49 patients with suspected VGI, seven false-positive cases were found, five of them showing a patchy FDG uptake pattern. In all these cases, adhesives had been applied during surgery [30]. Similar results were found in a study by Spacek et al. and in two cases reported by Schouten [31, 32].

A possible cause of false-negative results is the prolonged use of antibiotics. This may be explained by reduced chemotaxis of leukocytes to the infection site and lower metabolic activity of both inflammatory cells and microorganisms in the treated or partially treated infection site [7, 15]. In a meta-analysis by Rojoa et al., this was found as the prevalent reason for false-negative cases. However, in another study by Kagna et al. investigating the diagnostic performance of FDG PET/CT in infective processes during ongoing antibiotic treatment, no false-negative cases were detected in the group of patients receiving antimicrobial treatment, thus demonstrating that the accuracy of this modality is not influenced by antibiotic administration [33]. Einspieler et al. also found that antibiotic treatment did not have a substantial impact on the sensitivity of FDG PET/CT in their study of 50 suspected aortic VGI [25]. Hyperglycemia and uncontrolled diabetes may potentially cause false-negative results due to their influence on the distribution of FDG. However, a study by Rabkin et al. found no significant impact of either diabetes or hyperglycemia on false-negative rates in FDG PET/CT of patients with suspected infection or inflammation [34]. This is in contrast with oncological applications which were found to be significantly affected by elevated blood glucose levels at the time of FDG administration. The EANM/SNMMI Guideline for FDG use in inflammation and infection recommends that efforts be made to decrease blood glucose to the lowest possible level but hyperglycemia should not represent an absolute contraindication for performing FDG PET/CT in the investigation of infectious etiologies [21].

Monitoring Therapy

Very little data are available on the performance of FDG PET/CT in monitoring response to antibiotic therapy in VGI. A study by Husmann et al. including 25 patients with proved VGI showed that C-reactive protein levels correlated with

SUV during follow-up. They also found that the results of FDG PET/CT scans had an impact on the management of all patients with an increase or decrease in SUV measurements in areas of focal uptake found at diagnosis. The authors concluded that FDG PET/CT has the potential to differentiate between responders and nonresponders. Further investigations are necessary for understanding the role of FDG PET/CT in this indication [35].

Conclusion

Graft infection, is associated with significant morbidity and mortality. Prompt and accurate diagnosis of the prosthesis involvement by an infectious process is mandatory. PET/CT using FDG is a useful tool for the noninvasive diagnosis of vascular graft infection with high diagnostic accuracy. A negative PET/CT can rule out infection, but a positive result should be interpreted with caution to avoid possible pitfalls and false positive results. Well-controlled studies including large numbers of patients need to further confirm and validate the role of PET/CT in the management of patients with the challenging clinical dilemma of vascular graft infections.

References

1. Gharamti A, Kanafani ZA. Vascular graft infections: an update. Infect Dis Clin North Am. 2018;32(4):789–809.
2. Grabenwoger M, Alfonso F, Bachet J, Bonser R, Czerny M, Eggebrecht H, et al. Thoracic endovascular aortic repair (TEVAR) for the treatment of aortic diseases: a position statement from the European Association for Cardio-Thoracic Surgery (EACTS) and the European Society of Cardiology (ESC), in collaboration with the European Assoc. Eur Heart J. 2012;33(13):1558–63.
3. Buja LM, Schoen FJ. The pathology of cardiovascular interventions and devices for coronary artery disease, vascular disease, heart failure, and arrhythmias. In: Cardiovascular pathology. Amsterdam: Elsevier; 2016. p. 577–610.
4. Wilson WR, Bower TC, Creager MA, Amin-Hanjani S, O'Gara PT, Lockhart PB, et al. Vascular graft infections, mycotic aneurysms, and endovascular infections: a scientific statement from the American Heart Association. Circulation. 2016;134(20):e412–60.
5. Lyons OTA, Baguneid M, Barwick TD, Bell RE, Foster N, Homer-Vanniasinkam S, et al. Diagnosis of aortic graft infection: a case definition by the Management of Aortic Graft Infection Collaboration (MAGIC). Eur J Vasc Endovasc Surg. 2016;52(6):758–63.
6. Leroy O, Meybeck A, Sarraz-Bournet B, D'Elia P, Legout L. Vascular graft infections. Curr Opin Infect Dis. 2012;25(2):154–8.
7. Lauri C, Iezzi R, Rossi M, Tinelli G, Sica S, Signore A, et al. Imaging modalities for the diagnosis of vascular graft infections: a consensus paper amongst different specialists. J Clin Med. 2020;9(5):1510.
8. Vicaretti M. Pathophysiology of vascular graft infections. In: Mechanisms of vascular disease: a reference book for vascular specialists. Adelaide: University of Adelaide Press; 2011. p. 29.
9. Chakfé N, Diener H, Lejay A, Assadian O, Berard X, Caillon J, et al. Editor's choice—European Society for Vascular Surgery (ESVS) 2020 clinical practice guidelines on the Management of Vascular Graft and Endograft Infections. Eur J Vasc Endovasc Surg. 2020;59(3):339–84.
10. Coselli JS, Köksoy C, LeMaire SA. Management of thoracic aortic graft infections. Ann Thorac Surg. 1999;67(6):1990–3.
11. Reinders Folmer EI, Von Meijenfeldt GCI, Van der Laan MJ, Glaudemans AWJM, Slart RHJA, Saleem BR, et al. Diagnostic imaging in vascular graft infection: a systematic review and meta-analysis. Eur J Vasc Endovasc Surg. 2018;56(5):719–29.
12. Signore A, Jamar F, Israel O, Buscombe J, Martin-Comin J, Lazzeri E. Clinical indications, image acquisition and data interpretation for white blood cells and anti-granulocyte monoclonal antibody scintigraphy: an EANM procedural guideline. Eur J Nucl Med Mol Imaging. 2018;45(10):1816–31.
13. Puges M, Bérard X, Ruiz J-B, Debordeaux F, Desclaux A, Stecken L, et al. Retrospective study comparing WBC scan and 18F-FDG PET/CT in patients with suspected prosthetic vascular graft infection. Eur J Vasc Endovasc Surg. 2019;57(6):876–84.
14. Mochizuki T, Tsukamoto E, Kuge Y, Kanegae K, Zhao S, Hikosaka K, et al. FDG uptake and glucose transporter subtype expressions in experimental tumor and inflammation models. J Nucl Med. 2001;42(10):1551–5.
15. Rojoa D, Kontopodis N, Antoniou SA, Ioannou CV, Antoniou GA. 18F-FDG PET in the diagnosis of vascular prosthetic graft infection: a diagnostic test accuracy meta-analysis. Eur J Vasc Endovasc Surg. 2019;57(2):292–301.
16. Kim S-J, Lee S-W, Jeong SY, Pak K, Kim K. A systematic review and meta-analysis of 18F-fluorodeoxyglucose positron emission tomography or positron emission tomography/computed

tomography for detection of infected prosthetic vascular grafts. J Vasc Surg. 2019;70(1):307–13.

17. Khaja MS, Sildiroglu O, Hagspiel K, Rehm PK, Cherry KJ, Turba UC. Prosthetic vascular graft infection imaging. Clin Imaging. 2013;37(2):239–44.

18. Guenther SPW, Cyran CC, Rominger A, Saam T, Kazmierzcak PM, Bagaev E, et al. The relevance of 18F-fluorodeoxyglucose positron emission tomography/computed tomography imaging in diagnosing prosthetic graft infections post cardiac and proximal thoracic aortic surgery. Interact Cardiovasc Thorac Surg. 2015;21(4):450–8.

19. Dong W, Jinghong X, Linlin H, Xiaofen X, Mi H, Hacker M, et al. 18F-FDG-PET/CT imaging for detection of infected thoracic aortic prosthetic grafts. J Nucl Med. 2019;60(supplement 1):1436.

20. Lucinian YA, Lamarche Y, Demers P, Martineau P, Harel F, Pelletier-Galarneau M. FDG-PET/CT for the detection of infection following aortic root replacement surgery. JACC Cardiovasc Imaging. 2020;13(6):1447–9.

21. Jamar F, Buscombe J, Chiti A, Christian PE, Delbeke D, Donohoe KJ, et al. EANM/SNMMI guideline for 18F-FDG use in inflammation and infection. J Nucl Med. 2013;54(4):647–58.

22. Bruggink JLM, Glaudemans AWJM, Saleem BR, Meerwaldt R, Alkefaji H, Prins TR, et al. Accuracy of FDG-PET–CT in the diagnostic work-up of vascular prosthetic graft infection. Eur J Vasc Endovasc Surg. 2010;40(3):348–54.

23. Reinders Folmer EI, von Meijenfeldt GCI, Te Riet Ook Genaamd Scholten RS, van der Laan MJ, Glaudemans AWJM, Slart RHJA, et al. A systematic review and meta-analysis of 18F-fluoro-d-deoxyglucose positron emission tomography interpretation methods in vascular graft and endograft infection. J Vasc Surg. 2020;72(6):2174–2185.e2.

24. Saleem BR, Beukinga RJ, Boellaard R, Glaudemans AWJM, Reijnen MMPJ, Zeebregts CJ, et al. Textural features of 18F-fluorodeoxyglucose positron emission tomography scanning in diagnosing aortic prosthetic graft infection. Eur J Nucl Med Mol Imaging. 2017;44(5):886–94.

25. Einspieler I, Mergen V, Wendorff H, Haller B, Eiber M, Schwaiger M, et al. Diagnostic performance of quantitative and qualitative parameters for the diagnosis of aortic graft infection using [¹⁸F]-FDG PET/CT. J Nucl Cardiol. 2020;28(5):2220–8.

26. Keidar Z, Engel A, Hoffman A, Israel O, Nitecki S. Prosthetic vascular graft infection: the role of 18F-FDG PET/CT. J Nucl Med. 2007;48(8):1230–6.

27. Sah B-R, Husmann L, Mayer D, Scherrer A, Rancic Z, Puippe G, et al. Diagnostic performance of 18F-FDG-PET/CT in vascular graft infections. Eur J Vasc Endovasc Surg. 2015;49(4):455–64.

28. Keidar Z, Pirmisashvili N, Leiderman M, Nitecki S, Israel O. 18F-FDG uptake in noninfected prosthetic vascular grafts: incidence, patterns, and changes over time. J Nucl Med. 2014;55(3):392–5.

29. Wasselius J, Malmstedt J, Kalin B, Larsson S, Sundin A, Hedin U, et al. High 18F-FDG uptake in synthetic aortic vascular grafts on PET/CT in symptomatic and asymptomatic patients. J Nucl Med. 2008;49(10):1601–5.

30. Bowles H, Ambrosioni J, Mestres G, Hernández-Meneses M, Sánchez N, Llopis J, et al. Diagnostic yield of 18F-FDG PET/CT in suspected diagnosis of vascular graft infection: a prospective cohort study. J Nucl Cardiol. 2020;27(1):294–302.

31. Spacek M, Belohlavek O, Votrubova J, Sebesta P, Stadler P. Diagnostics of "non-acute" vascular prosthesis infection using 18F-FDG PET/CT: our experience with 96 prostheses. Eur J Nucl Med Mol Imaging. 2009;36(5):850–8.

32. Schouten L. Surgical glue for repair of the aortic root as a possible explanation for increased F-18 FDG uptake. J Nucl Cardiol. 2008;15(1):146–7.

33. Kagna O, Kurash M, Ghanem-Zoubi N, Keidar Z, Israel O. Does antibiotic treatment affect the diagnostic accuracy of 18 F-FDG PET/CT studies in patients with suspected infectious processes? J Nucl Med. 2017;58(11):1827–30.

34. Rabkin Z, Israel O, Keidar Z. Do hyperglycemia and diabetes affect the incidence of false-negative 18F-FDG PET/CT studies in patients evaluated for infection or inflammation and cancer? A comparative analysis. J Nucl Med. 2010;51(7):1015–20.

35. Husmann L, Ledergerber B, Anagnostopoulos A, Stolzmann P, Sah B-R, Burger IA, et al. The role of FDG PET/CT in therapy control of aortic graft infection. Eur J Nucl Med Mol Imaging. 2018;45(11):1987–97.

Left Ventricular Assist Device Infection

Chaitanya Madamanchi, Sami El-Dalati,
Marty Tam, Venkatesh L. Murthy,
and Richard L. Weinberg

Left ventricular assist devices (LVADs) improve survival and quality of life for end-stage heart failure patients [1]. Unfortunately, infection is a critical and common complication in patients with LVADs [2]. Diagnosis of LVAD infection in a timely fashion enables the selection and prompt initiation of therapy. However, because of the multiple internal and external components of LVADs, diagnosis and characterization of the extent of infection is particularly challenging. Furthermore, many patients may have other cardiac and extracardiac prosthetic devices. In addition to a comprehensive evaluation including history and physical, cultures, and biomarkers, imaging tests have an important role in the diagnosis of LVAD infections. In particular, FDG-PET/CT has emerged as a powerful imaging technique with high sensitivity and clinical value for diagnosing LVAD infections when added to a thorough clinical evaluation [3]. This chapter will review the epidemiology, and pathophysiology of LVAD infections, present diagnostic strategies, and offer a case-based discussion illustrating the utility of FDG-PET/CT in diagnosing LVAD infections.

Epidemiology

Over six million adults in the United States suffer from heart failure [4]. Individuals with end-stage heart failure may be considered for advanced life-prolonging therapies such as durable left ventricular assist devices (LVADs). Based on data from a national registry of patients who have undergone VAD placement (INTERMACS) [5], use of LVAD therapy is increasing, with more than 3000 patients undergoing implantation in 2019. Although improved survival and quality of life is well established [1, 6], adverse events related to LVAD devices remain common, with major bleeding and infection being among the most frequent [7]. LVAD-specific infections are categorized based on the time since implantation: early ($\leq$90 days, 0.159 events per patient-year) and late (>90 days, 0.165 events per patient-year). Infections occur most commonly at the driveline site but can also involve the pump, pump pocket, inflow cannula, and outflow cannula [8]. LVAD infections have also been associated with substantial mortality [9, 10].

C. Madamanchi · M. Tam · V. L. Murthy
Division of Cardiovascular Medicine, Department of Internal Medicine, Frankel Cardiovascular Center, University of Michigan, Ann Arbor, MI, USA

S. El-Dalati
Division of Infectious Diseases, University of Kentucky, Lexington, KY, USA

R. L. Weinberg (✉)
Division of Cardiology, Feinberg School of Medicine, Northwestern University, Chicago, IL, USA
e-mail: richard.weinberg@nm.org

Risk factors for LVAD-related infections identified for contemporary continuous flow devices include patient-related risk factors such as obesity [11–13] and younger age [14, 15]. Additional risk factors include prolonged critical illness post-LVAD implant (mechanical ventilation days, intensive care unit days) [14], total duration of LVAD support [11, 14, 16, 17], device revisions for bleeding [14], and trauma at the driveline exit site [16]. Standardized driveline care to ensure a sterile exit site and reduced site trauma has been associated with the reduction of infections [18, 19]. Specific surgical techniques such as double tunneling of the driveline [20–22] and internalizing the entire velour-covered portion of the driveline [23, 24] have been associated with lower rates of infection.

Pathophysiology

Ventricular assist device (VAD) infection is broadly defined by the International Society for Heart and Lung Transplantation (ISHLT) as "any infection that occurs in the presence of a ventricular assist device" [25]. In 2011 the ISHLT published more detailed classifications of LVAD infections which were divided into three categories: VAD-specific infections, VAD-related infections, and non-VAD infections. VAD-specific infections are those unique to patients with VADs, are related to the presence of device hardware, and do not occur in patients without VADs. VAD-specific infections can be further subclassified into three categories: percutaneous driveline infections, pocket infections, and pump and/or cannula infections. VAD-related infections include infections that can also occur in patients who do not have VADs but may have unique considerations for patients with VADs (e.g., blood-stream infection). Finally, non-VAD infections are infections that are not affected by the presence of the VAD and are unlikely to be related to the device [8]. This chapter will focus on VAD-specific and VAD-related infections.

VAD-Specific Infection: Percutaneous Driveline Infections

Left ventricular assist devices (LVADs) connect to an external power source through a subcutaneously tunneled cable known as a driveline, which typically exits the skin overlying the abdomen. The exit site is covered by a sterile dressing that is changed regularly by the patient [25]. Consequently, the driveline has direct exposure to the external environment and can serve as a nidus for infection. Owing to their external exposure, driveline infections are the most common VAD-specific infections, accounting for nearly half of all VAD infections. About 12–35% of VAD patients experience driveline infections, with the risk of infection increasing as the duration of device support lengthens [8, 17, 25, 26]. Driveline infections are further subcategorized by the ISHLT into superficial and deep infections and are rated as proven, probable, and possible. Proven superficial driveline infections are defined by purulent discharge from the incision site with associated erythema or warmth, positive aseptic skin culture, and surgical or histological involvement of tissues superficial to the fascia and muscle layers of the incision [8]. In contrast, proven deep driveline infections also involve the deep soft tissue and/or the presence of an abscess. Probable and possible driveline infections are characterized only by clinical and microbiologic findings in the absence of surgical debridement [8, 27] (see Tables 16.1, 16.2, 16.3, and 16.4).

Table 16.1 Definition of terms used for the diagnosis of ventricular assist device-specific pump and/or cannula infections[a] [8]

Major clinical criteria
- If the VAD is not removed, then an indistinguishable organism (genus, species, and antimicrobial susceptibility pattern) recovered from 2 or more peripheral blood cultures taken >12 h apart with no other focus of infection or

All of 3 or a majority of ≥4 separate positive blood cultures (with the first and last sample drawn at least 1 h apart) with no other focus of infection

- When 2 or more positive blood cultures are taken from the CVC and peripherally at the same time, and defined by criteria in Table 16.3 as either BSI-VAD-related or presumed VAD-related
- Echocardiogram positive for VAD-related IE (TEE recommended for patients with prosthetic valves, rated at least "possible IE" by clinical criteria, or complicated IE [paravalvular abscess] and in any patient in whom VAD-related infection is suspected and TTE is nondiagnostic; TTE as first test in other patients) defined as follows: intracardiac mass suspected to be vegetation adjacent to or in the outflow cannula, or in an area of turbulent flow such as regurgitant jets, or consistent with a vegetation on implanted material, or abscess, or new partial dehiscence of outflow cannula

Minor clinical criteria
- Fever ≥38 °C
- Vascular phenomena, major arterial emboli, septic pulmonary infarcts, mycotic aneurysm, intracerebral or visceral, conjunctival hemorrhage, and Janeway's lesions
- Immunologic phenomena: glomerulonephritis, Osler's nodes, Roth spot
- Microbiologic evidence: positive blood culture that does not meet criteria as noted above (excluding single-positive culture for coagulase-negative staphylococci excluding *Staphylococcus lugdunensis*)

CVC central venous cannula, *BSI* blood stream infection, *IE* infective endocarditis, *TEE* transesophageal echocardiogram, *TTE* transthoracic echocardiogram, *VAD* ventricular assist device

[a]Adapted from the Modified Duke's Criteria [28]. *Reprinted from The Journal of Heart and Lung Transplantation*, Vol 30/Number 4, Hannan MM, Husain S, Mattner F, Danziger-Isakov L, Drew RJ, Corey GR, et al. *Working formulation for the standardization of definitions of infections in patients using ventricular assist devices.* Page 379. Copyright (2011) [8]

Table 16.2 Definitions of ventricular assist device-specific pump infections and/or cannula infection [8]

Proven
- Microbiology. Isolation of indistinguishable organism (genus, species, antimicrobial susceptibility pattern) at explantation or intra-operatively from
  - ≥2 positive internal aspect culture samples from pump and/or cannula or
  - 1 positive peripheral blood culture and 1 positive culture from VAD internal aspect aspirate or endovascular brushings (internal aspect refers to the inner lumen of the cannula) or
  - In the case of coagulase-negative staphylococci excluding *Staphylococcus lugdunensis*; 2 or more positive sets of peripheral blood cultures and a positive internal aspect culture of pump and/or cannula
- Histologic features of infection from heart tissue samples from around the VAD pump and/or cannula at explantation or intra-operatively
- Clinical criteria (see Table 16.1)
- 2 major criteria

Probable
- 1 major criterion and 3 minor criteria or
- 4 minor criteria

Possible
- 1 major and 1 minor or
- 3 minor

Rejected
- Firm alternative diagnosis explaining the clinical findings
- Resolution of evidence of pump and/or cannula infection with antibiotic therapy for ≤4 days or
- No pathologic evidence of pump and/or cannula infection at surgery or autopsy with antibiotic therapy for ≤4 days or
- Does not meet criteria for possible pump and/or cannula infection

Reprinted from The Journal of Heart and Lung Transplantation, Vol 30/Number 4, Hannan MM, Husain S, Mattner F, Danziger-Isakov L, Drew RJ, Corey GR, et al. *Working formulation for the standardization of definitions of infections in patients using ventricular assist devices.* Page 379. Copyright (2011) [8]

Table 16.3 Definition of terms used for the diagnosis of ventricular assist device-specific pocket infection [8]

Major clinical criteria
- Microbiologic: aspirated fluid culture positive or fluid/pus diagnostic of infection[a]
- Radiologic: New fluid collection by radiologic criteria-CT/US/Indium (enhancement or gas or sinus tract or leukocyte migration)

Minor clinical criteria
- Fever ≥38 °C with no other recognized cause
- New local erythema over the pocket site
- Local pain and tenderness
- Induration or swelling
- Radiologic evidence: lymphangitis seen radiologically or
- New fluid collection without major criteria (above) and without diagnostic culture but not explained by other clinical conditions such as failure/anasarca/seroma

---

Reprinted from The Journal of Heart and Lung Transplantation, Vol 30/Number 4, Hannan MM, Husain S, Mattner F, Danziger-Isakov L, Drew RJ, Corey GR, et al. *Working formulation for the standardization of definitions of infections in patients using ventricular assist devices*. Page 380. Copyright (2011) [8]

[a] Image-guided aspiration

VAD-Specific Infection: Pump Pocket and Cannula Infections

The ISHLT has previously defined the LVAD pocket as the space that holds the pump inside the patient's body [8]. First-generation LVAD models utilizing pulsatile flow pumps required formation of this pocket, typically created within the abdominal wall or near the pericardium and diaphragm. Second-generation LVADs simplified the pump components which allowed for placement of the pump within cavities such as the pericardium or left ventricle. Third-generation devices utilize more compact centrifugal pumps which obviate the need for a pocket, thereby decreasing the amount of implanted prosthetic material susceptible to infection. Both the pump and pump pockets (in first- and second-generation LVADs) may become infected in 2–10% of patients [25, 26, 29, 30]. Infections within 30 days of device implantation are more likely to

Table 16.4 Definitions of ventricular assist device-specific percutaneous driveline infection [8]

	Surgical/histology	Microbiology	Clinical	General wound appearance
A. Superficial VAD-specific percutaneous driveline infection				
Proven = Surgical/ histology criteria ± other criteria	• Involvement of tissues superficial to the fascia and muscle layers of the incision documented	• Aseptic skin culture positive or not cultured	• Local increase in temperature around the exit site	• Purulent discharge from the incision but not involving fascia or muscle layers or • Erythema spreading around the exit site[a]
Probable = No surgical/ histology criteria with purulent discharge ± other criteria	• Surgical debridement not performed • No histology	• Aseptic skin culture positive or negative but patient already on antibiotic or had antiseptic used to clean wound	• Local increase in temperature around the exit site and • Treated as superficial infection with clinical response	• Purulent discharge from the incision but not involving fascia or muscle layers or • Erythema spreading around the exit site[a]

Table 16.4 (continued)

	Surgical/histology	Microbiology	Clinical	General wound appearance
Possible = No surgical/ histology or purulent discharge ± other criteria	· Surgical debridement not performed · No histology	· Aseptic skin culture positive or negative and patient not on antibiotics or had antiseptic used to clean the wound	· Local increase in temperature around the exit site and. · Treated as superficial infection with clinical response	· No discharge · Erythema spreading around the exit site[a]
B. Deep VAD-specific percutaneous driveline infection				
Proven = Surgical/ histology criteria ± other criteria	· Involves deep soft tissue (e.g., fascial and muscle layers) on direct examination or on direct examination during reoperation · An abscess is found on direct examination during reoperation	· Culture positive or histology puncture positive for infection	· Temperature >38 °C · Localized pain or tenderness	· A deep incision spontaneous dehiscence · Abscess deep to the incision around the driveline
Probable = No surgical/ histology criteria with spontaneous dehiscence ± other criteria	· No surgical debridement · No histology	· Culture negative but patients already on antibiotics or had antiseptic used on exit site	· Temperature >38 °C or · Localized pain or tenderness and · Treated as a deep infection	· An incision spontaneous dehiscence
Possible = No surgical/ histology criteria with positive ultrasound ± other clinical criteria	· No surgical debridement · No histology	· Cultures not reserved	· Localized pain or tenderness and · Treated as a deep infection with clinical response	· Positive ultrasound

VAD ventricular assist device
[a]Erythema excluding stitch abscess (minimal inflammation and discharge confined to the points of suture penetration). *Reprinted from The Journal of Heart and Lung Transplantation*, Vol 30/Number 4, Hannan MM, Husain S, Mattner F, Danziger-Isakov L, Drew RJ, Corey GR, et al. *Working formulation for the standardization of definitions of infections in patients using ventricular assist devices.* Page 381. Copyright (2011) [8]

be secondary to direct inoculation at the time of surgery, whereas infections acquired >30 days postoperatively are typically secondary to extension from a driveline infection [26].

In addition to infection of the pump and/or pocket, the inflow cannula connecting the left ventricle to the VAD pump and the outflow cannula connecting the pump to the aorta may also become infected. This relatively uncommon complication occurs in <1% of LVAD patients but is associated with significant morbidity and mortality. Analogous to driveline infections, pump, pump pocket, and cannula infections are subcategorized into proven, probable, and possible. Proven infection relies on isolation of organisms intra-operatively directly from the pump, the pocket, or the cannula or by identifying an abscess on imaging. Probable and possible pump, pocket, and cannula infections are diagnosed using major and minor clinical criteria that were adapted by the IHSLT from the Modified Duke Criteria [8, 28] (see Tables 16.1, 16.2, 16.3, and 16.4).

VAD-Related Infections

VAD-related infections include infective endocarditis (in ~1% of patients), blood-stream infection, mediastinitis, and sternal wound infections (in ~2% of patients) [8, 25, 31]. All cases of endocarditis are considered VAD-related per the ISHLT definitions. Bloodstream infections are presumed VAD-related unless a clear alternative source of infection can be identified. Similarly, mediastinitis and sternal wound infections are also considered VAD-related unless they are definitively proven to have another cause.

Microbiology

Skin flora, primarily Gram-positive cocci, are the most common microorganisms identified in all types of VAD-specific and VAD-related infection [25, 26]. *Staphylococcus aureus*, both methicillin-susceptible and methicillin-resistant, and coagulase-negative *Staphylococci* species are isolated in 17–75% of driveline infections and 25–75% of pump pocket infections [25, 26, 32]. Additionally, enterococcus species are isolated in 5–29% of VAD-specific infections, followed by Gram-negative rods including *Pseudomonas aeruginosa, Escherichia coli,* and *Klebsiella* species which comprise 7–43% of VAD-specific infections. Fungal pathogens, most notably *Candida* species, while less common than bacterial organisms, account for 2–8% of VAD-specific infections [25, 26]. Notably, the incidence of LVAD infections has decreased in second- and third-generation LVADs [33–35].

Treatment

A detailed review of the treatment of VAD-specific and VAD-related infections is beyond the scope of this chapter. However, there are certain general considerations that are important in this patient population. By definition, VAD-specific infections involve the device hardware, and the most common etiologic pathogens produce biofilms which make their eradication from prosthetic material challenging. Given the potential for ascending driveline infection resulting in the highly morbid contamination of the pump or cannula, most VAD-specific infections as well as VAD-related endocarditis or recurrent VAD-related bloodstream infections caused by the same organism will require some duration of intravenous antibiotic treatment in conjunction with either definitive surgical debridement or device explantation followed by long-term oral antibiotic suppression until transplant. The notable exception to this approach is superficial driveline infections caused by non-*Staphylococcus,* non-*Pseudomonas*, and non-fungal species for which a shorter 2-week course of therapy without long-term antibiotic suppression can be considered [25–27].

Diagnostic Strategies

Drawing from endocarditis literature, major and minor criteria have been proposed to help determine the likelihood of LVAD infection (see Tables 16.1 and 16.3). Using these clinical, pathological, and imaging criteria, suspected cases can be classified as either proven, probable, possible, or unlikely for LVAD infection (see Tables 16.2 and 16.4) [36]. Proven infection requires definitive microbiology, or histologic confirmation at explants, or two major clinical criteria [36, 37]. Infection is considered probable in the setting of one major and three minor criteria, or four minor criteria [36, 37]. Possible infection requires one major and one minor criteria, or three minor criteria [36, 37]. Infection is considered unlikely in the presence of an alternative diagnosis or resolution after less than or equal to 4 days of antibiotics, or no pathologic evidence at surgery after less than or equal to 4 days of antibiotics, or negative cultures from fluid during surgery or aspiration, or not meeting the criteria above [36, 37].

LVAD infections are difficult to diagnose as there are multiple external and internal components of the LVAD which can become infected. In addition, many of these patients have other prosthetic devices, including pacemakers, defibrillators, and valve replacements. These other devices can also become infected and should be evaluated in LVAD patients in whom infection is suspected.

Evaluation of all patients who are suspected of having an LVAD infection should include the following: white blood cell count, C-reactive protein, erythrocyte sedimentation rate, sterile aspirate for Gram stain, KOH preparation, routine bacterial and fungal culture of driveline at exit site if pus is present, echocardiogram including TEE if TTE is without findings consistent with infection, at least three sets of blood cultures drawn at different times over 24 h (two sets from peripheral sites), and chest radiograph [8].

Echocardiography is the first-line screening imaging modality for cardiac prosthetic device infections as it is readily available, provides both functional and anatomic information, does not require radiation, and can detect valvular vegetations and other sequelae of infection including paravalvular abscesses [38]. Transthoracic echocardiography (TTE) should be pursued first as it is noninvasive, and if it reveals findings consistent with endocarditis, then in some instances can obviate the need for further imaging. However, TTE has limited sensitivity in detecting prosthetic valve endocarditis [39]. In cases where TTE is inconclusive, then transesophageal echocardiography (TEE) should be pursued as it has significantly higher sensitivity in diagnosing endocarditis, specifically in patients with prosthetic devices. Limitations of echocardiography include artifacts related to prosthetic material, limited ability to detect perivalvular extension of infection in the setting of prosthetic valves, inability to detect peripheral complications of infection or clinically important extracardiac sequelae of infection, and, in some patients, contraindications that may make transesophageal echocardiography difficult or impossible [38].

In addition, if there is concern for pocket infection, then abdominal ultrasound and CT with contrast of chest/abdomen may be helpful [8]. Nonetheless, serum biomarkers of infection, TEE, and CT have been found to be poor predictors of LVAD infection when used in isolation [3]. Further, there is currently no gold standard for the diagnosis of LVAD infections. Despite this, a timely diagnosis is essential in the care of LVAD patients who typically have multiple comorbidities placing them at increased risk of mortality [3].

FDG-PET/CT is useful in the evaluation of patients suspected of having prosthetic device infection. It has high sensitivity and specificity in the evaluation of prosthetic valve endocarditis (sensitivity of 86% and specificity of 84%) and cardiac implantable electronic device (CIED) endocarditis (sensitivity of 72% and specificity of 83%) [40]. In addition, FDG-PET/CT can detect perivalvular complications of infection and characterize regional extent of infection [40]. Whole-body FDG-PET/CT imaging can identify embolic phenomenon and other etiologies for the source of infection [38]. Some of the limitations of FDG-PET/CT include the inability to detect small vegetations, false positives from postsurgical (sterile) inflammation, false positives from inflammation induced by certain surgical adhesives, and the reduced sensitivity to detect infection in patients who have been on long-term antimicrobial therapy prior to imaging. Furthermore, the performance of FDG-PET/CT is predicated on achieving adequate myocardial suppression of endogenous glucose uptake with metabolic preparation, necessitating a low-carbohydrate, high-fat diet [41–43]. Interpretation of FDG-PET/CT for cardiac infection requires specialized training and knowledge of the aforementioned caveats and the ability to distinguish normal versus pathological FDG uptake patterns.

There is a nascent but growing body of literature which supports the use of FDG-PET/CT in aiding the diagnosis of LVAD infection. A meta-analysis examined the utility of FDG-PET in the evaluation of LVAD infections [3]. A total of 119 scans were included across four centers, and the authors found that when added to a comprehensive evaluation including biomarkers of infection and other imaging studies, FDG-PET had a pooled sensitivity of 92% in the diagnosis of LVAD infection [3] (see Fig. 16.1). Specificity, on the other hand, was only 83% with wide confidence intervals [3]. Some of the limitations of the study included the lack of a gold standard test in diagnosing infections in cases where patients did not undergo surgery, variations in protocols and metabolic preparations for patients across the four centers, and selection bias as not all patients suspected of having LVAD infections are referred to have FDG-PET/CTs [3]. Overall, the use of FDG-PET/CT in the evaluation of LVAD infections is promising with high sensitivity, but specificity is lacking and requires further investigation.

FDG-PET/CT has been shown to be useful not only in the diagnosis of LVAD infection but also for prognosis of these patients based on the presence and site of infection [44]. In one study, FDG-PET/CTs were obtained in 35 patients with LVAD including 24 patients who were suspected of having LVAD infections and 11 who were not suspected of being infected [44]. After a mean follow-up of 23 months, none of the patients without evidence of infection on FDG-PET died. In contrast, 50 % of patients with evidence of infection on FDG-PET/CT died [44]. Among those, 86% had evidence of infection involving central components of the LVAD, whereas 14% had evidence of infection involving peripheral components of the LVAD [44]. This study highlights the importance of detecting and treating LVAD infections early—before the infection spreads to involve central components of the LVAD [44].

A diagnostic algorithm for the evaluation of patients suspected of having an LVAD infection is outlined in Fig. 16.2. Based on the criteria listed above, if patients have proven infection, they should be treated appropriately. If infection is deemed unlikely, then alterative diagnoses can be evaluated. In cases where a patient has probable or possible LVAD infection and is at high risk for surgical intervention, then FDG-PET/CT should be considered to aid in diagnosis and treatment selection [3].

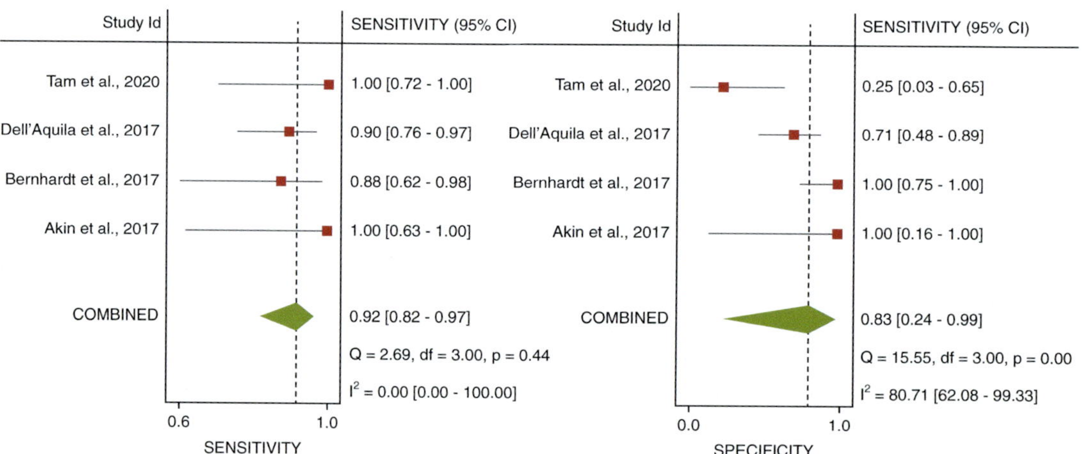

Fig. 16.1 Forest Plot. (Reprinted from *JACC: Cardiovascular Imaging, Vol 13/Number 5, Tam MC, Patel VN, Weinberg RL, Hulten EA, Aaronson KD, Pagani FD, Corbett JR, Murthy VL. Diagnostic Accuracy of FDG-PET/CT in Suspected LVAD Infections: A Case Series, Systematic Review, and Meta-Analysis*. Page 1199. Copyright (2020)) [3]. The pooled sensitivity and specificity of individual studies assessing diagnostic accuracy of fluorine-18 fluorodeoxyglucose positron emission tomography/computed tomography for left ventricular assist device infections with measures of heterogeneity. *CI* confidence interval

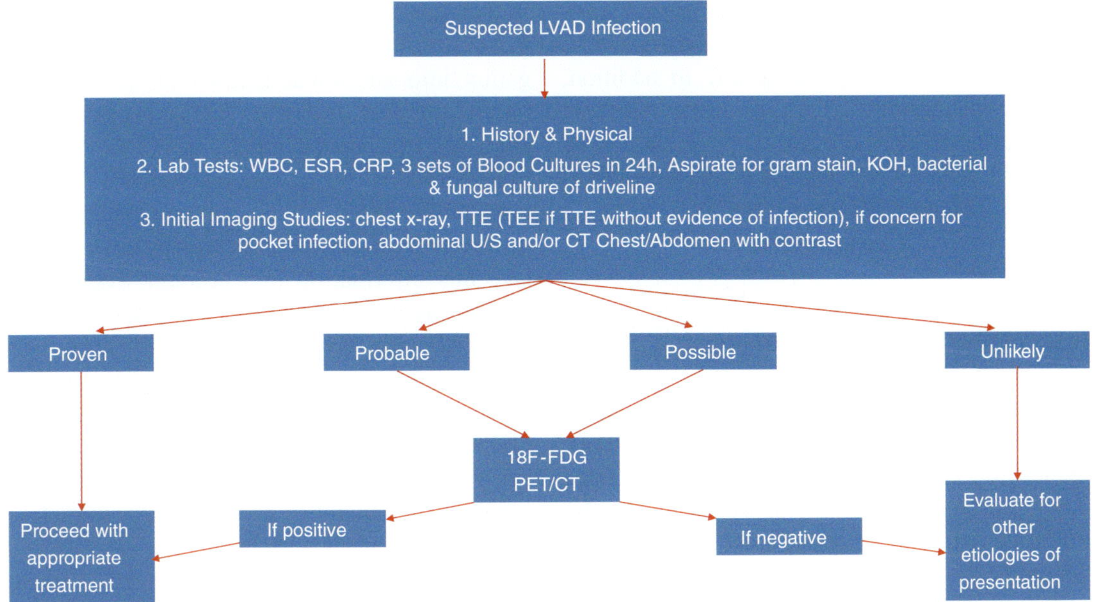

Fig. 16.2 Diagnostic approach for the evaluation of patients suspected of having an LVAD infection

Factors That Affect Image Quality and Interpretation

Preparation and Image Acquisition

One of the most important factors that affects image quality and interpretation of FDG-PET/CT for cardiac infection is the degree of suppression of endogenous myocardial glucose uptake [41–43]. Prior to undergoing FDG-PET/CT scanning, metabolic preparation is necessary to shift the energy source of the myocardium to free fatty acids (i.e., to minimize the chance that FDG signal seen in the myocardium is due to normal cardiac myocytes metabolizing glucose for energy). If proper suppression is not achieved, it can be very difficult to distinguish between physiologic and pathologic FDG uptake. In order to achieve adequate myocardial suppression of glucose uptake, it is imperative that patients adhere to a high fat, no carbohydrate diet for 24 h prior to the test followed by fasting for several hours including overnight prior to the day of the test (see Chap. 4 for further details).

Whole-body FDG/PET CT imaging obtained at the time of the cardiac PET/CT scan can identify embolic phenomenon that are sequelae of infective endocarditis [38, 45]. It can also be useful in determining other causes of inflammation (see Case 16.1) including other infections or neoplasms [38]. This information is essential in the evaluation of infective endocarditis as it can modify treatment plans, including prolonging the duration of antimicrobial therapy, lead to referral for surgical procedures, and prevent unnecessary device extraction [45].

CT attenuation correction images are used to improve PET image quality and interpretation by providing anatomic localization of radiotracer uptake and attenuation correction of PET images. In select cases, ECG-gated cardiac CTs can identify anatomic lesions including pseudoaneurysms, fistulas, and thrombosis [46]. Pizzi et al. demonstrated that fusing FDG images with ECG-gated CTA images reduced the number of doubtful studies on PET/nonenhanced CT from 20 to 8%, primarily by reclassifying doubtful cases to negative cases [46]. However, they did not find significant differences in the sensitivity and specificity of Duke Criteria + PET/CTA vs. Duke Criteria + PET/Nonenhanced CT. In addition, contrast-enhanced CT requires more radiation [46]. Furthermore, iodinated contrast can create artifacts on the CT attenuation images leading to the appearance of false-positive FDG uptake on the corrected PET images [47].

Interpretation and Reporting

The qualitative approach to interpretation relies on visual assessment of abnormal FDG activity related to various components of the LVAD or other prosthetic devices. This approach can be bolstered by a semi-quantitative approach in which increased FDG uptake involving any component of the LVAD is compared to background LV blood pool FDG uptake using standardized uptake value (SUV) to illustrate the intensity of inflammation.

The focality, intensity, and location of FDG signal are important factors to report when interpreting FDG-PET/CT studies in the evaluation of LVAD infection. FDG uptake that is very focal and intense suggests significant inflammation, more strongly suggesting infection. On the other hand, FDG uptake that is diffuse and mild may represent low-level inflammation. This low-level degree of inflammation can be seen in the post-surgical state [48]. The location of FDG uptake is important to report as it offers information on the extent of infection including involvement of driveline, inflow cannula, outflow graft, and any other intracardiac prosthetic devices (e.g., ICDs).

It is important to recognize that FDG uptake is non-specific and can be seen in infectious and noninfectious inflammatory conditions including sarcoidosis, myocarditis, postoperative state, and malignancy [3, 49, 50]. In the postoperative state, wound healing occurs via the formation of granulation tissue (the action of fibroblasts and inflammatory cells) [49]. If FDG-PET imaging is performed shortly following surgery, there may be residual low-level inflammation which can appear as mild, diffuse FDG uptake surrounding the surgical site and any graft material.

In fact, low-grade FDG signal can be seen for up to 1 year following surgery [48]. Further investigation into additional metrics of normality is required in these instances. This must be considered in the interpretation of FDG-PET/CT images relative to the time of surgery. In addition, certain surgical adhesives can lead to false-positive FDG scans [51]; thus, it is important to take this information into account when interpreting studies. Furthermore, it is not uncommon for LVAD patients to be treated with long courses of antibiotics for various infections. Long-term antimicrobial therapy prior to obtaining an FDG-PET/CT can alter FDG uptake and lead to false-negative studies, although the rate of false negatives is thought to be low at approximately 5% [3].

Attenuation correction images are used to improve PET image quality and interpretation as mentioned above. However, CT attenuation correction in the presence of high-density metallic implants can overcorrect for attenuation and lead to overestimation of FDG activity in the vicinity of an LVAD or other metallic objects [3, 52]. Thus, any FDG uptake noted on attenuation correction images should be compared with the non-attenuation corrected (uncorrected) images, with the thought that FDG signal that is not due to artifact should be present on both the sets of images.

Acknowledgement of common imaging pitfalls as described above, combined with integration of the clinical presentation, is of key importance when interpreting FDG-PET/CT studies for suspected LVAD infection. In addition, collaborative reading involving nuclear cardiologists and nuclear medicine specialists is beneficial in cases of abnormal peripheral FDG uptake. A comprehensive interpretation can accurately characterize LVAD infections and help influence treatment decisions.

Clinical Cases

Case 16.1

A 72-year-old man with ischemic cardiomyopathy, ICD, and HeartMate II Left Ventricular Assist Device (LVAD) implantation presented with fevers, leukocytosis, hypotension, chest pain, and elevated lactate dehydrogenase. Blood cultures remained negative, chest X-ray did not reveal any acute abnormalities, and transthoracic echocardiogram did not reveal any vegetations. FDG-PET/CT was obtained to evaluate for device infection. It revealed no evidence of FDG uptake in the myocardium, LVAD inflow or outflow cannulas (Fig. 16.3, red arrows), driveline, ICD leads, or generator. There was no imaging evidence of LVAD infection. However, FDG-PET/CT identified a rim of FDG uptake surrounding the gallbladder (Fig. 16.3, yellow arrows), indicating hypermetabolic activity which was suspicious for cholecystitis.

The patient was treated with antimicrobial therapy for acute cholecystitis. This case helps illustrate an important role of FDG-PET/CT in suspected LVAD infection, namely that the modality not only is useful in detecting device-related infection but also can reveal other etiologies for the patient's presentation, including infection or inflammation located elsewhere in the body [38, 45].

Case 16.2

A 64-year-old man with atrial fibrillation treated with ablation and ultimately left atrial appendage exclusion (left atrial appendage clip), nonischemic cardiomyopathy with ICD, and HeartMate 3 LVAD presented with nausea, vomiting, diarrhea, and generalized malaise. Blood cultures revealed *Streptococcus viridans* bacteremia. Chest X-ray did not reveal any acute abnormalities, and transthoracic echocardiogram did not reveal any vegetations. Transesophageal echocardiogram revealed two small linear, mobile echodensities attached to the aortic valve which were believed to represent Lambl's excrescences or atypical appearance of vegetations. FDG-PET/CT was obtained to evaluate for LVAD infection. It revealed focal, intense FDG uptake at the site of the LVAD inflow cannula (Fig. 16.4a, yellow arrows) with SUV_{max} of 5.0, as well as FDG uptake at the insertion of the outflow graft to the ascending aorta with SUV_{max} of 3.3 (Fig. 16.4b, orange arrows). In addition, FDG uptake was noted on the left atrial appendage clip with SUV_{max} of 4.5 (Fig. 16.4b, yellow arrows), compared to background FDG uptake of LV blood pool with SUVmean of 2.0. These findings were concerning for infection of the LVAD inflow and outflow cannulas, and left atrial appendage clip.

Although no FDG uptake was noted in generator pocket or ICD leads, the ICD was explanted in setting of bacteremia and the patient was

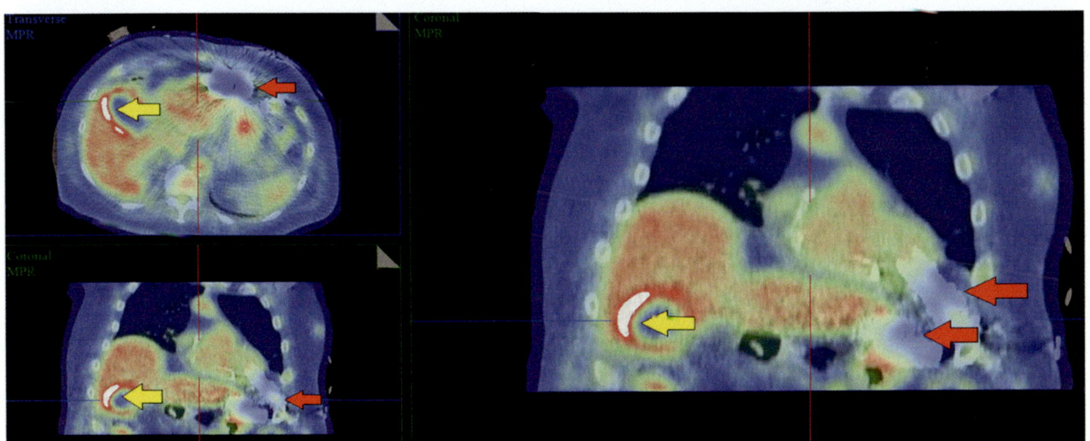

Fig. 16.3 True-negative scan for LVAD infection. FDG PET/CT images demonstrated no significant FDG uptake around the device pump, cannula, or driveline (red arrows). There was intense uptake along the gallbladder (yellow arrows), indicating high metabolic activity and possible infection. There was no clinical evidence of device infection, and the patient was treated for purulent cholecystitis. (Adapted from JACC:Cardiovascular Imaging, vol. 13, no. 5, 2020. Page 1195.)

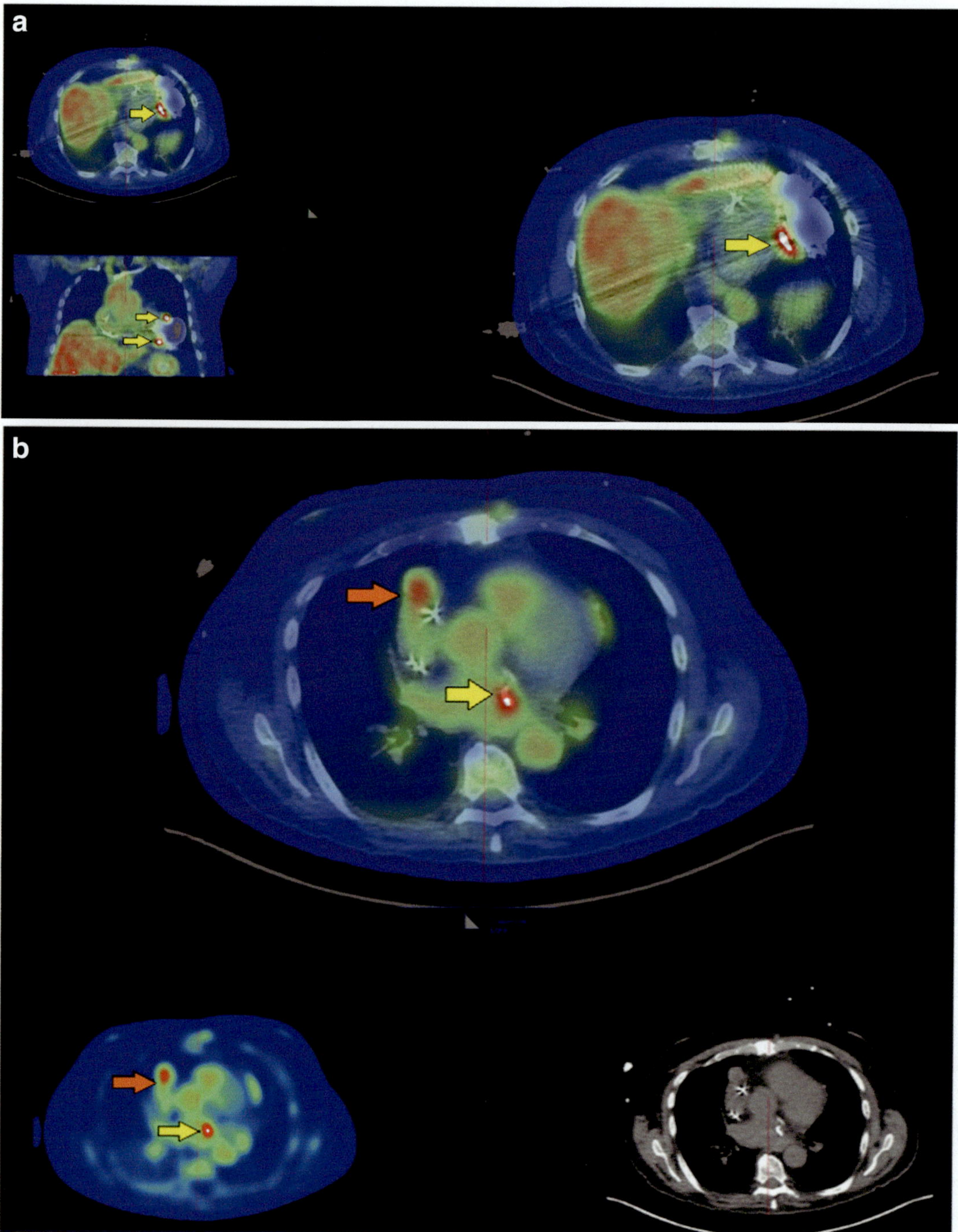

Fig. 16.4 Inflammation of LVAD inflow cannula (**a**, yellow arrows), outflow graft (**b**, orange arrows), and left atrial appendage clip (**b**, yellow arrows)

treated with an extended course of antimicrobial therapy for bacteremia and LVAD infection. This case illustrates that FDG-PET/CT can detect infection of various components of the LVAD including inflow cannulas, outflow grafts, and other prosthetic devices in the heart, such as the left atrial appendage clip.

Case 16.3

A 73-year-old man with nonischemic cardiomyopathy and ventricular tachycardia with ICD and Heartware LVAD presented with bilateral flank pain, fevers, and rigors. On physical examination, there was no drainage at the driveline site, but there was mild erythema. Blood cultures revealed *Staphylococcus aureus* bacteremia. Chest X-ray and CTA chest/abdomen/pelvis did not reveal any acute abnormalities. Transesophageal echocardiogram did not reveal any obvious vegetations. FDG-PET/CT was obtained to evaluate for LVAD infection. It revealed intense FDG uptake involving the inflow cannula (Fig. 16.5a, yellow arrows) with SUV_{max} of 3.4 and outflow graft (Fig. 16.5b, yellow arrows) with SUV_{max} of 3.6, compared to background FDG uptake of LV blood pool of 1.7. These findings were concerning for LVAD infection.

The patient was deemed a prohibitive risk for reoperation and was treated with long-term antimicrobial therapy. This case illustrates that FDG-PET/CT can help detect the extent of infection as nearly the entire outflow graft had intense, focal FDG uptake concerning for infection. The Standardized Uptake Value (SUV) units are a semiquantitative assessment of intensity of FDG uptake, which are reported along with a description of the focality and sites of involvement. Together, this information can be helpful in clinical decision-making for patients who are at high risk of surgical intervention.

Case 16.4

A 59-year-old man with ischemic cardiomyopathy with ICD and HeartMate II LVAD presented with generalized fatigue, elevated lactate dehydrogenase, and itching and discharge from his driveline site. Driveline cultures were positive for *Staphylococcus aureus*. Peripheral blood cultures remained negative. Transesophageal echocardiogram did not reveal any obvious vegetations. FDG-PET/CT was obtained to evaluate for LVAD infection. It revealed FDG uptake at the inflow cannula with SUV_{max} of 2.4 compared to LV blood pool of 1.1 (Fig. 16.6a, yellow arrows). It

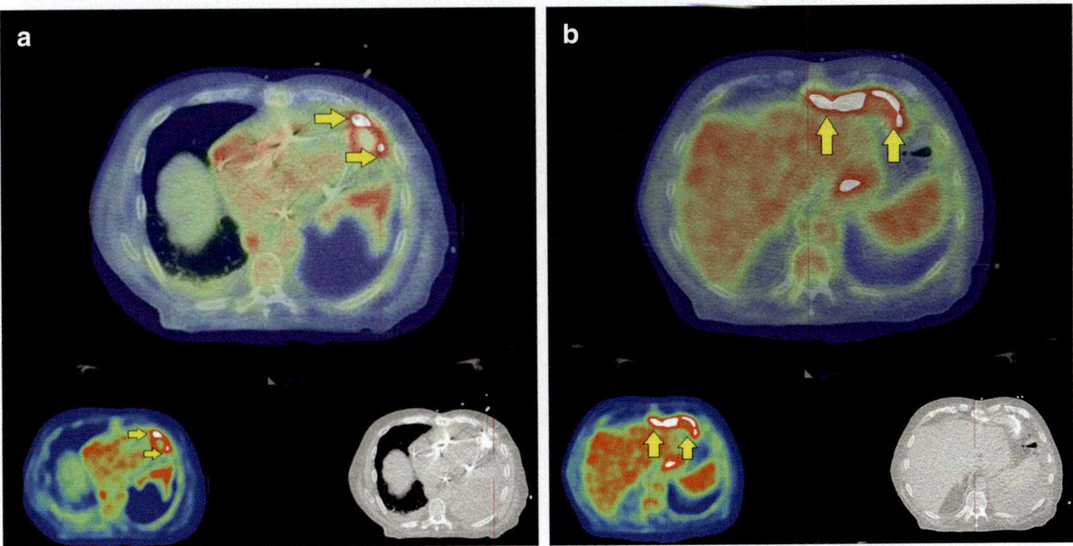

Fig. 16.5 Inflammation of LVAD inflow cannula (**a**, yellow arrows) and entire outflow graft (**b**, yellow arrows)

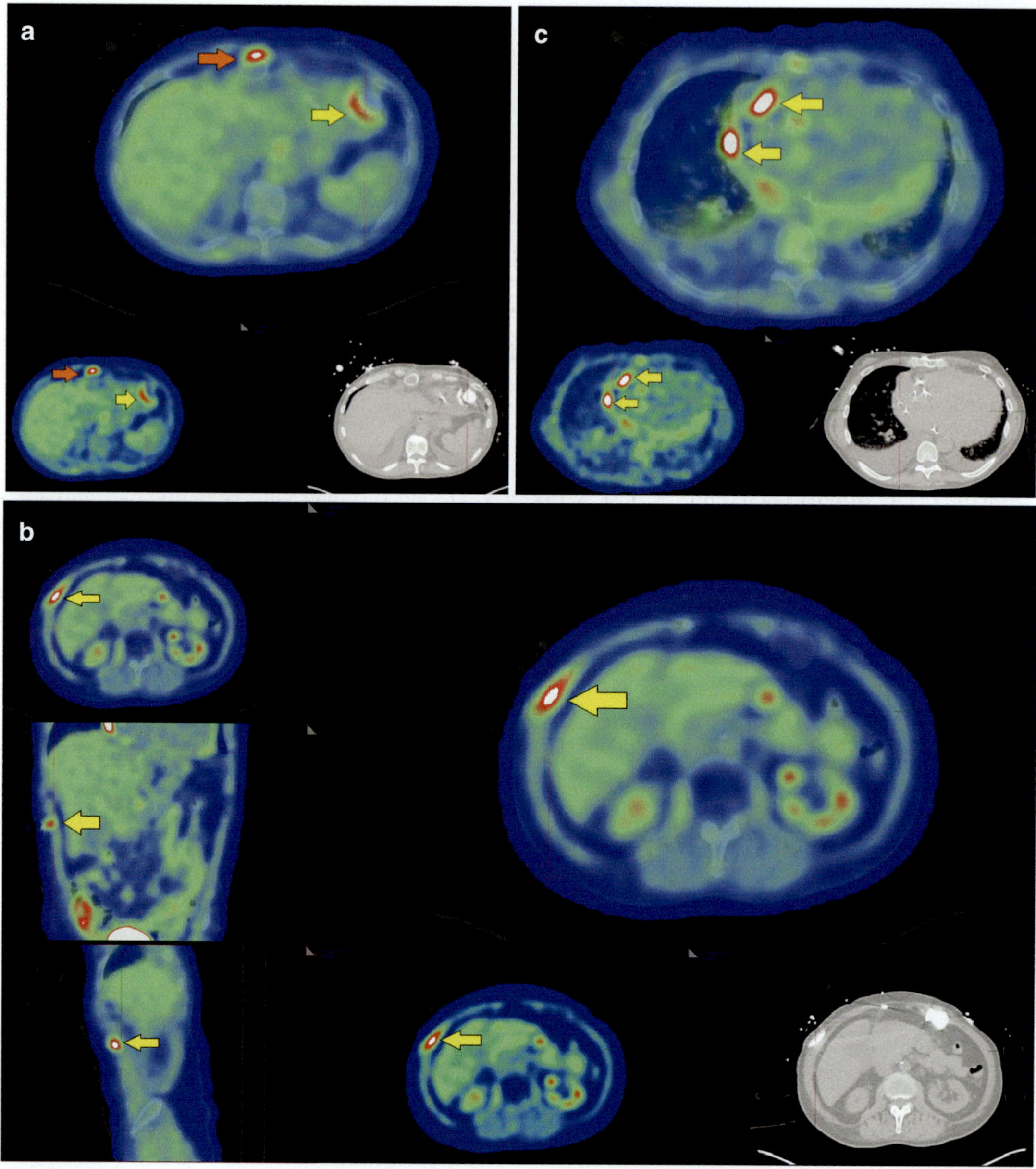

Fig. 16.6 Inflammation of LVAD inflow cannula (**a**, yellow arrows), outflow graft (**a**, orange arrows), driveline (**b**, yellow arrows), and pacemaker leads (**c**, yellow arrows)

also revealed FDG uptake at the outflow graft with SUV_{max} of 2.7 (Fig. 16.6a, orange arrows). In addition, there was FDG uptake along the driveline just inside the insertion point into the skin with SUV_{max} of 3.1 (Fig. 16.6b, yellow arrows). There was also FDG uptake involving the pacemaker leads in the right atrium with

SUV_{max} of 2.5 (Fig. 16.6c, yellow arrows). Overall, these findings are consistent with infection involving the LVAD inflow cannula, outflow graft, driveline, and pacemaker leads.

The patient was treated with long-term antimicrobial therapy and underwent pump exchange as he also had LVAD pump thrombosis. This case

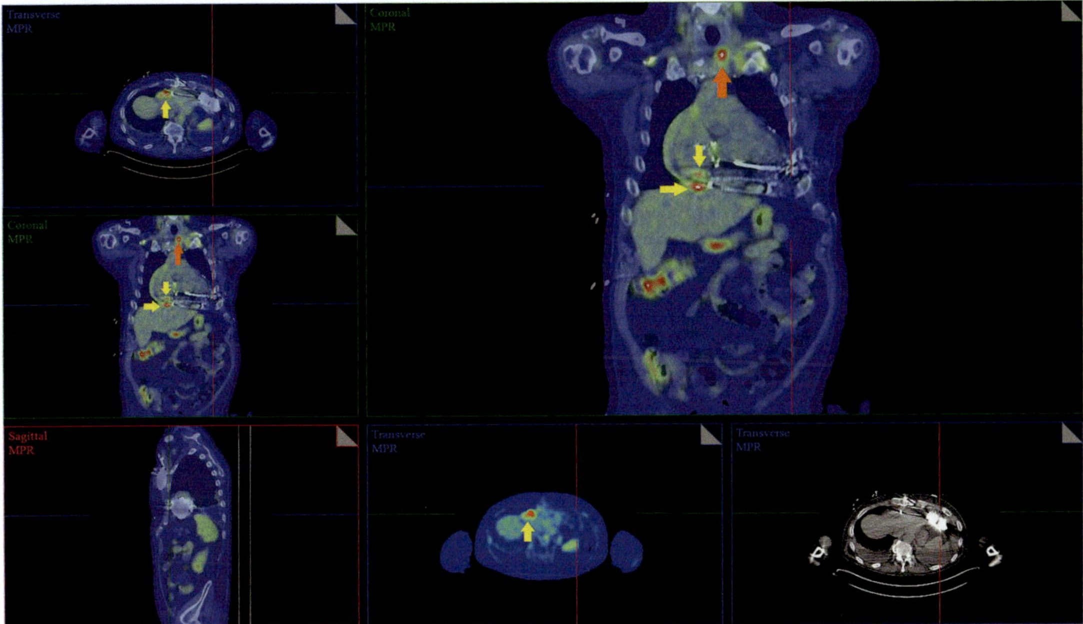

Fig. 16.7 Inflammation of LVAD outflow graft (yellow arrows) and left sternoclavicular joint (orange arrows)

illustrates the utility of FDG-PET/CT in detecting infection of various components of the LVAD including the driveline in addition to evaluating the inflow and outflow grafts and pacemaker leads.

Case 16.5

A 65-year-old man with a history of ischemic cardiomyopathy with ICD and HeartMate 3 LVAD implantation, presented with fever, fatigue, and left shoulder pain. Blood cultures revealed MSSA bacteremia, and treatment with oxacillin was initiated. Chest X-ray revealed no acute abnormalities. Transthoracic echocardiogram and subsequent transesophageal echocardiogram did not reveal any findings suggestive of infection. FDG-PET/CT was obtained to evaluate for LVAD infection. It revealed focal, intense FDG uptake involving the LVAD outflow graft with SUV_{max} of 5.6 compared to LV blood pool with SUVmean 1.7 (Fig. 16.7, yellow arrows). It also revealed focal, intense FDG uptake involving the left sternoclavicular joint (Fig. 16.7, orange arrows). These findings are consistent with infection involving the LVAD outflow graft and left sternoclavicular joint. The patient underwent sur-

gical exploration with sternoclavicular joint resection and was treated with long-term antimicrobial therapy. This case illustrates the importance of whole-body imaging in patients suspected of having LVAD infection, as FDG-PET/CT can detect infection of components of the LVAD as well as other sites of infection in the body.

Conclusion

FDG-PET/CT is being used more frequently to diagnose and manage patients suspected of having LVAD infection. This promising modality has high sensitivity for LVAD infection; however, specificity varies widely [3]. Proper patient preparation to achieve suppression of endogenous myocardial glucose uptake is a key component to ensure high-quality images. FDG-PET/CT is useful not only for the diagnosis of LVAD infections but also for the prognosis of these patients [44]. Readers should be aware of common pitfalls for false positives and negatives in FDG LVAD imaging as detailed in this review. Finally, FDG-PET/CT studies should be interpreted in clinical context and ideally in a multidisciplinary endocarditis team with involvement of cardiovascular imagers, heart failure cardiologists, infectious disease specialists, cardiac surgeons, and neurologists. A team-based approach may improve the ability to select and deliver effective healthcare to this population with high burden of risk factors and potential for adverse outcomes.

References

1. Rose EA, Gelijns AC, Moskowitz AJ, Heitjan DF, Stevenson LW, Dembitsky W, et al. Long-term use of a left ventricular assist device for end-stage heart failure. N Engl J Med. 2001;345(20):1435–43.
2. Califano S, Pagani FD, Malani PN. Left ventricular assist device-associated infections. Infect Dis Clin North Am. 2012;26(1):77–87.
3. Tam MC, Patel VN, Weinberg RL, Hulten EA, Aaronson KD, Pagani FD, et al. Diagnostic accuracy of FDG PET/CT in suspected LVAD infections: a case series, systematic review, and meta-analysis. JACC Cardiovasc Imaging. 2020;13(5):1191–202.
4. Virani SS, Alonso A, Aparicio HJ, Benjamin EJ, Bittencourt MS, Callaway CW, et al. heart disease and stroke statistics-2021 update: a report from the American Heart Association. Circulation. 2021;143(8):e254–743.
5. Molina EJ, Shah P, Kiernan MS, Cornwell WK, Copeland H, Takeda K, et al. The Society of Thoracic Surgeons Intermacs 2020 Annual Report. Ann Thorac Surg. 2021;111(3):778–92.
6. Frazier OH, Rose EA, McCarthy P, Burton NA, Tector A, Levin H, et al. Improved mortality and rehabilitation of transplant candidates treated with a long-term implantable left ventricular assist system. Ann Surg. 1995;222(3):327–36.
7. Kilic A, Acker MA, Atluri P. Dealing with surgical left ventricular assist device complications. J Thorac Dis. 2015;7(12):2158–64.
8. Hannan MM, Husain S, Mattner F, Danziger-Isakov L, Drew RJ, Corey GR, et al. Working formulation for the standardization of definitions of infections in patients using ventricular assist devices. J Heart Lung Transplant. 2011;30(4):375–84.
9. Kirklin JK, Naftel DC, Kormos RL, Pagani FD, Myers SL, Stevenson LW, et al. Interagency Registry for Mechanically Assisted Circulatory Support (INTERMACS) analysis of pump thrombosis in the HeartMate II left ventricular assist device. J Heart Lung Transplant. 2014;33(1):12–22.
10. Trachtenberg BH, Cordero-Reyes A, Elias B, Loebe M. A review of infections in patients with left ventricular assist devices: prevention, diagnosis and management. Methodist Debakey Cardiovasc J. 2015;11(1):28–32.
11. Raymond AL, Kfoury AG, Bishop CJ, Davis ES, Goebel KM, Stoker S, et al. Obesity and left ventricular assist device driveline exit site infection. ASAIO J. 2010;56(1):57–60.
12. Zahr F, Genovese E, Mathier M, Shullo M, Lockard K, Zomak R, et al. Obese patients and mechanical circulatory support: weight loss, adverse events, and outcomes. Ann Thorac Surg. 2011;92(4):1420–6.
13. Clerkin KJ, Naka Y, Mancini DM, Colombo PC, Topkara VK. the impact of obesity on patients bridged to transplantation with continuous-flow left ventricular assist devices. JACC Heart Fail. 2016;4(10):761–8.
14. Bejko J, Toto F, Gregori D, Gerosa G, Bottio T. Left ventricle assist devices and driveline's infection incidence: a single-centre experience. J Artif Organs. 2018;21(1):52–60.
15. Goldstein DJ, Naftel D, Holman W, Bellumkonda L, Pamboukian SV, Pagani FD, et al. Continuous-flow devices and percutaneous site infections: clinical outcomes. J Heart Lung Transplant. 2012;31(11):1151–7.
16. Zierer A, Melby SJ, Voeller RK, Guthrie TJ, Ewald GA, Shelton K, et al. Late-onset driveline infections: the Achilles' heel of prolonged left ventricular assist device support. Ann Thorac Surg. 2007;84(2):515–20.
17. Sharma V, Deo SV, Stulak JM, Durham LA 3rd, Daly RC, Park SJ, et al. Driveline infections in left ventricular assist devices: implications for destination therapy. Ann Thorac Surg. 2012;94(5):1381–6.
18. Cagliostro B, Levin AP, Fried J, Stewart S, Parkis G, Mody KP, et al. Continuous-flow left ventricular assist devices and usefulness of a standardized strategy to reduce drive-line infections. J Heart Lung Transplant. 2016;35(1):108–14.
19. Menon AK, Baranski SK, Unterkofler J, Autschbach R, Moza AK, Goetzenich A, et al. Special treatment and wound care of the driveline exit site after left ventricular assist device implantation. Thorac Cardiovasc Surg. 2015;63(8):670–4.
20. Schibilsky D, Benk C, Haller C, Berchtold-Herz M, Siepe M, Beyersdorf F, et al. Double tunnel technique for the LVAD driveline: improved management regarding driveline infections. J Artif Organs. 2012;15(1):44–8.
21. Fleissner F, Avsar M, Malehsa D, Strueber M, Haverich A, Schmitto JD. Reduction of driveline infections through doubled driveline tunneling of left ventricular assist devices. Artif Organs. 2013;37(1):102–7.
22. Wert L, Hanke JS, Dogan G, Ricklefs M, Fleissner F, Chatterjee A, et al. Reduction of driveline infections through doubled driveline tunneling of left ventricular assist devices-5-year follow-up. J Thorac Dis. 2018;10(Suppl 15):S1703–S10.
23. Singh A, Russo MJ, Valeroso TB, Anderson AS, Rich JD, Jeevanandam V, et al. Modified HeartMate II driveline externalization technique significantly

decreases incidence of infection and improves long-term survival. ASAIO J. 2014;60(6):613–6.

24. Dean D, Kallel F, Ewald GA, Tatooles A, Sheridan BC, Brewer RJ, et al. Reduction in driveline infection rates: results from the HeartMate II Multicenter Driveline Silicone Skin Interface (SSI) Registry. J Heart Lung Transplant. 2015;34(6):781–9.

25. Zinoviev R, Lippincott CK, Keller SC, Gilotra NA. In full flow: left ventricular assist device infections in the modern era. open forum. Infect Dis. 2020;7(5):ofaa124.

26. Nienaber JJ, Kusne S, Riaz T, Walker RC, Baddour LM, Wright AJ, et al. Clinical manifestations and management of left ventricular assist device-associated infections. Clin Infect Dis. 2013;57(10):1438–48.

27. Kusne S, Mooney M, Danziger-Isakov L, Kaan A, Lund LH, Lyster H, et al. An ISHLT consensus document for prevention and management strategies for mechanical circulatory support infection. J Heart Lung Transplant. 2017;36(10):1137–53.

28. Li JS, Sexton DJ, Mick N, Nettles R, Fowler VG Jr, Ryan T, et al. Proposed modifications to the duke criteria for the diagnosis of infective endocarditis. Clin Infect Dis. 2000;30(4):633–8.

29. Topkara VK, Kondareddy S, Malik F, Wang IW, Mann DL, Ewald GA, et al. Infectious complications in patients with left ventricular assist device: etiology and outcomes in the continuous-flow era. Ann Thorac Surg. 2010;90(4):1270–7.

30. Tong MZ, Smedira NG, Soltesz EG, Starling RC, Koval CE, Porepa L, et al. Outcomes of heart transplant after left ventricular assist device specific and related infection. Ann Thorac Surg. 2015;100(4):1292–7.

31. Pieri M, Müller M, Scandroglio AM, Pergantis P, Kretzschmar A, Kaufmann F, et al. surgical treatment of mediastinitis with omentoplasty in ventricular assist device patients: report of referral center experience. ASAIO J. 2016;62(6):666–70.

32. Gordon RJ, Weinberg AD, Pagani FD, Slaughter MS, Pappas PS, Naka Y, et al. Prospective, multicenter study of ventricular assist device infections. Circulation. 2013;127(6):691–702.

33. Martin SI, Wellington L, Stevenson KB, Mangino JE, Sai-Sudhakar CB, Firstenberg MS, et al. Effect of body mass index and device type on infection in left ventricular assist device support beyond 30 days. Interact Cardiovasc Thorac Surg. 2010;11(1):20–3.

34. Schulman AR, Martens TP, Christos PJ, Russo MJ, Comas GM, Cheema FH, et al. Comparisons of infection complications between continuous flow and pulsatile flow left ventricular assist devices. J Thorac Cardiovasc Surg. 2007;133(3):841–2.

35. Aaronson KD, Slaughter MS, McGee E, Cotts WG, Acker MA, Jessup ML. Evaluation of the HeartWare HVAD left ventricular assist device system for the treatment of advanced heart failure: results of the advance bridge to transplant trial. Circulation. 2010;122:2215–26.

36. Feldman D, Pamboukian SV, Teuteberg JJ, Birks E, Lietz K, Moore SA, et al. The 2013 international society for heart and lung transplantation guidelines for mechanical circulatory support: executive summary. J Heart Lung Transplant. 2013;32(2):157–87.

37. Hernandez GA, Breton JDN, Chaparro SV. Driveline infection in ventricular assist devices and its implication in the present era of destination therapy. Open J Cardiovasc Surg. 2017;9:1179065217714216.

38. Erba PA, Pizzi MN, Roque A, Salaun E, Lancellotti P, Tornos P, et al. Multimodality imaging in infective endocarditis: an imaging team within the endocarditis team. Circulation. 2019;140(21):1753–65.

39. Habets J, Tanis W, Reitsma JB, van den Brink RBA, Mali WPTM, Chamuleau SAJ, et al. Are novel non-invasive imaging techniques needed in patients with suspected prosthetic heart valve endocarditis? a systematic review and meta-analysis. Eur Radiol. 2015;25(7):2125–33.

40. Wang TKM, Sánchez-Nadales A, Igbinomwanhia E, Cremer P, Griffin B, Xu B. Diagnosis of infective endocarditis by subtype using (18)f-fluorodeoxyglucose positron emission tomography/computed tomography: a contemporary meta-analysis. Circ Cardiovasc Imaging. 2020;13(6):e010600.

41. Osborne MT, Hulten EA, Murthy VL, Skali H, Taqueti VR, Dorbala S, et al. Patient preparation for cardiac fluorine-18 fluorodeoxyglucose positron emission tomography imaging of inflammation. J Nucl Cardiol. 2017;24(1):86–99.

42. Chareonthaitawee P, Beanlands RS, Chen W, Dorbala S, Miller EJ, Murthy VL, et al. Joint SNMMI–ASNC expert consensus document on the role of & 18F-FDG PET/CT in cardiac sarcoid detection and therapy monitoring. J Nucl Med. 2017;58(8):1341.

43. Osborne M, Hulten E, Murthy V, Skali H, Taqueti V, Dorbala S, et al. Patient preparation for cardiac fluorine-18 fluorodeoxyglucose positron emission tomography imaging of inflammation. J Nucl Cardiol. 2016;24:86–99.

44. Kim J, Feller ED, Chen W, Liang Y, Dilsizian V. FDG PET/CT for early detection and localization of left ventricular assist device infection: impact on Patient management and outcome. JACC Cardiovasc Imaging. 2019;12(4):722–9.

45. Orvin K, Goldberg E, Bernstine H, Groshar D, Sagie A, Kornowski R, et al. The role of FDG-PET/CT imaging in early detection of extra-cardiac complications of infective endocarditis. Clin Microbiol Infect. 2015;21(1):69–76.

46. Pizzi MN, Roque A, Fernández-Hidalgo N, Cuéllar-Calabria H, Ferreira-González I, González-Alujas MT, et al. Improving the diagnosis of infective endocarditis in prosthetic valves and intracardiac devices with 18f-fluorodeoxyglucose positron emission tomography/computed tomography angiography: initial results at an infective endocarditis referral center. Circulation. 2015;132(12):1113–26.

47. Büther F, Stegger L, Dawood M, Range F, Schäfers M, Fischbach R, et al. Effective methods to correct contrast agent-induced errors in PET quantification in cardiac PET/CT. J Nucl Med. 2007;48(7): 1060–8.

48. Roque A, Pizzi MN, Fernández-Hidalgo N, Permanyer E, Cuellar-Calabria H, Romero-Farina G, et al. Morpho-metabolic post-surgical patterns of non-infected prosthetic heart valves by [18F]FDG PET/CTA: "normality" is a possible diagnosis. Eur Heart J Cardiovasc Imaging. 2020;21(1):24–33.

49. Garg G, Benchekroun MT, Abraham T. FDG-PET/CT in the postoperative period: utility, expected findings, complications, and pitfalls. Semin Nucl Med. 2017;47(6):579–94.

50. Kircher M, Lapa C. Novel noninvasive nuclear medicine imaging techniques for cardiac inflammation. Curr Cardiovasc Imaging Rep. 2017;10(2):6.

51. Ruiz-Zafra J, Rodriguez-Fernandez A, Sanchez-Palencia A, Cueto A. Surgical adhesive may cause false positives in integrated positron emission tomography and computed tomography after lung cancer resection. Eur J Cardiothorac Surg. 2013;43(6):1251–3.

52. Sureshbabu W, Mawlawi O. PET/CT imaging artifacts. J Nucl Med Technol. 2005;33(3):156–61; quiz 63-4.

Matthieu Pelletier-Galarneau, Stephanie Tan, Yoan Lamarche, Francois Harel, and Patrick Martineau

Introduction

Heart disease remains the leading cause of death in Western countries [1]. Despite advances in percutaneous interventions for coronary artery disease (CAD) and valvular diseases, cardiac surgery remains necessary in a large proportion of cases, with approximately 500,000 open-heart surgeries performed each year in the United States alone [1]. As with all surgical interventions, these surgeries are associated with a degree of morbidity and mortality resulting from various possible attendant complications. In particular, sternal wound infection (SWI) is a relatively frequent complication of open-heart surgery. SWI can constitute a surgical emergency and the identification of high-risk patients is essential in order to determine those requiring debridement surgery. This chapter provides an overview of the pathophysiology and epidemiology of SWIs. The role of computed tomography (CT), mag-

netic resonance (MR), and fluorodeoxyglucose-positron emission tomography (FDG-PET) for the diagnosis and follow-up of SWIs will be reviewed.

Epidemiology

SWIs are the leading cause of surgical site infections following cardiac surgery [2]. SWIs are subdivided into two separate categories based on the structures involved: superficial SWIs (SSWIs) and deep SWIs (DSWIs). SSWIs are limited to the skin, subcutaneous tissues, and pectoralis fascia and are relatively common complications of cardiac surgery with the reported incidence ranging from 0.5% to 8% [3–5]. Distinct from these are DSWIs which involve the sternum, substernal space, and/or mediastinum. By definition, both mediastinitis and sternal osteitis are considered DSWIs. Less frequent than SSWIs, DSWIs have a reported incidence ranging between 0.5% and 2% but are associated with higher morbidity and mortality, as well as prolonged hospitalization duration and significant costs [2, 3, 5]. In particular, patients with DSWIs following cardiac surgery have 4 times greater 1-year mortality compared to those without infection [6]. Treatment of DSWIs involves surgical debridement, with or without chest wall reconstruction, and successful surgery necessitates adequate debridement of infected areas to avoid the need

M. Pelletier-Galarneau (✉) · S. Tan · Y. Lamarche
F. Harel
Montreal Heart Institute, Montréal, QC, Canada
e-mail: Matthieu.pelletier-galarneau@icm-mhi.org

P. Martineau
BC Cancer, Vancouver, BC, Canada

© The Author(s), under exclusive license to Springer Nature Switzerland AG 2022
M. Pelletier-Galarneau, P. Martineau (eds.), *FDG-PET/CT and PET/MR in Cardiovascular Diseases*, https://doi.org/10.1007/978-3-031-09807-9_17

for repeated surgery. As therapeutic approaches and outcomes differ significantly between SSWIs and DSWIs, the ability to distinguish between the two is critical. In that context, FDG-PET/CT can guide surgery by revealing the extent of disease since areas of infection can be hidden or missed during debridement surgery [7]. In addition to providing disease extent, FDG-PET/CT can be useful to monitor response to therapy.

Pathogenesis

SWIs are usually the consequence of wound contamination during the procedure, which can occur despite optimal precautions, especially in long interventions. The vast majority of SWIs are caused by bacteria, with the most frequent organisms being *Staphylococcus aureus* followed by Gram-negative bacilli and streptococci [8, 9]. Infections with fungus and mycobacterium are rare and represent only a small fraction of SWI cases. *Mycobacterium chimaera* infections have been associated with contamination of heater-cooler devices [10]. In addition, *Candida* mediastinitis accounts for a very small fraction (<10%) of DSWIs but is fatal in nearly half of cases [11]. *Aspergillus* mediastinitis, which can occur in both immunosuppressed and immunocompetent patients, often results from airborne contamination by spores, especially in cases of prolonged chest opening after surgery [12]. Fungal and mycobacterial DSWIs represent a clinical challenge given their high mortality rates, the difficulty to culture organisms, and their atypical presentations, which is often paucisymptomatic.

Several factors, related to the patient or to the surgical procedure itself, have been associated with an increased risk of SWIs (Table 17.1) [2, 13]. In particular, factors associated with poor wound healing in general, such as diabetes, obe-

Table 17.1 Risk factors associated with sternal wound infection

Patient-related risk factors	Procedure-related risk factors
Diabetes	Sternal edge not aligned properly
Obesity	
Advanced age	Ischemic sternum
Smoking	Emergency surgery
Renal Failure	Reoperation for tamponade or bleeding
Prior cardiac surgery	
Immunosuppression	Intra-aortic balloon pump support
Coronary artery disease	
Abnormal underlying sternal bone	Post operative ventilator support
	Prolonged surgery

sity, and smoking, are all associated with increased risks of SWI. Of note, several of these factors are also associated with CAD and are therefore highly prevalent in the population of patients undergoing coronary artery bypass graft (CABG) surgery. Procedure-related risk factors include elements that may contribute to suboptimal sternal union such as misalignment of the sternal edges and asymmetric sternotomy. Further, maneuvers which can promote sternal ischemia, including bilateral harvesting of the mammary arteries and excessive cauterization, are associated with increased risk of SWIs [14]. The type of procedure also affects the risk of SWIs, with heart transplant and CABG (with the use of internal mammary artery) being associated with higher incidence of both SSWIs and DSWIs compared to other procedures such as valve replacement surgery [11]. The use of minimally invasive methods such as robot-assisted surgeries are associated with lower incidences of mediastinitis [15]. Various classification systems for SWIs have been proposed but have seen limited use in clinical settings and in research. One of the most cited is the Jones classification, presented in Table 17.2, which classifies SWI based on the anatomical extent and disease severity [16].

Table 17.2 Jones classification of sternal wound infection

Type	Depth	Description
1a	Superficial	Skin and subcutaneous dehiscence
1b	Superficial	Exposure of sutured deep fascia
2a	Deep	Bone exposure with stable sternotomy
2b	Deep	Bone exposure with unstable sternotomy
3a	Deep	Exposed necrotic or fractured bone, exposed heart
3b	Deep	Type 2 or 3 with septicemia

Adapted from [16]

Treatments

SSWI is typically treated with antibiotics. Incision and drainage of purulent material, wound packing, and negative pressure wound therapy may also be used [17]. On the other hand, DSWI treatment is more aggressive and relies on debridement of necrotic tissue, drainage and irrigation of infected spaces, and various sternal closure techniques [17]. When primary sternal wound closure is not possible, sternal wound flap closure with muscle or omental flaps may be considered. When sternal closure is delayed, negative pressure wound therapy should be considered. In cases of extensive sternal osteitis, debridement of the sternum and occasionally adjacent cartilage may be required and may also require extensive chest wall reconstruction.

Clinical Presentation

The clinical presentation of SWI varies depending on the extent and depth of tissue involvement, and whether the mediastinum is affected. SSWIs may present as local discomfort, cellulitis, and wound drainage. Patients may also present with fever and tachycardia, although these symptoms are more typically seen in cases of DSWIs. The most severe form of SWI, mediastinitis, typically occurs in the 2 weeks following surgery; however, presentation can be delayed with symptoms appearing several months after surgery [18].

Symptoms of mediastinitis include fever, tachycardia, sternal wound dehiscence, chest discomfort, sternal instability, wound drainage, and cellulitis. Fever preceding the appearance of cellulitis or wound drainage should raise the suspicion of mediastinitis. Nonetheless, drawing a distinction between SSWI and DSWI is not always straightforward on the basis of symptomology. Given the important differences in management and prognosis, being able to distinguish accurately and rapidly superficial from deep SWI is critical. The United States Centers for Disease Control and Prevention criteria are often reported in the literature to confirm the diagnosis of DSWI (Table 17.3) [19]. Although these criteria can be useful to confirm infection following interventions and can serve as gold standard in clinical trials, they are often met only after debridement surgery is performed and are therefore of limited use for the initial diagnosis and guiding therapeutic decisions in patients with suspected DSWI.

In addition, serologic biomarkers are of limited utility in the investigation of SWIs. Leukocytosis is frequent but is nonspecific. Inflammatory markers such as C-reactive protein (CRP) and erythrocyte sedimentation rate (ESR) are often elevated due to the recent surgery. Blood cultures may reveal the presence of microorganisms but are not specific for SWI and negative blood cultures do not exclude DSWI. Therefore, DSWI is primarily a clinical diagnosis, based on physical examination, vital signs, and symptoms. In cases where DSWI is not clinically evident but

Table 17.3 Centre for Disease Control (CDC) mediastinitis criteria

At least one of the following criteria must be met:
1. Patient has organisms cultured from mediastinal tissue or fluid obtained during a surgical operation or needle aspiration
2. Patient has evidence of mediastinitis seen during a surgical operation or histopathologic examination
3. Patient has at least one of the following signs or symptoms with no other recognized cause: (a) Fever (b) Chest pain (c) Sternal instability and at least one of the following: (a) Purulent discharge from mediastinal area (b) Organisms cultured from blood or discharge from mediastinal area (c) Mediastinal widening on X-ray
4. Patient ≤1 year of age has at least one of the following signs or symptoms with no other recognized cause: (a) Fever (b) Hypothermia (c) Apnea (d) Bradycardia (e) Sternal instability and at least one of the following: (a) Purulent discharge from mediastinal area (b) Organisms cultured from blood or discharge from mediastinal area (c) Mediastinal widening on X-ray

suspected, further testing, including CT and PET imaging may be helpful as it may provide valuable information with regard to infection extent and severity, and aid in surgical planning [20].

Computed Tomography

CT is a widely accessible modality to evaluate for sternal wound complication. It can also identify alternate diagnoses when the clinical presentation is nonspecific. In the early postoperative period, distinguishing normal postsurgical changes from sternal wound infection can be challenging on CT. In general, changes related to recent cardiac surgery including presternal and retrosternal soft tissue edema and hemorrhage, pneumomediastinum, pleural and pericardial effusions, as well as sternal gaps, which may persist for 2–3 weeks [21]. When prior imaging studies are available, resolving soft tissue and mediastinal findings favor normal postoperative changes. However, a new or progressive fluid collection is highly suggestive for DSWI [22] (Fig. 17.1). CT has a reported sensitivity and specificity of 88% and 91%, respectively, for the

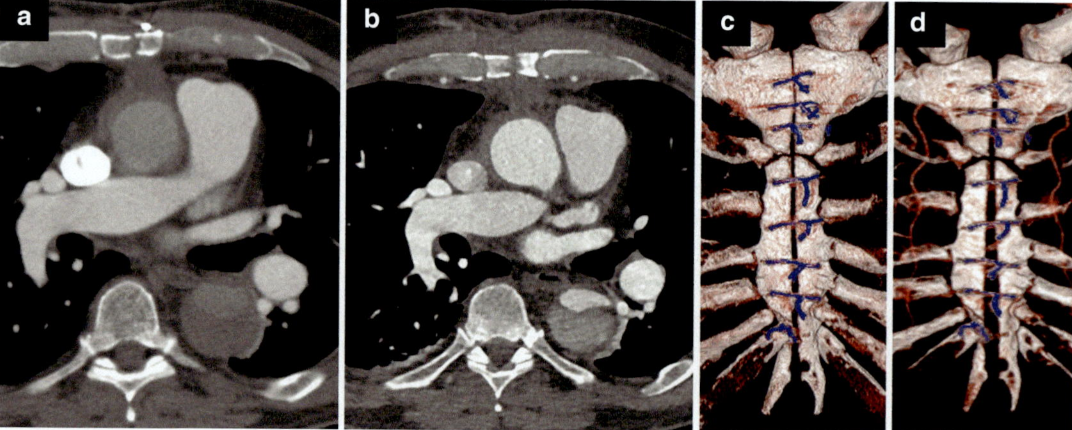

Fig. 17.1 Chest CT images obtained 2 weeks after median sternotomy for replacement of the ascending aorta. Axial image (**a**) demonstrates nonfusion of the median sternotomy which may represent a normal postoperative finding. A CT obtained 24 h later (**b**) shows increased diastasis of the sternotomy and increased pre- and retro-sternal soft tissue infiltration, highly suggestive of mediastinitis. Corresponding 3D reconstruction of CTs performed 24 h apart (**c** and **d**) demonstrates progressive diastasis of the sternum with intact sternotomy wires

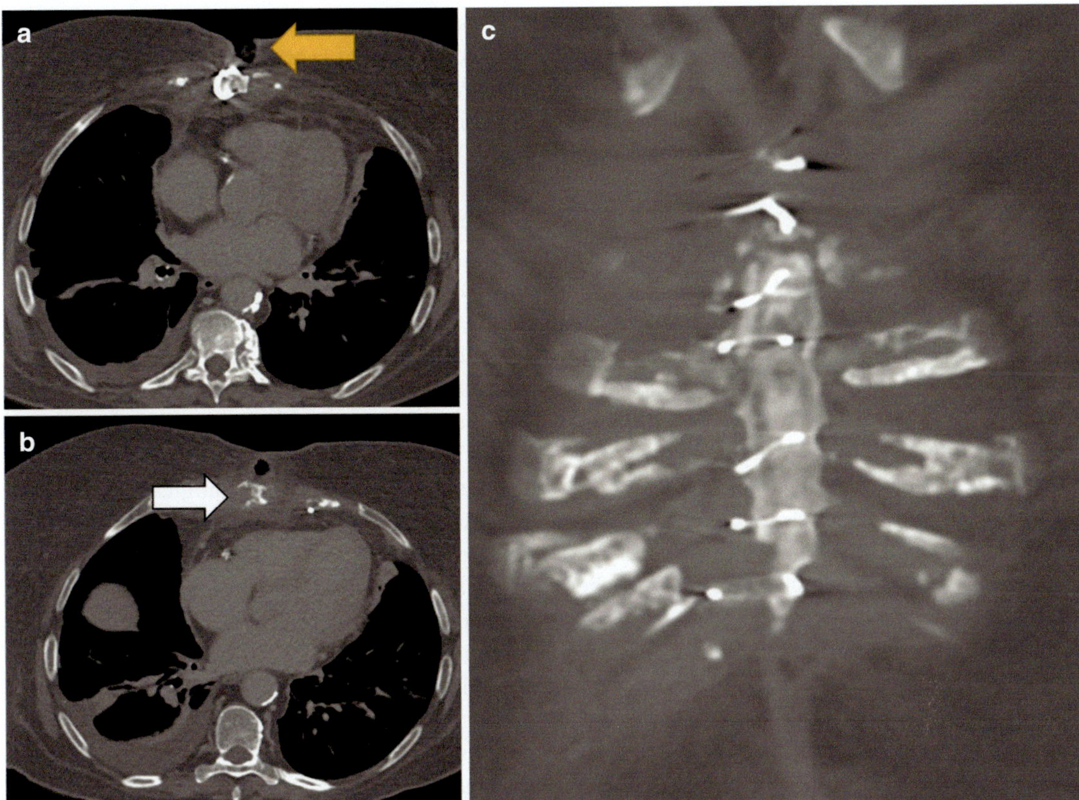

Fig. 17.2 Chest CT obtained 3 months post coronary artery bypass grafts. Axial images (**a** and **b**) shows a mesh inserted within a cutaneous dehiscence where purulent exudate was noted clinically (yellow arrow). There is pre- and retro-sternal soft tissue infiltration and right pleural effusion. Bone erosion (white arrow) is noted on the right side of the sternotomy, also noted on the coronal reconstruction (**c**), consistent with osteomyelitis

diagnosis of mediastinitis in the weeks following surgery [23]. In addition, sternal dehiscence can precede SWI and is recognized when sternotomy wires are displaced, when a side of the sternotomy is no longer held by the wires, or when there is a widening sternal gap. Sternal osteomyelitis is suspected when there is evidence of cortical erosion, for which CT has a sensitivity of 93% and specificity of 86–96% [23] (Fig. 17.2).

Deep sternal abscesses are suspected on unenhanced studies when there is a well-defined encapsulated fluid collection sometimes containing foci of air produced from gas-forming bacteria [22]. If intravenous contrast is administered, the collection can show thick, irregular peripheral enhancement [24]. Occasionally, a sinus tract is noted from the sternum or the retrosternal area leading up to the skin. In rare but serious cases, there may be vascular dissection or pseudoaneurysm which can also involve a coronary artery bypass graft [25].

Magnetic Resonance Imaging

Magnetic resonance imaging (MRI) can identify similar findings as CT and faces the same challenges during the immediate postoperative period. Mediastinal edema appears as fat stranding and increased T2 signal, while pneumomediastinum appears as susceptibility artifacts on MRI. Hematoma can have variable appearance depending on its age. In a relatively acute setting, blood presents as iso- to hyper-intense signal on T1-weighted images and hypo- to iso-intense signal on T2-weighted images. Chronic blood shows hypointense signal on both T1- and T2-weighted images [26]. Mediastinal abscesses manifest as hyperintense T2-weighted collections showing, similar to computed tomography, a thick and irregular enhancing wall. Gas bubbles within the abscess appears as foci of susceptibility artifact on MRI [27].

MRI surpasses CT for the identification of early signs of osteomyelitis with its ability to demonstrate bone marrow edema [28]. Edema appears as hypointense signal on T1-weighted images and hyperintense signal on T2-weighted images on MRI. Irregularity or loss of the hypointense cortex on T1- and T2-weighted images corresponds to cortical erosion seen on CT. A sinus tract appears as a tract with hyperintense T2-signal leading to the skin [27]. DSWI can also manifest as myositis, which is suspected when there is muscle edema on MRI, or pyomyositis if abscess develops within the muscle.

Positron Emission Tomography

FDG-PET imaging is playing an increasing role in the evaluation of patients with suspected infection, with whole-body PET enabling better assessment of the disease extent. In the specific case of SWI, FDG-PET may be useful for surgical planning as well as for therapy response monitoring (Table 17.4). However, just like CT and MRI, accuracy of FDG-PET may be affected by postsurgical changes in the immediate postoperative period.

Zhang et al. retrospectively analyzed 73 patients who underwent FDG-PET/CT study for suspicion of DSWI 1 month or more following surgery [29]. Of the 73 patients, one had superficial SWI, 64 had sternal osteomyelitis, 54 had

Table 17.4 Potential roles of FDG-PET/CT in sternal wound infection (SWI)

Initial diagnosis of SWI
Differentiation between deep and superficial SWI
Evaluation of disease extent
Aid in surgical planning
Assessment of response to antibiotic therapy
Assessment of effect of surgical debridement

mediastinitis, and 28 had costal chondritis. In addition, 6 out of 6 patients with vascular grafts had vascular graft infection. They observed a sensitivity and specificity of 98% and 78% for sternal osteomyelitis, 100% and 95% for mediastinitis, and 82% and 100% for costal chondritis, respectively. They used a 4-level visual scale to rate tracer uptake in the sternum, the mediastinum, the costal cartilage, and the vascular prosthesis. The grading system was as follows: Grade I, uptake similar to fat; Grade II, uptake greater than fat but inferior to vertebra; Grade III, moderate uptake greater than vertebra and below physiological myocardium; and Grade IV, intense uptake greater than physiological myocardial uptake. Grade IV uptake was only observed in infected tissue. Low-grade uptake (I and II) was associated with a high negative predictive value for mediastinal, sternal, and vascular prosthesis infection. Of note, 5/28 (18%) subjects with confirmed costal cartilage infection showed low grade uptake (I and II) [29]. Despite the good performance reported, this grading system is limited by the fact that myocardial uptake is highly variable. In addition, this system does not take into account the distribution of uptake, which may prove more useful to distinguish between sterile postsurgical inflammation and infection [30–32].

Yin et al. retrospectively analyzed the prospectively collected data of 108 patients who underwent CT and FDG-PET/CT for suspicion of DSWI [33]. They evaluated the diagnostic performance of FDG-PET/CT for DSWI and compared it to that of unenhanced CT for three separate sites consisting of the sternum, ribs/costal cartilage, and mediastinum. Focal or diffuse uptake greater than "surrounding structures" was considered infected while mild uptake was considered benign inflammation. They reported a 100% sensitivity of FDG-PET/CT for the detection of sternal and mediastinal infection compared to 91% and 17% for unenhanced CT, respectively. Specificity of FDG-PET/CT was inferior to CT for the detection of mediastinitis (62% vs. 94%) but higher than CT for sternal osteitis (100% vs. 50%). As for rib and cartilage infection, FDG-PET/CT was more sensitive than

CT (79% vs. 16%), with comparable specificity (99% vs. 98%). Evidently, the sensitivity and specificity reported in these studies is highly dependent on the interpretation criteria used. Nonetheless, it appears that identification of cartilage infection is more challenging with both CT and PET, as infection can be present with mild or minimal increased uptake [29, 33].

In a retrospective study of 40 subjects who underwent FDG-PET/CT following open-heart surgery, Hariri et al. reported a sensitivity and specificity of 91% and 97%, respectively, for the diagnosis of SWI [32]. They showed that uptake patterns (e.g., heterogeneous vs. homogeneous) were superior to uptake intensity (SUV_{max}) for differentiating between SWI and inflammation, especially in the first 6 months following surgery (Fig. 17.3).

Interestingly, Liu et al. reported that utilization of FDG-PET/CT was associated with fewer recurrences following debridement surgery compared to CT alone (21% vs. 41%, $p = 0.03$) and

shorter hospital stays following surgery (18 vs. 29 days, $p < 0.001$) [33]. These results highlight the ability of FDG-PET/CT to accurately delineate the areas of infection in various tissues, which can guide surgeons for optimal debridement. In addition, 10 subjects underwent repeated FDG-PET/CT to assess response to therapy. Of these, six subjects showed progression of infection as evidenced by an increase in uptake intensity or more extensive uptake on follow-up scans compared to the baseline study, all of which had recurrent infection requiring additional surgery (excluding one subject who died) while the remaining four subjects without evidence of progression on FDG-PET/CT did not have recurrence. These results suggest that FDG-PET/CT could be used to assess debridement success. However, caution must be taken when interpreting studies following recent debridement as postsurgical inflammation may mimic infection progression.

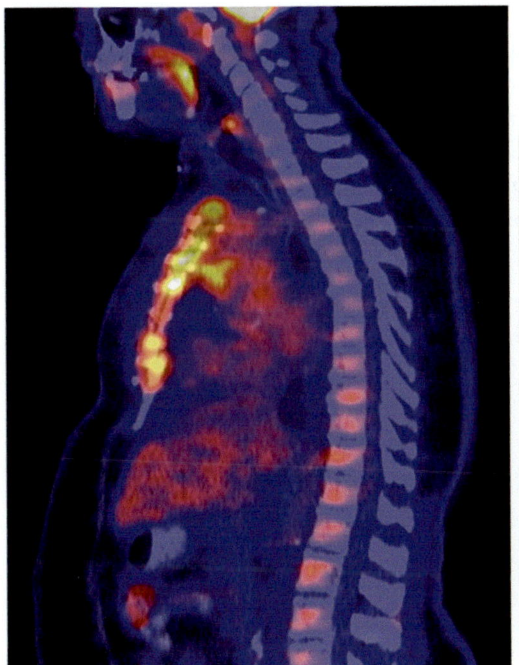

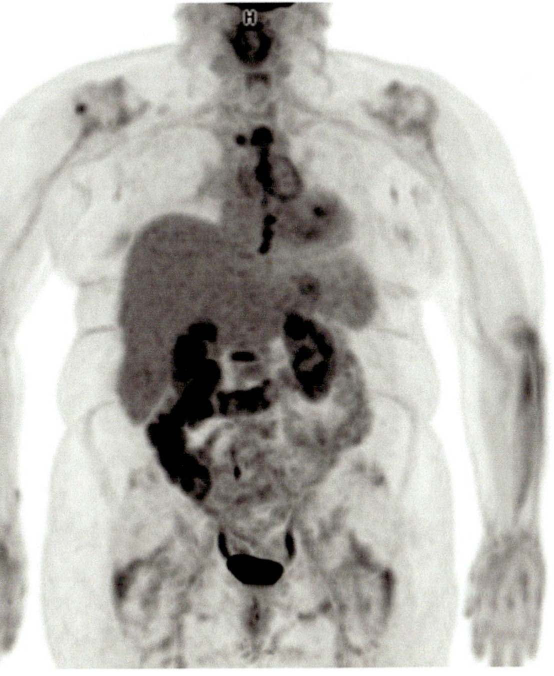

Fig. 17.3 Sagittal and maximal intensity projection FDG-PET/CT images of a 55 year-old female without SWI who underwent medial sternotomy for a Ross procedure 6 months prior to the study. Despite the intense linear uptake (with an SUV_{max} of 6.0) along the sternum, the activity is relatively homogeneous and compatible with sterile postsurgical changes

Imaging Protocol

Use of a myocardial suppression protocol is not always necessary in cases of suspected SWI, as physiological myocardial uptake should not interfere with study interpretation. However, a suppression protocol should be used whenever possible in patients who underwent valve replacement surgery or ascending aorta repair for optimal assessment of these structures. Furthermore, for patients with nonspecific presentations (e.g., fever of unknown origin) and in whom IE is not excluded, suppression protocols should be used. Approximately 185–370 MBq of FDG is injected intravenously. Whole-body PET/CT images are acquired from the base of the skull to the mid-thigh 60–90 min post tracer injection.

Image Interpretation

Distinction between benign postoperative inflammation and infection can be challenging, especially early after surgery. Hariri et al. showed that uptake intensity alone is not sufficient in order to accurately differentiate between infection and inflammation [32]. When PET imaging was performed within 6 months following surgery, sternal SUV_{max} was not significantly different between patients with sternal osteitis and those without infection (8.4 vs. 7.8 $p = 0.72$). On the other hand, in subjects with remote surgery (>6 months), sternal SUV_{max} was significantly higher in patients with sternal osteitis compared to noninfected subjects (8.5 vs. 1.3, $p < 0.0001$) [32]. In noninfected sterna, uptake intensity varied significantly in the first 6 months following sternotomy, with SUV_{max} ranging from 3.2 to 18.6, highlighting the limited value of this metric to distinguish infection from inflammation [32].

For the evaluation of SWI, FDG-PET interpretation should integrate information on tracer uptake pattern, especially in the early postoperative period, similar to evaluation of prosthetic valves and vascular graft infections [31, 34, 35]. Diffuse uptake limited to the sternotomy site, regardless of its intensity, is associated with sterile inflammation in most cases (Fig. 17.4). On the other hand, focal uptake, uptake associated with sternal wires, and heterogeneous uptake extending into the adjacent soft tissues is compatible with infection (Figs. 17.5, 17.6 and 17.7).

In some cases, focal uptake may be seen even in the absence of infection. For instance, utilization of biological glue has been associated with intense focal uptake which may persist for months after surgery [34, 36]. In addition, focal uptake may be seen around sternal wires, especially in the presence of mechanical strain [32].

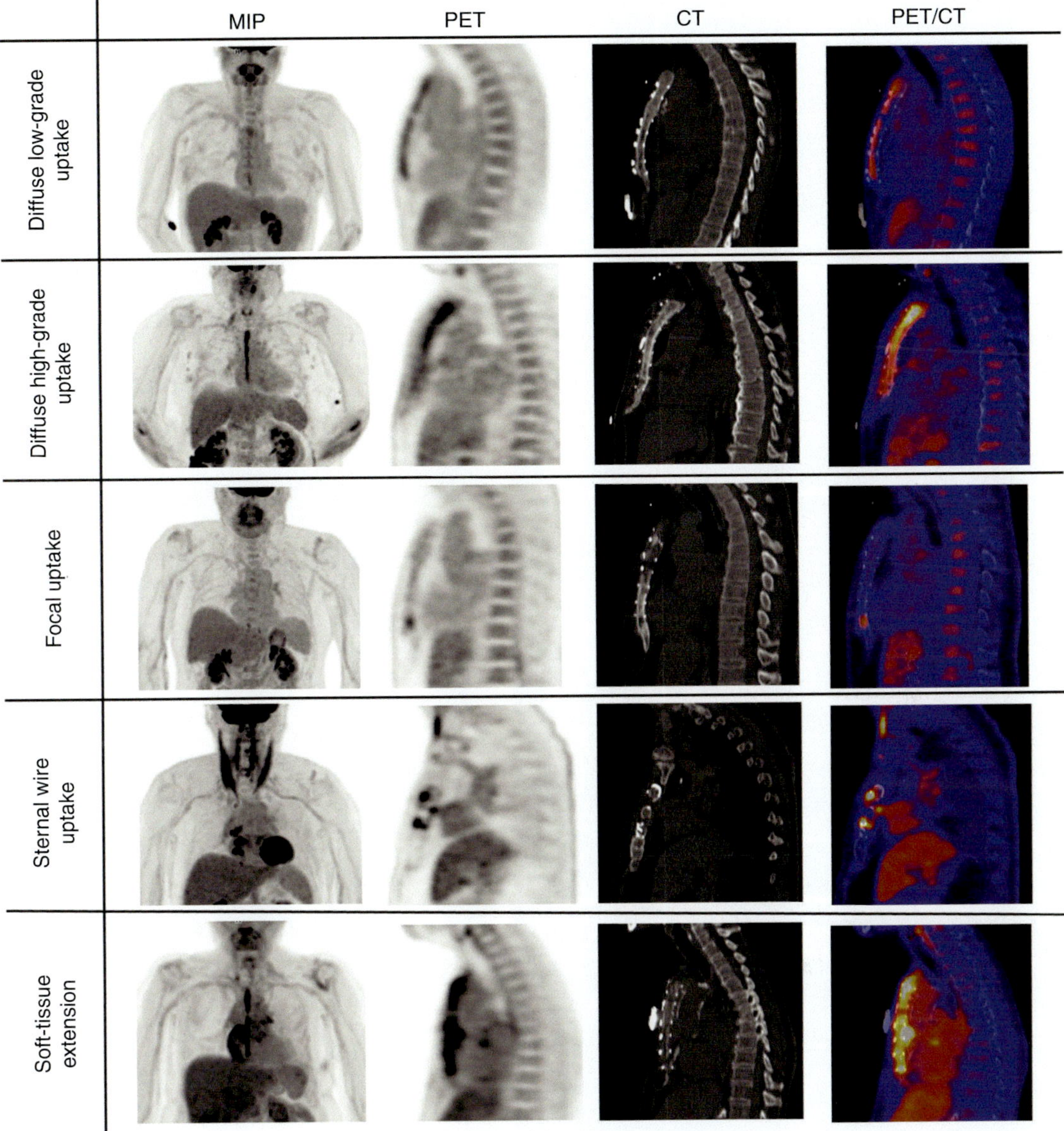

Fig. 17.4 Anterior maximal intensity projection (MIP) images, sagittal PET, CT, and fused PET/CT images of the FDG sternotomy uptake patterns. Diffuse uptake is associated with benign postsurgical changes while focal uptake and soft tissue uptake are suggestive of infection. Reproduced with permission from [32]

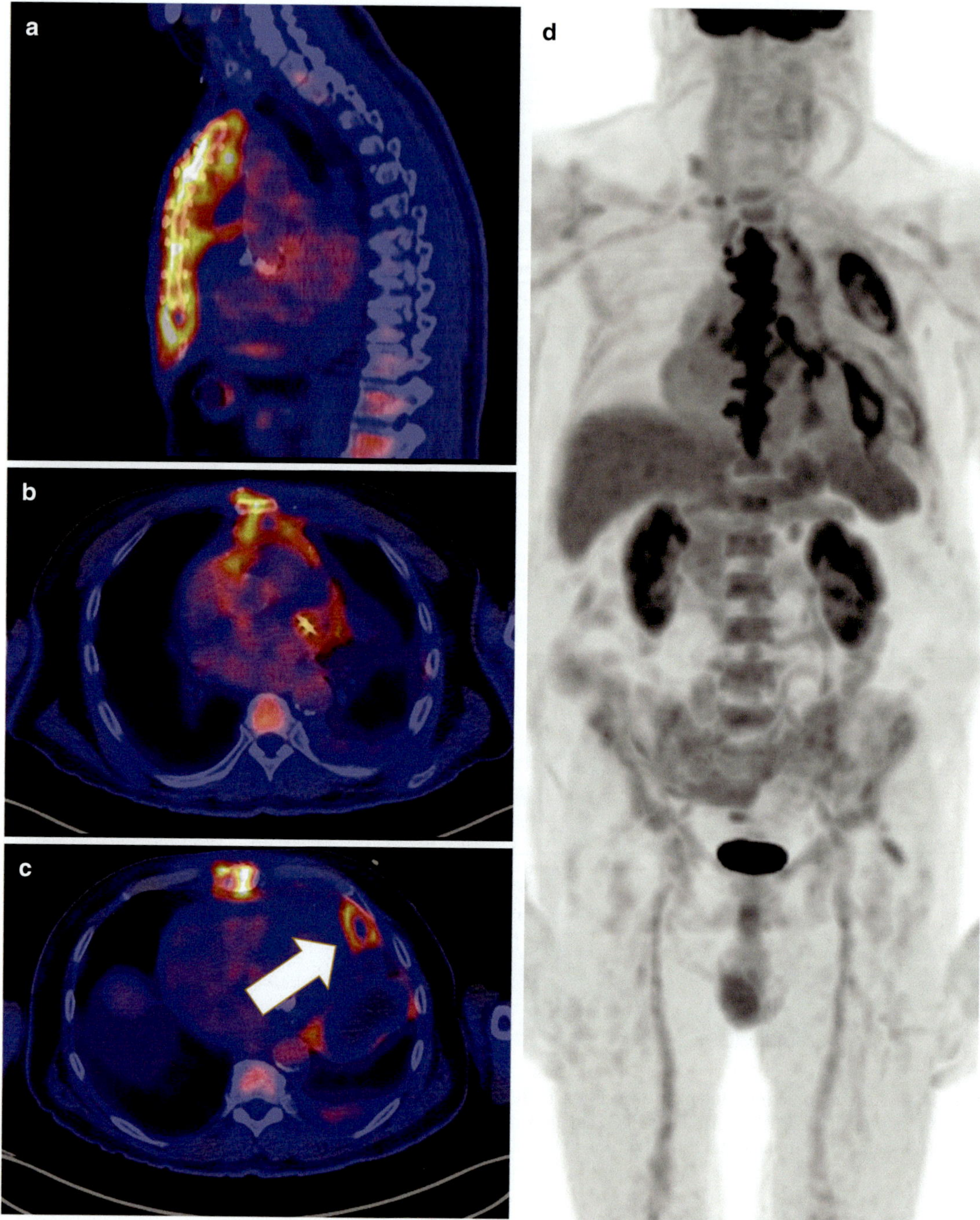

Fig. 17.5 A 78-year-old diabetic male, who underwent a CABG and aortic valve replacement with medial sternotomy 3 weeks prior to imaging, was clinically suspected of having mediastinitis. Sagittal (**a**) and axial (**b**, **c**) FDG-PET/CT images as well as maximal projection images (**d**) demonstrate intense uptake extending into the anterior mediastinum and retro-sternal region, compatible with mediastinitis. In addition, a pericardial fluid collection with circumferential FDG uptake (arrow) is compatible with an abscess

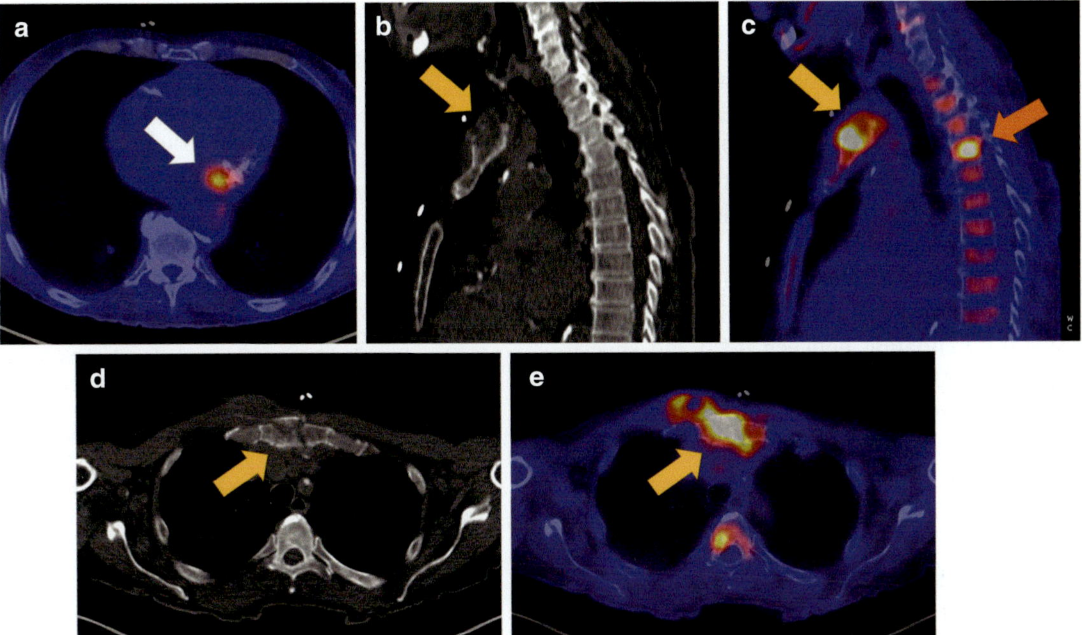

Fig. 17.6 Sternal osteitis can also be seen in patients without sternotomy. This 78-year-old male with mitral valve endocarditis (**a**, white arrow) with septic emboli causing spondylitis as seen on the sagittal CT (**b**) and fused FDG-PET/CT (**c**) images (orange arrow). Axial CT (**d**) and fused FDG-PET/CT images (**e**) also show extensive destruction of the manubrium (yellow arrow) associated with intense FDG uptake extending in the soft tissues anteriorly, consistent with osteomyelitis

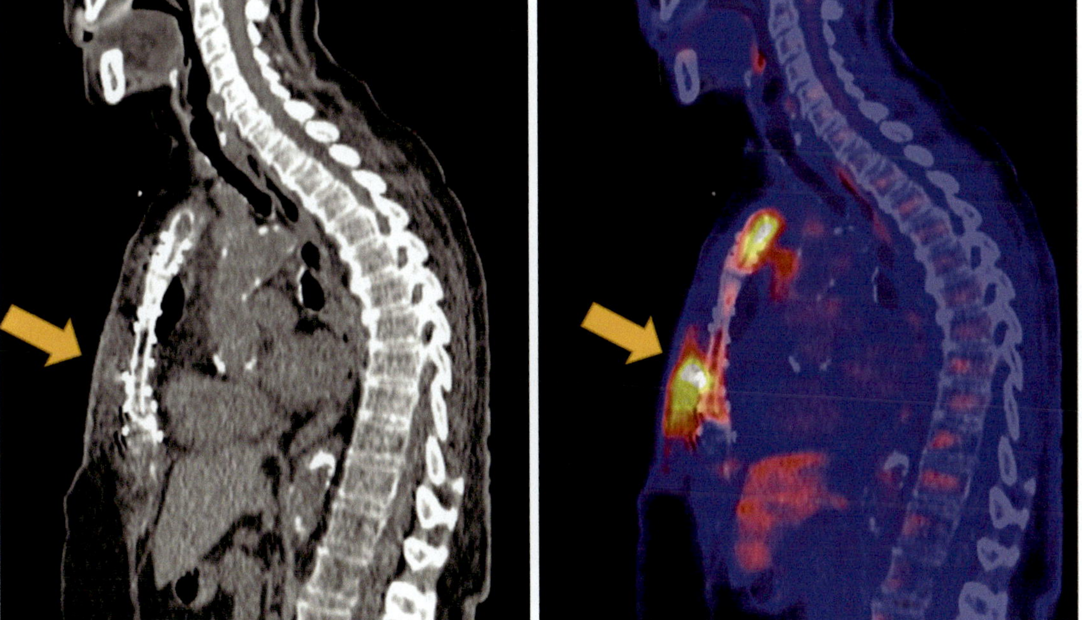

Fig. 17.7 Example of a patient with superficial sternal wound infection with (left) a sagittal CT image demonstrating fat infiltration and a soft tissue collection anterior to the sternum and (right) a sagittal FDG-PET/CT image demonstrating intense uptake limited to the soft tissue. Manubrium uptake, although intense, is linear and contained within the sternal body, consistent with postoperative changes

Conclusion

SWIs are the most important cause of surgical site infections following open-heart surgery. The distinction between SSWI and DSWI is critical, as the treatment and prognosis of these two entities differs significantly. The role of FDG-PET for the investigation of patients with suspected SWI is growing, and this modality may provide valuable information for the initial diagnosis of SWI, differentiating between deep and superficial SWI, evaluating disease extent, aiding in surgical planning, as well as assessing response to antibiotic therapy and the effects of surgical debridement.

References

1. Benjamin EJ, Paul M, Alvaro A, Bittencourt MS, Callaway CW, Carson AP, et al. Heart disease and stroke statistics—2019 update: a report from the American Heart Association. Circulation. 2019;139(10):e56–528.
2. Cove ME, Spelman DW, MacLaren G. Infectious complications of cardiac surgery: a clinical review. J Cardiothorac Vasc Anesth. 2012;26(6):1094–100.
3. Singh K, Anderson E, Harper JG. Overview and management of sternal wound infection. Semin Plast Surg. 2011;25(1):25–33.
4. Salehi Omran A, Karimi A, Ahmadi SH, Davoodi S, Marzban M, Movahedi N, et al. Superficial and deep sternal wound infection after more than 9000 coronary artery bypass graft (CABG): incidence, risk factors and mortality. BMC Infect Dis. 2007;7:112.
5. Ridderstolpe L, Gill H, Granfeldt H, Ahlfeldt H, Rutberg H. Superficial and deep sternal wound complications: incidence, risk factors and mortality. Eur J Cardiothorac Surg. 2001;20(6):1168–75.
6. Sears ED, Wu L, Waljee JF, Momoh AO, Zhong L, Chung KC. The impact of deep sternal wound infection on mortality and resource utilization: a population-based study. World J Surg. 2016;40(11):2673–80.
7. Read C, Branford OA, Verjee LS, Wood SH. PET-CT imaging in patients with chronic sternal wound infections prior to reconstructive surgery: a case series. J Plast Reconstr Aesthet Surg. 2015;68(8):1132–7.
8. Raad I, Kassar R, Ghannam D, Chaftari AM, Hachem R, Jiang Y. Management of the catheter in documented catheter-related coagulase-negative staphylococcal bacteremia: remove or retain? Clin Infect Dis. 2009;49(8):1187–94.
9. Trouillet J-L, Vuagnat A, Combes A, Bors V, Chastre J, Gandjbakhch I, et al. Acute poststernotomy mediastinitis managed with debridement and closed-drainage aspiration: factors associated with death in the intensive care unit. J Thorac Cardiovasc Surg. 2005;129(3):518–24.
10. Ogunremi T, Taylor G, Johnston L, Amaratunga K, Muller M, Coady A, et al. Mycobacterium chimaera infections in post–operative patients exposed to heater–cooler devices: an overview. Can Commun Dis Rep. 2017;43(5):107–13.
11. Lepelletier D, Perron S, Bizouarn P, Caillon J, Drugeon H, Michaud J-L, et al. Surgical-site infection after cardiac surgery: incidence, microbiology, and risk factors. Infect Control Hosp Epidemiol. 2005;26(5):466–72.
12. Caballero M-J, Mongardon N, Haouache H, Vodovar D, Ben Ayed I, Auvergne L, et al. Aspergillus mediastinitis after cardiac surgery. Int J Infect Dis. 2016;44:16–9.
13. Meszaros K, Fuehrer U, Grogg S, Sodeck G, Czerny M, Marschall J, et al. Risk factors for sternal wound infection after open heart operations vary according to type of operation. Ann Thorac Surg. 2016;101(4):1418–25.
14. Borger MA, Rao V, Weisel RD, Ivanov J, Cohen G, Scully HE, et al. Deep sternal wound infection: risk factors and outcomes. Ann Thorac Surg. 1998;65(4):1050–6.
15. McClure RS, Cohn LH, Wiegerinck E, Couper GS, Aranki SF, Bolman RM, et al. Early and late outcomes in minimally invasive mitral valve repair: an eleven-year experience in 707 patients. J Thorac Cardiovasc Surg. 2009;137(1):70–5.
16. Jones G, Jurkiewicz MJ, Bostwick J, Wood R, Bried JT, Culbertson J, et al. Management of the infected median sternotomy wound with muscle flaps. The Emory 20-year experience. Ann Surg. 1997;225(6):766–76. discussion 776-778
17. Lazar HL, Salm TV, Engelman R, Orgill D, Gordon S. Prevention and management of sternal wound infections. J Thorac Cardiovasc Surg. 2016;152(4):962–72.
18. Fariñas MC, Gald Peralta F, Bernal JM, Rabasa JM, Revuelta JM, González-Macías J. Suppurative mediastinitis after open-heart surgery: a case-control study covering a seven-year period in Santander, Spain. Clin Infect Dis. 1995;20(2):272–9.
19. Horan TC, Andrus M, Dudeck MA. CDC/NHSN surveillance definition of health care-associated infection and criteria for specific types of infections in the acute care setting. Am J Infect Control. 2008;36(5):309–32.
20. Gaudreau G, Costache V, Houde C, Cloutier D, Montalin L, Voisine P, et al. Recurrent sternal infection following treatment with negative pressure wound therapy and titanium transverse plate fixation. Eur J Cardiothorac Surg. 2010;37(4):888–92.
21. Li AE, Fishman EK. Evaluation of complications after sternotomy using single- and multidetector CT with three-dimensional volume rendering. Am J Roentgenol. 2003;181(4):1065–70.
22. Yamashiro T, Kamiya H, Murayama S, Unten S, Nakayama T, Gibo M, et al. Infectious mediastinitis after cardiovascular surgery: role of computed tomography. Radiat Med. 2008;26(6):343–7.

23. Gur E, Stern D, Weiss J, Herman O, Wertheym E, Cohen M, et al. Clinical-radiological evaluation of poststernotomy wound infection. Plast Reconstr Surg. 1998;101(2):348–55.
24. Glazer H, Siegel M, Sagel S. Low-attenuation mediastinal masses on CT. Am J Roentgenol. 1989;152(6):1173–7.
25. Sullivan K, Steiner R, Smullens S, Griska L, Meister S. Pseudoaneurysm of the ascending aorta following cardiac surgery. Chest. 1988;93:138–43.
26. Kang BK, Na DG, Ryoo JW, Byun HS, Roh HG, Pyeun YS. Diffusion-weighted mr imaging of intracerebral hemorrhage. Korean J Radiol. 2001;2(4):183–91.
27. Hota P, Dass C, Erkmen C, Donuru A, Kumaran M. Poststernotomy complications: a multimodal review of normal and abnormal postoperative imaging findings. Am J Roentgenol. 2018;211(6):1194–205.
28. Friebe B, Apostolova I, Ricke J. Radiological Diagnostics of Postoperative Sternal Osteomyelitis. In: Horch RE, Willy C, Kutschka I, editors. Deep sternal wound infections. Berlin, Heidelberg: Springer; 2016. p. 21–7. https://doi.org/10.1007/978-3-662-49766-1_5.
29. Zhang R, Feng Z, Zhang Y, Tan H, Wang J, Qi F. Diagnostic value of fluorine-18 deoxyglucose positron emission tomography/computed tomography in deep sternal wound infection. J Plast Reconstr Aesthet Surg. 2018;71(12):1768–76.
30. Juneau D, Pelletier-Galarneau M. Revisiting the relevance of the 3-month safety period in the evaluation of prosthetic valve endocarditis with FDG-PET/CT. J Nucl Cardiol. 2020;28(5):2269–71.
31. Lucinian YA, Lamarche Y, Demers P, Martineau P, Harel F, Pelletier-Galarneau M. FDG-PET/CT for the detection of infection following aortic root replacement surgery. JACC Cardiovasc Imaging. 2020;13(6):1447–9.
32. Hariri H, Tan S, Martineau P, Lamarche Y, Carrier M, Finnerty V, et al. Utility of FDG-PET/CT for the detection and characterization of sternal wound infection following sternotomy. Nucl Med Mol Imaging. 2019;53(4):253–62.
33. Liu S, Zhang J, Yin H, Pang L, Wu B, Shi H. The value of 18 F-FDG PET/CT in diagnosing and localising deep sternal wound infection to guide surgical debridement. Int Wound J. 2020;17(4):1019–27.
34. Pelletier-Galarneau M, Abikhzer G, Harel F, Dilsizian V. Detection of native and prosthetic valve endocarditis: incremental attributes of functional fdg pet/ct over morphologic imaging. Curr Cardiol Rep. 2020;22(9):93.
35. Pelletier-Galarneau M, Juneau D. Vascular graft infection: improving diagnosis with functional imaging. J Nucl Cardiol. 2020.
36. Ruiz-Zafra J, Rodríguez-Fernández A, Sánchez-Palencia A, Cueto A. Surgical adhesive may cause false positives in integrated positron emission tomography and computed tomography after lung cancer resection. Eur J Cardiothorac Surg. 2013;43(6):1251–3.

Azar Radfar, Shady Abohashem,
Michael T. Osborne, and Ahmed Tawakol

Introduction

Cardiovascular disease (CVD) is the chief cause of mortality worldwide [1]. Though previously depicted as a monotonous process of subendothelial accumulation of gruel, atherosclerosis is now understood to be a progressive inflammatory process [2–4]. Inflammation is the major pathological driver of several human maladies, including CVD and malignancies. Notably, both acute and chronic inflammation play important roles in the pathogenesis of numerous CVDs, of which atherosclerosis is of paramount importance [3].

Imaging atherosclerotic inflammation and other biological processes related to plaque formation and progression may provide important insights that could facilitate the development of

new strategies to mitigate CVD. Further, it is hoped that molecular imaging may potentially improve current tools of risk stratification for atherosclerotic diseases, allowing more personalized disease management. In this chapter, we focus on molecular imaging techniques used to assess atherosclerotic plaque biology.

Atherosclerotic Plaque Biology

Atherosclerosis involves several distinct disease pathways that collude to initiate and propagate biologically active atheromatous plaques. The disease is instigated by subendothelial accumulation of oxidized LDL, mostly in areas with disturbed laminar flow, which prompts a chronic inflammatory response in the affected arterial wall. The local activated endothelial cells express leukocyte adhesion molecules which help recruit additional inflammatory cells (i.e., monocytes and T-lymphocytes). Monocytes then differentiate into resident lipid-laden foam cells. Monocyte-derived macrophages, T cells, B cells, dendritic cells, mast cells, and smooth muscle cells with myofibroblast characteristics constitute the main cellular components of atheroma. The subsequent release of inflammatory mediators and cytokines perpetuates the inflammatory cascade, leading to further accumulation of cellular and lipid material and plaque enlargement. The apoptotic death of macrophages and smooth

A. Radfar
Cardiology Division, Massachusetts General Hospital, Harvard Medical School, Boston, MA, USA

S. Abohashem
Cardiovascular Imaging Research Center, Massachusetts General Hospital, Harvard Medical School, Boston, MA, USA

M. T. Osborne · A. Tawakol (✉)
Cardiology Division, Massachusetts General Hospital, Harvard Medical School, Boston, MA, USA

Cardiovascular Imaging Research Center, Massachusetts General Hospital, Harvard Medical School, Boston, MA, USA
e-mail: atawakol@mgh.harvard.edu

M. Pelletier-Galarneau, P. Martineau (eds.), *FDG-PET/CT and PET/MR in Cardiovascular Diseases*, https://doi.org/10.1007/978-3-031-09807-9_18

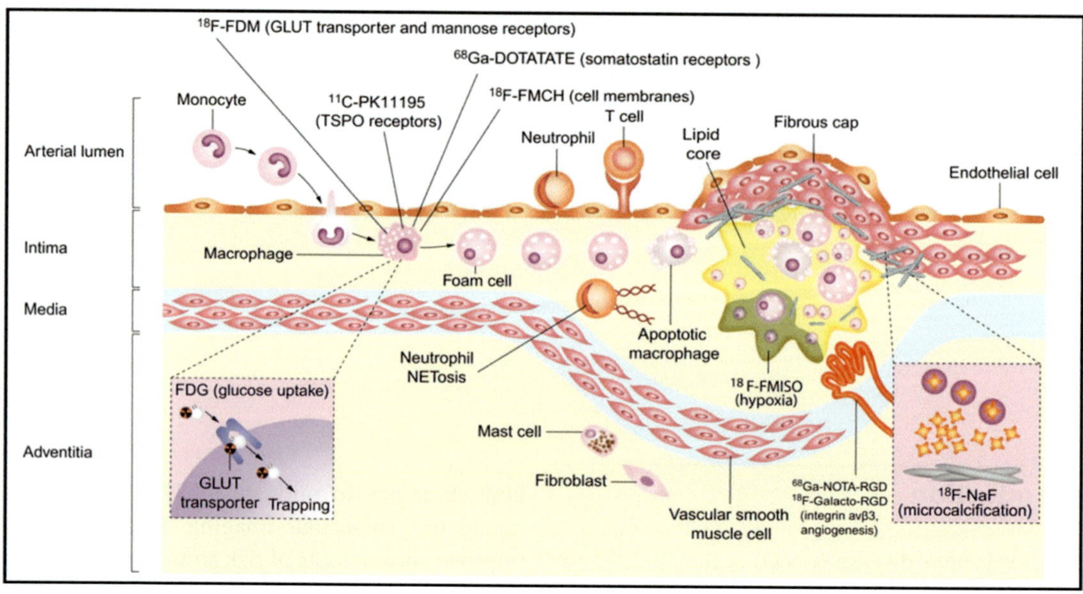

Fig. 18.1 Molecular targets for imaging of atherosclerosis using PET. Macrophages, as critical cellular constituents of atherosclerotic plaques, actively utilize glucose. Accordingly, ^{18}F-FDG and ^{18}F-FDM, isomers of glucose, are also taken up by macrophages. Several other receptors are expressed on macrophages and act as targets for PET tracers, including somatostatin receptors (^{68}Ga-DOTATATE), translocator protein receptors (^{11}C-PK11195), and macrophage cell membranes (^{18}F-FMCH). Additional radiotracers target other hallmarks of atherosclerotic inflammation, such as microcalcification (^{18}F-sodium fluoride), neoangiogenesis (^{68}Ga-NOTA-RGD and ^{18}F-Galacto-RGD), and cellular hypoxia (^{18}F-FMISO). *FDG* fluorodeoxyglucose, *FDM* fluoro-deoxymannose, *PET* positron emission tomography. (Reprinted with permission [6])

muscle cells further contribute to necrotic core formation within advanced plaques. Subsequently, thinning of the atheromatous fibrous cap is then induced by the increased matrix metalloproteinases activity secreted by recruited inflammatory cells along with microcalcifications (i.e., calcifications <50 μm in size) in the arterial intima. The necrotic lipid core, thinning of the fibrous cap, microcalcification, and heightened inflammatory state are all factors that predispose high-risk vulnerable plaque to rupture resulting in atherothrombotic events [5]. Several of these biological processes are attractive targets for molecular imaging of atherosclerosis (Fig. 18.1) [6].

Inflammation in Atherosclerosis

Inflammation is at the crossroads of the pathways that promote the progression of atherosclerotic CVD. In fact, basic science and human autopsy studies of atherosclerotic diseases have demonstrated that inflammation plays an important role in several phases of atherosclerosis, from plaque initiation to plaque progression and the potentiation of atherothrombotic events [7].

This important role for inflammation in atherosclerotic CVD has long been supported by the well-established association between inflammatory biomarkers and subsequent atherothrombotic events. Postmortem serum analysis of patients with severe coronary artery disease and sudden death revealed significant elevation of high-sensitivity C-reactive protein (hsCRP). There was also a robust association between hsCRP levels, superficial foam cells, expanded necrotic cores, and thin cap atheromatous plaques [8]. Moreover, inflammatory biomarkers (e.g., hsCRP) have been independently associated with CVD risk, which can be particularly useful for refining risk among individuals with intermediate risk by traditional criteria [9].

Additional evidence for an important role of inflammation in atherosclerosis comes from statin therapeutic studies. Statins efficiently reduce cardiovascular risk through lowering low-density lipoprotein (LDL). Such trials show that statins reduce inflammation (as determined by CRP) and that such reductions in inflammation associate with improvements in CVD risk [10]. Further, statin-induced changes in LDL and inflammation vary independently, suggesting that LDL and inflammation may represent distinct therapeutic targets [11]. Large-scale clinical trials provided further evidence for the importance of targeting inflammation to prevent atherosclerotic events. The JUPITER (Justification for the Use of Statins in Prevention: An Intervention Trial Evaluating Rosuvastatin) trial enrolled more than 17,000 subjects without known CVD who had elevated CRP levels (hsCRP >2 mg/L) and what was at the time considered "lower" LDL concentrations (LDL <130 mg/dL). In JUPITER, statin therapy resulted in a 47% relative risk reduction in first myocardial infarction, stroke, or cardiovascular death among individuals with "lower" LDL and elevated CRP [10]. PROVE-IT (Pravastatin or Atorvastatin Evaluation and Infection Therapy) and IMPROVE-IT (Improved Reduction of Outcomes: Vytorin Efficacy International) trials provided additional data demonstrating the relevance of lowering hsCRP in the context of lipid lowering [12, 13]. Together, those studies show that individuals who achieved lower values for both LDL and hsCRP experienced lower event rates compared to those with a reduction in one biomarker alone. These observations led to the concept of "residual inflammatory risk" to describe the CVD risk that remains among individuals with low LDL values, yet persistently elevated inflammatory markers [14]. Based on the aforementioned studies, current guidelines support the use of hsCRP to refine risk assessment while deliberating on whether to initiate statins for primary prevention of CVD [15].

More recently, the CANTOS (Canakinumab Anti-inflammatory Thrombosis Outcomes Study), Colcot (Colchicine Cardiovascular Outcomes Trial), and LoDoCo2 (Low Dose Colchicine for secondary prevention of cardiovascular disease) trials provided robust novel clinical evidence supporting the inflammatory hypothesis of atherosclerosis. CANTOS tested whether a selective anti-inflammatory agent (i.e., canakinumab, an IL-1β monoclonal antibody that has not been FDA-approved) would improve CVD outcomes in the absence of cholesterol lowering [16]. In this study, Ridker et al. reported that canakinumab resulted in a 15–20% reduction in the rate of recurrent CVD events despite no change in lipid concentrations [16]. With these results and the knowledge that the target of canakinumab, IL-1β, induces IL-6 production, a key cytokine of innate immunity, IL-6's role in atherosclerosis was placed directly in the spotlight. This interest was augmented by the fact that CANTOS participants who received canakinumab and achieved on-treatment IL-6 levels below the study median value demonstrated a 36% relative risk reduction in CVD events [17]. Considering these findings, it was assumed that inhibition of inflammation by targeting the innate immunity pathway of IL-1β to IL-6 to hsCRP might be the underlying cause of canakinumab's significant CVD reduction independent of lipid lowering and identify IL-6 as a possible primary focus of atherothrombosis prevention. In addition, Colcot demonstrated that daily low-dose colchicine, an effective anti-inflammatory medication, significantly lowered the risk of ischemic cardiovascular events in individuals post recent myocardial infarction [18]. Further, LoDoCo2 also endorsed the benefits of colchicine 0.5 mg daily in reducing recurrent coronary events in patients with chronic coronary disease [19]. Collectively, the above-mentioned trials provide supportive evidence of a causal role for inflammation in atherosclerotic CVD.

Noninvasive Molecular Imaging of Atherosclerosis Inflammation with ^{18}F-FDG

[18]F-Fluorodeoxyglucose (^{18}F-FDG) positron emission tomography/computed tomography (PET/CT) imaging is a widely employed imaging modality to assess inflammation in humans. ^{18}F-FDG-PET/CT is used to identify and characterize metabolically active tissues such as tumors and inflamed or infected tissues. ^{18}F-FDG is an FDA-approved radioactive analogue of glucose, which accumulates within tissues in proportion to their tissue glycolytic rates [6]. Since inflammatory cells, especially pro-inflammatory macrophages (e.g., subtype M1), have relatively high glycolytic rates, inflamed tissues tend to accumulate substantially more ^{18}F-FDG than surrounding tissues without inflammation [20].

Indeed, ^{18}F-FDG-PET/CT imaging has been used extensively to assess burden of the inflammatory atherosclerosis [21]. Several studies have shown that ^{18}F-FDG accumulates within the arterial wall in proportion to the density of atherosclerotic macrophages (Table 18.1) [22]. Furthermore, arterial ^{18}F-FDG uptake has been shown to increase in proportion to risk scores [23–26] and among individuals with CVD events [21, 27]. Additionally, arterial locations manifesting higher inflammation are more likely to subsequently manifest progression of the underlying atheroma [28, 29]. Additional human studies demonstrated that arterial ^{18}F-FDG uptake independently predicts subsequent incident atherothrombotic events beyond clinical risk score or the extent of coronary calcification (Figs. 18.2 and 18.3) [22, 30].

Table 18.1 The list of clinical studies assessing the correlation between ^{18}F-FDG uptake by PET/CT and arterial inflammation on histological analysis of the specimens from carotid endarterectomy

Study	Sample size (N)	Histological measure	Imaging Parameter	r	p-value
Tawakol et al. 2006	17	Absolute CD68 staining (mm^2)	SUV	0.49	<0.0001
			TBR	0.68	<0.0001
		% CD68 staining (most inflamed half of the vessel wall)	SUV	0.58	<0.0001
			TBR	0.7	<0.0001
Graebe et al. 2009	9	mRNA expression of CD68	TBR	0.71	0.02
Font et al. 2009	15	% CD68 staining	TBR	0.8	<0.005
Menezes et al. 2011	21	% CD68 staining	TBR	0.55	0.011
Saito et al. 2013	25	Grade (I, II, or III) CD68 staining	SUV	NA	0.006
Taqueti et al. 2014	25	% CD68 staining	TBR	0.64	<0.001
Skagen et al. 2015	36	% inflammatory cell staining (macrophages and leukocytes)	SUV	0.52	0.003
			TBR	NA	0.002
Cocker et al. 2018	49	% CD68 staining	SUV	0.45	0.001
			TBR	0.51	<0.0001
		Number of CD45 + pixels	SUV	0.88	<0.001
			TBR	0.63	0.009
Johnsrud et al. 2019	30	% area of inflammatory cells	SUV	0.54	0.008
			TBR	0.58	0.002

(*N*) number of patients who underwent carotid endarterectomy, *CD45* cluster of differentiation 45, *CD68* cluster of differentiation 68, *NA* not available, *SUV*, standardized uptake value, *TBR* target-to-background ratio. (Reprinted with permission [22])

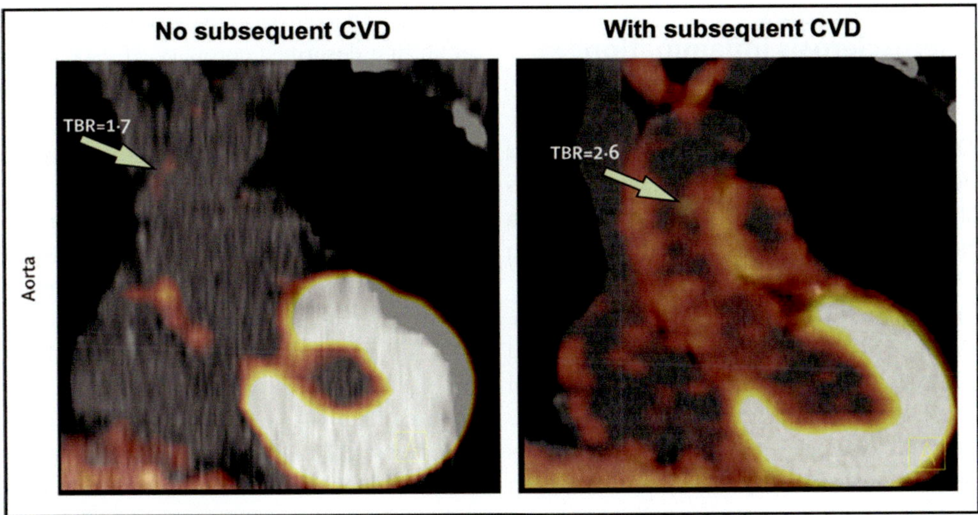

Fig. 18.2 Arterial inflammation predicts CVD events. Aortic ^{18}F-FDG uptake is higher in an individual who experienced a subsequent CVD event (right) compared with another patient with lower uptake (left). *CVD* cardiovascular disease, *FDG* fluorodeoxyglucose, *TBR* tissue-to-background ratio. (Adapted with permission [31])

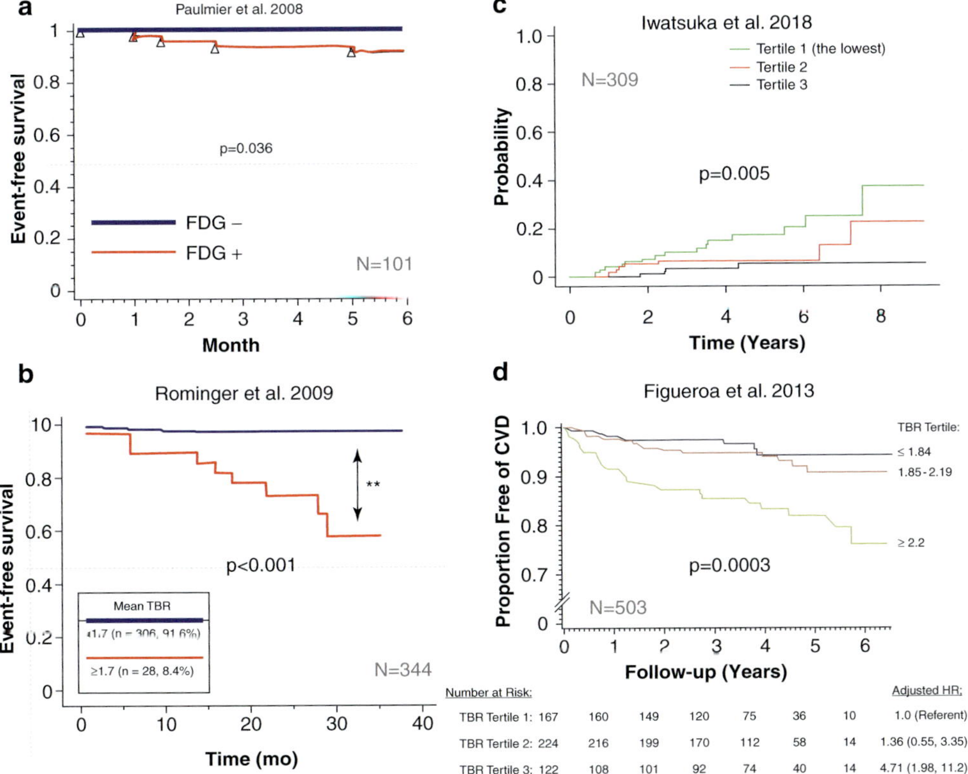

Number at Risk:							Adjusted HR:
TBR Tertile 1: 167	160	149	120	75	36	10	1.0 (Referent)
TBR Tertile 2: 224	216	199	170	112	58	14	1.36 (0.55, 3.35)
TBR Tertile 3: 122	108	101	92	74	40	14	4.71 (1.98, 11.2)

Fig. 18.3 Significant relationship between heightened arterial wall ^{18}F-FDG uptake and decreased cardiovascular event-free survival has been shown in several studies with distinct populations. *TBR* target-to-background ratio. (Reprinted with permission [22, 32])

Impact of Therapies on Atherosclerosis Inflammation Measured with ^{18}F-FDG

^{18}F-FDG-PET/CT imaging of atherosclerosis has been repeatedly applied to test therapies targeting atherosclerotic inflammation in research studies. Five drug classes have been evaluated in both ^{18}F-FDG-PET imaging and clinical endpoint trials [33, 34]. For each of those five drugs, there was concordance between directional changes seen on arterial imaging and clinical benefit observed in large clinical trials. The imaging and clinical endpoint trials' findings have been concordantly positive for two drug classes (i.e., statins and thiazolidinediones) where they reduced both plaque inflammation and clinical cardiovascular events [35, 36]. On the other hand, three drug classes (i.e., LPPLA2, CETP, and P38 MAP Kinase inhibitors) resulted in no reduction in pre-specified ^{18}F-FDG-PET imaging endpoints or in clinical endpoints [37–41]. Accordingly, relatively small, and brief ^{18}F-FDG-PET/CT imaging trials (e.g., 100–200 individuals studied for 3–6 months) have the potential to provide insights into the eventual clinical efficacy of drugs targeting atherosclerotic inflammation.

Molecular Imaging of Coronary Inflammation

Most ^{18}F-FDG-PET/CT arterial imaging studies have focused on larger arteries such as the aorta and the carotids. However, ^{18}F-FDG-PET/CT imaging of the coronary arteries has also been reported. In a retrospective study, Wykrzykowska et al. first described coronary ^{18}F-FDG uptake in subjects placed on a low-carbohydrate, high-fat diet designed to suppress physiologic myocardial ^{18}F-FDG uptake [42]. Subsequently, Rogers et al. [43] and Cheng et al. [34] demonstrated increased ^{18}F-FDG uptake within coronary culprit lesions in individuals with acute coronary syndrome (ACS) versus individuals with stable angina. Further work has shown that higher coronary ^{18}F-FDG uptake associates with high-risk plaque features, such as positive remodeling and increased lipid content [44]. More recently, Galiuto et al. demonstrated high correlations between coronary ^{18}F-FDG uptake and high-risk morphological features on coronary optical coherence tomography (OCT) [45].

However, unlike imaging of larger vessels, coronary ^{18}F-FDG-PET imaging is much more challenging. Despite great efforts to minimize background myocardial uptake of tracer, excess myocardial tracer uptake often impedes evaluation of coronary ^{18}F-FDG uptake and limits the practical utility of this imaging approach. To overcome this, new inroads are being made using alternative tracers, such as ^{68}Ga-DOTATATE (Fig. 18.4), that are more specific for inflammatory cells and are less impacted by adjacent myocardial background uptake [46]. In addition, PET imaging of coronary plaques faces other technical challenges (i.e., the limited spatial resolution of PET and motion of coronary arteries) that further limit the clinical utility of the approach. As such, it is likely that reliable molecular imaging of coronary inflammation imaging will require combines advances in tracers as well as imaging technologies.

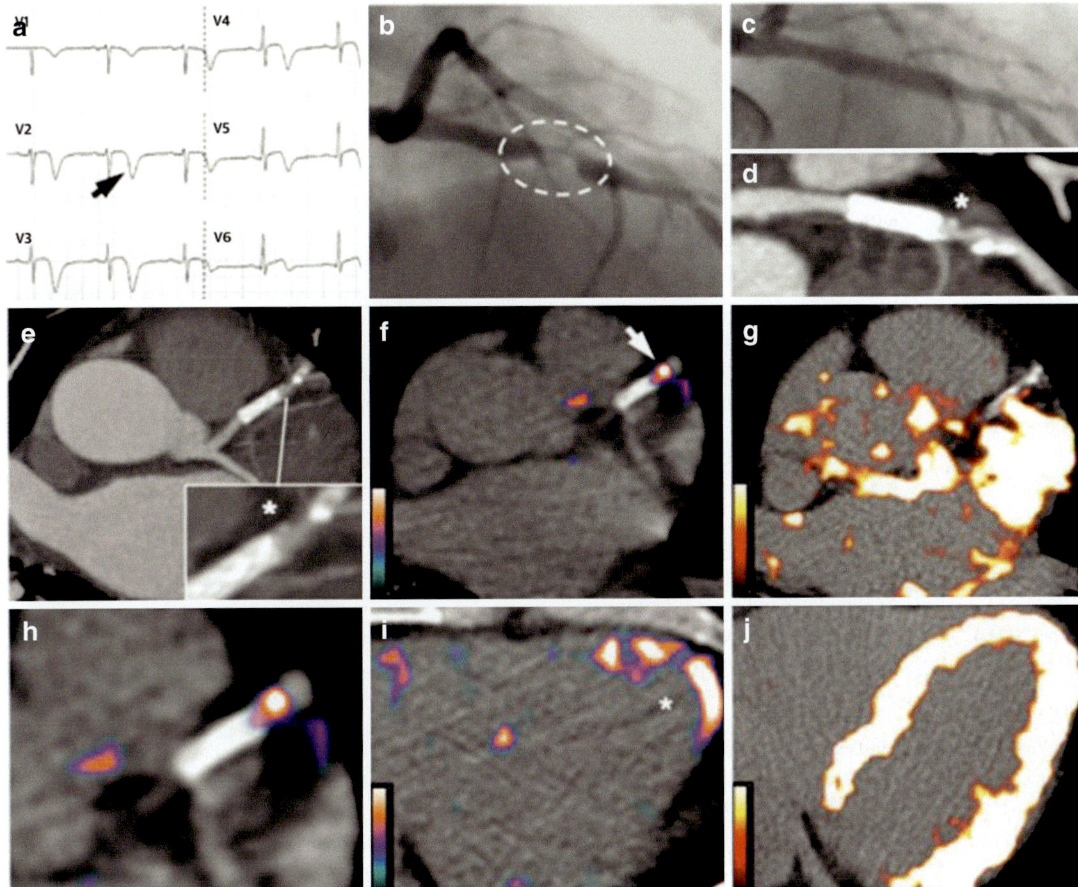

Fig. 18.4 Comparison between gallium-68-labeled DOTATATE (^{68}Ga-DOTATATE) and ^{18}F-FDG-PET imaging of coronary inflammation. Images belong to a patient with ACS and an electrocardiogram showing deep anterolateral T-wave inversions (**a**). Coronary angiography shows the culprit left anterior descending artery stenosis noted by dashed oval (**b**). A stent was placed (**c**). Coronary CT angiography revealed a residual coronary plaque (*inset) at the distal end of the stent with high-risk features such as low attenuation and spotty calcification (**d**, **e**). ^{68}Ga-DOTATATE PET (**f**, **h**, **i**) clearly spotted intense inflammation at the distal residual plaque (**f**, arrow) as well as the recently infarcted myocardium (**i**, *). However, ^{18}F-FDG-PET (**g**, **j**) showed intense background myocardial uptake, which entirely obscured uptake within the coronary arteries. *ACS* acute coronary syndrome, *CT* computed tomography, *^{18}F-FDG* fluorodeoxyglucose, *PET* positron emission tomography. (Reprinted with permission [46])

Microcalcification Activity and Other Targets for Molecular Imaging of Atherosclerotic Plaque

Several additional plaque features besides inflammation represent attractive targets for molecular imaging (Fig. 18.1). Such features include increased oxidative stress, hypoxia, hypoxia-induced angiogenesis, dysregulation of matrix metalloproteinase activity, and microcalcification activity. In an animal study, increased ^{18}F-fluoromisonidazole (^{18}F-FMISO) uptake has been associated with plaque hypoxia [47]. In separate studies, ^{68}Ga-NOTA-RGD and ^{18}F-Galacto-RGD targeted (integrin avb3) expression on activated endothelial cells correlated with neoangiogenesis in advanced atheromatous lesions [48, 49] (Fig. 18.1, Table 18.2).

One tracer of note, ^{18}F-sodium fluoride (^{18}F-NaF) incorporates into hydroxyapatite during osteogenesis and accumulates within areas of

Table 18.2 A list of current PET agents targeting atherosclerotic inflammation and their potential mechanisms of uptake

Agent	Potential mechanism of uptake
[18]F-Macroflor	Has affinity for cardiovascular resident macrophages
[18]F-Cerezyme	Has affinity for mannose receptors on macrophages
^{18}F-FMCH	Targets macrophage cell membrane
[18]F-Galacto-RGD	Binds to integrin avb3 expressed by macrophages and activated endothelial cells (associated with angiogenesis)
^{18}F-FDM	An isomer of ^{18}F-FDG that accumulates within inflamed tissues with possibly greater affinity for M2-polarized macrophages
^{18}F-FOL	Binds to the folate receptor β (FR-β) that is selectively expressed by macrophages
[11]C-PK11195	Has affinity for translocator protein, which is upregulated on inflammatory cells
^{68}Ga-CXCR4	Binds to inflammatory cells expressing the CXCR4 receptor
^{68}Ga-DOTA-octreotate	Binds to inflammatory cells expressing somatostatin receptors that are highly expressed on macrophages
^{18}F-FDG	A glucose analogue that accumulates within cells in proportion to glycolysis
[18]F–NaF	Accumulates within areas of active micro-calcification that are indirectly related to inflammation
[18]F-choline	Identifies heightened cell wall synthesis within atheroma
[64]Cu-ATSM	Accumulates in hypoxic regions
^{18}F-MISO	Accumulates in hypoxic regions
^{68}Ga-NOTA-RGD	Binds to integrin avb3 expressed by macrophages and activated endothelial cells that are associated with angiogenesis
[64]Cu-DOTA-CANF	Has affinity to natriuretic peptide receptor and is used in imaging neoangiogenesis
[18]F-A85380	Binds arterial nicotinic acetylcholine receptors that are possibly related to vascular damage
^{18}F-FLT	A labeled thymidine analogue that can identify myelopoiesis in the bone marrow and myelocyte turnover in the blood vessel wall

[11]C-PK11195 [11]C-(2-chlorophenyl)-N-methyl-N-(1-methylpropyl)-3-isoquinolinecarboxamide, *A85380* 3-([2S]-azetidinyl-methoxy) pyridine dihydrochloride, *ATSM* diacetyl-bis(N-methyl-thiosemicarbazone, *CXCR4* C-X-C chemokine receptor type 4, *DOTA-CANF* 1,4,7,10-tetraazacyclododecane-1,4,7,10-tetraacetic acid atrial natriuretic factor, *FDG* fluorodeoxyglucose, *FDM* fluoro-deoxymannose, *FLT* fluoro-thymidine, *MISO* fluoro-misonidazole, *NaF* sodium fluoride, *NOTA-RGD* 1,4,7-triazacyclononane-N,N0,N00-triacetic acid arginine-glycine-aspartate. (Adapted with permission [50])

active calcification. Clinically, ^{18}F-NaF has long been used to evaluate bone pathologies. More recently, it has been leveraged to identify areas of active microcalcification (i.e., calcifications <50 μm in size), a feature of biologically active high-risk plaques that is beneath the threshold of detection by CT imaging (i.e., coronary artery calcium [CAC]) [51, 52]. Notably, ^{18}F-NaF activity can be more readily measured in the coronaries (as compared to ^{18}F-FDG), owing to the relatively low background activity and lack of myocardial spill-over [51].

Importantly, culprit coronary and carotid plaques have shown higher ^{18}F-NaF uptake than asymptomatic atheroma [53] (Fig. 18.5). Moreover, in patients with established coronary artery disease, ^{18}F-NaF uptake throughout the coronary arteries quantified as coronary microcalcification activity (CMA) independently predicts coronary events beyond traditional risk stratification methods [54] (Fig. 18.6). ^{18}F-NaF uptake also identifies coronary segments which subsequently showed rapid progression of coronary calcification [55]. Further, higher ^{18}F-NaF uptake predicts peripheral arterial restenosis after percutaneous transluminal angioplasty [56]. Additionally, ^{18}F-NaF has demonstrated promise in the evaluation of abdominal aortic aneurysms in which it has been shown to independently predict aneurysm growth and future clinical events [57].

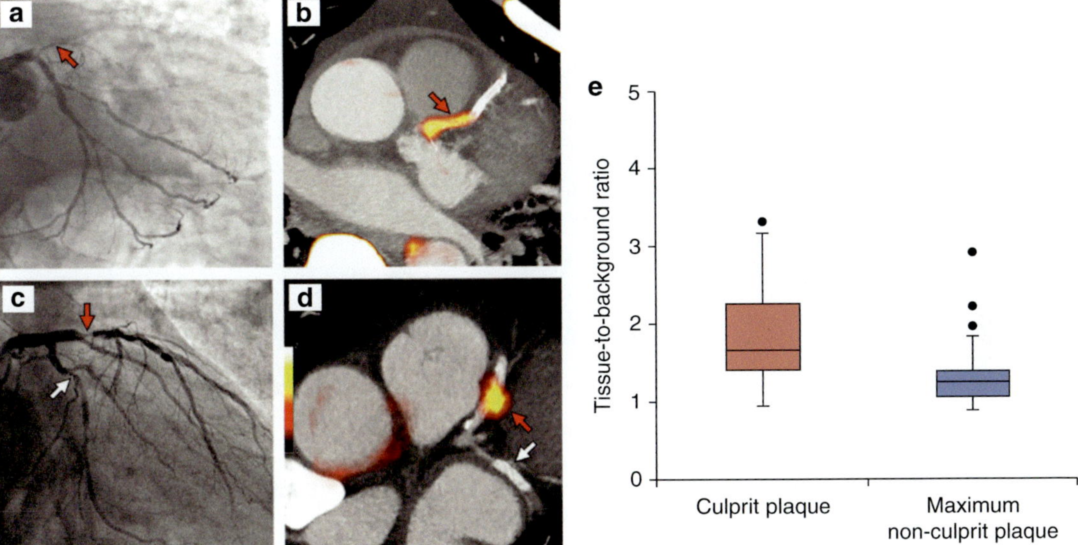

Fig. 18.5 Increased ^{18}F-NaF uptake in culprit coronary lesions. Individuals with recent myocardial infarction (MI) underwent ^{18}F-NaF-PET/CT. Coronary angiograms show culprit left anterior descending artery lesions (red arrows) in two individuals (**a** and **c**) with recent MI. Intense radiotracer uptake has been shown in the same locations of the same patients (**b** and **d**) who underwent ^{18}F-NaF-PET/CT. Higher ^{18}F-NaF activity was noted in the culprit lesions compared with nonculprit lesions in the same individuals (**e**). (Reprinted with permission [58])

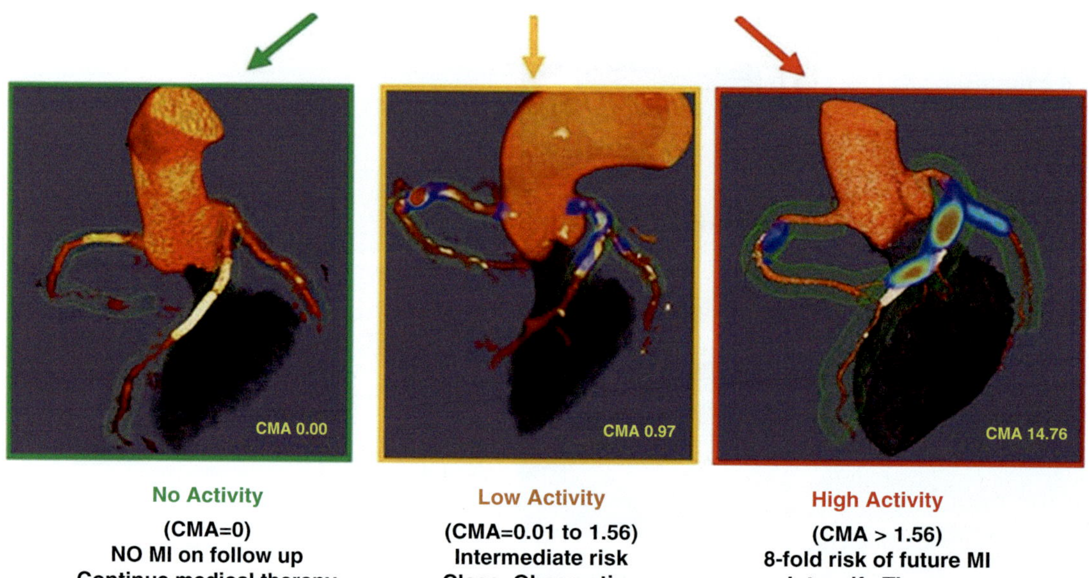

Fig. 18.6 ^{18}F-NaF-PET imaging of coronary calcification to assess disease activity. In patients with known CAD, the burden of coronary ^{18}F-NaF uptake predicts future coronary atherosclerotic events. Coronary microcalcification activity (CMA) was assessed by using ^{18}F-NaF-PET. Based on the amount of tracer uptake, individuals were categorized into no, low, and high disease activity. Those with higher ^{18}F-NaF uptake (i.e., CMA >1.56) exhibited an eightfold risk of future MI. Despite having advanced CAD, individuals with no ^{18}F-NaF uptake (i.e., CMA = 0) had no MI during the study follow-up. *CAD* coronary artery disease, *CMA* coronary microcalcification activity, *CT* computed tomography, *[18]F-NaF* ^{18}F-sodium fluoride, *MI* myocardial infarction, *PET* positron emission tomography. (Reprinted with permission [54])

Hybrid PET/Magnetic Resonance Imaging (MRI) Systems

PET/MRI is an emerging imaging technology that may provide advantages over PET/CT in certain applications. Potential advantages include enhanced soft tissue characterization, improved ability to evaluate cardiac structure, better assessment of ventricular function, and reduced exposure to ionizing radiation by omitting CT imaging. Further, MRI data are acquired simultaneously along PET data, allowing for better registration of the two datasets.

Several groups have demonstrated the feasibility of PET/MRI for the evaluation of atherosclerosis [59]. Robson et al. outlined a specialized approach to using PET/MRI to assess inflammation and microcalcification in the coronary arteries [60]. In an animal study, Calcagno et al. presented an integrated PET dynamic contrast-enhanced MRI (PET-DCE/MRI) protocol to measure rabbit aortic plaque inflammation, neoangiogenesis, permeability as well as test the efficacy of an experimental drug [61]. In addition, Senders et al. employed an integrative PET/MRI protocol in rabbits for plaque phenotyping by targeting vascular cell adhesion molecule (VCAM)-1, lectin-like oxidized low-density lipoprotein receptor (LOX)-1, and macrophage mannose receptor (MMR). The study was conducted in concordance with using other clinically approved modalities such as ^{18}F-FDG, ^{18}F-NaF, and MRI [62]. PET/MRI has the potential to facilitate multiparametric analysis of atherosclerosis, including plaque stenosis severity, hemodynamic markers, plaque composition, and activity along with the evaluation of myocardial viability. Accordingly, such information derived from this unified imaging modality seems to offer a unique approach to assess anti-atherosclerotic drug efficacy in the early phases of clinical trials.

Multimodality Molecular Imaging Approaches

Multimodality molecular imaging has been developed to obtain detailed structural, functional, and molecular data. Combining the capability of various imaging modalities (e.g., PET/CT, PET/MRI) offers the feasibility to derive pathobiological insights and potential translation into the clinical realm.

Importantly, multimodal, multiorgan imaging uniquely allows for the evaluation of disease processes that span multiple organ systems. Several animal studies show that bone marrow myelopoietic activity accelerates atherosclerosis [63]. For instance, Emami et al. leveraged ^{18}F-FDG-PET/CT to study the role of hematopoietic tissues (i.e., bone marrow, spleen) in human atherosclerotic disease [64]. The investigators quantified ^{18}F-FDG uptake in hematopoietic tissues and observed that the signal is: 1) heightened among individuals with recent acute coronary syndrome and 2) associated with circulating inflammatory biomarkers as well as arterial inflammation. Moreover, in a complementary study of 513 individuals without prior CVD, hematopoietic activity independently predicted the risk of future CVD events, illuminating the presence of a hematopoietic-arterial axis in humans. The link between hematopoietic tissues and atherosclerosis has been further studied using the PET tracer 3′-deoxy-3′-[^{18}F]-fluoro-thymidine (^{18}F-FLT), a thymidine analogue which accumulates in proliferating cells [65]. Using ^{18}F-FLT PET, myelopoietic stem and progenitor cell proliferation were found to be greater among individuals with atherosclerosis with increased tracer uptake in atherosclerotic plaques within macrophages in the above-mentioned cells and lesions. Further, multiorgan ^{18}F-FDG-PET/CT imaging has been employed to demonstrate a link between chronic stress, a known CVD risk factor, and CVD via the aforementioned hematopoietic-arterial axis [66, 67]. A recent study showed that stress-associated neural activity involving the amygdala, a crucial constituent of the brain's salience network, independently and robustly associated with the risk of subsequent CVD events. Moreover, mediation analysis suggested that it did so in part via the following pathway: ↑amygdalar activity → ↑bone marrow activity → ↑arterial inflammation → ↑CVD risk [31]. Hence, molecular imaging can also be leveraged provide unique and important insights into multi-system biological mechanisms.

Clinical Applications

Current clinical applications for arterial molecular imaging are limited. ^{18}F-FDG-PET imaging is used clinically to evaluate arterial inflammation in the context of known or suspected arteritis, where this application is supported by the clinical guidelines [68]. Yet, arterial molecular imaging to evaluate CVD risk is not widely performed. Before broad clinical implementation is possible, large prospective trials are needed to define the incremental value of the approach to predict subsequent CVD events. One such trial, "Prognostic Value of Arterial ^{18}F-FDG PET Imaging in Patients with History of Myocardial Infarction: PIAF" (funded by the International Atomic Energy Agency) is assessing the relationship between arterial ^{18}F-FDG uptake and subsequent CVD events in >1200 individuals. The relationship between tracer uptake and CVD risk will similarly need to be evaluated for other tracers before they are used broadly. Until those data are available, arterial molecular imaging of atherosclerosis will remain largely a research tool.

Conclusion

Atheromatous plaque biology represents an exciting target for molecular imaging of atherosclerosis, offering functional information to improve our understanding of the underlying pathophysiology. Current imaging techniques targeting pathobiological processes, such as inflammation, improve risk assessment and may lead to improved clinical decision making. The continued evolution of molecular imaging to assess inflammation and other important pathobiological processes in atherosclerosis has the potential to enhance the personalization of therapies and improve outcomes.

References

1. Barquera S, Pedroza-Tobías A, Medina C, Hernández-Barrera L, Bibbins-Domingo K, Lozano R, et al. Global overview of the epidemiology of atherosclerotic cardiovascular disease. Arch Med Res. 2015;46(5):328–38.
2. Libby P, Ridker PM, Maseri A. Inflammation and atherosclerosis. Circulation. 2002;105(9):1135–43.
3. Ross R. Atherosclerosis—an inflammatory disease. N Engl J Med. 1999;340(2):115–26.
4. Kuiper J, van Puijvelde GHM, van Wanrooij EJA, van Es T, Habets K, Hauer AD, et al. Immunomodulation of the inflammatory response in atherosclerosis. Curr Opin Lipidol. 2007 Oct;18(5):521–6.
5. Tabas I, García-Cardeña G, Owens GK. Recent insights into the cellular biology of atherosclerosis. J Cell Biol. 2015;209(1):13–22.
6. Joseph P, Tawakol A. Imaging atherosclerosis with positron emission tomography. Eur Heart J. 2016;37(39):2974–80.
7. Libby P. Inflammation in atherosclerosis. Arterioscler Thromb Vasc Biol. 2012;32(9):2045–51.
8. Burke AP, Tracy RP, Kolodgie F, Malcom GT, Zieske A, Kutys R, et al. Elevated C-reactive protein values and atherosclerosis in sudden coronary death: association with different pathologies. Circulation. 2002;105(17):2019–23.
9. Ridker PM, Buring JE, Rifai N, Cook NR. Development and validation of improved algorithms for the assessment of global cardiovascular risk in women: the Reynolds Risk Score. JAMA. 2007;297(6):611–9.
10. Ridker PM, Danielson E, Fonseca FAH, Genest J, Gotto AM Jr, Kastelein JJP, et al. Rosuvastatin to prevent vascular events in men and women with elevated C-reactive protein. N Engl J Med. 2008;359(21):2195–207.
11. Geovanini GR, Libby P. Atherosclerosis and inflammation: overview and updates. Clin Sci (Lond). 2018;132(12):1243–52.
12. Ridker PM, Cannon CP, Morrow D, Rifai N, Rose LM, McCabe CH, et al. C-reactive protein levels and outcomes after statin therapy. N Engl J Med. 2005;352(1):20–8.
13. Bohula EA, Giugliano RP, Cannon CP, Zhou J, Murphy SA, White JA, et al. Achievement of dual low-density lipoprotein cholesterol and high-sensitivity C-reactive protein targets more frequent with the addition of ezetimibe to simvastatin and associated with better outcomes in IMPROVE-IT. Circulation. 2015;132(13):1224–33.
14. Ridker PM. Clinician's guide to reducing inflammation to reduce atherothrombotic risk: JACC review topic of the week. J Am Coll Cardiol. 2018;72(25):3320–31.
15. Grundy SM, Stone NJ, Bailey AL, Beam C, Birtcher KK, Blumenthal RS, et al. 2018 AHA/ACC/AACVPR/AAPA/ABC/ACPM/ADA/AGS/APhA/ASPC/NLA/PCNA guideline on the management of blood cholesterol: executive summary: a report of the American College of Cardiology/American Heart Association Task Force on Clinical Practice Guidelines. J Am Coll Cardiol. 2019;73(24):3168–209.
16. Ridker PM, Everett BM, Thuren T, MacFadyen JG, Chang WH, Ballantyne C, et al. Antiinflammatory therapy with Canakinumab for atherosclerotic disease. N Engl J Med. 2017;377(12):1119–31.
17. Ridker PM, Libby P, MacFadyen JG, Thuren T, Ballantyne C, Fonseca F, et al. Modulation of the interleukin-6 signalling pathway and incidence rates of atherosclerotic events and all-cause mortality: analyses from the Canakinumab Anti-Inflammatory Thrombosis Outcomes Study (CANTOS). Eur Heart J. 2018;39(38):3499–507.
18. Tardif J-C, Kouz S, Waters DD, Bertrand OF, Diaz R, Maggioni AP, et al. Efficacy and safety of low-dose colchicine after myocardial infarction. N Engl J Med. 2019;381(26):2497–505.
19. Fischer BG. Colchicine in patients with chronic coronary disease. N Engl J Med. 2021;384(8):777.
20. Tawakol A, Singh P, Mojena M, Pimentel-Santillana M, Emami H, MacNabb M, et al. HIF-1α and PFKFB3 mediate a tight relationship between proinflammatory activation and anaerobic metabolism in atherosclerotic macrophages. Arterioscler Thromb Vasc Biol. 2015;35(6):1463–71.
21. Rudd JHF, Warburton EA, Fryer TD, Jones HA, Clark JC, Antoun N, et al. Imaging atherosclerotic

plaque inflammation with [18F]-fluorodeoxyglucose positron emission tomography. Circulation. 2002;105(23):2708–11.

22. Osborne MT, Abohashem S, Zureigat H, Abbasi TA, Tawakol A. Multimodality molecular imaging: gaining insights into the mechanisms linking chronic stress to cardiovascular disease. J Nucl Cardiol. 2021;28(3):955–66.

23. Bural GG, Torigian DA, Chamroonrat W, Houseni M, Chen W, Basu S, et al. FDG-PET is an effective imaging modality to detect and quantify age-related atherosclerosis in large arteries. Eur J Nucl Med Mol Imaging. 2008;35(3):562–9.

24. Joly L, Djaballah W, Koehl G, Mandry D, Dolivet G, Marie P-Y, et al. Aortic inflammation, as assessed by hybrid FDG-PET/CT imaging, is associated with enhanced aortic stiffness in addition to concurrent calcification. Eur J Nucl Med Mol Imaging. 2009;36(6):979–85.

25. Rudd JHF, Myers KS, Bansilal S, Machac J, Woodward M, Fuster V, et al. Relationships among regional arterial inflammation, calcification, risk factors, and biomarkers: a prospective fluorodeoxyglucose positron-emission tomography/computed tomography imaging study. Circ Cardiovasc Imaging. 2009;2(2):107–15.

26. Kim TN, Kim S, Yang SJ, Yoo HJ, Seo JA, Kim SG, et al. Vascular inflammation in patients with impaired glucose tolerance and type 2 diabetes: analysis with 18F-fluorodeoxyglucose positron emission tomography. Circ Cardiovasc Imaging. 2010;3(2):142–8.

27. Rogers IS, Tawakol A. Imaging of coronary inflammation with FDG-PET: feasibility and clinical hurdles. Curr Cardiol Rep. 2011;13(2):138–44.

28. Tawakol A, Migrino RQ, Bashian GG, Bedri S, Vermylen D, Cury RC, et al. In vivo 18F-fluorodeoxyglucose positron emission tomography imaging provides a noninvasive measure of carotid plaque inflammation in patients. J Am Coll Cardiol. 2006;48(9):1818–24.

29. Rudd JHF, Myers KS, Bansilal S, Machac J, Rafique A, Farkouh M, et al. (18)Fluorodeoxyglucose positron emission tomography imaging of atherosclerotic plaque inflammation is highly reproducible: implications for atherosclerosis therapy trials. J Am Coll Cardiol. 2007;50(9):892–6.

30. Figueroa AL, Abdelbaky A, Truong QA, Corsini E, MacNabb MH, Lavender ZR, et al. Measurement of arterial activity on routine FDG PET/CT images improves prediction of risk of future CV events. JACC Cardiovasc Imaging. 2013;6(12):1250–9.

31. Tawakol A, Ishai A, Takx RA, Figueroa AL, Ali A, Kaiser Y, et al. Relation between resting amygdalar activity and cardiovascular events: a longitudinal and cohort study. Lancet. 2017;389(10071):834–45.

32. Rominger A, Saam T, Wolpers S, Cyran CC, Schmidt M, Foerster S, et al. 18F-FDG PET/CT identifies patients at risk for future vascular events in an otherwise asymptomatic cohort with neoplastic disease. J Nucl Med. 2009;50(10):1611–20.

33. Cocker MS, Spence JD, Hammond R, deKemp RA, Lum C, Wells G, et al. [18F]-Fluorodeoxyglucose PET/CT imaging as a marker of carotid plaque inflammation: comparison to immunohistology and relationship to acuity of events. Int J Cardiol. 2018;271:378–86.

34. Cheng VY, Slomka PJ, Le Meunier L, Tamarappoo BK, Nakazato R, Dey D, et al. Coronary arterial 18F-FDG uptake by fusion of PET and coronary CT angiography at sites of percutaneous stenting for acute myocardial infarction and stable coronary artery disease. J Nucl Med. 2012;53(4):575–83.

35. Tawakol A, Fayad ZA, Mogg R, Alon A, Klimas MT, Dansky H, et al. Intensification of statin therapy results in a rapid reduction in atherosclerotic inflammation: results of a multicenter fluorodeoxyglucose-positron emission tomography/computed tomography feasibility study. J Am Coll Cardiol. 2013;62(10):909–17.

36. Mizoguchi M, Tahara N, Tahara A, Nitta Y, Kodama N, Oba T, et al. Pioglitazone attenuates atherosclerotic plaque inflammation in patients with impaired glucose tolerance or diabetes a prospective, randomized, comparator-controlled study using serial FDG PET/CT imaging study of carotid artery and ascending aorta. JACC Cardiovasc Imaging. 2011;4(10):1110–8.

37. Emami H, Vucic E, Subramanian S, Abdelbaky A, Fayad ZA, Du S, et al. The effect of BMS-582949, a P38 mitogen-activated protein kinase (P38 MAPK) inhibitor on arterial inflammation: a multicenter FDG-PET trial. Atherosclerosis. 2015;240(2):490–6.

38. STABILITY Investigators, White HD, Held C, Stewart R, Tarka E, Brown R, et al. Darapladib for preventing ischemic events in stable coronary heart disease. N Engl J Med. 2014;370(18):1702–11.

39. O'Donoghue ML, Glaser R, Cavender MA, Aylward PE, Bonaca MP, Budaj A, et al. Effect of Losmapimod on cardiovascular outcomes in patients hospitalized with acute myocardial infarction: a randomized clinical trial. JAMA. 2016;315(15):1591–9.

40. Schwartz GG, Olsson AG, Abt M, Ballantyne CM, Barter PJ, Brumm J, et al. Effects of dalcetrapib in patients with a recent acute coronary syndrome. N Engl J Med. 2012;367(22):2089–99.

41. Tawakol A, Singh P, Rudd JHF, Soffer J, Cai G, Vucic E, et al. Effect of treatment for 12 weeks with rilapladib, a lipoprotein-associated phospholipase A2 inhibitor, on arterial inflammation as assessed with 18F-fluorodeoxyglucose-positron emission tomography imaging. J Am Coll Cardiol. 2014;63(1):86–8.

42. Wykrzykowska J, Lehman S, Williams G, Parker JA, Palmer MR, Varkey S, et al. Imaging of inflamed and vulnerable plaque in coronary arteries with 18F-FDG PET/CT in patients with suppression of myocardial uptake using a low-carbohydrate, high-fat preparation. J Nucl Med. 2009;50(4):563–8.

43. Rogers IS, Nasir K, Figueroa AL, Cury RC, Hoffmann U, Vermylen DA, et al. Feasibility of FDG imaging of the coronary arteries: comparison between acute coronary syndrome and stable angina. JACC Cardiovasc Imaging. 2010;3(4):388–97.

44. Singh P, Emami H, Subramanian S, Maurovich-Horvat P, Marincheva-Savcheva G, Medina HM, et al. Coronary plaque morphology and the anti-inflammatory impact of Atorvastatin: a multi-center 18F-fluorodeoxyglucose positron emission tomographic/computed tomographic study. Circ Cardiovasc Imaging. 2016;9(12):e004195.

45. Galiuto L, Leccisotti L, Locorotondo G, Porto I, Burzotta F, Trani C, et al. Coronary plaque instability assessed by positron emission tomography and optical coherence tomography. Ann Nucl Med. 2021;35(10):1136–46.

46. Tarkin JM, Joshi FR, Evans NR, Chowdhury MM, Figg NL, Shah AV, et al. Detection of atherosclerotic inflammation by68Ga-DOTATATE PET compared to [18F]FDG PET imaging. J Am Coll Cardiol. 2017;69(14):1774–91.

47. Mateo J, Izquierdo-Garcia D, Badimon JJ, Fayad ZA, Fuster V. Noninvasive assessment of hypoxia in rabbit advanced atherosclerosis using 18F-fluoromisonidazole PET imaging. Circ Cardiovasc Imaging. 2014;7(2):312–20.

48. Paeng JC, Lee Y-S, Lee JS, Jeong JM, Kim K-B, Chung J-K, et al. Feasibility and kinetic characteristics of (68)Ga-NOTA-RGD PET for in vivo atherosclerosis imaging. Ann Nucl Med. 2013;27(9):847–54.

49. Beer AJ, Pelisek J, Heider P, Saraste A, Reeps C, Metz S, et al. PET/CT imaging of integrin αvβ3 expression in human carotid atherosclerosis. JACC Cardiovasc Imaging. 2014;7(2):178–87.

50. Teague HL, Ahlman MA, Alavi A, Wagner DD, Lichtman AH, Nahrendorf M, et al. Unraveling vascular inflammation: from immunology to imaging. J Am Coll Cardiol. 2017;70(11):1403–12.

51. Dweck MR, Chow MWL, Joshi NV, Williams MC, Jones C, Fletcher AM, et al. Coronary arterial 18F-sodium fluoride uptake: a novel marker of plaque biology. J Am Coll Cardiol. 2012;59(17):1539–48.

52. Wang Y, Osborne MT, Tung B, Li M, Li Y. Imaging cardiovascular calcification. J Am Heart Assoc. 2018;7(13):e008564.

53. Dweck MR, Aikawa E, Newby DE, Tarkin JM, Rudd JHF, Narula J, et al. Noninvasive molecular imaging of disease activity in atherosclerosis. Circ Res. 2016;119(2):330–40.

54. Kwiecinski J, Tzolos E, Adamson PD, Cadet S, Moss AJ, Joshi N, et al. Coronary 18F-sodium fluoride uptake predicts outcomes in patients with coronary artery disease. J Am Coll Cardiol. 2020;75(24):3061–74.

55. Delgado V, Saraste A, Dweck M, Bucciarelli-Ducci C, Bax JJ. Multimodality imaging: Bird's eye view from the European Society of Cardiology Congress 2019 Paris, August 31st–September 4th, 2019. J Nucl Cardiol. 2020;27(1):53–61.

56. Chowdhury MM, Tarkin JM, Albaghdadi MS, Evans NR, Le EPV, Berrett TB, et al. Vascular positron emission tomography and restenosis in symptomatic peripheral arterial disease. JACC Cardiovasc Imaging. 2020;13(4):1008–17.

57. Forsythe RO, Dweck MR, McBride OMB, Vesey AT, Semple SI, Shah ASV, et al. 18F-sodium fluoride uptake in abdominal aortic aneurysms: the SoFIA3Study. J Am Coll Cardiol. 2018;71(5):513–23.

58. Joshi NV, Vesey AT, Williams MC, Shah ASV, Calvert PA, Craighead FHM, et al. 18F-fluoride positron emission tomography for identification of ruptured and high-risk coronary atherosclerotic plaques: a prospective clinical trial. Lancet. 2014;383(9918):705–13.

59. Ripa RS, Pedersen SF, Kjær A. PET/MR imaging in vascular disease: atherosclerosis and inflammation. PET Clin. 2016;11(4):479–88.

60. Robson PM, Dweck MR, Trivieri MG, Abgral R, Karakatsanis NA, Contreras J, et al. Coronary artery PET/MR imaging: feasibility, limitations, and solutions. JACC Cardiovasc Imaging. 2017;10(10 Pt A):1103–12.

61. Calcagno C, Lairez O, Hawkins J, Kerr SW, Dugas MS, Simpson T, et al. Combined PET/DCE-MRI in a rabbit model of atherosclerosis: integrated quantification of plaque inflammation, permeability, and burden during treatment with a leukotriene A4 hydrolase inhibitor. JACC Cardiovasc Imaging. 2018;11(2 Pt 2):291–301.

62. Senders ML, Hernot S, Carlucci G, van de Voort JC, Fay F, Calcagno C, et al. Nanobody-facilitated multiparametric PET/MRI phenotyping of atherosclerosis. JACC Cardiovasc Imaging. 2019;12(10):2015–26.

63. Dutta P, Courties G, Wei Y, Leuschner F, Gorbatov R, Robbins C, et al. Myocardial infarction accelerates atherosclerosis. Nature. 2012;487(7407):325–9.

64. Emami H, Singh P, MacNabb M, Vucic E, Lavender Z, Rudd JHF, et al. Splenic metabolic activity predicts risk of future cardiovascular events: demonstration of a cardiosplenic axis in humans. JACC Cardiovasc Imaging. 2015;8(2):121–30.

65. Ye Y-X, Calcagno C, Binderup T, Courties G, Keliher EJ, Wojtkiewicz GR, et al. Imaging macrophage and hematopoietic progenitor proliferation in atherosclerosis. Circ Res. 2015;117(10):835–45.

66. Batty GD, Russ TC, Stamatakis E, Kivimäki M. Psychological distress and risk of peripheral vascular disease, abdominal aortic aneurysm, and heart failure: pooling of sixteen cohort studies. Atherosclerosis. 2014;236(2):385–8.

67. Nabi H, Kivimäki M, Batty GD, Shipley MJ, Britton A, Brunner EJ, et al. Increased risk of coronary heart disease among individuals reporting adverse impact of stress on their health: the Whitehall II prospective cohort study. Eur Heart J. 2013;34(34):2697–705.

68. Dejaco C, Ramiro S, Duftner C, Besson FL, Bley TA, Blockmans D, et al. EULAR recommendations for the use of imaging in large vessel vasculitis in clinical practice. Ann Rheum Dis. 2018;77(5):636–43.

James R. Pinney, Nandakumar Menon,
and René R. Sevag Packard

Abbreviations

^{18}F-NaF	^{18}F-Sodium fluoride
^{18}F-FDG	^{18}F-Fluorodeoxyglucose
^{18}F-FLT	^{18}F-Labeled thymidine
ACS	Acute coronary syndrome
CAC	Coronary artery calcium
CAD	Coronary artery disease
cMRI	Cardiac magnetic resonance imaging
CT	Computed tomography
CXCL12	CXC-motif chemokine ligand 12
CXCR4	CXC-motif chemokine receptor 4
HDL	High-density lipoprotein
LAD	Left anterior descending artery
LCx	Left circumflex artery
LDL	Low-density lipoprotein
NaF	^{18}F-Sodium fluoride
oxLDL	Oxidized low-density lipoprotein
PET	Positron emission tomography
RCA	Right coronary artery
STEMI	ST-Elevation myocardial infarction
SUV	Standardized uptake value
TBR	Target-to-background ratio

Introduction

Atherosclerosis is now established as a chronic inflammatory disease, with an early response to injury triggered by endothelial damage with sub-

J. R. Pinney
Division of Cardiology, Department of Medicine, David Geffen School of Medicine, University of California, Los Angeles, CA, USA

Division of Nuclear Medicine, Department of Radiology, Veterans Affairs Greater Los Angeles Healthcare System, Los Angeles, CA, USA

Ronald Reagan UCLA Medical Center, Los Angeles, CA, USA

N. Menon
Division of Nuclear Medicine, Department of Radiology, Veterans Affairs Greater Los Angeles Healthcare System, Los Angeles, CA, USA

Ronald Reagan UCLA Medical Center, Los Angeles, CA, USA

Veterans Affairs West Los Angeles Medical Center, Los Angeles, CA, USA

R. R. Sevag Packard (✉)
Division of Cardiology, Department of Medicine, David Geffen School of Medicine, University of California, Los Angeles, CA, USA

Division of Nuclear Medicine, Department of Radiology, Veterans Affairs Greater Los Angeles Healthcare System, Los Angeles, CA, USA

Ronald Reagan UCLA Medical Center, Los Angeles, CA, USA

Veterans Affairs West Los Angeles Medical Center, Los Angeles, CA, USA
e-mail: rpackard@mednet.ucla.edu

© The Author(s), under exclusive license to Springer Nature Switzerland AG 2022
M. Pelletier-Galarneau, P. Martineau (eds.), *FDG-PET/CT and PET/MR in Cardiovascular Diseases*, https://doi.org/10.1007/978-3-031-09807-9_19

sequent expression of vascular adhesion molecules and transmigration of leukocytes, particularly monocyte/macrophages, but also T-lymphocytes and dendritic cells, into the tunica intima, followed by the release of pro-inflammatory cytokines, proteases, and reactive oxygen species in response to modified lipids such as oxidized low-density lipoprotein cholesterol (oxLDL) [1–3]. The resulting pro-inflammatory cascade results in the formation of foam cells with the release of matrix metalloproteinases and other proteolytic enzymes such as cathepsins, leading to high-risk, rupture-prone atherosclerotic plaque development [4]. This includes a high macrophage to vascular smooth muscle cell ratio, intraplaque neo-angiogenesis, growth of a necrotic lipid core, outwards/positive remodeling, lesion growth in the shoulder region of the plaque, thinning of the fibroatheroma cap, and, ultimately, early microcalcification as a part of the body's innate response to stabilize and calcify areas marred by inflammation [5, 6]. All of these features ultimately lead to progressive inflammatory changes in atherosclerotic lesions in the coronary arteries, correlating directly with increased risk of plaque rupture and subsequent acute coronary syndrome (ACS).

Various modalities exist to characterize cardiovascular risk and evaluate coronary obstruction such as coronary computerized tomography (CT) angiography and positron emission tomography (PET) myocardial blood flow quantitation, now routinely used clinically. However, our improved understanding of the disease pathobiology has led to the development of molecular imaging approaches for improved diagnosis, prognosis, and even treatment of coronary artery disease (CAD) by the identification of inflammatorily active lesions, and thus patient selection for optimal medical therapy with or without invasive coronary angiography and revascularization. Indeed, to identify disease-specific cellular and molecular features, the last two decades have witnessed the development and implementation of nuclear medicine-based tracers to characterize high-risk CAD features. Here, we review the most established molecular tracers and present areas of ongoing research for CAD imaging-based risk assessment.

¹⁸F-Fluorodeoxyglucose (FDG) Imaging of Metabolic Activity

Initial studies in molecular CAD imaging were conducted with the glucose analog FDG. FDG is a positron-emitting radionuclide that has been widely used in molecular imaging for the assessment of inflammatory and neoplastic processes utilizing PET. After intravenous injection, FDG is absorbed by cells using glucose transporter proteins (primarily GLUT-1) and is phosphorylated by hexokinase to its final metabolite form, FDG-phosphate, which cannot be metabolized and thus remains trapped in cells. Thus, FDG serves as a marker for glucose metabolism and can label tissues with increased metabolic activity [7]. The exact cells responsible for FDG increase in atherosclerosis remain ill-defined. In vitro analyses of glucose utilization and metabolism in atheroma-bound cell populations showed that direct inflammatory activation by cytokines does not increase FDG metabolism in local macrophages, but rather in vascular smooth muscles and endothelial cells [8]. Moreover, cell studies simulating a hypoxic environment increased glucose transport, and thus FDG uptake, in macrophages [8]. Further studies are needed to dissect the cell types and pathways leading to increased GLUT-1 expression and FDG uptake in atherosclerotic lesions. Despite the incompletely understood biology, and due to its correlation with the relative increase in local macrophage metabolic activity, FDG-PET imaging quickly gained interest in applications for labeling atherosclerotic disease with active inflammation. The potential of FDG-PET to non-invasively detect highly metabolic macrophages and (likely) highly glycolytic smooth muscles very early in the atherosclerotic disease process offered a vital tool for CAD risk assessment [4, 9–16]. Additional investigations demonstrated FDG uptake in atherosclerotic plaques to be directly correlated with macrophage density and inflammation [14, 17, 18].

FDG Imaging for CAD Detection and Risk Prediction

Early work indicated a positive correlation between FDG uptake in large arteries and CAD [19]. Furthermore, increased FDG uptake is an effective proxy for the increased risk of major adverse cardiovascular events [20]. Additionally, FDG uptake is increased in culprit lesions shortly after an acute coronary syndrome (ACS) [16, 21], demonstrating the utility of this strategy to identify subsequent at-risk lesions and likely high-yield targets for staged revascularization. More recent studies have highlighted the FDG-PET-based prediction of ACS incidence compared to patients with no history of known CAD [22]. The group was subdivided into tertiles of target-to-background ratio (TBR) levels, and after 4 years it was shown that the highest TBR group had a more than fourfold increase in adverse coronary events [23]. Coronary artery calcium (CAC) scoring in the same subset of patients also showed high association with cardiovascular disease with a greater than threefold increased risk for calcium score greater than 100. However, when TBR tertiles were controlled for CAC score, the predictive valve of FDG-PET uptake was independent of CAC scoring, highlighting the unique value each approach can provide in characterizing atherosclerotic lesions [22].

Despite these promising features, the transformation of FDG-PET from a non-specific marker of inflammation to a reliable marker of coronary atherosclerosis has been challenged by limitations in resolution, development of standardized image processing protocols, and difficulty suppressing background signal from the surrounding myocardium. Early attempts to validate FDG-PET for the identification of atherosclerosis focused on static large arteries, demonstrating a direct correlation between tracer uptake in the carotid arteries and degree of inflammation and macrophage density by histology [24]. Notably, however, this study did not find reliable correlations between tracer uptake and plaque size or comorbidities such as hypertension, dyslipidemia, or diabetes mellitus [24].

Regardless of these challenges, these early studies demonstrated that vascular FDG uptake was repeatable on serial examinations with high interobserver reproducibility [25, 26] and modifiable by anti-inflammatory pharmacological agents such as statins [27]. By measuring maximum standardized uptake values (SUV) in four regions of the left main coronary artery to create an average coronary SUV and normalizing to the uptake in the superior vena cava to generate a quantitative target-to-background ratio (TBR), researchers were able to show a 20% decrease in arterial TBR after a 12-week treatment course with a high intensity statin [28]. This evaluation of the reliability of measuring FDG uptake in the proximal left main coronary artery offered promise that the application to downstream epicardial coronary arteries could help evaluate disease progression and treatment efficacy [29].

Subsequent studies validated FDG imaging in the coronary bed against the reference standard invasive angiography in patients with ACS. In patients that underwent FDG-PET after invasive angiography, increased tracer uptake was noted at the culprit site as well as in distal segments of the left main artery and even the ascending aorta [30], demonstrating the utility of FDG-PET in detecting local and systemic inflammation that can destabilize at-risk lesions and lead to adverse cardiovascular events. By highlighting these at-risk lesions in the days or weeks following infarct, FDG imaging may provide insight into patients with increased risk for subsequent ACS that could benefit from more aggressive therapies. Increased tracer uptake was also noted in atherosclerotic regions of patients with stable angina, highlighting the potential predictive value of FDG-PET in identifying patients at subsequent risk for major adverse cardiovascular events [30] (Fig. 19.1). Additional studies evaluating temporal change in FDG uptake after aggressive risk factor modification demonstrated up to 65% reduction in FDG-positive sites after a 17-month period of lifestyle modifications, including dietary counseling and physician-directed exercise and weight loss, suggesting a mechanism for plaque stabilization guided by nuclear imaging [4, 28, 31]. This correlated to a

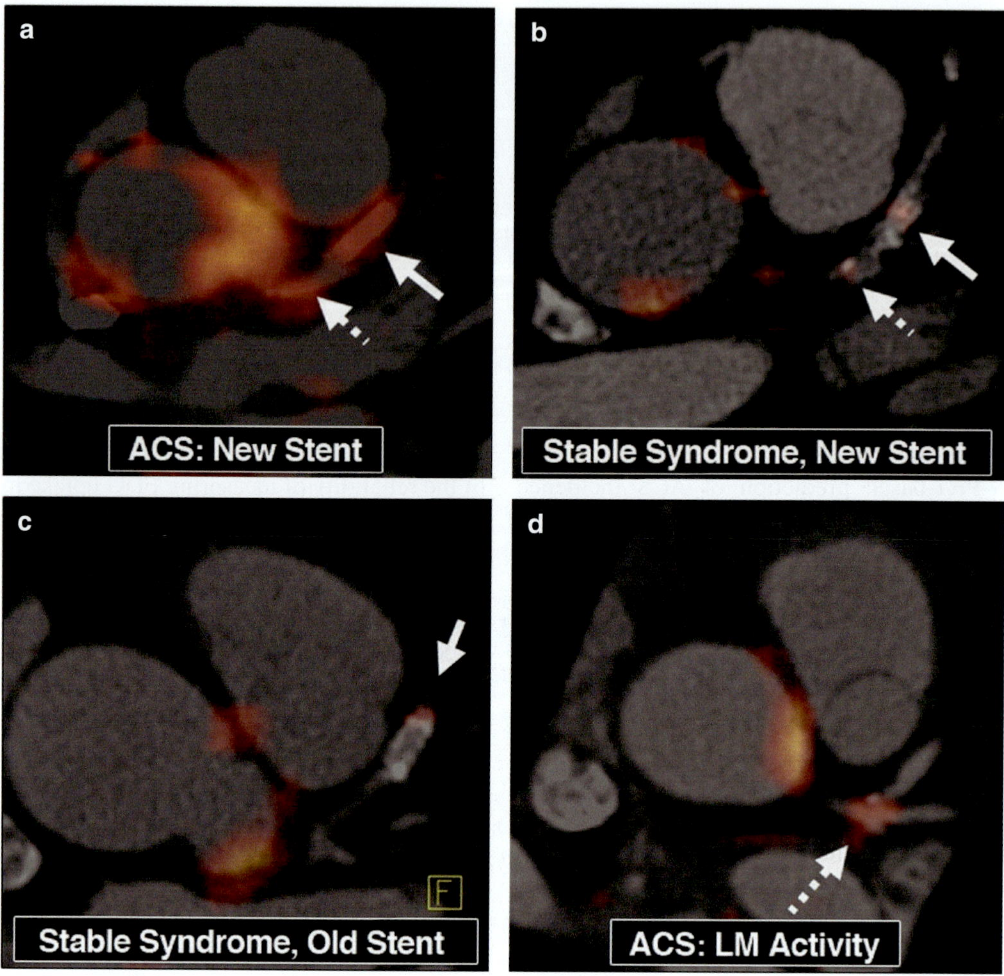

Fig. 19.1 Co-registered ^{18}F-FDG-PET/CT images showing FDG uptake in the coronary arteries. (**a**) Focal uptake in the left main artery (dashed arrow) and the stented portion of the LAD (solid arrow) in a patient with ACS. (**b**) Mild FDG uptake in a mixed plaque in the left main artery (dashed arrow) and stented portion of the LAD (solid arrow) in a patient with stable coronary disease. (**c**) Mild FDG uptake in the LAD stented several months prior to imaging. (**d**) Focal FDG uptake in the left main bifurcation in a patient with ACS. (Reproduced with permission from Rogers et al. [30])

significant, albeit small, decrease in total cholesterol, low-density lipoprotein (LDL) cholesterol, diastolic blood pressure, and body mass index, with a small increase in high-density lipoprotein (HDL) cholesterol [31].

Limitations of FDG Imaging in Coronary Atherosclerosis

FDG-PET evaluation of coronary atherosclerosis carries several technological challenges. Most notably, PET imaging is limited by a finite resolution of photon detection that achieves ranges from 4 to 6 mm [32]. FDG uptake in atherosclerosis is precisely observed and easily quantified in large vessels (≥ 1 cm) such as the aorta and carotid arteries [33]. Conversely, epicardial coronary arteries typically measure 2–4 mm in diameter and progressively taper toward the distal vessel, limiting the geographic reliability of this technology to identify small or distal vessel lesions [4]. Co-registration with computed tomography (CT) imaging can help improve lesion identification and localization; however, this can be further challenged by inherent motion artifact in the coronary vasculature. Early efforts at integrating PET scanners with magnetic resonance imaging have also shown promising improvements in resolution [34, 35].

These challenges are particularly relevant in imaging the right coronary artery (RCA), which is subjected to significant motion during the cardiac cycle [21]. Studies evaluating ideal ECG-gating algorithms demonstrated average RCA displacement in-plane of 24.1 mm compared to 3.6 mm and 15.0 mm in the left anterior descending (LAD) and left circumflex (LCx) arteries, respectively [36]. As a result, lesion identification in the RCA has been shown to be less reproducible with higher signal-to-noise ratio [21]. One study sought to co-register FDG-PET with CT angiography after percutaneous intervention in patients with stable CAD or in the setting of ACS to validate the ability of FDG-PET to identify coronary artery inflammation. The FDG-PET signal was not increased in the culprit lesion of half the patients who experienced ACS, raising concern about the sensitivity of this non-specific marker to reliably detect at-risk atherosclerotic lesions [16] (Fig. 19.2). Plaque FDG uptake is dependent on the microenvironmental milieu and predominant cell types present [15] and is the subject of ongoing research to distinguish quiescent from metabolically active lesions [37].

While low spatial resolution, motion artifacts, and limited tracer specificity interfere with reliable coronary plaque detection using FDG-PET imaging, a frequent technical challenge that has decreased its clinical utility is the intense myocardial uptake of FDG [13, 19, 27, 38]. Dietary factors and available energy sources can also affect cardiomyocyte metabolism, with lack of available blood glucose diverting energy streams to the consumption of free fatty acids with a compensatory decrease in oxidative metabolism [39]. However, distinguishing physiologic myocardial glucose uptake from the pathologic metabolic activity of intra-coronary macrophages is challenging in practice and requires appropriate acquisition and patient preparation protocols.

Addressing this requires optimizing the TBR of FDG uptake in the arterial wall. Furthermore, these protocols must be standardized to allow them to be interpretable across different scanners and detectors as well as temporally with changes in patient condition, comorbidities, and medical treatment. Standardization of imaging protocols that includes adequate dietary preparation to suppress myocardial FDG uptake, consistent FDG dose administration, improved data acquisition hardware and processing algorithms, and regulated imaging time should substantially enhance the ability of FDG-PET to detect coronary atherosclerosis [13, 19, 27]. This necessitates establishing a standardized uptake value (SUV) to objectively quantify FDG binding and signal intensity to generate reproducible results. The SUV is a mathematical ratio of the concentration of tissue radioactivity normalized to injected dose and patient weight

$$\left(SUV = \frac{\text{Regional Radioactivity Concentration}}{\left(\text{Injected Dose of FDG}\right) \times \left(\text{Patient Weight}\right)} \right).$$

From this, the TBR is calculated as a ratio of the SUV of a region of interest and the SUV of a previously defined background region of interest. The standardization of the determination of SUV has been challenged by protocol variability across imaging systems and institutions. General practice involves choosing a region of maximum or mean SUV in the region of interest by averaging pixel counts in a target arterial wall, then subsequently normalizing to a blood pool uptake by measuring SUV, generally in the venous blood pool [40, 41]. This method of systematic quantification is also limited by the natural variability of FDG uptake over time, as well as patient factors and variabilities in metabolism or tracer distribution [19]. Furthermore, due to PET's susceptibility to partial volume effects from limited detector spatial resolution, FDG uptake in the distal coronary arteries becomes difficult to estimate as the artery size approaches the finite pixel resolution [42, 43]. This is further exacerbated by user-biased factors such as variability in image partitioning and identification of the regions of interest.

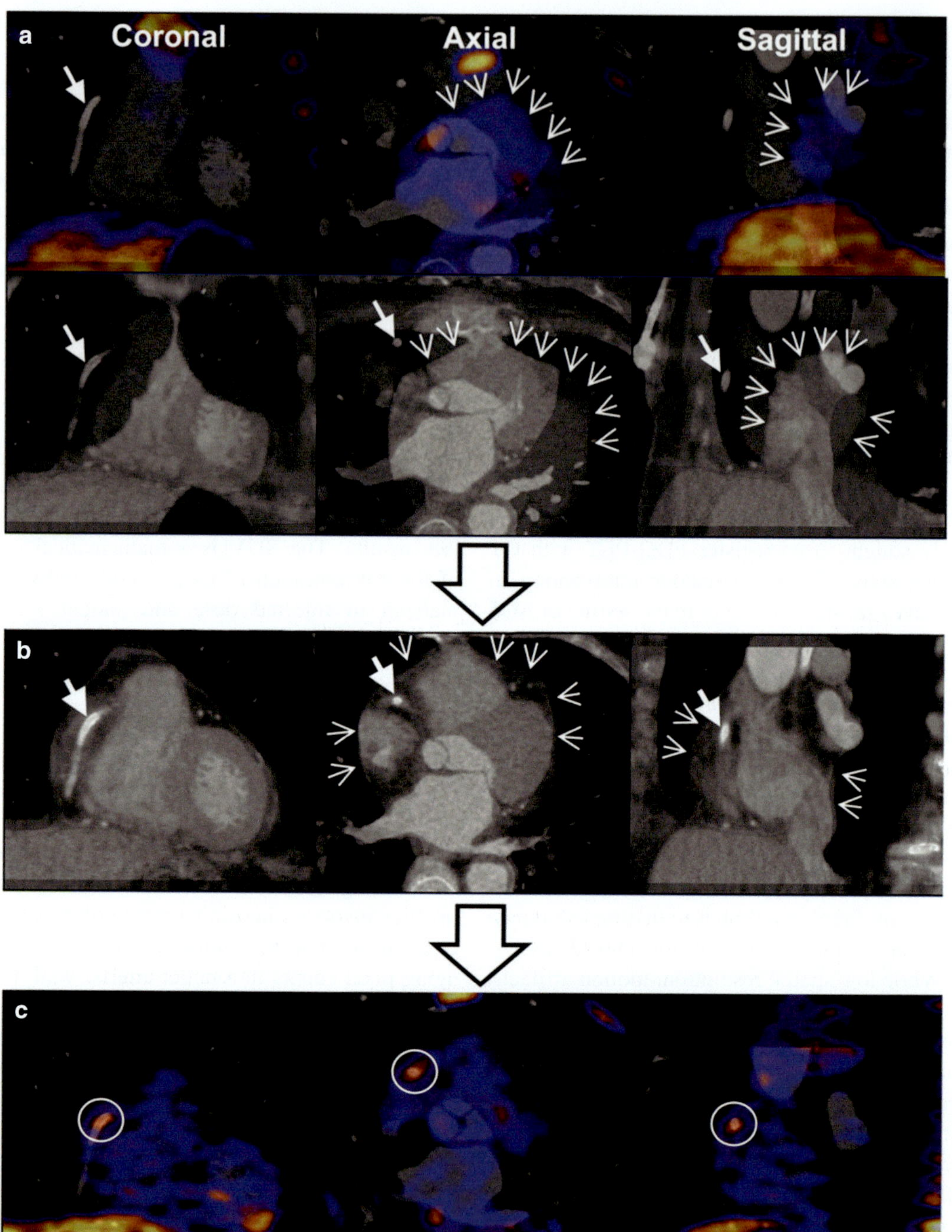

Fig. 19.2 Co-registered images of a coronary CT angiogram and ^{18}F-FDG-PET from a patient with a stented proximal RCA STEMI. (**a**) Top row shows overlayed coronary CT angiogram with FDG-PET uptake. Bottom row shows overlayed coronary CT angiogram with non-contrast cardiac CT. Arrow denotes RCA stent. Arrowheads denote silhouette of heart from FDG-PET or non-contrast cardiac CT compared to CT angiogram demonstrating offset of images. (**b**) Coronary CT angiogram and non-contrast cardiac CT are co-registered using the stent position as a coordinate marker (arrow) with improved overlay (arrowheads). (**c**) Superimposed FDG-PET on this co-registered image now show improved co-localization with FDG uptake at the stent site (circle). (Reproduced with permission from Cheng et al. [16])

Standardizing FDG Protocols for Improved Imaging of Coronary Atherosclerosis

In an effort to overcome these technical limitations, a variety of coronary FDG-PET protocols have been proposed to standardize outputs. These including reducing blurring from cardiac and respiratory motion by computational motion correction techniques [44], instituting cardiac and respiratory gating [45, 46], and by developing 3D and 4D PET imaging protocols [47, 48], which, together, have enabled millimeter-level accuracy in controlled phantom studies [48]. Of note, however, each of these approaches has tradeoffs of artificially introduced signal bias or decrease in signal detection limits.

Adequate patient preparation is critical. This implicates strict patient preparation with a high-fat, low-carbohydrate diet to induce fatty acid metabolism and suppress undesirable myocardial FDG uptake, thereby enhancing the detection of coronary atherosclerotic FDG [49–51]. To obtain high signal-to-noise ratios, protocols call for complete abstinence from all carbohydrate sources including fruits, vegetables, breads and starches, and any sweetened foods while favoring meals high in protein and fat for 1–3 days prior to the exam followed by a temporary fast for up to 12 h prior [52]. These protocols are challenging to monitor in an outpatient setting and can lead to variable results that rely on strict patient adherence to complicated protocols. However, one group demonstrated a sixfold improvement in study quality by providing patients with structured meal regimens prior to the exam [53].

While many technical challenges such as non-specific uptake by the myocardium, smooth muscles, and other inflammatory conditions may limit FDG's utility, it will remain a viable alternative to monitor and detect progressive coronary atherosclerotic disease in at-risk patient populations.

^{18}F-NaF Imaging of Microcalcification

Of particular interest has been the recent work studying ^{18}F-sodium fluoride (NaF) as a molecular PET tracer for coronary atherosclerosis evaluation. Used for decades to diagnose bone turnover and osseous metastases, the incidental finding of the localization of NaF to calcified intramural atherosclerotic lesions in the aorta offered novel opportunities, beyond the well-established CT-based CAC scoring which has demonstrated a clear association with adverse cardiovascular outcomes [54].

NaF binds its molecular target by replacing hydroxyl groups on hydroxyapatite-calcium salt crystals, enabling it to adsorb to the surface of calcium deposits [55]. In binding to susceptible molecular targets in the arterial tree, NaF may offer insight into lesion-specific risk of plaque rupture and adverse cardiovascular outcomes, thereby helping to identify patients at elevated risk of ACS. Indeed, the ability of NaF to identify culprit plaques or plaques at risk of destabilization and rupture could transform the landscape of individual risk assessment and medical and interventional therapies for patients. Furthermore, it is apparent that lesions characterized by NaF imaging are distinct from areas of heightened metabolic activity identified by FDG, demonstrated by regional coincident uptake of NaF and FDG in only 6.5% of 215 arterial (non-coronary) lesions [56], thus suggesting a potentially complementary role of the two approaches. Further advantages of NaF are a relatively simple production process, a favorable 110-min half-life, rapid distribution and clearance from the blood pool, and, most importantly, negligible myocardial uptake, which facilitate visualization of target arterial binding sites [1].

One study of system-wide arterial calcifications demonstrated colocalization of CT-based calcification with PET-based NaF signal in 88%

of 254 arterial lesions with tracer uptake. By contrast, however, only 12% of the total sites of calcification demarcated by CT were found to uptake NaF, indicating that NaF tracer uptake depends on more than just the presence of arterial calcium deposits [57]. The demonstration that some calcified lesions do not show significant NaF uptake and that signal can also be detected in regions without visible calcification on traditional CT imaging modalities suggests that the degree of binding of NaF to vascular calcifications is proportional to the surface area of calcium crystals available for binding. Indeed, microcalcifications, defined as plaque-embedded deposits $\leq$60 μm in diameter, have a higher surface area to volume ratio available for binding, as compared to macrocalcifications [5, 58]. These early microcalcifications are composed of nanocrystalline nucleations of hydroxyapatite, indicative of metabolically active atherosclerotic lesions, and provide a high surface area for NaF binding [5]. Over time, coalescence of calcium deposits into more stable macrocalcifications in a thickened fibrous layer. These mature lesions show decreased risk of rupture and, although bulky and potentially flow-limiting, are considered to be lower risk sites for plaque rupture [58]. Additionally, bulky macrocalcifications offer less surface-available hydroxyapatite for binding of NaF molecules, illuminating why these more stable, mature lesions are relatively quiescent on molecular imaging studies using NaF [58].

This critical qualitative distinction has helped spark further studies into the characterization of calcified, mature lesions that may be at lower risk for adverse cardiovascular events due to the lack of active inflammation as opposed to microcalcifications that can promote plaque rupture [58, 59] (Fig. 19.3). It is the earlier stages of inflammation marred by punctate, rigid microcalcifications which act as a nidus for local stress concentration through this focal gradient in elastic modulus, increasing circumferential stress and risk of intimal tear and plaque rupture [60]. The relatively increased availability of hydroxyapatite nucleation sites in the nanocrystalline structure promotes NaF binding and suggests the value of NaF imaging as a lesion-specific marker of high-risk inflammatory plaque growth [61].

Clinical Utility of NaF in Coronary Atherosclerotic Imaging

More recently, several studies have sought to correlate NaF binding with known culprit lesions from patients with anginal symptoms or recent myocardial infarction. In a study of coronary and carotid NaF uptake in 92 patients who underwent invasive angiography for stable angina ($n = 40$), acute myocardial infarction ($n = 40$), or patients undergoing carotid endarterectomy for symptomatic carotid artery disease ($n = 12$), 100% of carotid plaque ruptures and 93% of culprit lesions causing ACS were found to have increased uptake of NaF [1]. When compared to results from intravascular ultrasound assessments, 45% of the patients that presented with stable angina had focal uptake of NaF that was positively associated with high-risk features including remodeling, microcalcification, and necrotic core size [1]. Furthermore, 72% of these lesions were considered non-obstructive with <70% angiographic stenosis, suggesting a role for NaF in identifying high-risk lesions prior to the development of hemodynamically significant flow-limiting stenosis [1]. In the same study, FDG imaging was performed which highlighted the limitations of this traditional molecular tracer, which was unable to be interpreted in the vascular territories of nearly half of the patients studied, despite adequate suppression of myocardial tissue uptake, and only showed focal uptake in 10% of the patients post infarction [1] (Fig. 19.4).

Co-registration with invasive intravascular ultrasound has also shown strong association of NaF uptake with known high-risk features. NaF uptake was increased in the border zones of high-intensity calcifications where it was associated with microcalcifications and calcified fibroatheroma, as well as increased remodeling and necrotic tissue [62]. Further studies have also identified complementary imaging features that help identify high-risk plaques. For example, NaF uptake

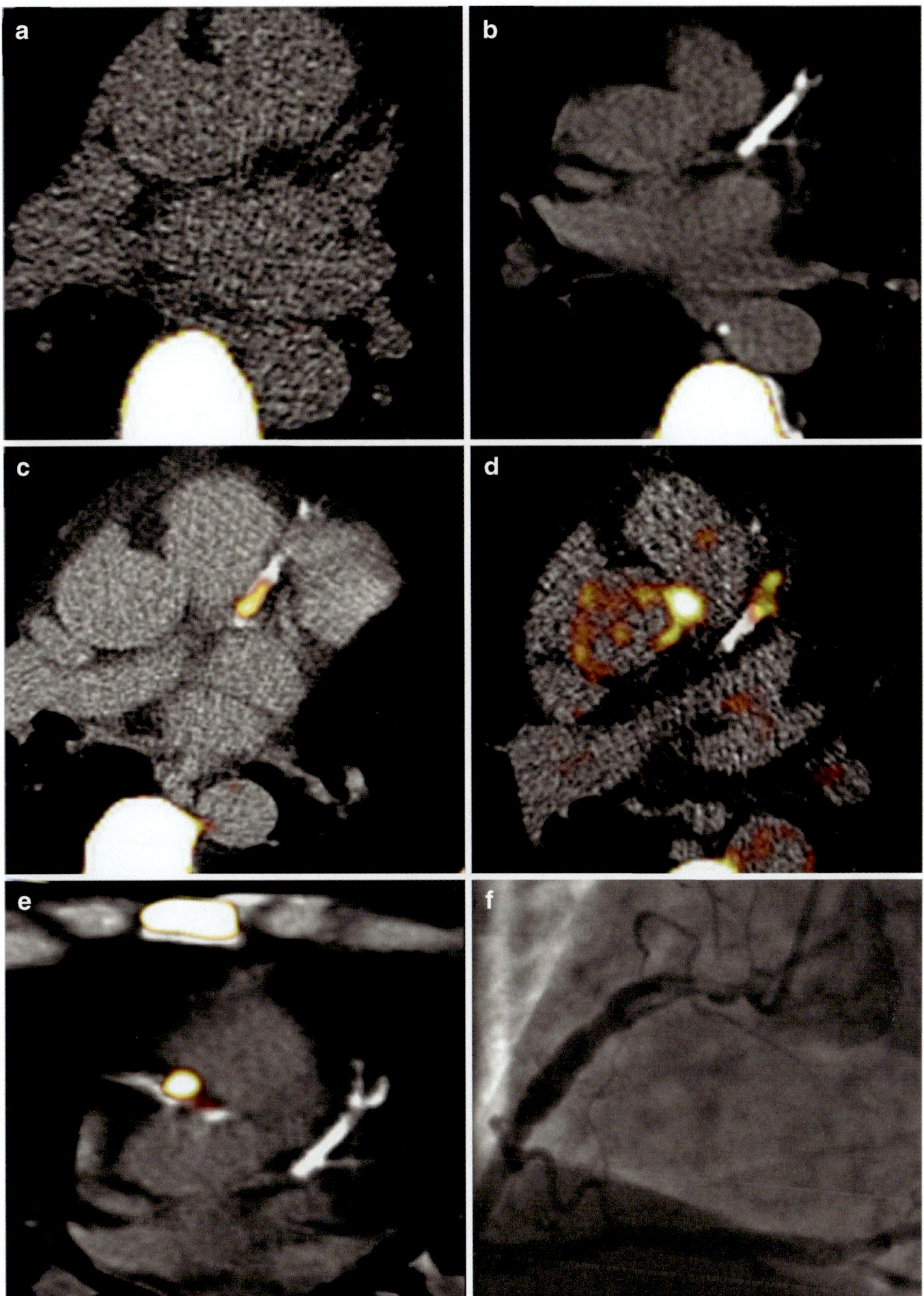

Fig. 19.3 Co-registered ^{18}F-NaF-PET/CT images showing uptake in the coronary arteries. (**a**) No uptake seen in patient without coronary calcium. (**b**) Patient with extensive LAD calcification without NaF uptake. (**c**) Patient with extensive LAD calcification with focal NaF uptake. (**d**) Patient with LAD calcification with NaF uptake adjacent to the calcified segment suggesting expanding microcalcification. (**e**) Patient with recent ACS in the RCA territory with corresponding NaF uptake in the proximal RCA. (**f**) Angiogram of patient from (**e**) showing ulcerated plaque and thrombus in the proximal RCA corresponding to the area of NaF uptake. (Reproduced with permission from Dweck et al. [59])

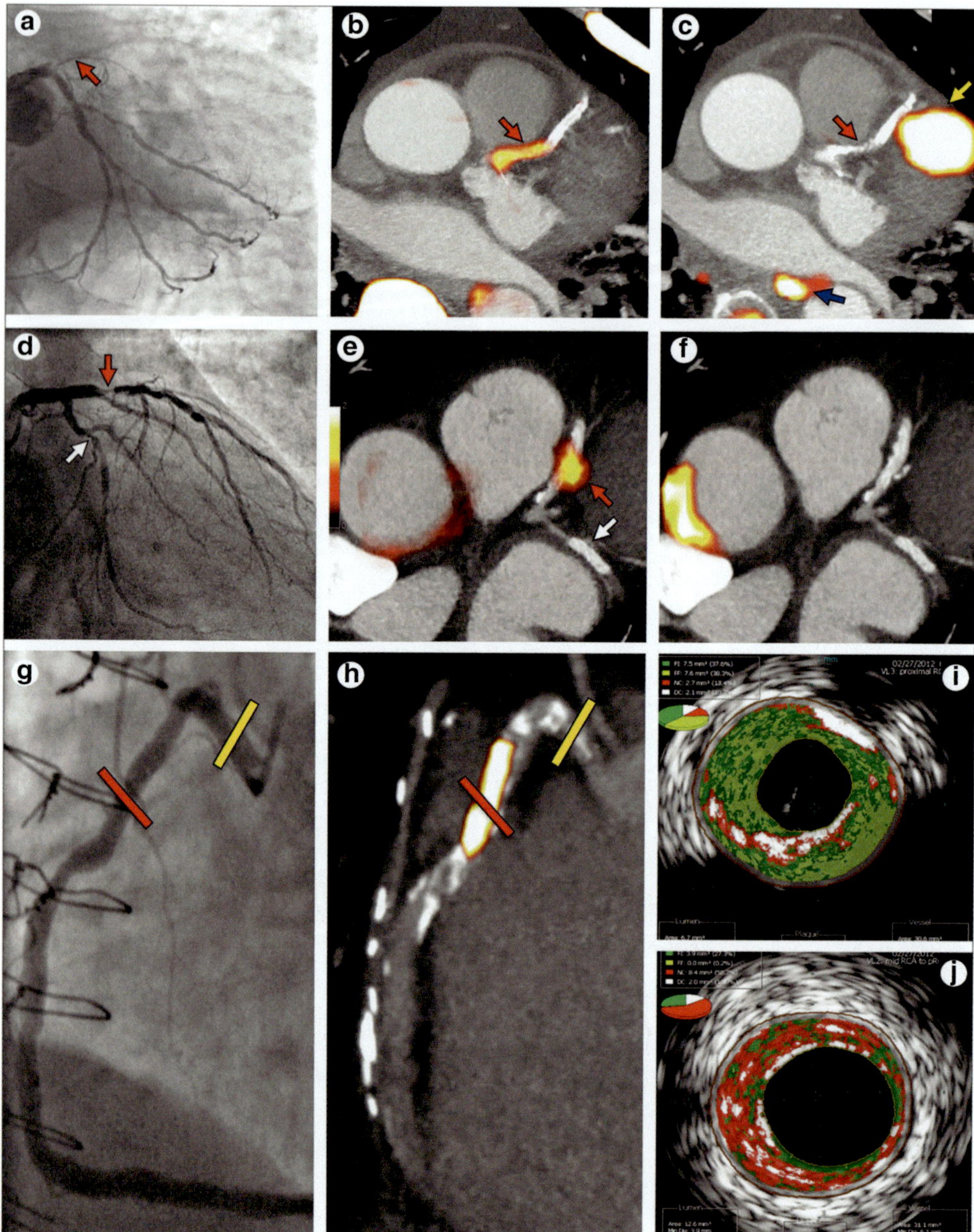

Fig. 19.4 Comparison of ^{18}F-NaF and ^{18}F-FDG uptake in patients with CAD. (**a**) Coronary angiogram of patient with proximal LAD STEMI. (**b**) NaF-PET showing intense proximal LAD uptake. (**c**) FDG-PET without significant focal uptake at the culprit proximal LAD lesion. Yellow arrow denotes myocardial uptake in the LAD distribution. Blue arrow denotes esophageal uptake. (**d**) Coronary angiogram of patient with proximal LAD ACS (non-STEMI) (red arrow) and bystander non-culprit CAD in the LCx (white arrow), both of which were stented. (**e**) NaF uptake shown in the culprit stented LAD without significant uptake in the bystander stented LCx. (**f**) FDG-PET without tracer uptake in either the culprit LAD or the bystander LCx in the same patient. (**g**) Coronary angiogram showing non-obstructive disease in the proximal to mid RCA in a patient with stable angina. (**h**) NaF-PET showing tracer uptake in the mid RCA lesions (red) but not in the proximal RCA (yellow). (**i**) Intravascular ultrasound of the NaF-negative lesion showing predominantly fibrofatty infiltration (green) and confluent macrocalcifications (white) without significant necrosis (red). (**j**) Intravascular ultrasound of the NaF-positive lesion shows microcalcifications (white) and significant necrotic core (red), consistent with high-risk features. (Reproduced with permission from Joshi et al. [1])

colocalizes with peri-coronary adipose tissue as recognized by low-attention plaques on coronary CT and often identified in proximity to culprit lesions of ACS [63]. Although both elevated CAC score and presence of high-risk, partially calcified or low-attenuation plaques on coronary CT are proportional to the uptake of NaF, the presence of obstructive disease (>70% stenosis or >50% stenosis of the left main or proximal left anterior descending (LAD) arteries) was not predictive of increased maximum TBR of NaF, highlighting its complementary qualitative information in personalized risk assessment [55].

NaF Imaging in Prospective Risk Assessment

Additional work has sought to identify the utility of NaF imaging in prospective trials to predict lesions at impending risk of rupture and subsequent myocardial infarction. Initial reports of association of age, male sex, and low HDL serum concentrations with increased NaF uptake provided evidence of a direct correlation of signal intensity with risk for adverse cardiovascular outcomes [59].

A study evaluated 293 patients who underwent NaF imaging, coronary CT co-registration, and invasive coronary angiography for either symptomatic stable angina or recent myocardial infarction [64]. By quantifying global NaF uptake in the coronary vascular tree, 69% of subjects were found to have a non-zero NaF signal. Over 42 months, 7% of the subjects experienced a fatal or non-fatal myocardial infarction, all of whom had increased NaF uptake, with zero subjects without positive NaF signal experiencing an adverse cardiovascular outcome. Although the overall event number was low during the period of the study, it is notable that neither CAC score nor the presence of obstructive lesions on coronary CT was predictive of subsequent myocardial infarction. Indeed, in this study only NaF uptake emerged as a statistically significant predictor of adverse cardiovascular events with several standard clinical scoring systems failing to demonstrate a reliable prognostic linkage. Furthermore,

elevated NaF TBR carried a statistically significant hazard ratio of 4.6 for the risk of subsequent infarction [64].

A second, smaller study looked at the co-registration of NaF-PET imaging with coronary CT for the prospective evaluation of adverse coronary events over 2 years of follow-up [65]. Coronary events occurred in 11 of the 32 patients that completed follow-up, with analysis demonstrating a significantly increased uptake of NaF imaging during the initial evaluation. Furthermore, correlation with increased CAC score as well as the presence of partially calcified or high-risk plaque features on coronary CT (defined as low density <30 Hounsfield Units, or with a remodeling index of >1.1) were found in all patients that had increased NaF uptake. While most patients in this study had baseline obstructive lesions identified on coronary CT, defined as a 2 mm segment with ≥50% stenosis, in two of the noted coronary events coronary CT did not reveal obstructive stenosis of the culprit lesion while NaF uptake was increased at the culprit site prior to intervention, implicating the potential complementary role of molecular NaF imaging in high-risk patients [65].

An NaF-based strategy may also help differentiate patients identified as high-risk by modalities such as CAC scoring into patients with stable, mature coronary calcifications as opposed to those with active inflammation and concomitant microcalcification that may benefit from more aggressive interventions [59]. However, robust prospective clinical studies will need to be performed to establish the proposed ability of NaF to identify metabolically active, high-risk coronary atherosclerotic lesions.

Limitations and Future Directions

Although early results and imaging correlations with NaF have been promising, other studies have shown less significant associations with increased tracer uptake. Indeed, a study of 88 patients with diabetes mellitus imaged prospectively with NaF PET failed to identify a significant number of potentially high-risk plaques as would be expected in such an at-risk population. Additional studies are underway with improved long-term clinical monitoring after imaging to identify subjects with cardiac events to better elucidate this potential [66]. Increased radiation exposure may also be restrictive in some clinical centers with baseline NaF-PET/CT scans associated with 8–9 mSv of radiation [67]. The PET spatial resolution limitation of 3–4 mm may also impede the utility of NaF for individualized assessment of smaller, focal atherosclerotic lesions [68]. Ultimately, longer term prospective clinical studies will need to be undertaken to better understand the prognostic utility of NaF-PET imaging in atherosclerotic disease and the promising role that NaF-PET may play as a complementary tool in the screening and serial evaluation of high-risk patient populations.

⁶⁸Ga-Pentixafor Imaging of CXCR4 Inflammation

There has been continued progress in identifying targeted tracers that provide more specific and potentially predictive data in regard to CAD activity and risk for adverse clinical outcomes. One of the most promising developments from this work has been the identification of the CXC-motif chemokine receptor 4 (CXCR4) which, when bound to the associated ligand CXC-motif chemokine ligand 12 (CXCL12), is associated with leukocyte-mediated inflammatory processes that are seen in models of ischemic injury [69]. Histologic evaluation of inflammatory coronary plaques has revealed CXCR4-positive leukocyte populations, primarily monocyte/macrophages, although populations of smooth muscle cells, endothelial cells, T-cells, B-cells, and thrombocytes have also shown significant CXCR4 expression in atherosclerotic zones [69, 70].

The CXCR4 Signaling Pathway

CXCR4 is a transmembrane G-protein-coupled chemokine receptor that has been implicated in a variety of inflammatory and autoimmune diseases, as well as in cancer progression where it has been studied as a potential therapeutic target to interrupt metastasis [70]. Additionally, the CXCR4 signaling axis has been implicated in the evolution of coronary plaque through its role in development and growth of smooth muscle and endothelial progenitor cells. The precise pathways through which endothelial and smooth muscle cells are integrated into the CXCR4 signaling pathway are incompletely characterized, but it appears to play a homeostatic role in helping to recruit inflammatory populations to areas of vascular microinjury, ultimately leading to endothelial proliferation and repair of the vascular bed [69]. CXCR4 is implicated in the activation and recruitment of intralesional macrophages in atherosclerotic plaques and in the early post myocardial infarction period [69, 70] (Fig. 19.5). Indeed, this process is cumulative throughout the development of atherosclerotic plaques and, as such, offers promise as a targeted molecule for evaluation of patients with high-risk for cardiovascular disease [69]. As the density of macrophages increases, the risk of thrombotic events increases due to the release of cytokines and macrophage-associated proteases such as matrix metalloproteases, compromising the thin fibrous cap and leading to further local inflammation. By targeting one of the key cell types that is integral to the progression of advanced atherosclerotic plaques, CXCR4 offers increased specificity with a narrower bandwidth signal than currently more established tracers such as FDG and NaF [69]. Even more intriguingly, early animal studies have evaluated the therapeutic potential of CXCR4 blockade with small molecules such as the allo-

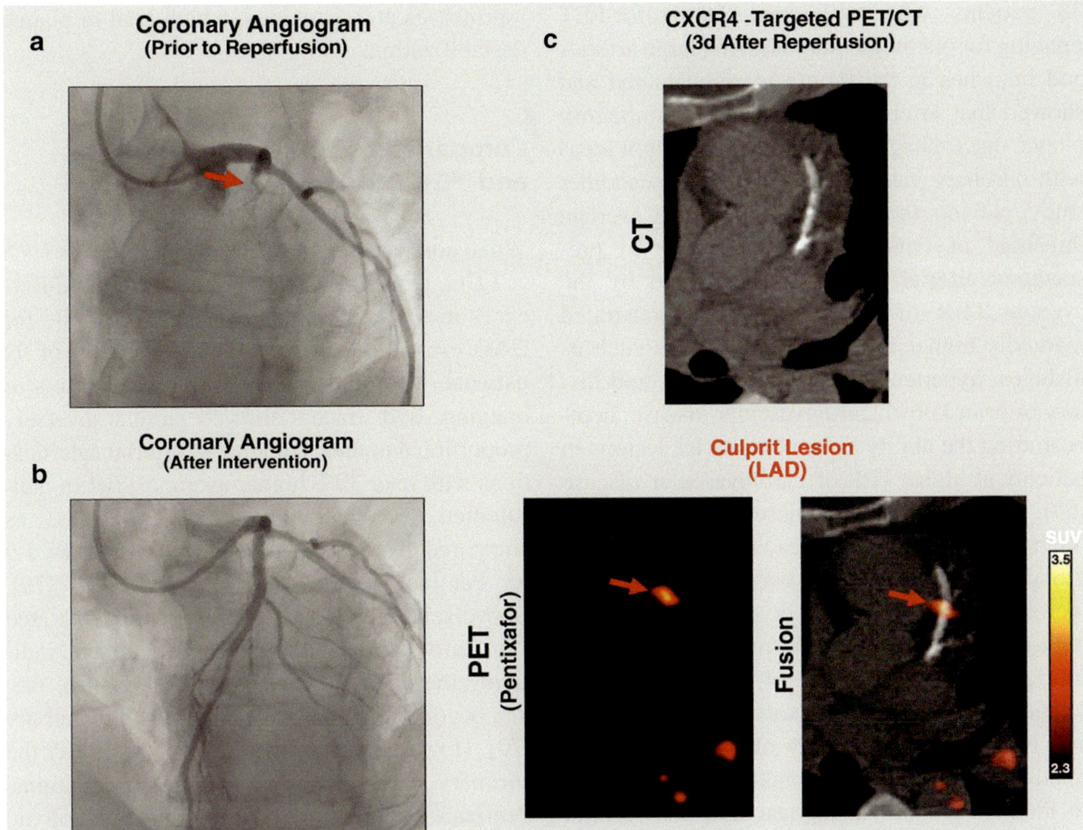

Fig. 19.5 ^{68}Ga-Pentixafor uptake in a patient with ACS after reperfusion. (**a**) Coronary angiogram with acute LAD occlusion (red arrow). (**b**) Coronary angiogram showing reperfusion of the LAD after stenting. (**c**) Fused Pentixafor-PET/CT scan showing focal tracer uptake at the mid-site of the LAD stent (red arrow). (Reproduced with permission from Derlin et al. [74])

steric antagonist AMD3100 (Plerixafor) that can even lead to improved function and recovery after acute myocardial infarction when delivered within a narrow therapeutic window of time post infarct [71].

Nuclear Imaging of CXCR4 in Coronary Atherosclerosis

To take advantage of this promising molecular target, the radiotracer ^{68}Ga-pentixafor was developed as a highly specific ligand of CXCR4. Early studies demonstrated the potential clinical utility of this targeted radiotracer by comparing the con-

cordance of Pentixafor uptake in patients recently diagnosed with ACS with myocardial inflammation on cardiac magnetic resonance imaging (cMRI), suggesting a role for CXCR4 signaling to promote inflammatory remodeling. Although tracer uptake was not ubiquitous across all subjects in this population, all Pentixafor positive segments corresponded to regions of infarct on cMRI, and uptake appeared to be proportional to the extent of infarct as measured by troponin elevation level, serving as an early proof of concept on the clinical utility of Pentixafor imaging [72].

Further efforts were undertaken to study the association of Pentixafor uptake with high-risk patient demographics. In a retrospective study of

38 patients who underwent Pentixafor-PET imaging for oncologic purposes, the large arteries and branches in the thorax were evaluated and showed that arterial uptake from inflammatory plaque macrophages may serve to highlight areas with coronary vascular disease [73]. In another study, patients that surpassed a defined average threshold of Pentixafor tracer uptake in pre-specified arterial segments, as defined by the average TBR of tracer uptake, demonstrated markedly higher rates of comorbidities such as diabetes, hypertension, hyperlipidemia, and history of prior known cardiovascular disease, demonstrating the ability to identify at-risk lesions in patients at higher risk of cardiovascular disease [69]. The prevalence of these risk factors was often at least four times greater in the high TBR group, and indeed, there was an overall 12% increase in tracer uptake in patients with any high-risk demographic features for atherosclerotic disease [69]. This type of "dose-dependent" relationship between Pentixafor signal intensity and high-risk features may also help establish relative cut-offs in tracer uptake that can be used to identify plaques at highest risk of potential rupture.

More specifically than association with clinical syndromes, considerable study has gone into the evaluation of the colocalization of Pentixafor uptake with arterial neo-intimal calcifications [15]. A retrospective analysis of patients that underwent Pentixafor-PET/CT imaging showed that nearly 34% of sites with Pentixafor uptake were also found to have calcifications on CT, but conversely, only 7% of the total calcified arterial lesions showed Pentixafor uptake [69]. This underlines the hypothesis that CXCR4 may be more associated with early plaque development through its role in the recruitment of macrophages and subsequent release of metalloproteases and cytokines, which lead to plaque destabilization.

Comparison of ^{18}F-FDG and ^{68}Ga-Pentixafor Imaging

When compared to more established tracers such as FDG, there are notable similarities and differences in the Pentixafor tracer uptake profile for CAD evaluation. In a retrospective study of 92 patients who underwent FDG and Pentixafor imaging, both tracers showed similar inversely proportional uptake to degree of arterial calcifications with over 30% higher average TBR in non-calcified, metabolically active lesions as compared to severely calcified lesions (1.4 vs. 1.9 for Pentixafor and 1.1 vs. 1.5 for FDG) [70]. Conversely, 35% of patients demonstrated Pentixafor uptake without any FDG uptake, indicating the utility of this tracer to recognize factors beyond focal macrophage metabolic activity [70]. However, due to the inability to biopsy the coronary vasculature in clinical evaluations, Pentixafor studies to date lack histopathologic corroboration of the cell populations responsible for uptake of the tracer. Efforts to address this have included evaluation of cadaveric heart samples or explants from carotid endarterectomies [74]. These studies have been able to confirm the high density of CXCR4-positive cells in areas of atherosclerosis without significant CXCR4 expression in healthy vascular segments (5% CXCR4-positive cells vs. negligible number in healthy segments). Interestingly, these ex vivo analyses have also identified direct correlations between Pentixafor uptake intensity and symptomatic carotid artery disease (15% CXCR4-positive cells in symptomatic lesions vs. 2% CXCR4-positive cells in asymptomatic lesions), further implicating the ability of CXCR4 targeting imaging to identify clinically relevant inflammatory regions in diseased arteries [74].

Clinical Applications of CXCR4-Targeted Imaging

In animal models of myocardial infarction designed for early testing of CXCR4 antagonists, Pentixafor uptake intensity was directly related to time after infarct, with highest signal intensity 3 days after infarct, consistent with the timing of inflammatory recruitment to the infarct zone [71]. Most recently, several groups have worked to demonstrate the clinical utility of CXCR4-targeted nuclear imaging in prospective studies of patients with known CAD or recent ACS. Evaluation of human subjects post infarction with Pentixafor imaging co-registered with cMRI demonstrated increased uptake in culprit arterial segments, with uptake intensity related to severity of ischemic burden as characterized by edema and late gadolinium enhancement [71]. However, the generalizability of this correlation as a predictor of ACS rather than a sequela continues to be studied. In one study of 37 patients imaged within 1 week of an acute ST-elevation myocardial infarction (STEMI) after undergoing stent-based reperfusion, Pentixafor uptake was quantified in both culprit lesions that were stented as well as non-culprit, non-stented regions [74] (Fig. 19.6). Although both demonstrated significant uptake, maximum SUV in the defined regions of interest was over 30% higher in stented culprit lesions compared to stented non-culprit lesions, and over 60% higher than non-stented non-culprit calcified lesions, suggesting that some CXCR4 activity

could also be attributed to direct intravascular injury from revascularization [74].

A theranostic approach, evaluating the potential use of CXCR4 pathways for treatment of acute infarction, is underway [75]. Pentixafor uptake after induced infarction in mice becomes measurable in the myocardial infarct zone within hours after infarct and peaks within 1–3 days, with a subsequent decline to baseline levels by 1 week [75]. Interestingly, subjects with catastrophic post-infarct complications such as ventricular rupture showed a 30% higher tracer uptake in the infarcted myocardium at 3 days post infarct as compared to surviving subjects, suggesting a pathologic consequence to sustained CXCR4 activation [75]. Indeed, the use of the competitive inhibitor of CXCR4 receptor binding, AMD3100, at day 3 after infarct demonstrated a threefold reduction (8% vs. 23%) in the incidence of ventricular rupture and improved long-term ventricular function as compared to untreated subjects [75]. Additionally, there was a 15% improvement in left ventricular ejection fraction without affecting infarct size [75]. However, as a testament to the dynamic and multifaceted role of the CXCR4 signaling cascade, subjects not treated until 7 days after infarction actually experience an increased risk of left ventricular rupture (31% vs. 8%) without the benefit of improved ventricular function seen in subjects treated at the day 3 inflammation peak [75]. These observations indicate CXCR4 can be used to identify subjects with sustained or severe inflammation that may benefit from more advanced therapies due to increased risk of delayed complications. In fact, retrospective evaluation of 50 patients after acute myocardial infarction demonstrated that the intensity of Pentixafor uptake 3–5 days after infarct was

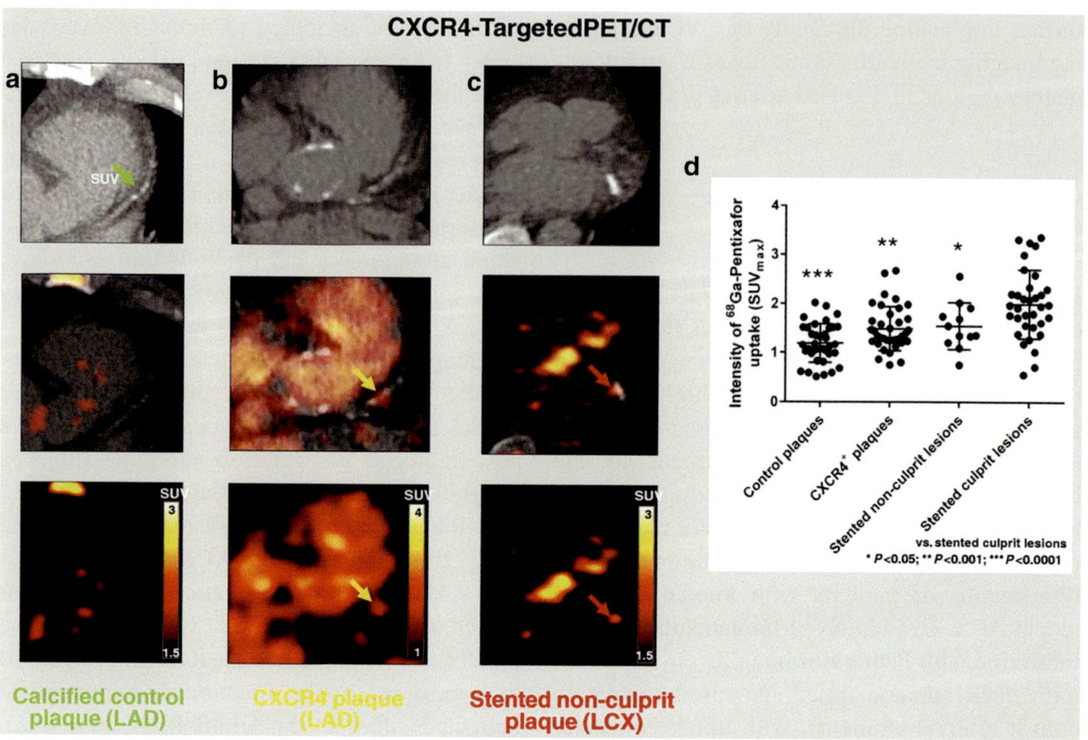

Fig. 19.6 ^{68}Ga-Pentixafor uptake in various coronary lesions (top row = CT scan, bottom row = Pentixafor-PET, middle row = fused image). (**a**) Calcified LAD plaque without Pentixafor uptake. (**b**) Partially calcified lesion with Pentixafor uptake in the proximal LAD (yellow arrow). (**c**) Pentixafor uptake in the stented portion of a non-culprit LCx lesion. (**d**) Scatter plot of Pentixafor uptake intensity in control calcified plaques versus Pentixafor-positive plaques showing highest uptake in culprit stented lesions with modest uptake in non-culprit stented lesions and lowest uptake in stable calcified plaques. (Reproduced with permission from Derlin et al. [74])

inversely proportional to resultant ventricular function several months later (correlation coefficient of -0.41 comparing ejection fraction versus maximum CXCR4 SUV) [75].

Although the specificity of the CXCR4 signaling pathway has shown promise in targeted identification of at-risk atherosclerotic lesions, the incompletely understood and diverse functions that CXCR4 plays in other local cell types merit further studies. CXCR4 expression in mature endothelial and smooth muscle cells has been associated with maintenance of arterial wall integrity and endothelial barrier function in animal models, highlighting the importance of evaluating clinical context and complementary data when interpreting Pentixafor-based imaging in the evaluation of CAD [69].

Emerging Tracers

Continued understanding of the disease pathobiology, identification of novel molecular tracers, as well as improvement in imaging techniques will continue to advance the utility of PET imaging of atherosclerosis using targeted molecular tracers. Additionally, this may allow the development of predictive algorithms determining risk of adverse events in a lesion-specific manner, and surveillance methods for plaque stabilization. Several additional PET radiotracers are being studied that target atherosclerosis through metabolic pathways such as biosynthesis of nucleotides [76] and phospholipids [77, 78], and markers of endothelium activation and immune cell recruitment [79].

In response to atherosclerotic immune activation, cells entering the proliferative stage require nucleotides as building blocks [80]. One study in mice, rabbits, and humans demonstrated significantly higher uptake of ^{18}F-labeled thymidine (^{18}F-FLT) in subjects with atherosclerosis compared to controls [76]. Similarly, taking advantage of cholesterol, fatty acid, and phospholipid biosynthesis in proliferating macrophages, [11]C- and ^{18}F-labeled choline, a phospholipid precursor, has shown increased atherosclerotic plaque uptake in mice [77] and humans [78]. In addition to probes targeting metabolic pathways, investigators are also exploring cell surface molecules that are upregulated during atherosclerosis for molecular PET imaging. Evaluation of ^{68}Ga-DOTATATE, a derivative of the somatostatin analog octreotide that targets somatostatin receptor subtype-2, which is upregulated in macrophages, has shown excellent specificity and superior coronary lesion discriminating features compared to ^{18}F-FDG in mice [81] and humans [82]. Additional studies with ^{64}Cu-DOTATATE have also shown promising results in human studies [83]. Moreover, another tracer targeting upregulated translocator protein expression in macrophages, ^{11}C-PK11195, has also shown higher uptake in symptomatic carotid plaques of humans [84]. Finally, in an effort to further improve target specificity, smaller antibody fragment-based radiotracers or nano-tracers are being developed and investigated in atherosclerosis [85–87]. While prospective trials are required to firmly establish the clinical utility of these agents, molecular PET imaging holds the promise of providing a targeted approach to assist practitioners in the diagnosis and treatment of inflammatorily active coronary atherosclerotic lesions.

Acknowledgments VA Merit BX004558, UCLA Cardiovascular Discovery Fund/Lauren B. Leichtman and Arthur E. Levine Investigator Award.

References

1. Joshi NV, Vesey AT, Williams MC, Shah ASV, Calvert PA, Craighead FHM, et al. 18F-fluoride positron emission tomography for identification of ruptured and high-risk coronary atherosclerotic plaques: a prospective clinical trial. Lancet. 2014;383(9918):705–13.
2. Geovanini GR, Libby P. Atherosclerosis and inflammation: overview and updates. Clin Sci. 2018;132(12):1243–52.
3. Gisterå A, Hansson GK. The immunology of atherosclerosis. Nat Rev Nephrol. 2017;13(6):368–80.
4. Abdelbaky A, Tawakol A. Noninvasive positron emission tomography imaging of coronary arterial inflammation. Curr Cardiovasc Imaging Rep. 2011;4(1):41–9.
5. Bellinge JW, Francis RJ, Majeed K, Watts GF, Schultz CJ. In search of the vulnerable patient or the vulnerable plaque: 18F-sodium fluoride positron emission tomography for cardiovascular risk stratification. J Nucl Cardiol. 2018;25(5):1774–83.
6. Ehara S, Kobayashi Y, Yoshiyama M, Shimada K, Shimada Y, Fukuda D, et al. Spotty calcification typifies the culprit plaque in patients with acute myocardial infarction: an intravascular ultrasound study. Circulation. 2004;110(22):3424–9.
7. Mettler F, Guiberteau M. Essentials of nuclear medicine imaging. Amsterdam: Elsevier; 2012.
8. Folco EJ, Sheikine Y, Rocha VZ, Christen T, Shvartz E, Sukhova GK, et al. Hypoxia but not inflammation augments glucose uptake in human macrophages: implications for imaging atherosclerosis with 18fluorine-labeled 2-deoxy-D-glucose positron emission tomography. J Am Coll Cardiol. 2011;58(6):603–14.
9. Feil S, Fehrenbacher B, Lukowski R, Essmann F, Schulze-Osthoff K, Schaller M, et al. Transdifferentiation of vascular smooth muscle cells to macrophage-like cells during atherogenesis. Circ Res. 2014;115(7):662–7.
10. Basatemur GL, Jørgensen HF, Clarke MCH, Bennett MR, Mallat Z. Vascular smooth muscle cells in atherosclerosis. Nat Rev Cardiol. 2019;16(12):727–44.
11. Liu M, Gomez D. Smooth muscle cell phenotypic diversity. Arterioscler Thromb Vasc Biol. 2019;39(9):1715–23.
12. Yun M, Yeh D, Araujo LI, Jang S, Newberg A, Alavi A. F-18 FDG uptake in the large arteries: a new observation. Clin Nucl Med. 2001;26(4):314–9.
13. Mayer M, Borja AJ, Hancin EC, Auslander T, Revheim ME, Moghbel MC, et al. Imaging atherosclerosis by PET, with emphasis on the role of FDG and NaF as potential biomarkers for this disorder. Front Physiol. 2020;11:511391.

14. Tawakol A, Migrino RQ, Hoffmann U, Abbara S, Houser S, Gewirtz H, et al. Noninvasive in vivo measurement of vascular inflammation with F-18 fluorodeoxyglucose positron emission tomography. J Nucl Cardiol. 2005;12(3):294–301.

15. Krishnan S, Otaki Y, Doris M, Slipczuk L, Arnson Y, Rubeaux M, et al. Molecular imaging of vulnerable coronary plaque: a pathophysiologic perspective. J Nucl Med. 2017;58(3):359–64.

16. Cheng VY, Slomka PJ, Le Meunier L, Tamarappoo BK, Nakazato R, Dey D, et al. Coronary arterial 18F-FDG uptake by fusion of PET and coronary CT angiography at sites of percutaneous stenting for acute myocardial infarction and stable coronary artery disease. J Nucl Med. 2012;53(4):575–83.

17. Chen Q, Williams R, Healy CL, Wright CD, Wu SC, O'Connell TD. An association between gene expression and better survival in female mice following myocardial infarction. J Mol Cell Cardiol. 2010;49(5):801–11.

18. Ogawa M, Ishino S, Mukai T, Asano D, Teramoto N, Watabe H, et al. 18F-FDG accumulation in atherosclerotic plaques: immunohistochemical and PET imaging study. J Nucl Med. 2004;45(7):1245–50.

19. Sheikine Y, Akram K. FDG-PET imaging of atherosclerosis: do we know what we see? Atherosclerosis. 2010;211(2):371–80.

20. Gogia S, Kaiser Y, Tawakol A. Imaging high-risk atherosclerotic plaques with PET. Curr Treat Options Cardiovasc Med. 2016;18(12):76.

21. Rogers IS, Tawakol A. Imaging of coronary inflammation with FDG-PET: feasibility and clinical hurdles. Curr Cardiol Rep. 2011;13(2):138–44.

22. Figueroa AL, Abdelbaky A, Truong QA, Corsini E, MacNabb MH, Lavender ZR, et al. Measurement of arterial activity on routine FDG PET/CT images improves prediction of risk of future CV events. JACC Cardiovasc Imaging. 2013;6(12):1250–9.

23. Iwatsuka R, et al. Arterial inflammation measured by 18F-FDG-PET-CT to predict coronary events in older subjects. Atherosclerosis. 2017;268:49–54.

24. Tawakol A, Migrino RQ, Bashian GG, Bedri S, Vermylen D, Cury RC, et al. In vivo 18F-Fluorodeoxyglucose positron emission tomography imaging provides a noninvasive measure of carotid plaque inflammation in patients. J Am Coll Cardiol. 2006;48(9):1818–24.

25. Rudd JHF, Myers KS, Bansilal S, Machac J, Rafique A, Farkouh M, et al. 18Fluorodeoxyglucose positron emission tomography imaging of atherosclerotic plaque inflammation is highly reproducible. Implications for atherosclerosis therapy trials. J Am Coll Cardiol. 2007;50(9):892–6.

26. Rudd JHF, Myers KS, Bansilal S, Machac J, Pinto CA, Tong C, et al. Atherosclerosis inflammation imaging with 18F-FDG PET: carotid, iliac, and femoral uptake reproducibility, quantification methods, and recommendations. J Nucl Med. 2008;49(6):871–8.

27. Chen W, Dilsizian V. 18F-fluorodeoxyglucose pet imaging of coronary atherosclerosis and plaque inflammation. Curr Cardiol Rep. 2010;12(2):179–84.

28. Singh P, Emami H, Subramanian S, Maurovich-Horvat P, Marincheva-Savcheva G, Medina HM, et al. Coronary plaque morphology and the anti-inflammatory impact of atorvastatin. Circ Cardiovasc Imaging. 2016;9(12):1–9.

29. Ali A, Tawakol A. FDG PET/CT imaging of carotid atherosclerosis. Neuroimaging Clin N Am. 2016;26(1):45–54.

30. Rogers IS, Nasir K, Figueroa AL, Cury RC, Hoffmann U, Vermylen DA, et al. Feasibility of FDG imaging of the coronary arteries: comparison between acute coronary syndrome and stable angina. JACC Cardiovasc Imaging. 2010;3(4):388–97.

31. Lee SJ, Young KO, Eun JL, Joon YC, Kim BT, Lee KH. Reversal of vascular 18F-FDG uptake with plasma high-density lipoprotein elevation by atherogenic risk reduction. J Nucl Med. 2008;49(8):1277–82.

32. Wassélius JA, Larsson SA, Jacobsson H. FDG-accumulating atherosclerotic plaques identified with 18F-FDG-PET/CT in 141 patients. Mol Imaging Biol. 2009;11(6):455–9.

33. James OG, Christensen JD, Wong TZ, Neto SB, Koweek LM. Utility of FDG PET/CT in inflammatory cardiovascular disease. Radiographics. 2011;31(5):1271–86.

34. Munoz C, Kunze KP, Neji R, Vitadello T, Rischpler C, Botnar RM, et al. Motion-corrected whole-heart PET-MR for the simultaneous visualisation of coronary artery integrity and myocardial viability: an initial clinical validation. Eur J Nucl Med Mol Imaging. 2018;45(11):1975–86.

35. Robson PM, Dweck MR, Trivieri MG, Abgral R, Karakatsanis NA, Contreras J, et al. Coronary artery PET/MR imaging: feasibility, limitations, and solutions. JACC Cardiovasc Imaging. 2017;10(10):1103–12.

36. He S, Dai R, Chen Y, Bai H. Optimal electrocardiographically triggered phase for reducing motion artifact at electron-beam CT in the coronary artery. Acad Radiol. 2001;8(1):48–56.

37. Joseph P, Tawakol A. Imaging atherosclerosis with positron emission tomography. Eur Heart J. 2016;37(39):2974–2980b.

38. McKenney-Drake ML, Moghbel MC, Paydary K, Alloosh M, Houshmand S, Moe S, et al. 18F-NaF and 18F-FDG as molecular probes in the evaluation of atherosclerosis. Eur J Nucl Med Mol Imaging. 2018;45(12):2190–200.

39. Schelbert HR. PET contributions to understanding normal and abnormal cardiac perfusion and metabolism. Ann Biomed Eng. 2000;28(8):922–9.

40. Kim S, Lee S, Kim JB, Na JO, Choi CU, Lim H, et al. Concurrent carotid inflammation in acute coronary syndrome as assessed by 18 F-FDG PET / CT: a possible mechanistic link for ischemic stroke. J Stroke Cerebrovasc Dis. 2015;24(11):2547–54.

41. Thie A. SUVs: methods and implications for usage. J Nucl Med. 2004;45(9):1431–4.
42. Mayer J, Jin Y, Wurster TH, Makowski MR, Kolbitsch C. Evaluation of synergistic image registration for motion-corrected coronary NaF-PET-MR. Philos Trans R Soc A Math Phys Eng Sci. 2021;379(2200):20200202.
43. Soret M, Bacharach SL, Buvat I. Partial-volume effect in PET tumor imaging. J Nucl Med. 2007;48(6):932–45.
44. Rubeaux M, Joshi NV, Dweck MR, Fletcher A, Motwani M, Thomson LE, et al. Motion correction of ^{18}F-NaF PET for imaging coronary atherosclerotic plaques. J Nucl Med. 2016;57(1):54–9.
45. Büther F, Dawood M, Stegger L, Wübbeling F, Schäfers M, Schober O, et al. List mode-driven cardiac and respiratory gating in PET. J Nucl Med. 2009;50(5):674–81.
46. Teräs M, Kokki T, Durand-Schaefer N, Noponen T, Pietilä M, Kiss J, et al. Dual-gated cardiac PET-clinical feasibility study. Eur J Nucl Med Mol Imaging. 2010;37(3):505–16.
47. Park SJ, Ionascu D, Killoran J, Mamede M, Gerbaudo VH, Chin L, et al. Evaluation of the combined effects of target size, respiratory motion and background activity on 3D and 4D PET/CT images. Phys Med Biol. 2008;53(13):3661–79.
48. Lucignani G. Respiratory and cardiac motion correction with 4D PET imaging: shooting at moving targets. Eur J Nucl Med Mol Imaging. 2009;36(2):315–9.
49. Williams G, Kolodny GM. Suppression of myocardial 18F-FDG uptake by preparing patients with a high-fat, low-carbohydrate diet. AJR Am J Roentgenol. 2008;190(2):W151–6.
50. Wykrzykowska J, Lehman S, Williams G, Parker JA, Palmer MR, Varkey S, et al. Imaging of inflamed and vulnerable plaque in coronary arteries with 18F-FDG PET/CT in patients with suppression of myocardial uptake using a low-carbohydrate, high-fat preparation. J Nucl Med. 2009;50(4):563–8.
51. Dunphy MPS, Freiman A, Larson SM, Strauss HW. Association of vascular 18F-FDG uptake with vascular calcification. J Nucl Med. 2005;46(8):1278–84.
52. Lu Y, Grant C, Xie K, Sweiss NJ. Suppression of myocardial 18F-FDG uptake through prolonged high-fat, high-protein, and very-low-carbohydrate diet before FDG-PET/CT for evaluation of patients with suspected cardiac sarcoidosis. Clin Nucl Med. 2017;42(2):88–94.
53. Christopoulos G, Jouni H, Acharya GA, Blauwet LA, Kapa S, Bois J, et al. Suppressing physiologic 18-fluorodeoxyglucose uptake in patients undergoing positron emission tomography for cardiac sarcoidosis: the effect of a structured patient preparation protocol. J Nucl Cardiol. 2019;28(2):664–74.
54. Hou ZH, Lu B, Gao Y, Jiang SL, Wang Y, Li W, et al. Prognostic value of coronary CT angiography and calcium score for major adverse cardiac events in outpatients. JACC Cardiovasc Imaging. 2012;5(10):990–9.
55. Kitagawa T, Yamamoto H, Toshimitsu S, Sasaki K, Senoo A, Kubo Y, et al. 18F-sodium fluoride positron emission tomography for molecular imaging of coronary atherosclerosis based on computed tomography analysis. Atherosclerosis. 2017;263:385–92.
56. Derlin T, Tóth Z, Papp L, Wisotzki C, Apostolova I, Habermann CR, et al. Correlation of inflammation assessed by18F-FDG PET, active mineral deposition assessed by18F-fluoride PET, and vascular calcification in atherosclerotic plaque: a dual-tracer PET/CT study. J Nucl Med. 2011;52(7):1020–7.
57. Derlin T, Richter U, Bannas P, Begemann P, Buchert R, Mester J, et al. Feasibility of 18F-sodium fluoride PET/CT for imaging of atherosclerotic plaque. J Nucl Med. 2010;51(6):862–5.
58. Vancheri F, Longo G, Vancheri S, Danial JSH, Henein MY. Coronary artery microcalcification: imaging and clinical implications. Diagnostics (Basel). 2019;9(4):1–17.
59. Dweck MR, Chow MWL, Joshi NV, Williams MC, Jones C, Fletcher AM, et al. Coronary arterial 18F-sodium fluoride uptake: a novel marker of plaque biology. J Am Coll Cardiol. 2012;59(17):1539–48.
60. Vengrenyuk Y, Carlier S, Xanthos S, Cardoso L, Ganatos P, Virmnani R, et al. A hypothesis for vulnerable plaque rupture due to stress-induced debonding around cellular microcalcifications in thin fibrous caps. Proc Natl Acad Sci U S A. 2006;103(40):14678–83.
61. Høilund-Carlsen PF, Sturek M, Alavi A, Gerke O. Atherosclerosis imaging with 18F-sodium fluoride PET: state-of-the-art review. Eur J Nucl Med Mol Imaging. 2020;47:1538–51.
62. Li L, Li X, Jia Y, Fan J, Wang H, Fan C, et al. Sodium-fluoride PET-CT for the non-invasive evaluation of coronary plaques in symptomatic patients with coronary artery disease: a cross-correlation study with intravascular ultrasound. Eur J Nucl Med Mol Imaging. 2018;45(12):2181–9.
63. Kwiecinski J, Tzolos E, Adamson PD, Cadet S, Moss AJ, Joshi N, et al. Coronary 18F-sodium fluoride uptake predicts outcomes in patients with coronary artery disease. J Am Coll Cardiol. 2020;75(24):3061–74.
64. Kwiecinski J, Cadet S, Daghem M, Lassen ML, Dey D, Dweck MR, et al. Whole-vessel coronary 18F-sodium fluoride PET for assessment of the global coronary microcalcification burden. Eur J Nucl Med Mol Imaging. 2020;47(7):1736–45.
65. Kitagawa T, Yamamoto H, Nakamoto Y, Sasaki K, Toshimitsu S, Tatsugami F, et al. Predictive value of18F-sodium fluoride positron emission tomography in detecting high-risk coronary artery disease in combination with computed tomography. J Am Heart Assoc. 2018;7(20):e010224.
66. Raggi P, Senior P, Shahbaz S, Kaul P, Hung R, Coulden R, et al. 18F-sodium fluoride imaging of coronary atherosclerosis in ambulatory patients with diabetes mellitus. Arterioscler Thromb Vasc Biol. 2019;39(2):276–84.

67. Marafi F, Esmail A, Rasheed R, Alkandari F, Usmani S. Novel weight-based dose threshold for 18F-NAF PET-CCT imaging using advanced PET-Ct systems: a potential tool for reducing radiation burden. Nucl Med Commun. 2017;38(9):764–70.

68. Raynor W, Houshmand S, Gholami S, Emamzadehfard S, Rajapakse CS, Blomberg BA, et al. Evolving role of molecular imaging with 18F-sodium fluoride PET as a biomarker for calcium metabolism. Curr Osteoporos Rep. 2016;14:115–25.

69. Weiberg D, Thackeray JT, Daum G, Sohns JM, Kropf S, Wester HJ, et al. Clinical molecular imaging of chemokine receptor CXCR4 expression in atherosclerotic plaque using 68 Ga-Pentixafor PET: correlation with cardiovascular risk factors and calcified plaque burden. J Nucl Med. 2018;59(2):266–72.

70. Kircher M, Tran-Gia J, Kemmer L, Zhang X, Schirbel A, Werner RA, et al. Imaging inflammation in atherosclerosis with CXCR4-directed 68Ga-Pentixafor PET/CT: correlation with 18F-FDG PET/CT. J Nucl Med. 2020;61(5):751–6.

71. Thackeray JT, Derlin T, Haghikia A, Napp LC, Wang Y, Ross TL, et al. Molecular imaging of the chemokine receptor CXCR4 after acute myocardial infarction. JACC Cardiovasc Imaging. 2015;8(12):1417–26.

72. Lapa C, Reiter T, Werner RA, Ertl G, Wester HJ, Buck AK, et al. [68Ga]Pentixafor-PET/CT for imaging of chemokine receptor 4 expression after myocardial infarction. JACC Cardiovasc Imaging. 2015;8(12):1466–8.

73. Li X, Heber D, Leike T, Beitzke D, Lu X, Zhang X, et al. [68Ga]Pentixafor-PET/MRI for the detection of chemokine receptor 4 expression in atherosclerotic plaques. Eur J Nucl Med Mol Imaging. 2018;45(4):558–66.

74. Derlin T, Sedding DG, Dutzmann J, Haghikia A, König T, Napp LC, et al. Imaging of chemokine receptor CXCR4 expression in culprit and nonculprit coronary atherosclerotic plaque using motion-corrected [68Ga]Pentixafor PET/CT. Eur J Nucl Med Mol Imaging. 2018;45(11):1934–44.

75. Hess A, Derlin T, Koenig T, Diekmann J, Wittneben A, Wang Y, et al. Molecular imaging-guided repair after acute myocardial infarction by targeting the chemokine receptor CXCR4. Eur Heart J. 2020;41(37):3564–75.

76. Ye YX, Calcagno C, Binderup T, Courties G, Keliher EJ, Wojtkiewicz GR, et al. Imaging macrophage and hematopoietic progenitor proliferation in atherosclerosis. Circ Res. 2015;117(10):835–45.

77. Laitinen IEK, Luoto P, Någren K, Marjamäki PM, Silvola JMU, Hellberg S, et al. Uptake of 11C-choline in mouse atherosclerotic plaques. J Nucl Med. 2010;51(5):798–802.

78. Vöö S, Kwee RM, Sluimer JC, Schreuder FHBM, Wierts R, Bauwens M, et al. Imaging intraplaque inflammation in carotid atherosclerosis with 18F-fluorocholine positron emission tomography-computed tomography. Circ Cardiovasc Imaging. 2016;9(5):e004467.

79. Pérez-Medina C, Fayad ZA, Mulder WJM. Atherosclerosis Immunoimaging by positron emission tomography. Arterioscler Thromb Vasc Biol. 2020;40(4):865–73.

80. Koelwyn GJ, Corr EM, Erbay E, Moore KJ. Regulation of macrophage immunometabolism in atherosclerosis. Nat Immunol. 2018;19(6):526–37.

81. Rinne P, Hellberg S, Kiugel M, Virta J, Li XG, Käkelä M, et al. Comparison of somatostatin receptor 2-targeting PET tracers in the detection of mouse atherosclerotic plaques. Mol Imaging Biol. 2016;18(1):99–108.

82. Tarkin JM, Joshi FR, Evans NR, Chowdhury MM, Figg NL, Shah AV, et al. Detection of atherosclerotic inflammation by 68Ga-DOTATATE PET compared to [18F]FDG PET imaging. J Am Coll Cardiol. 2017;69(14):1774–91.

83. Pedersen SF, Sandholt BV, Keller SH, Hansen AE, Clemmensen AE, Sillesen H, et al. 64Cu-DOTATATE PET/MRI for detection of activated macrophages in carotid atherosclerotic plaques: studies in patients undergoing endarterectomy. Arterioscler Thromb Vasc Biol. 2015;35(7):1696–703.

84. Gaemperli O, Shalhoub J, Owen DRJ, Lamare F, Johansson S, Fouladi N, et al. Imaging intraplaque inflammation in carotid atherosclerosis with 11C-PK11195 positron emission tomography/computed tomography. Eur Heart J. 2012;33(15):1902–10.

85. Varasteh Z, Mohanta S, Li Y, López Armbruster N, Braeuer M, Nekolla SG, et al. Targeting mannose receptor expression on macrophages in atherosclerotic plaques of apolipoprotein E-knockout mice using 68 Ga-NOTA-anti-MMR nanobody: noninvasive imaging of atherosclerotic plaques. EJNMMI Res. 2019;9:5.

86. Ederle J, Dobson J, Featherstone RL, Bonati LH, van der Worp HB, de Borst GJ, et al. Carotid artery stenting compared with endarterectomy in patients with symptomatic carotid stenosis (international carotid stenting study): an interim analysis of a randomised controlled trial. Lancet. 2010;375(9719):985–97.

87. Broisat A, Hernot S, Toczek J, De Vos J, Riou LM, Martin S, et al. Nanobodies targeting mouse/human VCAM1 for the nuclear imaging of atherosclerotic lesions. Circ Res. 2012;110(7):927–37.

Kevin Emery Boczar, Christiane Wiefels,
Andrew M. Crean, Robert A. deKemp,
and Rob Beanlands

Introduction

Ischemic cardiomyopathy is a leading cause of morbidity and mortality worldwide [1]. It is a far-reaching condition, with incidence and prevalence that continue to rise. There were over 6.2 million American adults living with heart failure (HF) between the years of 2013 and 2016, compared with only 5.7 million between 2009 and 2012 [1]. Based on these data, projections show that there could be over eight million people living with heart failure by the year 2030 [1].

While medical advances continue to improve the survival of those with a diagnosis of HF, it unfortunately remains a disease with an extremely poor prognosis. Data suggest that the associated 5-year mortality approaches 50% for patients with this condition [2]. Thus, given the impact that ischemic HF places on patients and the health-care system, management strategies aimed at improving outcomes have been a prominent focus of research for many years. Specifically, the role that revascularization can play to improve patient outcomes has been widely investigated. In this regard, research on the utility of viability imaging to indicate which patients may benefit most from revascularization has demonstrated great potential in some studies, but not in others. As such, data is not uniformly consistent toward definitive conclusions on the role of viability detection.

This chapter will discuss the concept of myocardial viability, the multimodality imaging tools available to assess viable myocardium, the new advances through research in this field, the clinical applications of viability assessment, and future directions in the area.

K. E. Boczar (✉)
Division of Cardiology, Department of Medicine,
National Cardiac PET Centre, University of Ottawa
Heart Institute, Ottawa, ON, Canada

Department of Medicine, School of Epidemiology
and Public Health, University of Ottawa,
Ottawa, ON, Canada

University of Pennsylvania, Philadelphia, PA, USA
e-mail: kboczar@ottawaheart.ca

C. Wiefels
Division of Cardiology, Department of Medicine,
National Cardiac PET Centre, University of Ottawa
Heart Institute, Ottawa, ON, Canada

Department of Cardiovascular Sciences, Federal
Fluminense University, Niterói, Rio de Janeiro, Brazil

Division of Nuclear Medicine, Department of
Medicine, University of Ottawa, Ottawa, ON, Canada

A. M. Crean · R. A. deKemp · R. Beanlands
Division of Cardiology, Department of Medicine,
National Cardiac PET Centre, University of Ottawa
Heart Institute, Ottawa, ON, Canada

Viability: Back to Basics: Understanding the Terminology

The concept of myocardial viability and the terms surrounding its use are often misused and misunderstood. Thus, a discussion of viability imaging modalities would not be complete without a brief discussion of the correct definitions and understanding of these fundamental terms.

Myocardial ischemia is the result of an imbalance between myocardial oxygen supply and demand; this can result either from an acute coronary syndrome, or alternatively, from chronic ischemic heart disease. In patients with chronic ischemic heart disease, persistent ventricular dysfunction can result from repeated stress-induced ischemia—this dysfunction can either be due to stunning of the myocardium, hibernating myocardium, or scar. Prolonged ischemia-related myocardial injury results in cell death whereby scar replaces healthy myocardial tissue. To distill it to its simplest form, the term "viable myocardium" encompasses all tissue that is not scarred [3]. If the ischemia-related injury is not severe or prolonged enough to cause cell death, the myocardial tissue is considered viable. Dysfunctional myocardium that is viable has the potential to recover from injury, if myocardial flow is either maintained or restored [4–6]. However, there are several subcategories of viable myocardium that require clarification.

Stunned myocardium refers to left ventricle (LV) dysfunction that occurs after either one acute episode or multiple repetitive episodes of ischemia [3]. While the coronary blood flow was reduced and restored so that it is preserved at rest, the myocardial function remains impaired; with the capacity to recover with time (assuming resolution of the ongoing ischemic insult).

Repetitive ischemic insult that is ongoing over time can cause the myocardial tissue that has been repeatedly "stunned" to adapt by reducing its perfusion and contractile function to preserve cellular integrity; this adaptation of downregulation of flow and function is the so-called state of hibernating myocardium [3, 6]. If blood flow can be adequately restored before irreversible injury occurs, then LV function is potentially recoverable (either in whole or in part) [3]. This concept is central in the field of viability imaging and is illustrated in Table 20.1 [4–6].

There are several imaging modalities that are available to assess viability including cardiac PET, single-photon emission computed tomography (SPECT), dobutamine echocardiography (ECHO), dobutamine CMR, late gadolinium enhancement CMR (LGE-CMR), late iodine enhancement CT (LIE-CT) [4] and myocardial contrast ECHO [17, 18]. The nuclear methods and LGE-CMR techniques that are used clinically are summarized in more depth below.

Table 20.1 Characteristics of viable and nonviable myocardium

Myocardium	Flow/perfusion	Glucose metabolism ([18]FDG)	Function/contractile reserve	Structural changes	Potential to recover/clinical relevance
Viable					
Stunning	Preserved (after transitory ischemic insult)	Variable (normal, increased, or reduced)	Reduced	No	Likely to recover if ischemic injury does not persist or become repetitive; revascularization can prevent recurrent stunning
Hibernation	Reduced	Preserved or increased (=perfusion-metabolism mismatch)	Reduced	Yes some	May have partial/delayed or full recovery if adequate revascularization can be achieved
Ischemia	Preserved at rest, impaired at stress	Normal at rest, increased at stress	Preserved at rest, impaired at stress	No	May benefit from revascularization to prevent recurrent ischemia
Nonviable					
Scar	Reduced	Reduced	Absent	Fibrosis	Unlikely to recover with or without revascularization

Reproduced with permission from Kandolin et al., CJC 2019 [3]. Data obtained from multiple sources [3, 4, 7–16]
[18]FDG 18F-fluorodeoxyglucose

Clinical Applications for Viability

While it may be straightforward to understand the potential clinical importance of viability as a general concept, it can be less clear when viability imaging should be applied in specific clinical scenarios. Viability assessment is most useful when the decision to revascularize a patient is not "clear-cut", and where the treatment strategy is more nuanced. We consider imaging for viability to offer the biggest incremental value in patients with the following:

1. IHD (or where it is very strongly suspected).
2. Symptomatic heart failure (≥NYHA II).
3. Moderate to severe LV dysfunction (LVEF <40%).
4. Moderate to large persistent perfusion defects on stress perfusion imaging.

   *Of note, patients with LV dysfunction, should **not** already have significant ischemia identified, as this would indicate that myocardium is viable and they **would** likely benefit from revascularization, thus obviating the need for viability testing*

There are certainly other factors that would modify the decision-making to pursue (or not) revascularization (and would thereby modify the utility of viability imaging). Factors such as the following will alter the incremental utility of viability assessment (Table 20.2):

(a) Extensive patient comorbidities.
(b) Suitability of target vessels for coronary artery bypass surgery (CABG).
(c) Presence of CCS II or greater anginal symptoms (which would thereby strongly point toward the need for revascularization given the proven symptom and outcome benefit in such patients).

Table 20.2 Characteristics to consider in decision regarding which patients will benefit from viability imaging

Viability testing not needed/unlikely to add useful information	Viability testing may add useful information
Younger patients	Older patients
HFrEF with > class II angina	HFrEF without angina
Proven moderate-to-severe ischemia on other testing	No evidence of ischemia; moderate to large persistent perfusion defects suggesting scar (but may be hibernating)
Higher LVEF (>40%)	Lower LVEF (<40%)
Left main coronary artery disease	Chronic total occlusion
No or limited comorbidities	Severe/multiple comorbidities (renal insufficiency, COPD, previous CABG)

Reproduced with permission from Kandolin et al., CJC 2019 [3]. Data obtained from multiple sources [16, 19–21]
CABG coronary artery bypass graft, *CAD* coronary artery disease, *COPD* chronic obstructive pulmonary disease, *HFrEF* heart failure with reduced ejection fraction, *LVEF* left ventricular ejection fraction

Once it has been decided that a viability assessment is the right test for the patient, the next step is to decide on the correct means to assess viability. Ultimately, several techniques (^{18}FDG PET, dobutamine echocardiography, ^{201}Tl-SPECT, ^{99m}Tc-SPECT, and CMR) can be used for viability assessment, and each modality carries its own strengths and limitations (Table 20.3). Key factors that should be weighed in selecting a modality include patient contraindications to specific modalities (i.e., severe renal failure, pacemakers and implantable cardiac defibrillators for CMR), local center expertise, as well as availability of the modality.

Table 20.3 Imaging methods for assessing viability

Modality	Mechanism	Findings indicative of viability	Advantages/disadvantages
Dobutamine echocardiography/CMR	Contractile reserve[a]	Improvement by visual or strain rate imaging (echo)	A: Specific, widely available, without radiation, can detect ischemia, assess valvular disease D: interobserver variability, risk related to dobutamine[b]
SPECT Thallium-201	Perfusion: Sarcolemma membrane integrity (K+ analogue)	Tracer uptake: >50% maximum	A: Widely available, moderate cost D: radiation dose, moderate sensitivity with low specificity
SPECT Technetium-99 m-labelled tracers	Mitochondrial membrane integrity	Tracer uptake: >50–65% of maximum	A: Widely available, moderate cost D: moderate accuracy
PET Perfusion/metabolism	Perfusion: 13NH3, 82Rb, 15O-water Myocyte glucose utilization: FDG	Flow-metabolism mismatch = hibernation, (Match = nonviable)	A: Highly sensitive D: Limited availability, high cost, need for glucose load or insulin clamp in patients with diabetes
CMR	LGE Wall thickness	Scarring (LGE) <50% wall thickness Systolic thickening of a dyskinetic segment	A: Highly sensitive, without radiation, assess valvular disease D: Limited availability, high cost, risks in renal failure, cannot use with certain devices

Reproduced with permission from Kandolin et al., CJC 2019 [3]

[a]Biphasic response. Dobutamine low dose 5–10 mg/kg/min leads to improved contractility in hibernating myocardium. Dobutamine high dose up to 40 mg/kg/min (+ atropine) leads to increased oxygen consumption, induced ischemia, and decreased contractility

[b]Risk of potentially life-threatening complications 0.2% [22]

Nuclear Methods for Assessing Viability

SPECT

SPECT is a widely available imaging modality and has been well validated from a clinical perspective [23]. Both Thallium-201 (^{201}Tl) and Technetium-99 m-labelled agents (^{99m}Tc) can be used to assess myocardial viability [24].

^{99m}Tc-labelled agents

The ^{99m}Tc-labelled agents, ^{99m}Tc-sestamibi and ^{99m}Tc-tetrofosmin, have lipophilic properties that enable them to enter cells passively [25]. Despite this, their ability to remain within the cardiomyocyte is an active process that is reliant on the integrity of the mitochondrial membrane; it is this property which enables them to be utilized for viability imaging.

With a stress–rest protocol, if there is a reversible defect present, it indicates ischemia, which if moderate or severe, automatically negates the need for further viability testing (as the tissue must be viable and the patient may benefit from revascularization) [3]. However, the presence of a persistent ("fixed") defect cannot distinguish scar from hibernating myocardium—it is in this situation that viability imaging is sometimes warranted.

While it is technically possible to utilize rest-only ^{99m}Tc-based perfusion imaging for viability, it has been shown that the use of nitrates can improve detection [26–31]. Additionally, adding nitrates to ^{99m}Tc-based perfusion imaging better correlates with recovery of left ventricular function following revascularization [26–31]. The administration of nitrates prior to an additional rest imaging has the capacity to increase blood flow in the dilated epicardial and collateral vessels which can thereby increase the sensitivity to detect viable myocardium. A protocol that combines rest perfusion imaging and rest perfusion post-nitrate administration imaging (usually 10 mg of oral isosorbide nitrate given 10–15 min before the image acquisition) can be used. While dysfunctional myocardium that has normal perfusion is indicative of stunned myocardium (that is likely to recover with time), segments with reduced perfusion at rest that improve post-nitrate administration suggest hibernating myocardium and thus viability. When persistent defects with absence of tracer uptake are noted on both rest and post-nitrate images, it suggests a lack of viability; this is tissue that is unlikely to recover with revascularization.

Thallium-201

^{201}Tl is the oldest radiopharmaceutical available that is used to assess viability. ^{201}Tl is a potassium analogue, and as such, its uptake is dependent on membrane integrity. This is because it uses the Na+/K+ ATPase pump to penetrate the cell. The high first-pass extraction and capacity to redistribute in the myocardium with time makes this tracer suitable to assess both the presence of ischemia as well as the presence of hibernating myocardium.

There are different protocols available for viability assessment with ^{201}Tl. The most common protocol, similar to ^{99m}Tc-labelled agents, begins with performing stress/rest imaging. In this case, the protocol begins by giving one single injection of 2.5–3.5 mCi of ^{201}Tl during peak stress. Prompt image acquisition, up to 15 min post-stress will demonstrate the first distribution of the tracer, proportional to blood flow. After 30 min the redistribution phase starts, with a progressive washout from the myocardium; this is due to a concentration gradient between the myocyte and the blood. The first redistribution (rest) images are then acquired 2.5–4 h afterward. This allows

one to determine if there is a reversible or persistent defect. If rest perfusion thallium imaging shows a persistent defect, the defect may indicate scar or may still be viable. The options for distinguishing between these two include late redistribution or reinjection. In regions that initially had low Tl-201 uptake, the redistribution of Tl-201 into the blood over time leads to gradient reversal in tissues that initially had low Tl-201 uptake. If this tissue is viable, then it will take up Tl-201 over time and will appear reversible.

If the defect is persistent (or fixed) on both initial stress (or rest) and redistribution rest images, then late redistribution images at 18–24 h should be acquired and interpreted [32]. If the defect remains persistent on the late redistribution images, this suggests the myocardium is nonviable scar and unlikely to recover after revascularization. However, if the defect is reversible on the late redistribution images (or alternatively, on the delayed images of a rest-redistribution protocol), it indicates the presence of viable hibernating myocardium which could potentially benefit from revascularization.

A reversible defect is described as an increase in >10% of the maximum regional uptake, above 50–60% [33]. Viable hibernating cells have a slower washout, and will therefore have a greater relative uptake in delayed images when compared with viable nonischemic cells. ^{201}Tl redistribution is an ongoing, continuous process that requires blood supply to the viable tissue. Thus, its uptake is related both to perfusion as well as the degree of coronary artery narrowing in the vascular territory of interest [34]. Evidence has shown that in viability imaging with ^{201}Tl, viable myocardial tissue will show thallium redistribution (i.e., a reversible defect) on reinjection imaging after the 4 h redistribution images or late imaging (8–72 h), while nonviable tissue will appear as a persistent, or fixed, defect with no thallium uptake [34–37].

A rest-only viability assessment can also be performed with the injection of 2.5–3.5 mCi of ^{201}Tl injected at rest, followed by redistribution imaging either 3–4 h later or 18–24 h later; this eliminates the stress-imaging component altogether. An alternative to the late redistribution

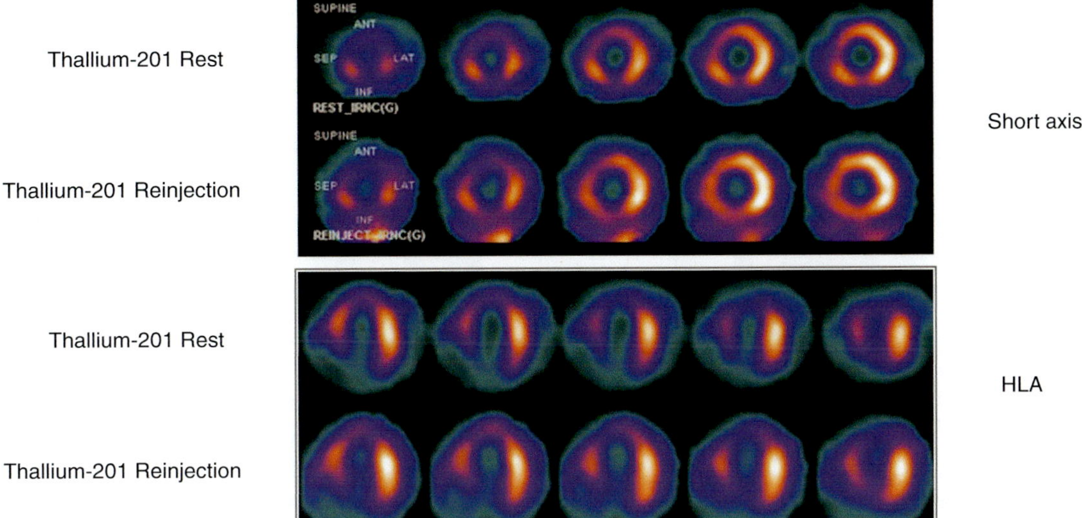

Fig. 20.1 Example of rest and reinjection short-axis and horizontal long-axis thallium tomogram images in a patient with known coronary artery disease. An apparently irreversible distal anterior defect on rest images improves after reinjection indicating viable myocardium

image is a reinjection of 1 mCi of ^{201}Tl after the rest redistribution at 4 h, followed by prompt image reacquisition (Figs. 20.1, 20.2, and 20.3).

PET

Fluorine-18-fluorodeoxyglucose (^{18}FDG) is a glucose analogue and is used clinically to assess and quantify myocardial glucose utilization [3]. The use of ^{18}FDG PET for viability assessment relies on the underlying principles of myocardial metabolic function. Cardiomyocytes can utilize many different substrates for energy metabolism including free fatty acids (FFA), glucose, lactate, pyruvate, and ketones; however, FFA and glucose form the primary energy substrates of choice of cardiomyocytes [39–41]. Adrenergic stimulation, ischemia and insulin can all shift the body's myocardial energy substrate-use toward the preferential utilization of glucose, whereas fasting shifts energy metabolite use toward FFA utilization [42–45].

During periods of ischemia or states with increased plasma insulin levels, glucose transporters 1 and 4 (GLUT 1 and 4) are transported from intracellular storage to the plasma membrane, and lead to increased glucose uptake (and the preferential utilization of glucose as an energy substrate) by the cardiomyocyte [46, 47]. Furthermore, conditions of adrenergic stimulation or myocardial ischemia cause the process of FFA oxidation to decrease or even stop; hence, under these states, anaerobic glycolysis facilitates the use of glucose as the main substrate of myocardial energy [42, 44]. Thus, in hibernating myocardium, glucose is preferentially used as the primary energy substrate of choice, and forms the basis of our ability to utilize ^{18}FDG PET for viability assessment.

While ^{18}FDG PET is often thought of as an assessment of myocardial glucose metabolism, more accurately, it is a surrogate marker for exogenous glucose uptake [48]. Once ^{18}FDG is transported into the cardiomyocyte, it is converted into ^{18}FDG-6-phosphate as part of the cellular metabolic pathway [49]. After this step occurs, the metabolite is then trapped and cannot continue further down the metabolic pathway, and the tracer thereby remains trapped within the cardiomyocyte [49].

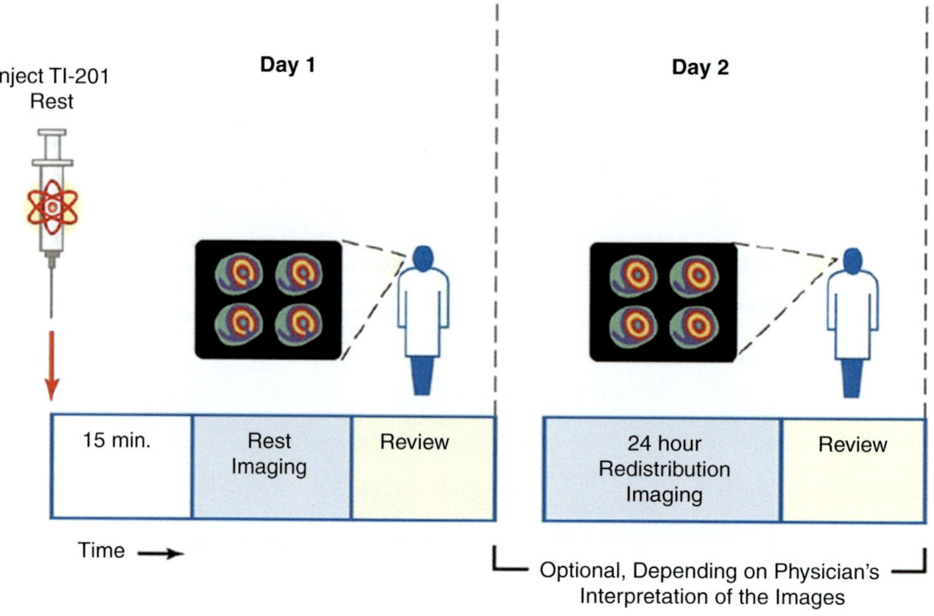

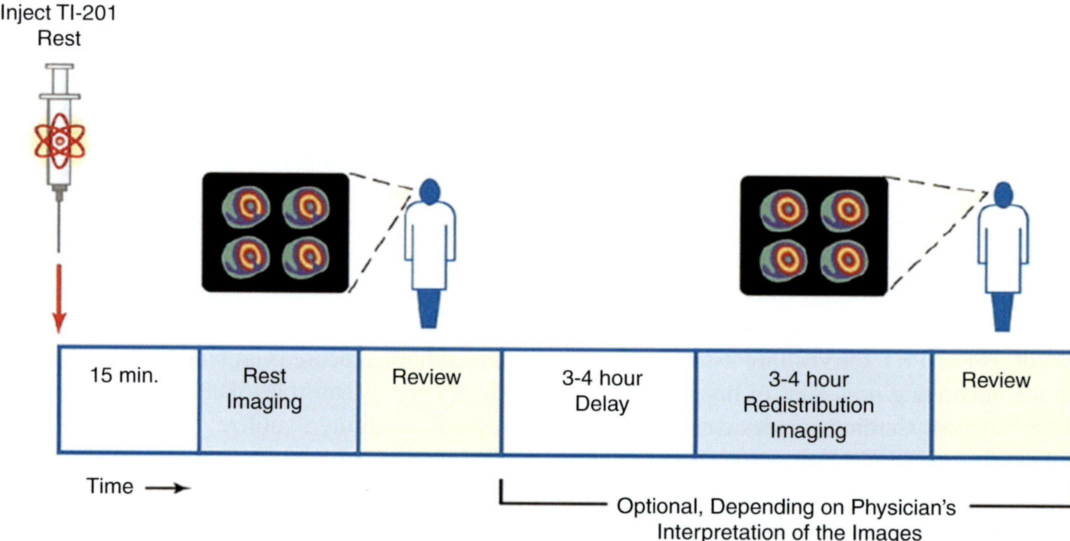

Fig. 20.2 ^{201}Tl rest-redistribution protocol for viability assessment, with permission from Henzlova et al. [38]. *Tl-201* Thallium-201

FDG PET Imaging Protocols

The imaging protocols to assess myocardial viability using PET are normally composed of two distinct and important components: (1) rest perfusion imaging performed with either nitrogen-13-ammonia (^{13}NH$_3$) or rubidium-82 (^{82}Rb) in North America; (oxygen-15-water is also used in Europe and Asia) and (2) metabolic imaging with ^{18}FDG [3]. Notably, if PET perfusion tracers are not available, then SPECT rest perfusion images

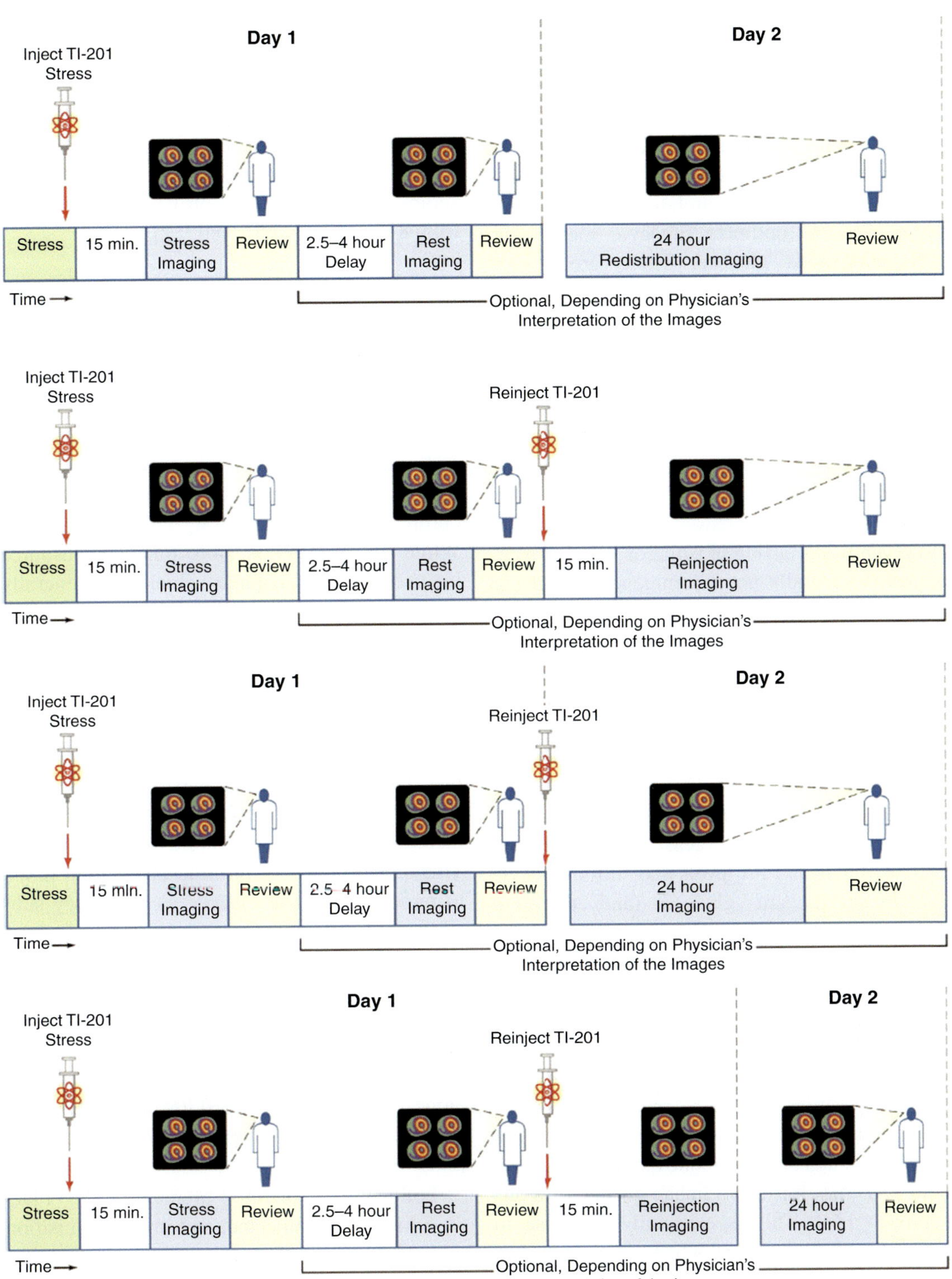

Fig. 20.3 ^{201}Tl stress–rest imaging protocols, with permission from Henzlova et al. [38]. *Tl-201* Thallium-201

(preferably with CT attenuation correction) can be used in their stead to compare with metabolic [18]FDG PET images [50].

Ensuring adequate and meticulous patient preparation for [18]FDG PET viability imaging is of the utmost importance to insure high-quality images for viability interpretation. Patient preparation aims to optimize myocyte metabolism with exogenous glucose. There are several options to achieve this:

Fasting Of the methods available to optimize the cardiomyocyte shift to glucose metabolism, fasting is the easiest from a technical-perspective. Under fasting conditions, normal myocardium consumes FFAs, while ischemic myocardium will preferentially use [18]FDG and will thereby appear as an area of increased uptake on imaging. However, using fasting in isolation of other techniques is generally not recommended, as it can lead to inferior image quality overall since normal myocardium will not take up FDG [51]. Rather, it is commonly used as part of a combined strategy to optimize glucose metabolism, with fasting being completed prior to either a glucose +/− insulin load, as outlined below [32, 52].

Glucose Loading Higher levels of plasma glucose stimulate insulin release, which thereby decreases plasma FFA levels and shifts myocyte metabolism toward glucose (and therefore [18]FDG) utilization. Thus, glucose loading can be used as a means to prepare patients for [18]FDG viability imaging. Following a fasting period of 6–12 h, an intravenous or oral glucose load is given [52]. [18]FDG is administered approximately 1 h after the initial glucose load [53]. A limitation with preparation protocols involving glucose loading can also relate to image quality; it has been shown that upward of one quarter of patients with CAD may have poor image quality with this approach [32]. This is especially the case in patients with diabetes or patients with impaired glucose tolerance. Thus, in these cases, intravenous (IV) insulin may need to be coadministered with the glucose load according to a sliding scale. Generally, the IV insulin is given 45–60 min following glucose administration and these corrective boluses are repeated every 15 min until a serum glucose level between 100 and 140 mg/dL (5.5–8 mmol/L) is achieved [52].

Hyperinsulinemic/Euglycemic Clamp A protocol using the hyperinsulinemic/euglycemic clamp strategy involves the simultaneous IV administration of both glucose and insulin. During the protocol, blood glucose levels must be closely monitored, and the infusions of glucose and insulin are adjusted and tailored to each patient to maintain tight blood glucose control to optimize viability imaging quality [32, 52]. While this strategy is more time and resource intensive, the image quality obtained is generally superior to the standard glucose loading protocol [53, 54]. Thus, while some centers use this protocol routinely, others reserve it solely for patients with diabetes.

Acipimox Acipimox is a nicotinic acid derivative that acts by inhibiting peripheral lipolysis which thereby reduces FFA availability and increases the relative availability of glucose [55]. This has the effect of priming myocardial tissue to preferentially use glucose as its energy substrate [56]. Literature has shown that Acipimox utilization provides image quality that is comparable to the hyperinsulinemic/euglycemic clamp strategy [54, 57]. In comparison, administration of nicotinic acid itself, or Niacin, can improve upon oral loading with supplemental insulin alone, but has demonstrated lower image quality than the hyperinsulinemic/euglycemic clamp [53, 58].

Following patient preparation, [18]FDG (3–5 MBq/kg) is injected, and image acquisition then undertaken 40–60 min later. The actual image acquisition period typically lasts 10–30 min in static (ungated), ECG-gated, or list-mode. Attenuation correction is used and images are reconstructed using an iterative statistical method [32, 59].

It is extremely important to compare the CT and PET images to ensure they are properly aligned, as misalignment of these images will create artifacts which could cause misinterpretation of the study. Similar to SPECT imaging, the [18]FDG images are reoriented and displayed in short-axis (SA), horizontal long axis (HLA) and vertical long axis (VLA). The [18]FDG metabolism images are normalized according to rest perfusion images. When interpretating the image sets, [18]FDG metabolism images are compared with rest perfusion images, in an analogous manner to how SPECT rest and stress images are compared [52] (Fig. 20.4).

Image Interpretation of FDG

When interpreting a PET viability imaging study, the metabolism images with [18]FDG are concurrently compared with the rest PET perfusion images that used either ^{13}N or [82]Rb. Of note, [18]FDG PET images can also be compared with resting images that are acquired from SPECT MPI [61]. However, this must be done cautiously, as error can be introduced when a non–attenuation-corrected SPECT myocardial perfusion image is being compared with an attenuation-corrected [18]FDG PET image.

There are four specific patterns of flow/metabolism that are described (Table 20.4) [62]:

1. Normal myocardial perfusion at rest and normal glucose metabolism—indicates viable, nonischemic myocardium at rest (if it is also dysfunctional this could be stunned or remodelled myocardium but is still viable).
2. Reduced rest perfusion with preserved (or partly preserved) metabolism (perfusion/metabolism mismatch)—indicates hibernating/viable myocardium.
3. Reduced rest perfusion and reduced metabolism (perfusion/metabolism match)—indicates nonviable myocardium or scar.
4. Normal myocardial perfusion with reduced metabolism (reverse mismatch)—this scenario can be seen in several different clinical scenarios such as patients with left bundle branch block with altered septal metabolism, patients with diabetes where glucose uptake is impaired in nonischemic tissue [63], in repetitive stunning [62], and also in patients who are early postrevascularization after an acute myocardial infarction [64–66] (Figs. 20.5 and 20.6).

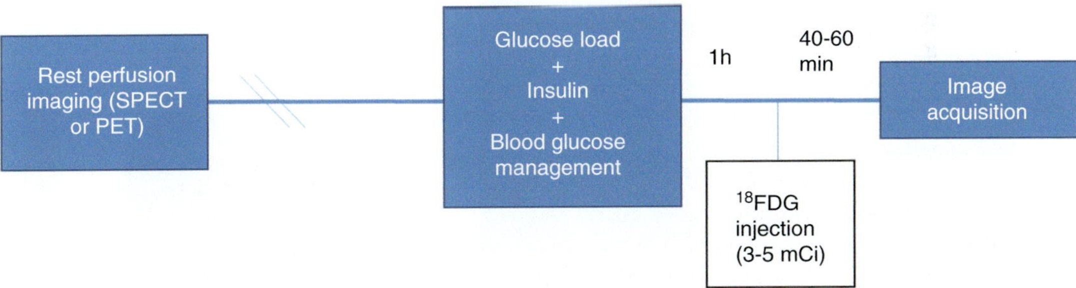

Fig. 20.4 PET viability protocol, with permission from Wiefels et al. [60]. *[18]FDG* 18F-fluorodeoxyglucose, *PET* positron emission tomography, *SPECT* single-photon emission computed tomography

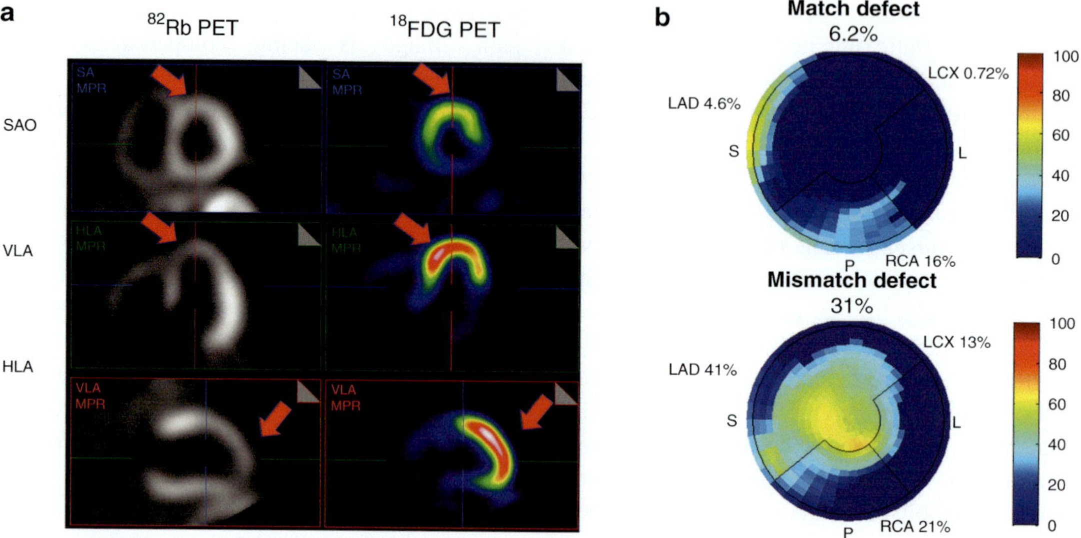

Fig. 20.5 (**a**) ^{13}N PET perfusion PET and [18]FDG metabolism PET in short axis, horizontal long axis and vertical long axis showing extensive area of mismatch in the mid to apical anteroseptal wall, inferoseptal wall and apex (red arrows). (**b**) Polar map with quantitative analysis of the amount of scar (match defect) (top) and hibernating myocardium (mismatch) (bottom). The patient was referred for revascularization

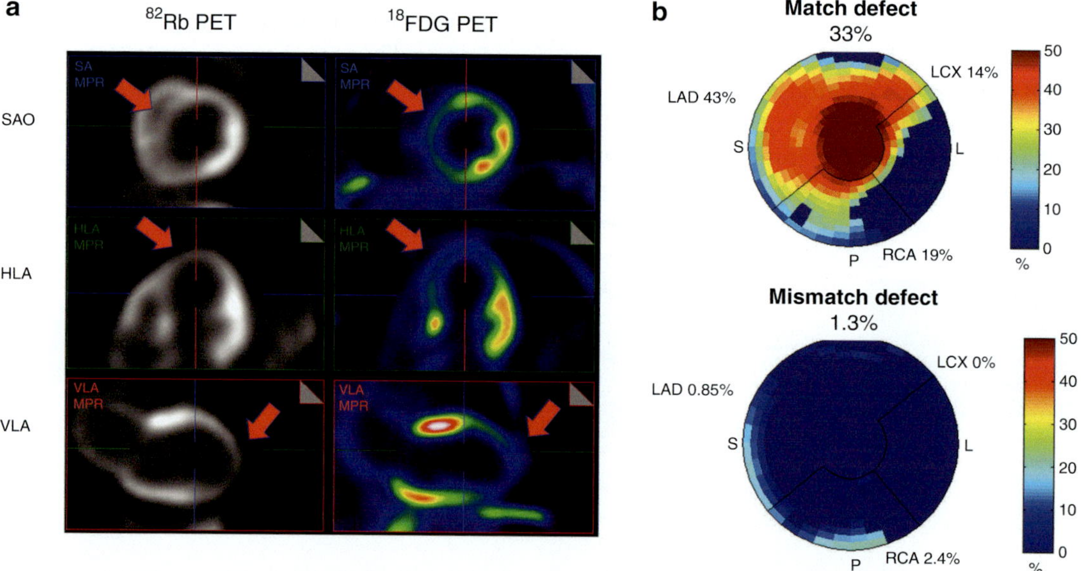

Fig. 20.6 (**a**) [82]Rb PET perfusion PET and [18]FDG metabolism PET in short axis (SAO), horizontal long axis (HLA) and vertical long axis (VLA) showing no significant mismatch (scar) in anterior wall and apex—24% of scar and <2% of hibernated myocardium. (**b**) Polar map with quantitative analysis of the amount of scar (match defect) (top) and hibernating myocardium (mismatch) (bottom)

Table 20.4 Imaging interpretation of FDG PET study

Perfusion	FDG uptake	Category	Clinical relevance
Preserved	Preserved	Normal—viable	Normal Stunning Ischemia (normal perfusion at rest and abnormal during stress—may benefit from revascularization)
Reduced	Preserved	Mismatch perfusion metabolism (hibernation myocardium)—viable	Likely to recover with adequate revascularization [4]; may be observed early post-MI or post-MI revascularization [67]
Reduced	Reduced	Scar (match)—nonviable	Unlikely to recover even with adequate revascularization [4]
Preserved	Reduced	Reverse mismatch	LBBB with altered septal metabolism in ischemic or nonischemic cardiomyopathy (may respond to CRT) [68], insulin resistance [69], repetitive stunning, may be observed post-MI revascularization [65]

Patterns of flow-glucose metabolism and clinical relevance
Adapted with permission from Erthal et al. [62]
CRT cardiac resynchronization therapy, *FDG* 18F-fluorodeoxyglucose, *LBBB* left bundle branch block, *MI* myocardial infarction

Cardiovascular Magnetic Resonance Imaging Methods for Assessing Viability

Cardiac magnetic resonance (CMR) imaging represents an emerging alternative tool to assess viability. CMR has the ability to assess a variety of markers that reflect myocardial viability including myocardial scar burden [70], coronary perfusion [71], and contractile reserve [72]. Assessment of coronary flow reserve, coronary anatomy and myocardial metabolism continue to be areas of active development [73].

CMR determines suspected hibernating myocardium by a combination of techniques including determining left ventricular end-diastolic thickness (LV EDWT), measuring the inotropic reserve of segmental contractile function, and using late-gadolinium enhancement agent to determine the extent of fibrosis [74].

End Diastolic Wall Thickness To Predict Functional Recovery

In the early days of CMR, neither perfusion nor late gadolinium enhancement (LGE) imaging were available. Viability assessments were necessarily crude and based on simple parameters such as wall motion and wall thickness, although neither were terribly reliable [75]. For example, the optimum sensitivity and specificity for a wall thickness of 8 mm or less to predict absence of metabolic activity on akinetic regions were 74% and 79% respectively. Other studies argued for a lower threshold of 5.4 mm, which had a 94% sensitivity but only 52% specificity for predicting segmental functional recovery after revascularization [76, 77].

Once LGE imaging became available at the start of the twenty-first century, investigators tried to refine the prediction rule by comparing total wall thickness and the extent of the unenhanced epicardial rim in infarct zones [78]. Doing so, Kuhl et al. were able to demonstrate that with a cutoff of wall thickness of 5.4 mm or below, sensitivity and specificity to exclude viability were 74% and 85%, respectively. However, prediction was improved further when looking at the extent of unenhanced epicardial rim, where a threshold of greater than 3 mm had a sensitivity and specificity to identify viability of 87% and 94%, respectively. In patients in whom there were divergent results at the segmental level between the two metrics, the unenhanced epicardial rim was the stronger predictor of viability, against a reference standard of FDG-PET.

Dobutamine CMR for Assessment of Contractile Reserve to Predict Functional Recovery

Low dose dobutamine (LDD) echo has already been mentioned. Similar attempts were made to employ LDD-CMR to establish contractile reserve in dysfunctional segments and hence further improve viability prediction. One early study from the mid 90s yielded diagnostic concordance of 89% for the presence of viability between dobutamine-induced contractile reserve (threshold >1 mm improvement) and FDG PET [77]. Again, dobutamine-induced wall thickening was a better predictor of residual metabolic activity (sensitivity, 81%; specificity, 95%; positive predictive accuracy, 96%) than was end-diastolic wall thickness (sensitivity, 72%; specificity, 89%; positive predictive accuracy, 91%).

Transmural Extent of Scar by LGE Imaging to Predict Functional Recovery

The development of gadolinium-based contrast agents, together with the inversion recovery imaging sequence for identifying scar, transformed the CMR world and redefined it from a niche academic pursuit to a clinical contender. Gadolinium is taken up into the extracellular space and washes out promptly under normal conditions. However, where the extracellular space is expanded due to edema or fibrosis from prior cell death, (or where contrast gains access to the intracellular space in the setting of cell death and ruptured cell membranes), then the usual temporal wash in/wash out dynamics are altered in these regions compared to healthy myocardium. The technique is therefore based upon administration of an IV gadolinium dose followed by a wait period of around 10 min prior to commencement of imaging. This allows for greater wash-out of gadolinium from healthy tissue, while injured myocardium retains relatively greater quantities due to both delayed wash-in and slower wash-out. An inversion recovery preparation pulse is then used to suppress the signal from healthy myocardium (often referred to as 'nulling') which appears dark/black. In comparison, irreversibly injured myocardium will be apparent as segmental regions of increased signal (white) which starts at the subendocardium with variable transmural extent toward the epicardium. Myocardium which is *dysfunctional* but does *not* show such increased signal (remains black) is therefore either stunned or hibernating. The transmural extent of scar from endo- to epicardium has been demonstrated to predict the likelihood of functional recovery of that segment following revascularization in a landmark paper by Judd and Kim in 2000. In essence, segments with little or minimal (<25%) transmural extent of scar have >90% chance of recovery if the subtending coronary artery is successfully grafted. Those dysfunctional segments with >50% transmural scar, on the other hand, have a <10% chance of recovery postrevascularization. Segments with 25–74% transmural scar are the most difficult to predict on an individual patient basis. Adding in LDD-CMR here may be useful, with a dobutamine contractile reserve of 1 grade improvement having a higher specificity to predict segmental recovery than transmural extent alone [79]. This seems to be a specific finding, but is less sensitive because even low dose dobutamine may induce ischemia and worsen wall motion, thereby confusing the overall picture. It may therefore be more reliable to use lower doses of dobutamine (2.5–5 µg/kg/min) over longer infusion periods to evoke recruitability without provoking ischemia. When comparing CMR techniques for overall accuracy in viability assessment, meta-analysis indicates that LGE transmural extent provides the highest sensitivity at 95%, whereas LDD is the most specific at 91% [80].

Future Prospects for Metabolic and Hybrid CMR to Predict Functional Recovery

There are ongoing attempts to further the field of viability imaging by CMR and these include imaging the resonance signal from nuclei other than hydrogen, including Na^{23}. At higher field strengths, sodium imaging may represent an option for assessing cellular metabolites and has been shown to be able to differentiate viable myocardium from infarcted muscle [81–83]. The primary limitations currently for the use of this technique is low signal-to-noise ratio, low spatial resolution, and exceedingly long time for acquisition [84]. Other areas under active exploration include metabolic imaging using hyperpolarization CMR, CMR spectroscopy and chemical exchange saturation transfer (CEST) CMR, often in combination with deep learning techniques to enhance the relatively limited signal inherent to these techniques [85]. As always, these techniques are more difficult to apply to the heart than to stationary tissues where most work has been focussed.

The success of PET/CT has also raised interest in the combination of CMR with PET imaging; this allows for the use of the metabolic information from PET associated with the superior soft tissue resolution and lower radiation from CMR [86]. Although it offers several theoretical advantages, accurate attenuation correction can prove challenging and the overall scan times are long, since most CMR sequences require breath-holding and therefore can not be run during the free breathing PET acquisition. More data is needed to evaluate this modality directly against PET-CT and to determine the clinical and economic impacts of its potential use [86].

Evidence for the Role of Viability Imaging

There is now robust data that has individually evaluated the ability of all different modalities of viability imaging to determine LV functional recovery. Observational data has shown that nuclear imaging, dobutamine echo, and MRI viability have all demonstrated the ability to predict LV functional recovery and outcome benefit. To this end, in a systematic review and meta-analysis that compared the various viability modalities that are commonly available, ^{18}FDG PET emerged as the most sensitive modality to predict functional recovery following revascularization when it was compared against ^{201}Tl and ^{99m}Tc scintigraphy, dobutamine echocardiography, and CMR [4]. The pooled analysis of 24 studies of 756 patients demonstrated a mean sensitivity of 92%, specificity of 63%, positive predictive value of 74%, and negative predictive value of 87% with ^{18}FDG PET [4]. Conversely, dobutamine echocardiography emerged as the most specific test for prediction of LV functional recovery [4]. Notably, CMR was underrepresented in this early systematic review, and more recent repeat studies have shown that DE-MRI is also highly sensitive, while low-dose dobutamine CMR retains greater specificity [80].

There is unfortunately a paucity of available prospective literature for the assessment of viability, as only a select handful of trials have been completed. However, we will cover the landmark trials and prospective literature that is available.

The PARR-2 trial (Positron emission tomography and recovery following revascularization Phase 2) is one of the largest prospective trials to date that evaluated a viability assessment modality in the ability to predict functional recovery postrevascularization. PARR-2 randomized 430 patients from 9 centers to undergo ^{18}FDG PET or standard of care before revascularization decisions [7]. Patients were followed for cardiac death, myocardial infarction (MI), and cardiac hospitalization at 1 year. While no statistically significant difference between the two groups was observed for the primary outcome (RR 0.82; $p = 0.16$, and HR 0.78; $p = 0.15$), a prespecified secondary analysis showed that patients who had not had recent angiography had a mortality benefit with therapy directed by FDG PET. In addition, for the primary outcome it was noted that recommendations from the viability imaging results were not used consistently in revascularization decisions in approximately 25% of patients [7]. Thus, the study results were reanalyzed in a post hoc analysis that evaluated the subgroup of patients where the revascularization decisions were indeed guided on the imaging results. In this analysis, it was discovered that there was a significant reduction in adverse outcomes in the [18]FDG arm (HR 0.62; $p = 0.019$) [7]. Another post hoc examination of the PARR-2 data showed that among 182 patients who underwent [18]FDG PET, patients with a larger burden of viable tissue derived greater benefit from revascularization. This finding was mirrored by Ling et al., who also found that an increasing size of hibernating myocardium territory was associated with increasing benefit of revascularization [12]. In the 5-year follow-up of PARR-2, data again demonstrated that when PET recommendations regarding revascularization decisions were followed, the primary outcome of cardiac death, myocardial infarction, or cardiac hospitalization was reduced, with an HR of 0.73 (95% CI 0.54–0.99; $p = 0.042$) (Figs. 20.7 and 20.8) [11].

The Ottawa-FIVE substudy was a further evaluation of the PARR2 data that examined 111 patients from a single recruiting center (Ottawa) which had a particular expertise in viability assessment, readily available access to [18]FDG PET viability imaging, and integration between the imaging, heart failure and revascularization teams [13]. In this substudy, it was shown that the proportion of events in the PET-assisted management group was greatly reduced compared to the standard care group (19% vs. 41% events, respectively) suggesting that outcome benefit can be achieved in an experienced center with a team-based approach [13, 87].

While a large body of literature does support the utility of viability imaging to guide revascularization decisions [7, 8, 13, 24, 88–90], there has also been evidence to the contrary. Siebelink et al. compared the ability of viability imaging with ^{13}N-ammonia/[18]FDG PET against ^{99m}Tc-sestamibi SPECT viability imaging to guide therapy in a small randomized trial of 112 patients [91]. They observed no difference in cardiac

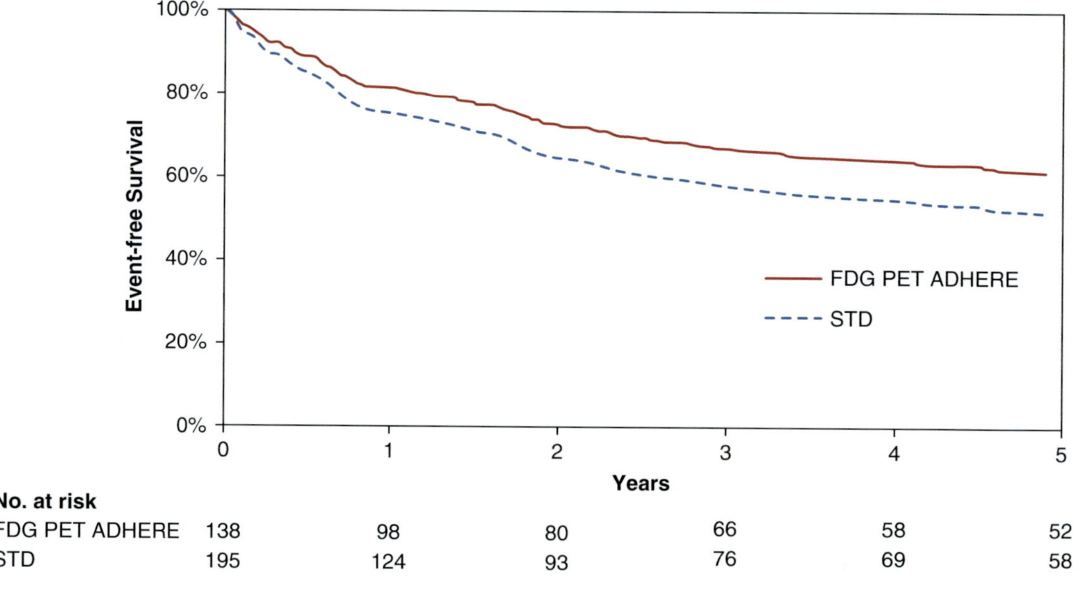

Fig. 20.7 5-year follow-up of PARR-2 data showing risk-adjusted, event-free survival curves for time-to-composite event for patients who adhered to PET imaging recommendations (FDG PET Adhere) versus standard care (STD) in patients randomized at sites participating in long-term follow-up. Hazard ratio = 0.73 (95% CI 0.54–0.99; $P = 0.042$). (With permission from McArdle et al. [11]). No at risk = number of patients who had not died, not been transplanted not dropped out, and not had events. Seven patients whose last follow-up date was within 10 days of 1825 days (5 years) were included in the 5-year total. *CI* indicates confidence interval, *FDG PET* F-18-fluorodeoxyglucose positron emission tomography, *STD* standard care

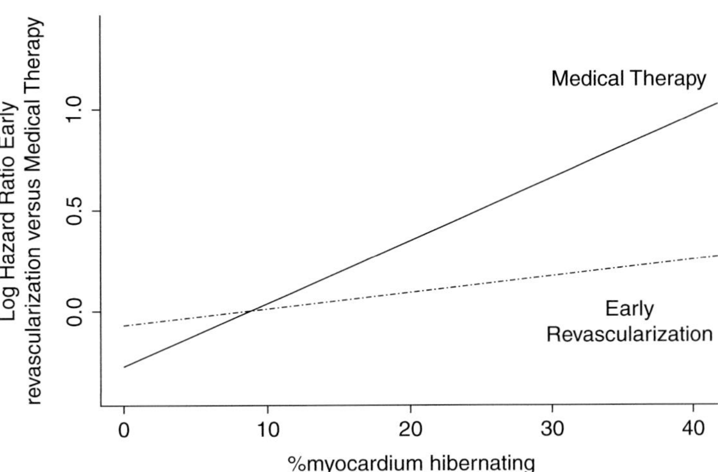

Fig. 20.8 Relationship between percent of myocardium that is hibernating and adjusted hazard ratio for patients treated with early revascularization vs. medical therapy. Risk increases as a function of percent myocardium hibernation in medically treated patients. Percent myocardium hibernation–treatment interaction; $P = 0.0009$. (Reproduced with permission from Ling et al. [12])

event-free survival (cardiac death, MI, and revascularization) between the PET and SPECT arms [91]. Importantly, it should be noted that only 35% of their trial population had severe LV dysfunction, and the study was also likely underpowered to detect any meaningful difference between the groups, given the low overall event rates [92].

The STICH trial randomized 1212 patients to either optimal medical therapy (OMT) or OMT plus revascularization [93]. Of these patients, roughly half underwent myocardial viability assessment with either SPECT or dobutamine echocardiography, but viability imaging was actually not part of randomization [93]. Although the unadjusted hazard ratio (HR) for mortality in the viable myocardial group was 0.64 ($p = 0.003$), after adjusting for the baseline characteristics of the participants, the association lost significance ($p = 0.21$), thereby suggesting a lack of benefit of myocardial viability assessment [93]. In the STICH Extension Study (STICHES), after 10 years, outcome benefit was demonstrated in the CABG arm [94]. As well, better outcomes were observed in patients who had myocardium viability on imaging if they had CABG [95]. The authors were not able to show that there was an interaction between revascularization and viability detection.

If one takes a cursory look at the "one-line conclusion" from PARR-2 and STICH, the results appear to yield conflicting results. However, care and nuance must be taken into consideration when properly interpreting the data in light of the methodologies of the studies. Firstly, the trial design and baseline study populations differed between these two trials. The PARR-2 trial was designed to randomize patients with uncertain revascularization strategies to either standard of care or viability assessment [7]. Thus, an assessment of myocardial viability was clinically used in these patients to assist in revascularization decision-making in the FDG arm. Conversely, while the STICH trial randomized to CABG versus medical therapy, viability imaging was not randomized per se; patients were already considered acceptable candidates for revascularization (and therefore had known suitable anatomy for revascularization). Therefore, these participants had no clinical need for viability imaging. Furthermore, the PARR-2 trial participants were more comorbid—specifically with a higher proportion of patients with renal dysfunction and a higher number of patients with previous CABG [93, 96]. One last additional, and major, limitation of the STICH trial was the fact that viability assessment did not include either PET or CMR—two methods that are considered to have the highest sensitivity in the detection of viable myocardium.

Both PARR2 and STICH(ES) point to the fact that viability imaging should not be used in most patients with ischemic cardiomyopathy. However, an argument can be made that viability imaging may be an additional factor to weigh in the clinical context of benefit and risk in patients where therapy decisions are most challenging. While current guidelines do support the use of viability imaging to assist in guiding decision-making with respect to revascularization in patients with CAD and LV dysfunction [97–99], further questions remain in the field. Both a multicenter trial [100] as well as a registry [101] may help answer some of these questions. The Alternative Imaging Modalities Ischemic Heart Failure (AIMI-HF) IMAGE HF trial includes centers from North America, Europe and Latin America and is comparing the use of SPECT imaging versus advanced imaging modalities (including PET and CMR) to guide HF therapy [100]. While a common scenario is for centers to rely on local expertise to guide therapy, it is clear that this process is subject to the bias and personal experience of the local imaging physician, cardiologist and cardiac surgeon. Thus, while many questions remain in the field, hopefully these current trials will help to shed light on the role that viability imaging can and should play in the revascularization decision-making algorithm for patients with ischemic heart disease.

Future Directions

The combination of PET with CMR imaging may allow for the utilization of the strength of each of these modalities in viability assessment. While CMR evaluates fibrotic tissue and/or myocardial contractile reserve, PET assessment focuses on metabolic markers and evaluates myocardial perfusion. Thus, by fusing PET/MRI, this information can be integrated together. However, the additional benefit of this strategy is not yet known. Early data suggests that this approach is feasible, and parameters can predict regional recovery, although the FDG uptake portion may be a better predictor early after MI [102]. However, for CTO, the combination of FDG PET and MRI appears better than either alone [103].

Research has demonstrated that hibernating myocardium may increase a patient's risk for sudden cardiac death [104], and this may be mediated through heterogeneity in sympathetic innervation (which can be measured by ^{11}C-hydroxyexphendrine (HED) PET or Tc-99 m MIBG SPECT–(tracers that are specific for sympathetic presynaptic nerve function) [105]. In the PAREPET study, it was demonstrated that HED PET done in conjunction with FDG PET for viability could successfully assess myocardial denervation and predict risk of sudden cardiac death [106]. However, future studies are needed in order to shed further light on the potential role that neurohormonal imaging could play in assisting revascularization-based decision-making. PAREPET II (clincialtrials.gov NCT03493516) evaluates F-18 flubrobenguane, another false neurotransmitter tracer that identifies sympathetic nerve function similar to HED [107] that could be more widely distributed as an F-18 tracer due to its longer half-life.

Viability imaging may play a role in optimizing patient selection for CTO revascularization [108]. However, the exact role of the testing and selection of patients who would benefit from a viability assessment as well as how the results could be best utilized is not clear at present. Two ongoing trials, NOBLE-CTO (The Nordic-Baltic Randomized Registry Study for the Evaluation of PCI in Chronic Total Coronary Occlusion; NCT03392415) and ISCHEMIA-CTO (Revascularization or Optimal Medical Therapy of CTO; NCT03564317 will help answer these questions. Also, a recent PET/MRI study suggests that the hybrid approach is more accurate to predict recovery than either approach alone [103].

Conclusion

Ischemic cardiomyopathy is a leading cause of morbidity and mortality worldwide [1]. Decision-making regarding revascularization for patients with ischemic cardiomyopathy is fraught with difficulties and nuances; patients with ischemic heart failure often have multiple comorbidities and have high risks associated with revascularization. Viability assessment with nuclear imaging can enable clinicians to individually tailor

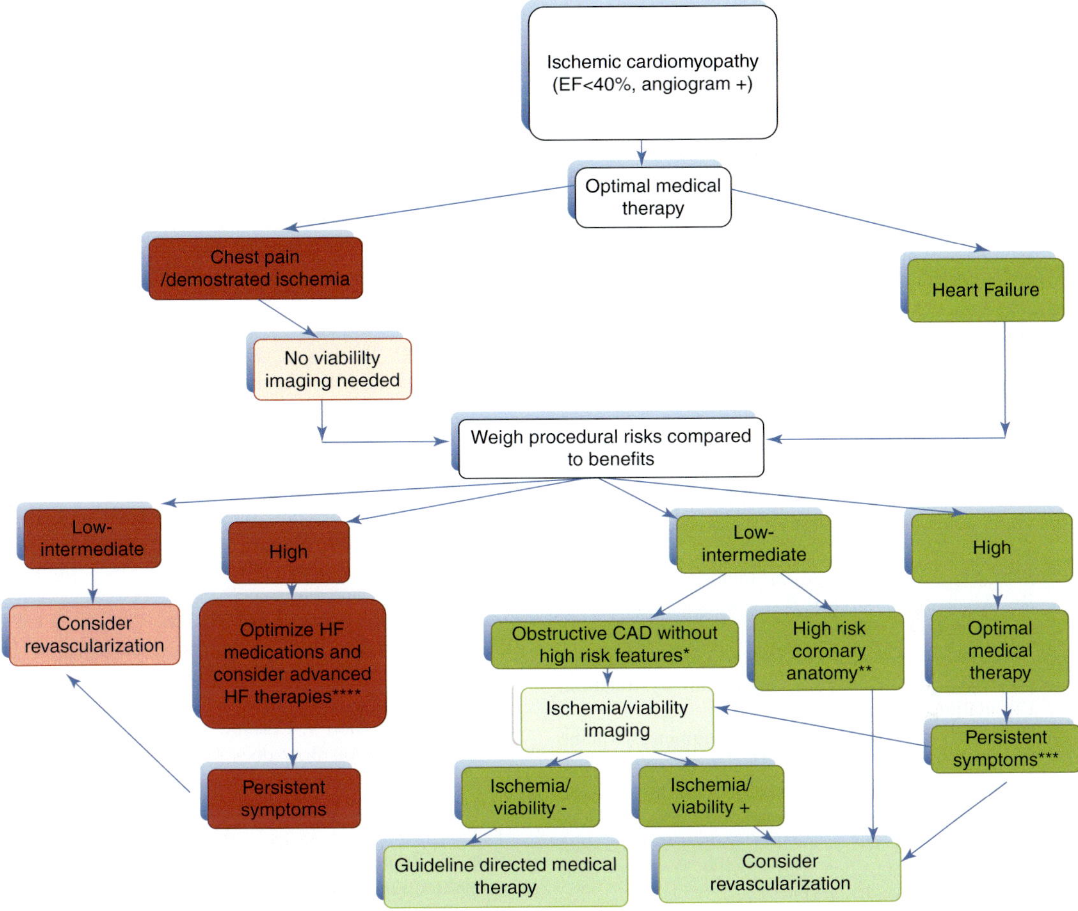

Fig. 20.9 Proposed algorithm for the integration of ischemia/viability testing in guiding revascularization decisions in ischemic cardiomyopathy. (Reproduced with permission from Kandolin et al., CJC 2019 [3]). Based on Neumann et al. [109] and the clinical evidence from observational data and guidelines discussed in this article. *including chronic total occlusions. ** >50% left main/ proximal left anterior descending (LAD) coronary artery stenosis. ***ischemia/viability testing may be considered depending on patient, anatomy, targets, and revascularization risk. ****For eligible candidates. *EF* ejection fraction, *CAD* coronary artery disease, (+) presence of, (−) absence of

recommendations for their patients and help guide choices between pursuing revascularization versus pursuing medical therapy alone. A suggested algorithm regarding patient selection for viability imaging is shown in Fig. 20.9.

Acknowledgments and Disclosures KEB is a cardiology resident at the University of Ottawa Heart Institute and holds a Canadian Institutes of Health Research Fellowship (FRN: **171284**).

RSB was a career investigator supported by the Heart and Stroke Foundation of Ontario; is a distinguished research chair supported by the University of Ottawa, and the University of Ottawa Heart Institute's Vered chair in cardiology. He receives research support and honoraria from Lantheus Medical Imaging, Jubilant DraxImage and GE.

AMC is a consultant cardiologist at the University of Ottawa Heart Institute and is on the speakers bureau for Bristol Myers Squibb on matters relating to hypertrophic cardiomyopathy.

CW was cardiac imaging fellow at the University of Ottawa Heart Institute and holds an UOHI Division of Cardiology Kaufman-Chan Endowed Fellowship.

RdK is a consultant for Jubilant DraxImage, and receives license revenues from Jubilant DraxImage and INVIA Medical Solutions.

References

1. Writing Group M, Mozaffarian D, Benjamin EJ, Go AS, Arnett DK, Blaha MJ, et al. Heart disease and stroke statistics-2016 update: a report from the American Heart Association. Circulation. 2016;133(4):e38–360.

2. Levy D, Kenchaiah S, Larson MG, Benjamin EJ, Kupka MJ, Ho KK, et al. Long-term trends in the incidence of and survival with heart failure. N Engl J Med. 2002;347(18):1397–402.

3. Kandolin RM, Wiefels CC, Mesquita CT, Chong AY, Boland P, Glineur D, et al. The current role of viability imaging to guide revascularization and therapy decisions in patients with heart failure and reduced left ventricular function. Can J Cardiol. 2019;35(8):1015–29.

4. Schinkel AF, Bax JJ, Poldermans D, Elhendy A, Ferrari R, Rahimtoola SH. Hibernating myocardium: diagnosis and patient outcomes. Curr Probl Cardiol. 2007;32(7):375–410.

5. Lim SP, Mc Ardle BA, Beanlands RS, Hessian RC. Myocardial viability: it is still alive. Semin Nucl Med. 2014;44(5):358–74.

6. Braunwald E, Kloner RA. The stunned myocardium: prolonged, postischemic ventricular dysfunction. Circulation. 1982;66(6):1146–9.

7. Beanlands RS, Nichol G, Huszti E, Humen D, Racine N, Freeman M, et al. F-18-fluorodeoxyglucose positron emission tomography imaging-assisted management of patients with severe left ventricular dysfunction and suspected coronary disease: a randomized, controlled trial (PARR-2). J Am Coll Cardiol. 2007;50(20):2002–12.

8. D'Egidio G, Nichol G, Williams KA, Guo A, Garrard L, deKemp R, et al. Increasing benefit from revascularization is associated with increasing amounts of myocardial hibernation: a substudy of the PARR-2 trial. JACC Cardiovasc Imaging. 2009;2(9):1060–8.

9. Canty JM Jr, Fallavollita JA. Hibernating myocardium. J Nucl Cardiol. 2005;12(1):104–19.

10. Camici PG, Dutka DP. Repetitive stunning, hibernation, and heart failure: contribution of PET to establishing a link. Am J Physiol Heart Circ Physiol. 2001;280(3):H929–36.

11. Mc Ardle B, Shukla T, Nichol G, deKemp RA, Bernick J, Guo A, et al. Long-term follow-up of outcomes with F-18-fluorodeoxyglucose positron emission tomography imaging-assisted management of patients with severe left ventricular dysfunction secondary to coronary disease. Circ Cardiovasc Imaging. 2016;9(9):e004331.

12. Ling LF, Marwick TH, Flores DR, Jaber WA, Brunken RC, Cerqueira MD, et al. Identification of therapeutic benefit from revascularization in patients with left ventricular systolic dysfunction: inducible ischemia versus hibernating myocardium. Circ Cardiovasc Imaging. 2013;6(3):363–72.

13. Abraham A, Nichol G, Williams KA, Guo A, deKemp RA, Garrard L, et al. 18F-FDG PET imaging of myocardial viability in an experienced center with access to 18F-FDG and integration with clinical management teams: the Ottawa-FIVE substudy of the PARR 2 trial. J Nucl Med. 2010;51(4):567–74.

14. Mc Ardle BA, Beanlands RS. Myocardial viability: whom, what, why, which, and how? Can J Cardiol. 2013;29(3):399–402.

15. Nihoyannopoulos P, Vanoverschelde JL. Myocardial ischaemia and viability: the pivotal role of echocardiography. Eur Heart J. 2011;32(7):810–9.

16. Erthal F, Wiefels C, Promislow S, Kandolin R, Stadnick E, Mielniczuk L, et al. Myocardial viability: from PARR-2 to IMAGE HF–current evidence and future directions. Int J Cardiovasc Sci. 2019;32(1):70–83.

17. Kaul S. Myocardial contrast echocardiography: a 25-year retrospective. Circulation. 2008;118(3):291–308.

18. Camici PG, Prasad SK, Rimoldi OE. Stunning, hibernation, and assessment of myocardial viability. Circulation. 2008;117(1):103–14.

19. Velazquez EJ, Bonow RO. Revascularization in severe left ventricular dysfunction. J Am Coll Cardiol. 2015;65(6):615–24.

20. Bax JJ, Delgado V. Chronic total occlusion without collateral blood flow does not exclude myocardial viability and subsequent recovery after revascularization. J Nucl Cardiol. 2019;26(5):1731–3.

21. Wang L, Lu MJ, Feng L, Wang J, Fang W, He ZX, et al. Relationship of myocardial hibernation, scar, and angiographic collateral flow in ischemic cardiomyopathy with coronary chronic total occlusion. J Nucl Cardiol. 2019;26(5):1720–30.

22. Geleijnse ML, Fioretti PM, Roelandt JR. Methodology, feasibility, safety and diagnostic accuracy of dobutamine stress echocardiography. J Am Coll Cardiol. 1997;30(3):595–606.

23. Underwood SR. Imaging techniques in the assessment of myocardial hibernation. Eur J Nucl Med Mol Imaging. 2004;31(8):1209; author reply 10-1.

24. Allman KC, Shaw LJ, Hachamovitch R, Udelson JE. Myocardial viability testing and impact of revascularization on prognosis in patients with coronary artery disease and left ventricular dysfunction: a meta-analysis. J Am Coll Cardiol. 2002;39(7):1151–8.

25. Grunwald AM, Watson DD, Holzgrefe HH Jr, Irving JF, Beller GA. Myocardial thallium-201 kinetics in normal and ischemic myocardium. Circulation. 1981;64(3):610–8.

26. Bisi G, Sciagra R, Santoro GM, Fazzini PF. Rest technetium-99m sestamibi tomography in combination with short-term administration of nitrates: feasibility and reliability for prediction of postrevascularization outcome of asynergic territories. J Am Coll Cardiol. 1994;24(5):1282–9.

27. Bisi G, Sciagra R, Santoro GM, Rossi V, Fazzini PF. Technetium-99m-sestamibi imaging with nitrate infusion to detect viable hibernating myocardium and predict postrevascularization recovery. J Nucl Med. 1995;36(11):1994–2000.

28. Sciagra R, Bisi G, Santoro GM, Zerauschek F, Sestini S, Pedenovi P, et al. Comparison of baseline-nitrate technetium-99m sestamibi with rest-redistribution thallium-201 tomography in detecting viable hibernating myocardium and predicting postrevascularization recovery. J Am Coll Cardiol. 1997;30(2):384–91.

29. Schneider CA, Voth E, Gawlich S, Baer FM, Horst M, Schicha H, et al. Significance of rest technetium-99m sestamibi imaging for the prediction of improvement of left ventricular dysfunction after Q wave myocardial infarction: importance of infarct location adjusted thresholds. J Am Coll Cardiol. 1998;32(3):648–54.

30. Maurea S, Cuocolo A, Soricelli A, Castelli L, Nappi A, Squame F, et al. Enhanced detection of viable myocardium by technetium-99m-MIBI imaging after nitrate administration in chronic coronary artery disease. J Nucl Med. 1995;36(11):1945–52.

31. Galli M, Marcassa C, Imparato A, Campini R, Orrego PS, Giannuzzi P. Effects of nitroglycerin by technetium-99m sestamibi tomoscintigraphy on resting regional myocardial hypoperfusion in stable patients with healed myocardial infarction. Am J Cardiol. 1994;74(9):843–8.

32. Hesse B, Tagil K, Cuocolo A, Anagnostopoulos C, Bardies M, Bax J, et al. EANM/ESC procedural guidelines for myocardial perfusion imaging in nuclear cardiology. Eur J Nucl Med Mol Imaging. 2005;32(7):855–97.

33. Bonow RO, Dilsizian V, Cuocolo A, Bacharach SL. Identification of viable myocardium in patients with chronic coronary artery disease and left ventricular dysfunction. Comparison of thallium scintigraphy with reinjection and PET imaging with 18F-fluorodeoxyglucose. Circulation. 1991;83(1):26–37.

34. Gutman J, Berman DS, Freeman M, Rozanski A, Maddahi J, Waxman A, et al. Time to completed redistribution of thallium-201 in exercise myocardial scintigraphy: relationship to the degree of coronary artery stenosis. Am Heart J. 1983;106(5 Pt 1):989–95.

35. Kiat H, Berman DS, Maddahi J, De Yang L, Van Train K, Rozanski A, et al. Late reversibility of tomographic myocardial thallium-201 defects: an accurate marker of myocardial viability. J Am Coll Cardiol. 1988;12(6):1456–63.

36. Cloninger KG, DePuey EG, Garcia EV, Roubin GS, Robbins WL, Nody A, et al. Incomplete redistribution in delayed thallium-201 single photon emission computed tomographic (SPECT) images: an overestimation of myocardial scarring. J Am Coll Cardiol. 1988;12(4):955–63.

37. Yang LD, Berman DS, Kiat H, Resser KJ, Friedman JD, Rozanski A, et al. The frequency of late reversibility in SPECT thallium-201 stress-redistribution studies. J Am Coll Cardiol. 1990;15(2):334–40.

38. Henzlova MJ, Duvall WL, Einstein AJ, Travin MI, Verberne HJ. ASNC imaging guidelines for SPECT nuclear cardiology procedures: stress, protocols, and tracers. J Nucl Cardiol. 2016;23(3):606–39.

39. Camici P, Ferrannini E, Opie LH. Myocardial metabolism in ischemic heart disease: basic principles and application to imaging by positron emission tomography. Prog Cardiovasc Dis. 1989;32(3):217–38.

40. Depre C, Vanoverschelde JL, Taegtmeyer H. Glucose for the heart. Circulation. 1999;99(4):578–88.

41. Neely JR, Morgan HE. Relationship between carbohydrate and lipid metabolism and the energy balance of heart muscle. Annu Rev Physiol. 1974;36:413–59.

42. Liedtke AJ. Alterations of carbohydrate and lipid metabolism in the acutely ischemic heart. Prog Cardiovasc Dis. 1981;23(5):321–36.

43. Stanley WC, Lopaschuk GD, Hall JL, McCormack JG. Regulation of myocardial carbohydrate metabolism under normal and ischaemic conditions: potential for pharmacological interventions. Cardiovasc Res. 1997;33(2):243–57.

44. Goodwin GW, Ahmad F, Doenst T, Taegtmeyer H. Energy provision from glycogen, glucose, and fatty acids on adrenergic stimulation of isolated working rat hearts. Am J Physiol. 1998;274(4):H1239–47.

45. Barger PM, Kelly DP. PPAR signaling in the control of cardiac energy metabolism. Trends Cardiovasc Med. 2000;10(6):238–45.

46. Mueckler M. Facilitative glucose transporters. Eur J Biochem. 1994;219(3):713–25.

47. Egert S, Nguyen N, Schwaiger M. Myocardial glucose transporter GLUT1: translocation induced by insulin and ischemia. J Mol Cell Cardiol. 1999;31(7):1337–44.

48. Dilsizian V. 18F-FDG uptake as a surrogate marker for antecedent ischemia. J Nucl Med. 2008;49(12):1909–11.

49. Avril N. GLUT1 expression in tissue and (18)F-FDG uptake. J Nucl Med. 2004;45(6):930–2.

50. Beanlands RS, Ruddy TD, deKemp RA, Iwanochko RM, Coates G, Freeman M, et al. Positron emission tomography and recovery following revascularization (PARR-1): the importance of scar and the development of a prediction rule for the degree of recovery of left ventricular function. J Am Coll Cardiol. 2002;40(10):1735–43.

51. Berry JJ, Baker JA, Pieper KS, Hanson MW, Hoffman JM, Coleman RE. The effect of metabolic milieu on cardiac PET imaging using fluorine-18-deoxyglucose and nitrogen-13-ammonia in normal volunteers. J Nucl Med. 1991;32(8):1518–25.

52. Bacharach SL, Bax JJ, Case J, Delbeke D, Kurdziel KA, Martin WH, et al. PET myocardial glucose metabolism and perfusion imaging: Part 1-Guidelines for data acquisition and patient preparation. J Nucl Cardiol. 2003;10(5):543–56.

53. Vitale GD, deKemp RA, Ruddy TD, Williams K, Beanlands RS. Myocardial glucose utilization and optimization of (18)F-FDG PET imaging in patients with non-insulin-dependent diabetes mellitus, coronary artery disease, and left ventricular dysfunction. J Nucl Med. 2001;42(12):1730–6.

54. Knuuti MJ, Yki-Jarvinen H, Voipio-Pulkki LM, Maki M, Ruotsalainen U, Harkonen R, et al. Enhancement of myocardial [fluorine-18]fluorodeoxyglucose uptake by a nicotinic acid derivative. J Nucl Med. 1994;35(6):989–98.

55. Vosper H. Niacin: a re-emerging pharmaceutical for the treatment of dyslipidaemia. Br J Pharmacol. 2009;158(2):429–41.

56. Hannah JS, Bodkin NL, Paidi MS, Anh-Le N, Howard BV, Hansen BC. Effects of Acipimox on the metabolism of free fatty acids and very low lipoprotein triglyceride. Acta Diabetol. 1995;32(4):279–83.

57. Bax JJ, Veening MA, Visser FC, van Lingen A, Heine RJ, Cornel JH, et al. Optimal metabolic conditions during fluorine-18 fluorodeoxyglucose imaging; a comparative study using different protocols. Eur J Nucl Med. 1997;24(1):35–41.

58. Knuuti MJ, Nuutila P, Ruotsalainen U, Saraste M, Harkonen R, Ahonen A, et al. Euglycemic hyperinsulinemic clamp and oral glucose load in stimulating myocardial glucose utilization during positron emission tomography. J Nucl Med. 1992;33(7):1255–62.

59. Dilsizian V, Bacharach SL, Beanlands RS, Bergmann SR, Delbeke D, Dorbala S, et al. ASNC imaging guidelines/SNMMI procedure standard for positron emission tomography (PET) nuclear cardiology procedures. J Nucl Cardiol. 2016;23(5):1187–226.

60. Wiefels C, Kandolin R, Small GR, Beanlands R. PET and SPECT evaluation of viable dysfunctional myocardium. In: Mesquita CT, Rezende MF, editors. Nuclear cardiology. Berlin: Springer; 2021.

61. Schelbert HR, Beanlands R, Bengel F, Knuuti J, Dicarli M, Machac J, et al. PET myocardial perfusion and glucose metabolism imaging: Part 2-Guidelines for interpretation and reporting. J Nucl Cardiol. 2003;10(5):557–71.

62. Erthal F, Aleksova N, Chong AY, de Kemp RA, Beanlands RSB. Microvascular function, is there a link to myocardial viability: is this another piece to the puzzle? J Nucl Cardiol. 2017;24(5):1651–6.

63. Paternostro G, Camici PG, Lammerstma AA, Marinho N, Baliga RR, Kooner JS, et al. Cardiac and skeletal muscle insulin resistance in patients with coronary heart disease. A study with positron emission tomography. J Clin Invest. 1996;98(9):2094–9.

64. Ghosh N, Rimoldi OE, Beanlands RS, Camici PG. Assessment of myocardial ischaemia and viability: role of positron emission tomography. Eur Heart J. 2010;31(24):2984–95.

65. Anselm DD, Anselm AH, Renaud J, Atkins HL, de Kemp R, Burwash IG, et al. Altered myocardial glucose utilization and the reverse mismatch pattern on rubidium-82 perfusion/F-18-FDG PET during the sub-acute phase following reperfusion of acute anterior myocardial infarction. J Nucl Cardiol. 2011;18(4):657–67.

66. Thompson K, Saab G, Birnie D, Chow BJ, Ukkonen H, Ananthasubramaniam K, et al. Is septal glucose metabolism altered in patients with left bundle branch block and ischemic cardiomyopathy? J Nucl Med. 2006;47(11):1763–8.

67. Fukuoka Y, Nakano A, Tama N, Hasegawa K, Ikeda H, Morishita T, et al. Impaired myocardial microcirculation in the flow-glucose metabolism mismatch regions in revascularized acute myocardial infarction. J Nucl Cardiol. 2017;24(5):1641–50.

68. Birnie D, de Kemp RA, Tang AS, Ruddy TD, Gollob MH, Guo A, et al. Reduced septal glucose metabolism predicts response to cardiac resynchronization therapy. J Nucl Cardiol. 2012;19(1):73–83.

69. Hansen AK, Gejl M, Bouchelouche K, Tolbod LP, Gormsen LC. Reverse mismatch pattern in cardiac 18F-FDG viability PET/CT is not associated with poor outcome of revascularization: a retrospective outcome study of 91 patients with heart failure. Clin Nucl Med. 2016;41(10):e428–35.

70. Marti V, Ballester M, Udina C, Carrio I, Alvarez E, Obrador D, et al. Evaluation of myocardial cell damage by In-111-monoclonal antimyosin antibodies in patients under chronic tricyclic antidepressant drug treatment. Circulation. 1995;91(6):1619–23.

71. Gewirtz H, Dilsizian V. Myocardial viability: survival mechanisms and molecular imaging targets in acute and chronic ischemia. Circ Res. 2017;120(7):1197–212.

72. Kalra DK, Zhu X, Ramchandani MK, Lawrie G, Reardon MJ, Lee-Jackson D, et al. Increased myocardial gene expression of tumor necrosis factor-alpha and nitric oxide synthase-2: a potential mechanism for depressed myocardial function in hibernating myocardium in humans. Circulation. 2002;105(13):1537–40.

73. Shan K, Constantine G, Sivananthan M, Flamm SD. Role of cardiac magnetic resonance imaging in the assessment of myocardial viability. Circulation. 2004;109(11):1328–34.

74. Garcia MJ, Kwong RY, Scherrer-Crosbie M, Taub CC, Blankstein R, Lima J, et al. State of the art: imaging for myocardial viability: a scientific statement from the American Heart Association. Circ Cardiovasc Imaging. 2020;13(7):e000053.

75. Perrone-Filardi P, Bacharach SL, Dilsizian V, Maurea S, Marin-Neto JA, Arrighi JA, et al. Metabolic evidence of viable myocardium in regions with reduced wall thickness and absent wall thickening in patients with chronic ischemic left ventricular dysfunction. J Am Coll Cardiol. 1992;20(1):161–8.

76. Baer FM, Smolarz K, Jungehulsing M, Beckwilm J, Theissen P, Sechtem U, et al. Chronic myocardial infarction: assessment of morphology, function, and perfusion by gradient echo magnetic resonance imaging and 99mTc-methoxyisobutyl-isonitrile SPECT. Am Heart J. 1992;123(3):636–45.

77. Baer FM, Voth E, Schneider CA, Theissen P, Schicha H, Sechtem U. Comparison of low-dose

dobutamine-gradient-echo magnetic resonance imaging and positron emission tomography with [18F]fluorodeoxyglucose in patients with chronic coronary artery disease. A functional and morphological approach to the detection of residual myocardial viability. Circulation. 1995;91(4):1006–15.

78. Kuhl HP, van der Weerdt A, Beek A, Visser F, Hanrath P, van Rossum A. Relation of end-diastolic wall thickness and the residual rim of viable myocardium by magnetic resonance imaging to myocardial viability assessed by fluorine-18 deoxyglucose positron emission tomography. Am J Cardiol. 2006;97(4):452–7.

79. Wellnhofer E, Olariu A, Klein C, Grafe M, Wahl A, Fleck E, et al. Magnetic resonance low-dose dobutamine test is superior to SCAR quantification for the prediction of functional recovery. Circulation. 2004;109(18):2172–4.

80. Romero J, Xue X, Gonzalez W, Garcia MJ. CMR imaging assessing viability in patients with chronic ventricular dysfunction due to coronary artery disease: a meta-analysis of prospective trials. JACC Cardiovasc Imaging. 2012;5(5):494–508.

81. Constantinides CD, Kraitchman DL, O'Brien KO, Boada FE, Gillen J, Bottomley PA. Noninvasive quantification of total sodium concentrations in acute reperfused myocardial infarction using 23Na MRI. Magn Reson Med. 2001;46(6):1144–51.

82. Kim RJ, Lima JA, Chen EL, Reeder SB, Klocke FJ, Zerhouni EA, et al. Fast 23Na magnetic resonance imaging of acute reperfused myocardial infarction. Potential to assess myocardial viability. Circulation. 1997;95(7):1877–85.

83. Kim RJ, Judd RM, Chen EL, Fieno DS, Parrish TB, Lima JA. Relationship of elevated 23Na magnetic resonance image intensity to infarct size after acute reperfused myocardial infarction. Circulation. 1999;100(2):185–92.

84. Souto ALM, Souto RM, Teixeira ICR, Nacif MS. Myocardial viability on cardiac magnetic resonance. Arq Bras Cardiol. 2017;108(5):458–69.

85. van Zijl PCM, Brindle K, Lu H, Barker PB, Edden R, Yadav N, et al. Hyperpolarized MRI, functional MRI, MR spectroscopy and CEST to provide metabolic information in vivo. Curr Opin Chem Biol. 2021;63:209–18.

86. Ramalho M, AlObaidy M, Catalano OA, Guimaraes AR, Salvatore M, Semelka RC. MR-PET of the body: early experience and insights. Eur J Radiol Open. 2014;1:28–39.

87. Juneau D, Chow BJW, Beanlands R, Crean AM. Heart teams for cardiac imaging: the right test at the right time for the right patient. Cham: Springer; 2019. p. 109–25.

88. Haas F, Haehnel CJ, Picker W, Nekolla S, Martinoff S, Meisner H, et al. Preoperative positron emission tomographic viability assessment and perioperative and postoperative risk in patients with advanced ischemic heart disease. J Am Coll Cardiol. 1997;30(7):1693–700.

89. Mule JD, Bax JJ, Zingone B, Martinelli F, Burelli C, Stefania A, et al. The beneficial effect of revascularization on jeopardized myocardium: reverse remodeling and improved long-term prognosis. Eur J Cardiothorac Surg. 2002;22(3):426–30.

90. Tamaki N, Yonekura Y, Yamashita K, Saji H, Magata Y, Senda M, et al. Positron emission tomography using fluorine-18 deoxyglucose in evaluation of coronary artery bypass grafting. Am J Cardiol. 1989;64(14):860–5.

91. Siebelink HM, Blanksma PK, Crijns HJ, Bax JJ, van Boven AJ, Kingma T, et al. No difference in cardiac event-free survival between positron emission tomography-guided and single-photon emission computed tomography-guided patient management: a prospective, randomized comparison of patients with suspicion of jeopardized myocardium. J Am Coll Cardiol. 2001;37(1):81–8.

92. Beanlands RS, Ruddy TD, Freeman M, Nichol G. Patient management guided by viability imaging. J Am Coll Cardiol. 2001;38(4):1271–3.

93. Bonow RO, Maurer G, Lee KL, Holly TA, Binkley PF, Desvigne-Nickens P, et al. Myocardial viability and survival in ischemic left ventricular dysfunction. N Engl J Med. 2011;364(17):1617–25.

94. Velazquez EJ, Lee KL, Jones RH, Al-Khalidi HR, Hill JA, Panza JA, et al. Coronary-artery bypass surgery in patients with ischemic cardiomyopathy. N Engl J Med. 2016;374(16):1511–20.

95. Panza JA, Ellis AM, Al-Khalidi HR, Holly TA, Berman DS, Oh JK, et al. Myocardial viability and long-term outcomes in ischemic cardiomyopathy. N Engl J Med. 2019;381(8):739–48.

96. Mielniczuk LM, Beanlands RS. Does imaging-guided selection of patients with ischemic heart failure for high risk revascularization improve identification of those with the highest clinical benefit?: Imaging-guided selection of patients with ischemic heart failure for high-risk revascularization improves identification of those with the highest clinical benefit. Circ Cardiovasc Imaging. 2012;5(2):262–70. discussion 70

97. Klocke FJ, Baird MG, Lorell BH, Bateman TM, Messer JV, Berman DS, et al. ACC/AHA/ASNC guidelines for the clinical use of cardiac radionuclide imaging—executive summary: a report of the American College of Cardiology/American Heart Association Task Force on Practice Guidelines (ACC/AHA/ASNC Committee to Revise the 1995 Guidelines for the Clinical Use of Cardiac Radionuclide Imaging). J Am Coll Cardiol. 2003;42(7):1318–33.

98. Hendel RC, Berman DS, Di Carli MF, Heidenreich PA, Henkin RE, Pellikka PA, et al. ACCF/ASNC/ACR/AHA/ASE/SCCT/SCMR/SNM 2009 Appropriate use criteria for cardiac radionuclide imaging: a report of the American College of Cardiology Foundation Appropriate Use Criteria Task Force, the American Society of Nuclear Cardiology, the American College of Radiology,

the American Heart Association, the American Society of Echocardiography, the Society of Cardiovascular Computed Tomography, the Society for Cardiovascular Magnetic Resonance, and the Society of Nuclear Medicine. J Am Coll Cardiol. 2009;53(23):2201–29.

99. Anavekar NS, Chareonthaitawee P, Narula J, Gersh BJ. Revascularization in patients with severe left ventricular dysfunction: is the assessment of viability still viable? J Am Coll Cardiol. 2016;67(24):2874–87.

100. O'Meara E, Mielniczuk LM, Wells GA, deKemp RA, Klein R, Coyle D, et al. Alternative imaging modalities in ischemic heart failure (AIMI-HF) IMAGE HF Project I-A: study protocol for a randomized controlled trial. Trials. 2013;14:218.

101. Hall AB, Ziadi MC, Guo A, Chen L, de Kemp R, Renaud J, et al. 516 Cardiac FDG PET results impact decisions and identify patients likely to benefit from revascularization in a multi-center provincial registry (CADRE). Can J Cardiol. 2021;27(5):S249–50.

102. Rischpler C, Langwieser N, Souvatzoglou M, Batrice A, van Marwick S, Snajberk J, et al. PET/MRI early after myocardial infarction: evaluation of viability with late gadolinium enhancement transmurality vs. 18F-FDG uptake. Eur Heart J Cardiovasc Imaging. 2015;16(6):661–9.

103. Vitadello T, Kunze KP, Nekolla SG, Langwieser N, Bradaric C, Weis F, et al. Hybrid PET/MR imaging for the prediction of left ventricular recovery after percutaneous revascularisation of coronary chronic total occlusions. Eur J Nucl Med Mol Imaging. 2020;47(13):3074–83.

104. Canty JM Jr, Suzuki G, Banas MD, Verheyen F, Borgers M, Fallavollita JA. Hibernating myocardium: chronically adapted to ischemia but vulnerable to sudden death. Circ Res. 2004;94(8):1142–9.

105. Luisi AJ Jr, Suzuki G, Dekemp R, Haka MS, Toorongian SA, Canty JM Jr, et al. Regional 11C-hydroxyephedrine retention in hibernating myocardium: chronic inhomogeneity of sympathetic innervation in the absence of infarction. J Nucl Med. 2005;46(8):1368–74.

106. Fallavollita JA, Heavey BM, Luisi AJ Jr, Michalek SM, Baldwa S, Mashtare TL Jr, et al. Regional myocardial sympathetic denervation predicts the risk of sudden cardiac arrest in ischemic cardiomyopathy. J Am Coll Cardiol. 2014;63(2):141–9.

107. Zelt JGE, Britt D, Mair BA, Rotstein BH, Quigley S, Walter O, et al. Regional distribution of fluorine-18-flubrobenguane and carbon-11-hydroxyephedrine for cardiac PET imaging of sympathetic innervation. JACC Cardiovasc Imaging. 2021;14(7):1425–36.

108. Wiefels C, Beanlands RSB, Chong AY. Imaging in CTO: should you look before you open? J Nucl Cardiol. 2020;28(6):2609–12.

109. Neumann FJ, Hochholzer W, Siepe M. ESC/EACTS guidelines on myocardial revascularization 2018: the most important innovations. Herz. 2018;43(8):689–94.

FDG-PET in Special Populations

Geneviève April, Sophie Turpin, Raymond Lambert, and Joaquim Miró

Introduction

^{18}F-FDG PET/CT is well established in the pediatric population for both oncologic and nononcologic indications. Among them, cardiac ^{18}F-FDG PET/CT represents a very polyvalent and specific niche, with particular considerations in children. The aim of this chapter is to review the features, particularities, and applications of pediatric cardiac ^{18}F-FDG PET/CT imaging, including protocol optimization and its role in the investigation of Kawasaki disease and anomalous coronaries, infection, congenital heart disease, and pericardial disease.

Minimization of Radiation Exposure

Cardiac ^{18}F-FDG PET/CT, although uncommonly performed in children, can be helpful in various clinical contexts. It can, however, represent an additional source of ionizing radiation and must therefore be used responsibly [1]. The typical effective dose of an ^{18}F-FDG PET/CT study is 3.5–8.6 mSv (0.10–0.14 mCi/kg) for the PET component. For the CT component, the effective dose is 0.3–2.2 mSv for a low-dose attenuation correction CT and 2–10 mSv for diagnostic CT. Absorbed dose (mGy) and effective dose (mSv/mCi) are typically higher for small children and infants compared to teenagers and adults [2]. This is mainly due to a more compact anatomical disposition of organs and a higher radiosensitivity of tissues. Some strategies for dose optimization of ^{18}F-FDG PET/CT include the following [2–5]:

Eliminating Unnecessary Examinations

When imaging is considered necessary, the ordering physician should choose the best modality to appropriately answer the underlying clinical question. Important factors include availability, cost, diagnostic accuracy, radiation exposure, and feasibility in children while minimizing risks and discomfort. Referring physicians should be aware of the limitations and diagnostic yield of the chosen imaging modality. In cases where ^{18}F-FDG PET/CT is considered appropriate, it should follow the best technical standards in order to optimize the diagnostic yield of the test.

Reducing Radiotracer Dose

Harmonized consensus guidelines have been developed by the European Association of

G. April (✉) · S. Turpin · R. Lambert · J. Miró
CHU Ste-Justine, Montreal, QC, Canada
e-mail: Joaquim.Miro.med@ssss.gouv.qc.ca

Nuclear Medicine (EANM) and the Society of Nuclear Medicine and Molecular Imaging (SNMMI) regarding optimal ^{18}F-FDG dosing in children. The 2021 guidelines recommend doses of 0.10–0.14 mCi/kg (3.7–5.2 MBq/kg) of ^{18}F-FDG for whole-body PET/CT imaging, with a minimum of 0.7 mCi (26 MBq) and a maximum of 10 mCi (370 MBq). The purpose of this weight-based dosing is to minimize radiation exposure without compromising diagnostic performance. A good overall strategy is to determine the longest reasonably achievable scan time per bed position and to adjust administered radio-tracer activity accordingly [6, 7].

Optimizing CT Imaging Parameters and Reducing Scan Range

Diagnostic CT in pediatrics is considered more challenging than in adults mainly because of lower intrinsic soft tissue contrast in children. The CT component of an ^{18}F-FDG PET/CT study is used for attenuation correction purposes and anatomical localization and can provide additional tissue characterization when iodinated contrast agents are used. Factors affecting radiation dose delivered during a CT include tube current time product (mAs), beam energy (kVp), helical pitch, and axial collimation. Child-specific CT protocols reduce CT radiation exposure by decreasing mAs, reducing kVp, and increasing pitch. One suggested approach is to categorized CT acquisition parameters by weight range. Attention must be focused on optimal patient positioning, as off-center positioning increases peripheral and surface CT dose indexes (CTDI) by as much as 10–50% [8, 9]. In addition, CT parameters should be tailored to the area of the body imaged.

^{18}F-FDG PET/CT Protocols

Typical ^{18}F-FDG PET/CT Imaging Session

For a typical ^{18}F-FDG PET/CT session, the patient is installed in a dark, quiet room, with a warm blanket, with or without premedication, to avoid activation of brown fat metabolism. Patient weight, height, and blood sugar level are measured. A fasting period of 4–6 h is typically required, and dextrose infusions can be stopped 90 min before injection. The use of short-acting insulin should also be avoided at least 4 h before radiotracer injection. The uptake period following radiotracer injection varies depending on indication but is usually between 30 and 90 min. Before the acquisition, the patient is asked to void and/or the diaper is changed. Acquisitions usually last between 10 and 50 min. After imaging, hydration is recommended to minimize bladder radiation dose [10].

Myocardial Viability

The main goal of a viability protocol is to maximize heart glucose consumption. The corollary being that viable cardiomyocytes, including hibernating myocardium, maintain the ability to metabolize glucose. Bringing the patient into a hyperglycemic state stimulates insulin production and release, which promotes entry of glucose into cardiomyocytes. As opposed to adult myocardial viability preparation, pediatric patients do not need to fast prior to imaging and no insulin injection is required. After measurement of blood sugar level, an oral glucose solution (1.5 g/kg up to a maximum of 50 g) is given. After 45 min, blood sugar level is reassessed and ^{18}F-FDG is injected. Imaging takes place approximately 45 min following radiotracer injection. Should oral intake be impossible, an intravenous glucose (25% or 50%, 0.3 g/kg, over a period of 15 min) can be employed [11].

Myocardial Suppression

The main goal of a suppression protocol is to minimize physiological heart glucose consumption by favoring fatty acid metabolism. When appropriately suppressed, myocardial glucose uptake should reflect inflammation or infection rather than physiological metabolism. Various suppression protocols emulating those used in adults have been proposed. These include a 24-h low-carbohydrate diet (including avoidance of dextrose infusion), a prolonged fast of 12 h or more, and administration of low-dose IV heparin 45 min (5 UI/kg IV) and 15 min (10 UI/kg IV) before ^{18}F-FDG injection. In breastfed or formula-fed infants, it is often not possible to perform a myocardial suppression study [12].

^{18}F-FDG PET/CT and Pediatric Sedation

Sedation is not a substitution for adequate child and parent preparation, as multiple nonpharmacologic strategies exist to help children cooperation. Optimization of the PET/CT or PET/MR environment is key. In neonates and infants, darker rooms, noise-reduction techniques, as well as feed-and-wrap techniques have been proven successful. In older children, the main goal is to decrease anxiety and to promote distraction using movies and music to reduce motion artifacts. Using these strategies, most ^{18}F-FDG PET/CT examinations can be performed without the use of sedation. However, in some cases, sedation remains necessary for reduction of patient motion, cooperation, and discomfort minimization considerations [13].

Sedation can be divided into conscious sedation, deep sedation, and general anesthesia, with some overlap between these levels of sedation. Patients who require more than conscious sedation necessitate appropriate monitoring. Risks associated with sedation include hypoventilation and apnea, airway obstruction, and sometimes morbidity related to gastrointestinal adverse effects, reactive airway disease, and risk of seizure [14].

Selecting the level of sedation should be made on a case-by-case basis. Guidelines recommend a minimum of 2 h of clear fluid fasting prior to elective procedures. However, prolonged fasting may be deleterious especially in infants. Therefore, ingestion of clear fluids up to 1 h before elective anesthesia or sedation is acceptable. Breastfeeding and milk preparations should be stopped 4 h, and solids minimally 6 h before procedure [15].

The choice of drugs and route of administration depends on multiple factors, including age, underlying comorbidities, institutional protocols, length and type of procedure, availability of reversal drugs, monitoring equipment and adequately trained practitioners to manage all levels of sedation [16]. The most frequently used sedative agents include chloral hydrate, phenobarbital sodium (Nembutal), midazolam, ketamine, dexmedetomidine, propofol, and nitrous oxide [17, 18].

Pediatric ^{18}F-FDG PET/MR Cardiovascular Imaging

Hybrid PET/MR systems offer several advantages in the pediatric population, allowing for the combination of PET functional information with the precise anatomical information and high-contrast structural resolution of MRI [19]. PET/MR does not require additional CT to perform attenuation correction or spatial coregistration, resulting in a more favorable dosimetry. However, whole-body PET/MR acquisitions are longer compared to a whole-body PET/CT and require optimal registration, which usually necessitates patient sedation. Furthermore, several devices such as pacemakers or mechanical heart valves, frequently present in children with congenital heart disease, are not MRI compatible or may lead to significant artifact. Finally, PET/MR is susceptible to artifacts related to field-of-view truncation, attenuation-correction, and motion [20, 21].

Cardiac MRI is technically challenging in children. Proper acquisition requires the use of

ECG gating, which may be technically challenging in infants with rapid heart rate or in patients with pacemakers. Sequences have to be adapted depending on the patient's ability to breathe hold and their size for proper contrast enhanced MRI angiography [22, 23]. When combined with MRI, respiratory gating of the PET component is possible, but the use of a respiratory belt remains more efficient than gating with MR-based navigators [24, 25].

In pediatric cardiology, potential applications of hybrid PET/MR include the evaluation of cardiac tumors and myopathies, where both modalities are complementary. In children for whom both PET and MRI are required, hybrid PET/MR allows imaging within a single session, minimizing discomfort and potentially avoiding additional sedation. Children could benefit from ^{18}F-FDG PET/MR for the evaluation of rare primary cardiac tumors or secondary invasion by either adjacent or metastatic neoplasms, with superior soft tissue characterization. PET/MR also provides anatomical precision for the evaluation of congenital cardiac abnormalities before surgery, as well as improved evaluation of soft tissue infection. PET/MR has the potential to assess flow, metabolism, and cardiac function in conditions such as Kawasaki disease, aberrant coronary arteries, and for the differentiation of ischemic and nonischemic cardiomyopathies. It can also be combined with ^{18}F-FDG for viability assessment, delineation of scar tissue by late gadolinium enhancement (LGE) imaging, identification of fat content, tissue edema and inflammation, as well as infiltrative diseases such as myocarditis [26, 27].

Kawasaki Disease

Kawasaki disease (KD) is an acute systemic vasculitis of unknown etiology. It affects mainly small and medium-sized arteries including the coronary arteries. When coronary arteries are involved, KD can lead to major complications such as acute myocardial infarction (AMI). It is one of the most frequent acquired heart diseases in children, especially in North America and Japan [28]. Classic KD presentation includes ongoing fever for 5 days or more, and at least 4 of the 5 following clinical features: mucosal changes, polymorphous exanthema, nonexudative conjunctivitis, skin alteration of the extremities, and lymphadenopathy.

Even with optimal treatment, which includes aspirin and intravenous immunoglobulins, coronary artery aneurysms and stenosis are relatively frequent in KD. While half to two-thirds of KD-induced coronary aneurysms regress spontaneously, some, mainly giant aneurysms (>8 mm), tend to persist and are associated with an increased risk of complications. Regression of lesions is more frequent in younger children, females, and in more distally located aneurysms. Approximately one-third of moderate-size lesions persist beyond 3 years after onset. Overall, coronary artery sequelae occur in approximately 20–25% of cases [29]. Since KD sequelae often present as multivessel disease, coronary revascularization is often necessary. A combination of a perfusion study, using ^{99m}Tc SPECT agents or PET tracers (e.g. NH$_3$ and ^{82}Rb), along with a ^{18}F-FDG PET viability study can be performed to evaluate viable myocardium (Fig. 21.1) [30].

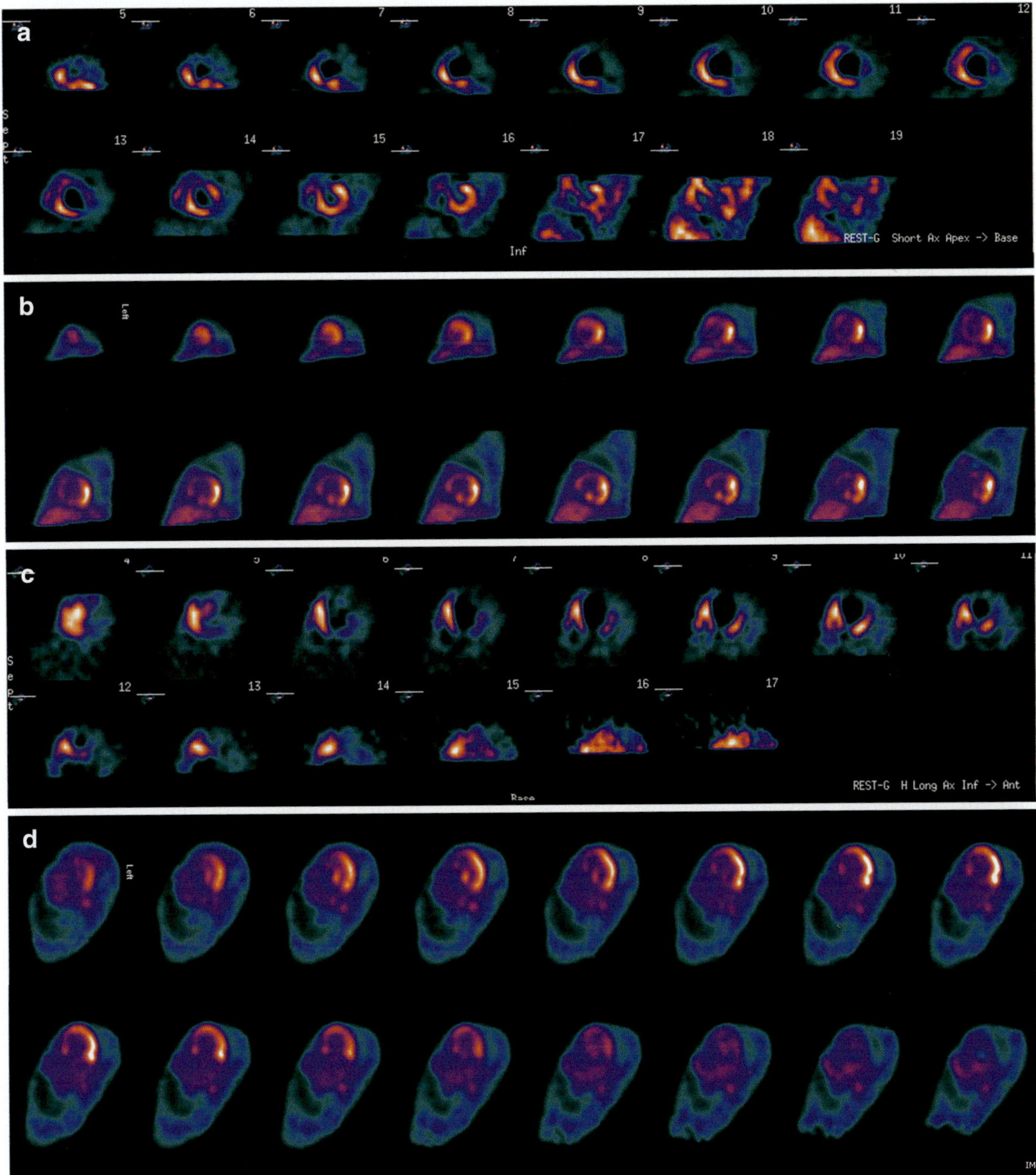

Fig. 21.1 ^{18}F-FDG PET/CT of a 5-year-old girl with a previous history of Kawasaki disease complicated by coronary aneurysm admitted with acute myocardial infarct. Tc99m myocardial rest perfusion study demonstrated extensive defects involving the anterior, anterolateral, and apical regions both on vertical short axis (**a**) and horizontal long axis (**c**). Post procedure evaluation of residual viable myocardium with ^{18}F-FDG PET/CT after glucose loading demonstrated myocardial hibernation and thus viability in the anterior, anterolateral, and apical regions both on vertical short axis (**b**) and horizontal long axis (**d**)

Anomalous Coronaries

Anomalous coronaries can be isolated or found in association with other cardiac malformations. Several classifications have been proposed based on the affected coronary, location of the anomalous origin, as well as its course in relation to the aorta and main pulmonary artery [31–33]. Native coronary anomalies are found in approximately 0.2–1.2% of the population [34, 35].

Anomalous origin of the left coronary artery from the pulmonary artery (ALCAPA) is a relatively prevalent congenital anomaly, usually seen as an isolated lesion and affecting 0.25–0.5% of the population. It is a well-known cause of myocardial ischemia and infarction in children and, if left untreated, can result in a mortality rate of up to 80–90% within the first year of life [36]. The typical clinical presentation, known as Bland–White–Garland syndrome, includes pallor, failure to thrive, sweating, and atypical chest pain while eating or crying. Neonatal pulmonary vascular resistance is high and pulmonary artery (PA) pressure ensure antegrade flow from the PA into the anomalous left coronary. With time, as pulmonary vascular resistance decreases, there is a consequent decrease in left coronary artery antegrade flow, with eventual reversal resulting in left-to-right shunting into the PA, causing the so-called coronary steal [37]. Infants have essentially no collateral circulation, leading to the rapid onset of severe myocardial ischemia, left ventricular dysfunction, and possible mitral valve regurgitation from papillary muscle ischemia. ALCAPA must be suspected in any infant or child presenting with myocardial dysfunction. Surgical correction is usually performed as soon as possible, regardless of age and degree of collateralization.

Imaging of coronary anomalies relies mainly on coronary computed tomographic angiography (CCTA), transthoracic echocardiography, and MRI [38, 39]. Perfusion and myocardial viability studies using PET can be used to assess for the presence of hibernating myocardium, which may influence surgical management in patients with massive infarction or aneurysm. Absence of via-ble tissue may indicate the need to consider heart transplant over revascularization. Resection of nonviable aneurysms may prevent malignant arrhythmias from developing and help prevent myocardial remodeling. Children with hibernating myocardium often show a significant recovery of function following revascularization. As well, mitral insufficiency frequently regresses after revascularization. Quantifying the amount of viable myocardium can also help predict surgical outcomes and the need for mechanical support bridging, as well as orienting postoperative follow-up [30].

Congenital Heart Disease

Congenital heart disease (CHD) is one of the most frequent congenital disorders and a leading cause of mortality associated with birth defects. Global prevalence of CHD is estimated to be 8 per 1000 live births. With improvement of surgical and medical management, survival is now possible for most patients, even with serious anomalies, although many patients have significant complications during adulthood. Approximately two third of adults with CHD eventually die from a cardiac cause, mainly heart failure and sudden death. Predictors of unfavorable prognosis are CHD severity, endocarditis, arrhythmias, myocardial infarction, and pulmonary hypertension [40]. As surgical techniques and patient survival continue to improve, more patients with repaired CHD may present with complications in adulthood. Thus, knowledge of the basic anatomy and physiology of CHD is critical for all cardiovascular imagers. The following sections provides a brief overview of the most frequent CHD and procedures.

Transposition of the Great Arteries

In transposition of the great arteries (TGA), the aorta and pulmonary artery connect to the inappropriate ventricles. In the majority of cases, this is an isolated anomaly, leading to profound cyanosis shortly after birth. The anatomy of the coronaries with regard to origin, proximal course, and branching is variable. One-year life expectancy without surgery is lower than 20%. Primary arterial switch operation is currently the treatment of choice. This intervention needs to be performed early in life, while the left ventricle is still exposed to high pressures and involves translocation of the coronary arteries to the neoaorta.

Single Ventricle and Hypoplastic Left Heart Syndrome

Univentricular CHD malformations are characterized by hypoplasia or absence of one of the ventricles or cardiac valves, leading to the impossibility of establishing normal serial circulation. The most severe form is hypoplastic left heart syndrome (HLHS), characterized by multiple levels of stenosis/hypoplasia of the structures of the left heart, and associated with aortic and mitral stenosis or atresia. As a consequence, the ascending aorta and aortic arch are hypoplastic, and systemic circulation is dependent on a patent ductus arteriosus. Other univentricular CHDs include double outlet right ventricle in which both the aorta and pulmonary artery arise from the right ventricle; hypoplastic right heart, the most severe form being secondary to tricuspid atresia; and the rare double inlet ventricle in which both atria are connected to a single ventricle. Univentricular CHD requires multiple staged surgical interventions to achieve serial circulation with one ventricle pumping the systemic circulation, while the pulmonary circulation depends on venous pressure, without any active pump (i.e. Fontan physiology).

Modified Blalock–Taussig Shunt

The modified Blalock–Taussig (BT) shunt is a palliative technique which uses a prosthetic graft to connect a subclavian artery to the ipsilateral pulmonary artery. It is commonly used in the neonatal period to augment pulmonary flow and relieve cyanosis, allowing the pulmonary arteries to grow and pulmonary resistances to drop, before corrective surgery or further palliation.

Bidirectional Glenn (Cavobipulmonary) Shunt

Bidirectional Glenn shunt is a palliative procedure which creates a shunt from the superior vena cava to the pulmonary arteries, in order to supply blood flow after neonatal pulmonary pressures have normalized. It is frequently used as a staging procedure in children with single-ventricle morphology who will eventually get a Fontan procedure. It results in one-half (from superior vena cava) of the systemic venous return going directly to the lungs, while the other half from the inferior vena cava returns directly to the heart.

Norwood Staged Procedures

The Norwood staged palliation for HLHS consists of three interventions. The first stage, performed shortly after birth, reestablishes an unobstructed systemic circulation using the right ventricle. To achieve this, the main pulmonary artery is transected and used to enlarge the hypoplastic aortic arch (the Damus–Kaye–Stansel procedure) (Fig. 21.2). The interatrial septum is excised to allow unobstructed pulmonary venous return to the systemic (right) ventricle. Since the pulmonary arteries are not connected to the right ventricle, an alternative source of pulmonary blood flow must be created, either by a modified BT shunt or a small conduit between the right ventricle and pulmonary arteries (Sano conduit) (Fig. 21.3). The second stage of the Norwood palliation consists of a bidirectional Glenn and is performed typically around 6 months of age, when pulmonary resistances have decreased. The third stage consist of a Fontan procedure, where the inferior vena cava is

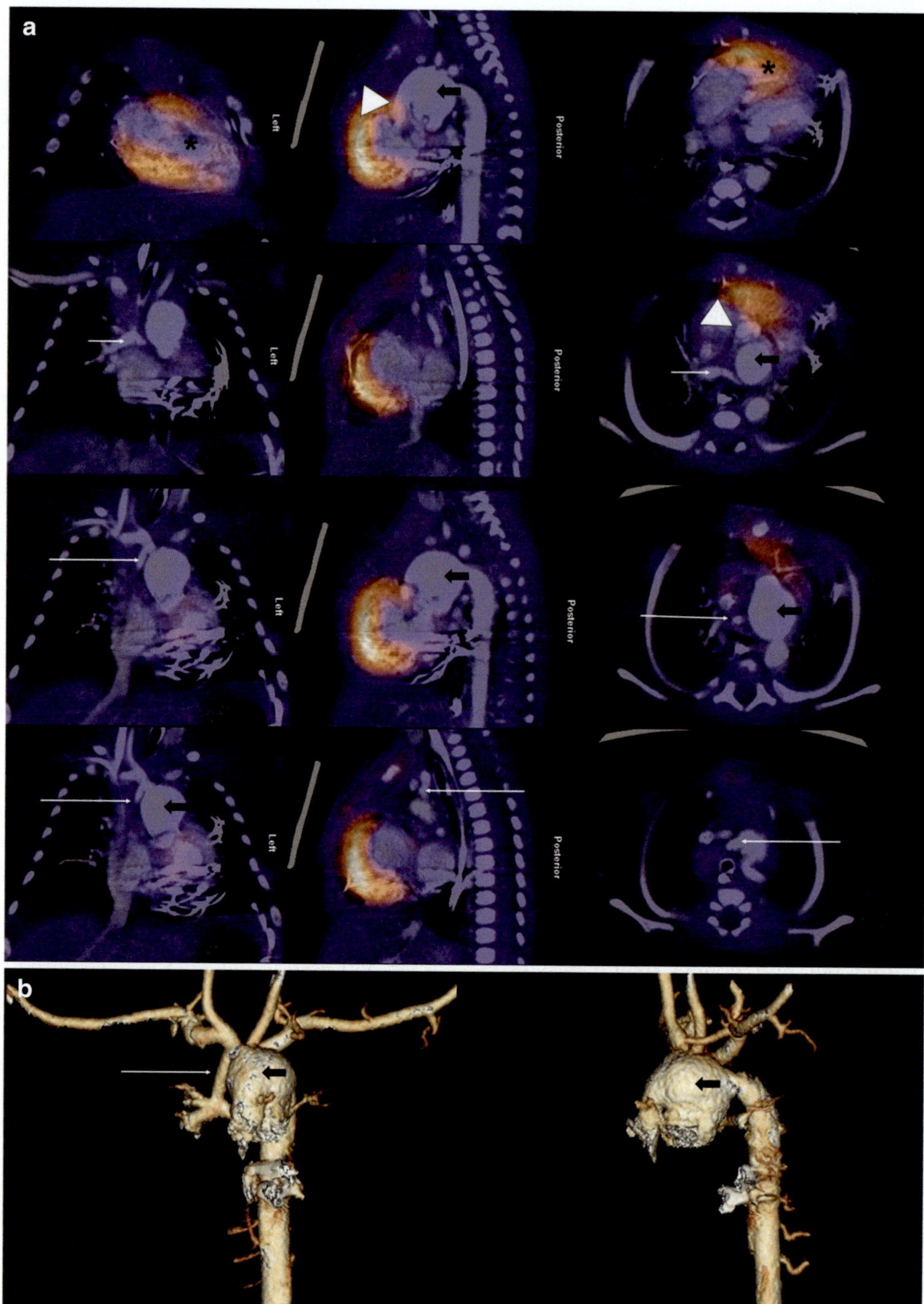

Fig. 21.2 ^{18}F-FDG PET/CT of a 1-month-old patient with left ventricle hypoplasia (*). ^{18}F-FDG CTAC images were fused with cardiac CT with contrast (**a**) and three-dimensional cardiac CT reconstructions (**b**). Norwood procedure with a Blalock–Taussig (BT) shunt (long thin arrow) between the right subclavian artery and right pulmonary artery (short thin arrow). Damus–Kaye–Stansel (DKS) procedure for creation of the neoaorta, with anastomosis of the main pulmonary artery (open arrow) and hypoplastic native aorta (arrow head)

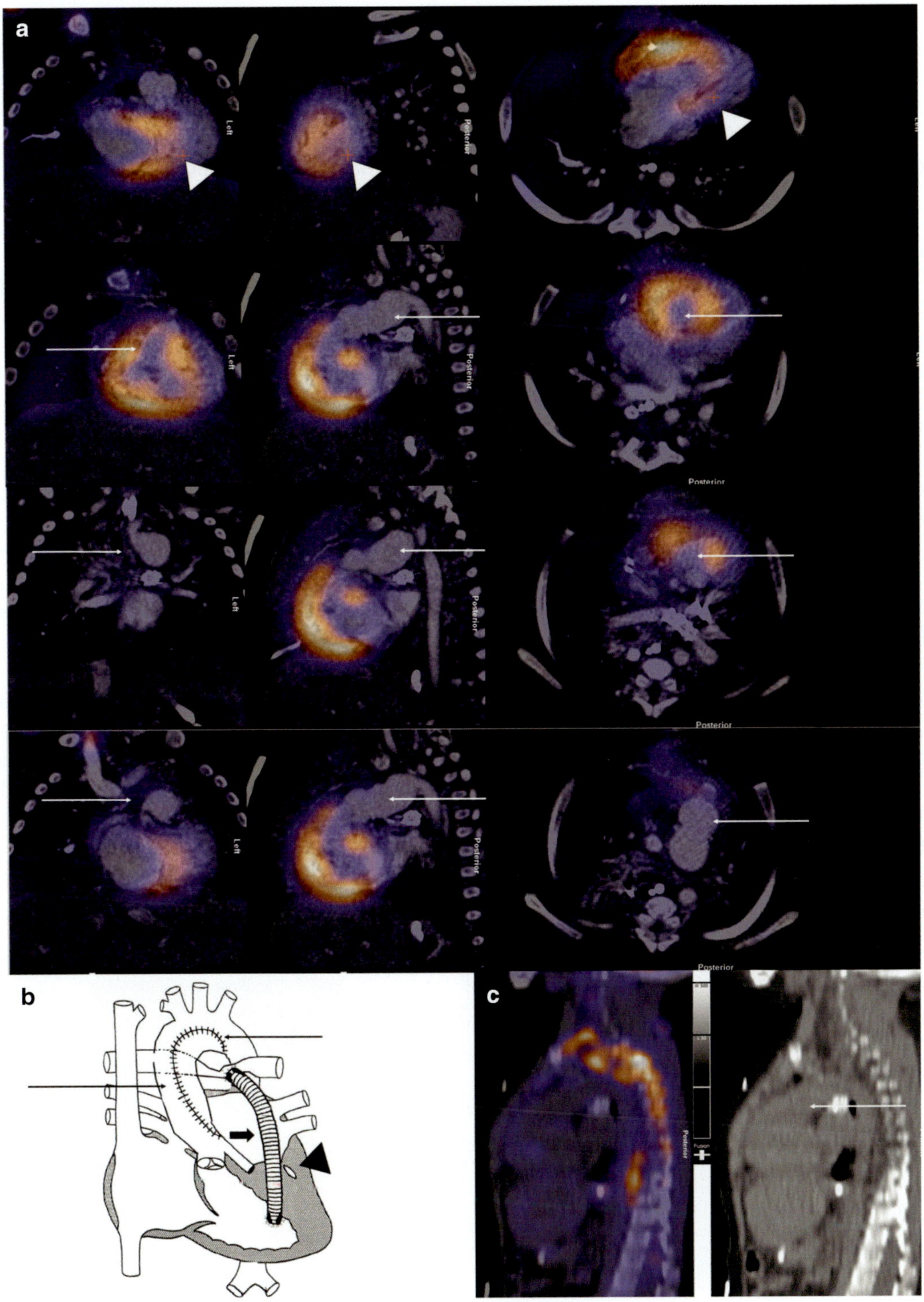

Fig. 21.3 ^{18}F-FDG PET/CT performed in a 2-year-old girl with left ventricular and aortic hypoplasia, status post Norwood–Sano procedure. ^{18}F-FDG CT AC images fused with: cardiac CT with contrast (**a**), cardiac catheterization image (**b**) and sagittal FDG CTAC PET/CT (**c**). Visible reconstructed aortic arch (long thin arrow), Sano shunt (open arrow) and hypoplastic left ventricle (arrowhead). When interpreting ^{18}F-FDG PET/CT, specifically in children with congenital heart disease, correlation with other modalities is paramount

connected to the pulmonary artery. Following this last stage, all deoxygenated blood from the venous system flows through the lungs. This last step is typically executed around 4 years of age, when the pulmonary arteries are mature enough to accommodate a large conduit [41].

Jatene Arterial Switch Procedure

This is the anatomical repair of transposition of great arteries performed to establish the left ventricle as the systemic arterial ventricle. If not possible in the neonatal period, it can sometimes be preceded by pulmonary artery banding, which places prosthetic material encircling the main pulmonary artery to "train" the left ventricle for systemic pressures.

Right Ventricle–Pulmonary Artery (RV-PA) Conduit

This technique uses, among different options, a valved prosthetic homograft material to create an artificial conduit between the right ventricle and pulmonary artery. Different surgical corrections can use this technique as a reconstruction of the right ventricular outflow tract (Fig. 21.4).

Tetralogy of Fallot

Although tetralogy of Fallot (ToF) and truncus arteriosus are distinct cyanotic congenital heart defects, they share some common characteristics. Both are a consequence of abnormal embryonic conotruncal development. They include a large septal defect at the ventricular outlet, with characteristic abnormalities of semilunar valves and great arteries. To be classified as ToF, CHD must fulfill specific requirements, including pulmonic stenosis, ventricular septal defect, overriding aorta, and right ventricular hypertrophy which represents a consequence of long-standing right ventricular pressure overload.

ToF are usually repaired using infundibulectomy and a patch repair of the RV outflow stenosis, which may involve the pulmonary valve. In cases where the pulmonary valve must be excised, a free pulmonary insufficiency is created, which may require future revalvulation. ToF repair frequently involves patch enlargement of the small pulmonary arteries, and even unifocalization, when the arteries are not in continuity (in this case, the pulmonary flow may come from aortopulmonary collaterals) or an RV-PA conduit. Complete ToF repair also involves closure of the ventricular septal defect using a patch allowing for septal realignment (Fig. 21.5).

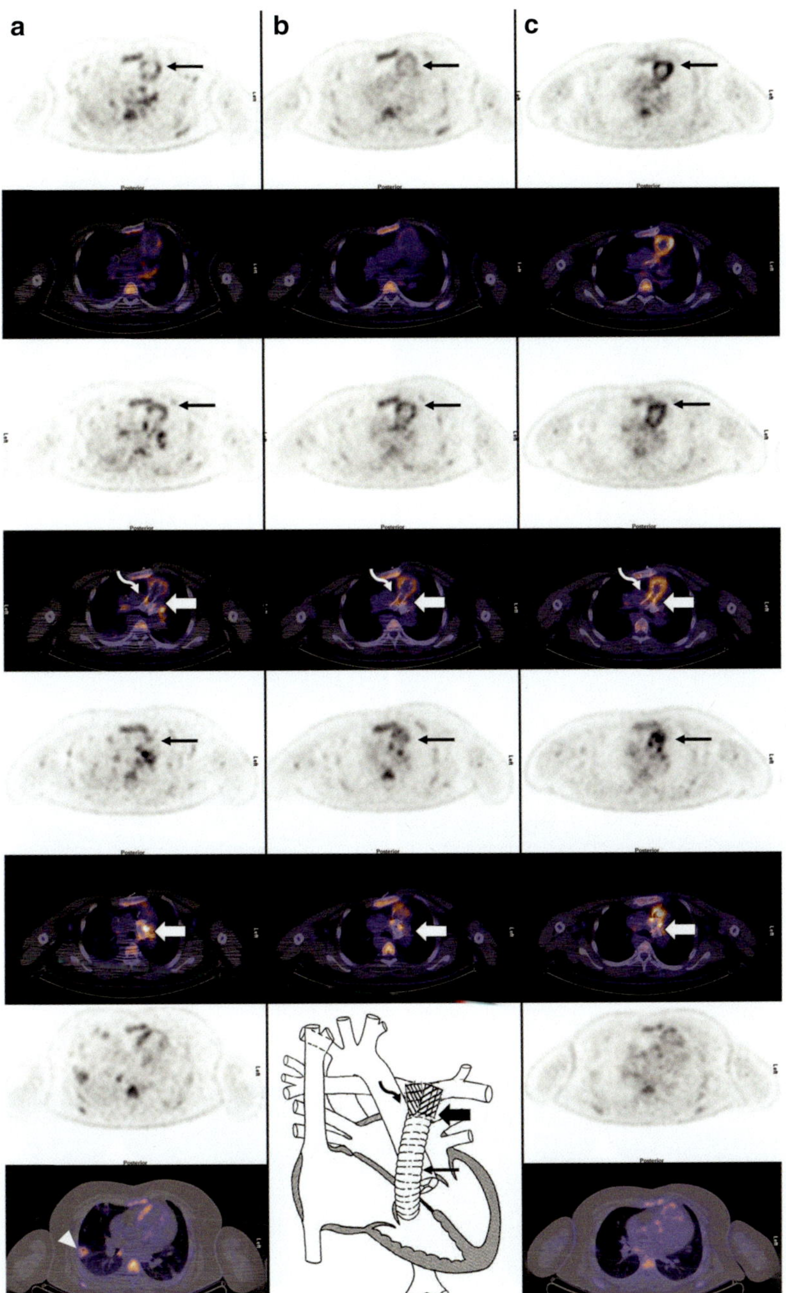

Fig. 21.4 ^{18}F-FDG PET/CT performed after a cardiac suppression protocol to assess extension of infection in a 15-year-old patient with truncus arteriosus status post RV-PA conduit (thin arrow), RPA (curvilinear arrow) and LPA (open arrow) stent placement. Clinically, the patient presented with *Staphylococcus aureus* septic shock following a toe infection. ^{18}F-FDG PET/CT demonstrating an active infectious process at the level of the RV-PA conduit, RPA and LPA stents, with lung septic emboli (arrow head) (**a**). Following 3 weeks of antibiotics, some improvement was noted (**b**), but during the following 2 weeks, despite aggressive antimicrobial treatment, the patient remained afebrile with increased inflammatory markers. A follow-up ^{18}F-FDG PET/CT study showed no further improvement at the levels of the LPA and RPA stents and progression of uptake surrounding the RV-PA conduit. Only resolution of the lung lesions was demonstrated (**c**). Shortly after, RV-PA conduit and both stents were surgically removed. Multiple vegetations, abscesses and *Staphylococcus aureus* were found on the material. A new RV-PA conduit was installed, the antibiotic treatment completed and patient's subsequent evolution was favorable

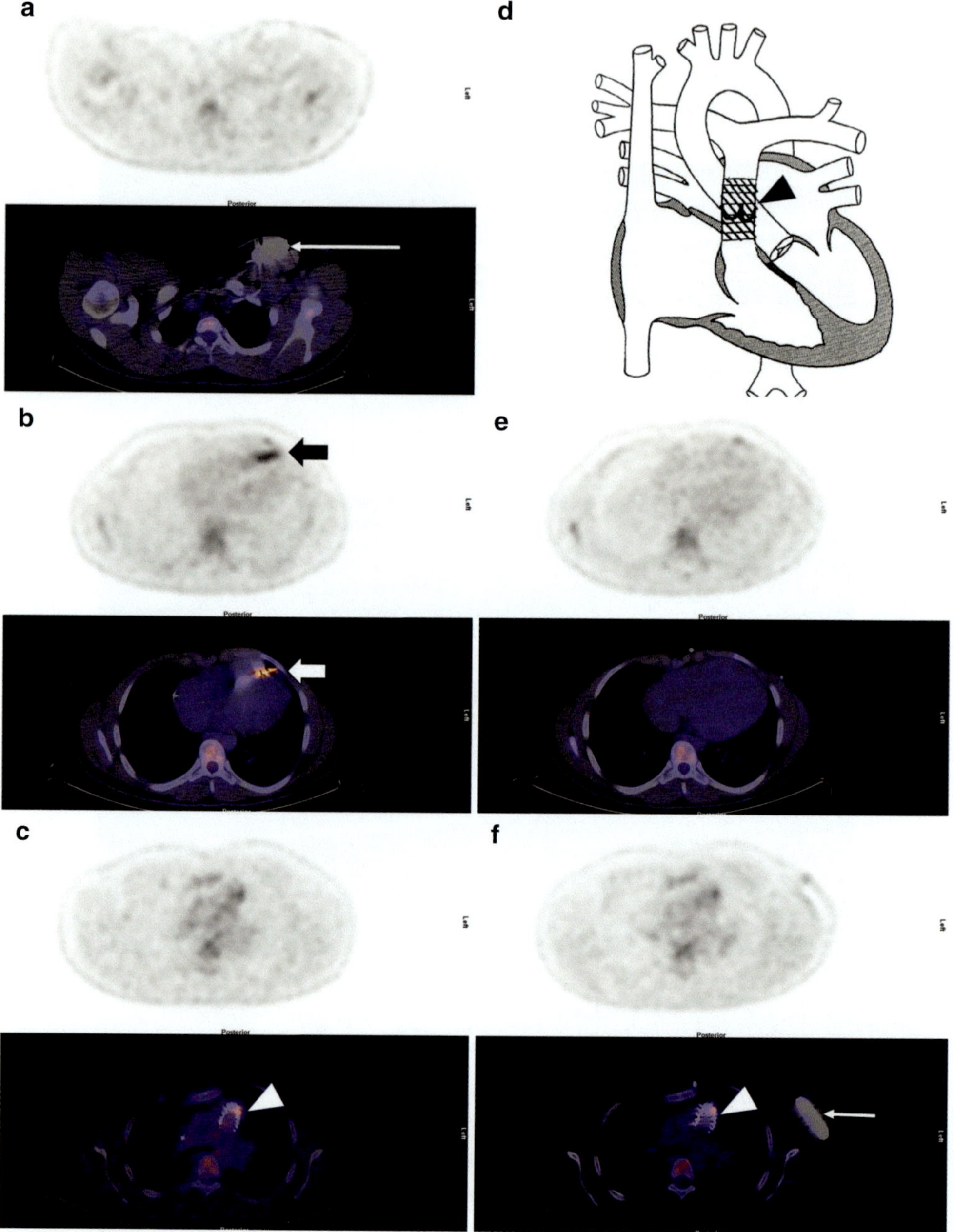

Fig. 21.5 ¹⁸F-FDG PET/CT performed after cardiac suppression protocol to assess the extent of infection in a 16-year-old patient status post Fallot tetralogy repair. Status post stent placement Main Pulmonary Artery with Melody valve; status post Fortify Assura cardioverter defibrillator device (CDD) implantation. Follow-up echocardiogram showing vegetations at the level of the intracavitary apical defibrillation lead. No FDG uptake around was seen at the casing (long thin arrow) (**a**) but there was visible FDG uptake at the level of the defibrilla-tion lead (short thick arrow) (**b**). Mild uptake at the level of the Melody valve (arrow head) but otherwise no FDG uptake at the level of the stent (**c**, **d**). The CDD was removed and cultures were positive for *Staphylococcus hominis*. Following antibiotic therapy, a second ¹⁸F-FDG PET/CT showed resolution of uptake in the left ventricle (**e**) and unchanged appearance of the Melody valve (arrow head) (**f**). No evidence of persistent infection during follow-up. New subcutaneous implantable defibrillator (EMBLEM MRI S-ICD) (short thin arrow)

Cardiovascular Infections

In 2013, a joint European Association of Nuclear Medicine (EANM)/Society of Nuclear Medicine and Molecular Imaging (SNMMI) guideline recommended the use of ^{18}F-FDG PET/CT in inflammation and infection indications such as sarcoidosis, peripheral bone osteomyelitis, suspected spinal infection, fever of unknown origin (FUO), metastatic infection of high-risk patients with bacteremia, and primary evaluation of vasculitis [42]. The latest joint collaboration of the EANM and European Association of Cardiovascular Imaging (EACVI) published in 2020 now includes interpretation and reporting criteria of prosthetic valve endocarditis, cardiac implantable electronic devices, left ventricular assist device, and vascular graft infections [43]. However, these guidelines mainly apply to the adult population and pediatric-specific literature and recommendations remain scarce.

Infections Related to Sternotomy

Delayed sternal closure after cardiac surgery is a common technique in pediatric cardiac surgery, when sternal closure can negatively affect cardiac and respiratory function in the immediate postoperative period. Factors associated with increased infection risks are prolonged skin barrier disruption, prolonged mechanical ventilation/sedation/neuromuscular blockade, complex surgical intervention, younger age, and repeated surgery. Although antibiotic prophylaxis and wound dressing care reduces infection rates, infections including mediastinitis have been reported in between 4 and 10% of patients and ^{18}F-FDG PET/CT can be useful for the evaluation of suspected infection [44–46]

Congenital Heart Disease Repair

Surgical repair of CHD also often requires prosthetic material, which can be a predisposing factor for infection. In addition to the sternotomy site, multiple sites of infection are possible, including prosthetic conduits, native or prosthetic valves, and cardiac implantable devices. Infectious endocarditis (IE) prevalence is higher in patients with CHD. The reliability of the modified Duke criteria, including echocardiography findings, is limited due to artifacts and complex anatomy. Imaging is critical, not only for diagnosis, but also for the evaluation of response to therapy. The latest guidelines have incorporated ^{18}F-FDG PET/CT findings as a major criterion in the diagnostic algorithms for IE. ^{18}F-FDG PET/CT is also useful for the demonstration of extracardiac complications of endocarditis. Specifically, it allows for the detection of concomitant or alternative infective thoracic foci, such as pericardial collections, mediastinitis, and pulmonary infections (Fig. 21.6). Endocarditis can be associated with septic emboli, with extracardiac foci of infection reported in 15–60% [47–51].

Fever of Unknown Origin

Fever is one of the chief complaints of children presenting at the hospital, estimated to account for 16–30% of cases. FUO refers to a prolonged febrile condition without an established etiology despite complete evaluation, and no definite cause is found in 10–20% of cases. Although no widespread consensus exists, most current definitions of FUO in children include: temperature ≥ 38.3°C for >1 week, no history of immunosuppression in the preceding 3 months, with no clear cause identified despite complete physical examination, labo-

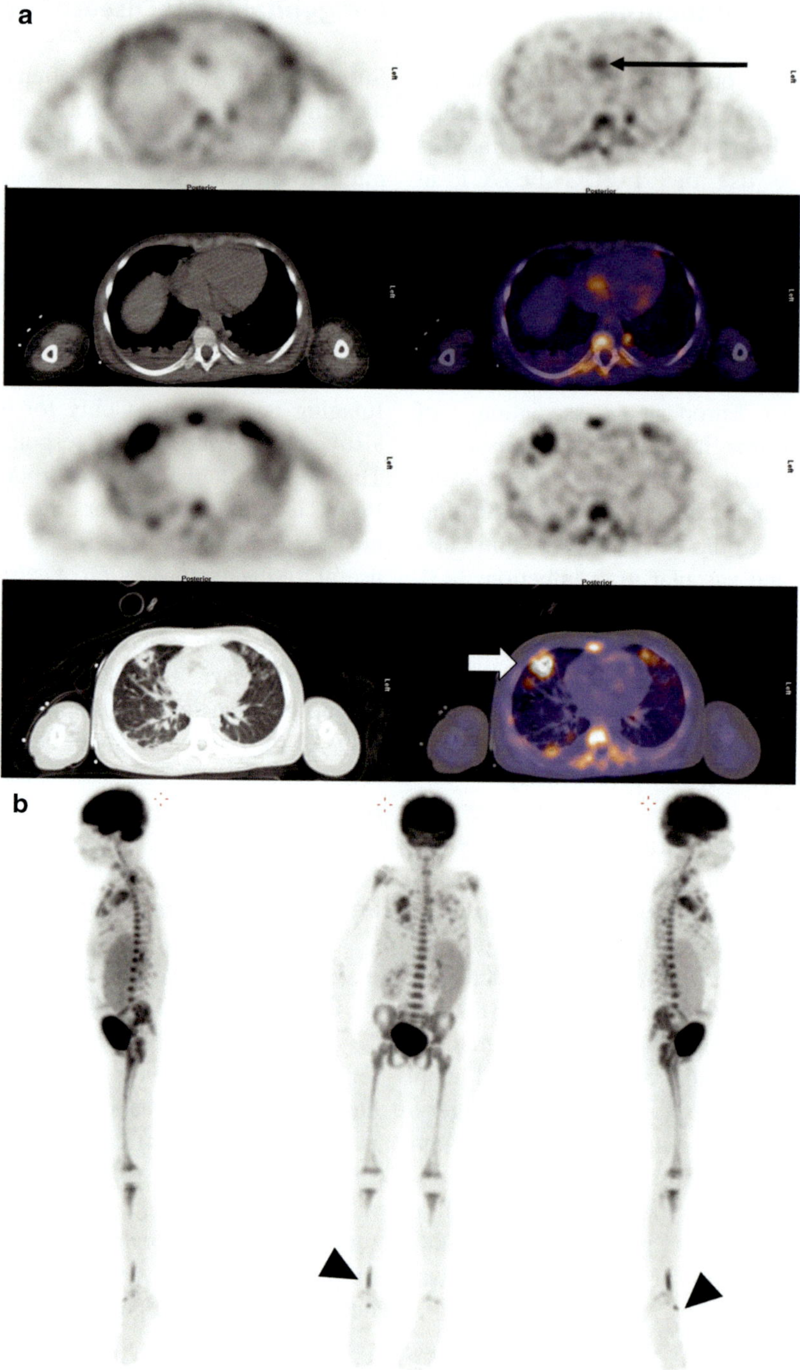

Fig. 21.6 ^{18}F-FDG PET/CT of a 10-year-old patient with indwelling central catheter for intravenous hyperalimentation admitted for septic shock. Tricuspid valve endocarditis and lung septic emboli were demonstrated on echocardiogram and chest CT. ^{18}F-FDG PET/CT was requested for the evaluation of left hip pain and performed with myocardial suppression protocol. Selected axial images (**a**) and Maximum Intensity Projections (**b**). FDG uptake was noted at the level of the tricuspid valve (long thin arrow). Lung septic emboli were present, some with cavitation (open arrow). Residual activity is seen at the FDG injection site (arrow head). No hip anomaly or other focus of infection was detected. The patient was known for splenomegaly

ratory and imaging workup. Causes of FUO include infection, malignancy, inflammatory disease, and other miscellaneous causes. ^{18}F-FDG PET/CT was found to have high sensitivity for several causes such as tumor (>90%), infection (89%), arthritis and vasculitis (65%), and is generally considered helpful in almost half of cases (25–75%), including chronic low-grade infections. ^{18}F-FDG PET/CT has good diagnostic accuracy in FUO, with reported sensitivity of ~85%, specificity of ~80%, PPV of ~70–85% and NPV of ~80–90%. ^{18}F-FDG PET/CT leads to modification of treatment in approximately half of cases, and has also proven useful in immunosuppressed children [52–54].

Ventricular Assist Devices

Infection affects nearly 15–20% of patients within a year of ventricular assist device (VAD) implantation, with infection at the driveline exit site seen most frequently. If isolated, the driveline can be debrided and revised, and the infection treated with antibiotics. Infection extending to internal components is associated with a high mortality rate and needs to be treated more aggressively. ^{18}F-FDG PET/CT has been shown useful in detecting infection of VADs in the adult population, with a pooled sensitivity of 92% and specificity of 83%, resulting in management changes in as much as 80% of patients [55–58] (Fig. 21.7).

Cardiac Implantable Electronic Devices

Cardiac Implantable Electronic Device (CIED) infections can present with superficial incisional infection, pocket infection, infection of thoracic leads, and endocarditis. Although less than 1% of all CIED are implanted in children, there are unique characteristics of the devices used in children. For instance, pacemaker stimulation is epicardial in smaller patients or patients with cavopulmonary connections, and the implantation chamber is often tunneled to the left upper abdominal quadrant (Fig. 21.8). Device dependence is more frequent with certain CHD (e.g., atrioventricular discordance), after open heart surgeries performed near the atrioventricular or the sinus node, and after complex heart surgeries, cardiomyopathies, or malignant ventricular arrhythmias. ^{18}F-FDG PET/CT enables diagnosis of infection, assessment of the extracardiac portion of leads, and localization of septic emboli foci. ^{18}F-FDG PET/CT is particularly effective in differentiating superficial tissue infection from deep pocket CIED infections requiring surgical excision (Fig. 21.9). A recent meta-analysis revealed a pooled sensitivity of 96% and pooled specificity of 97% for local pocket infection. Accuracy was slightly lower for lead infection, with a pooled sensitivity of 76% and specificity of 83% [59, 60].

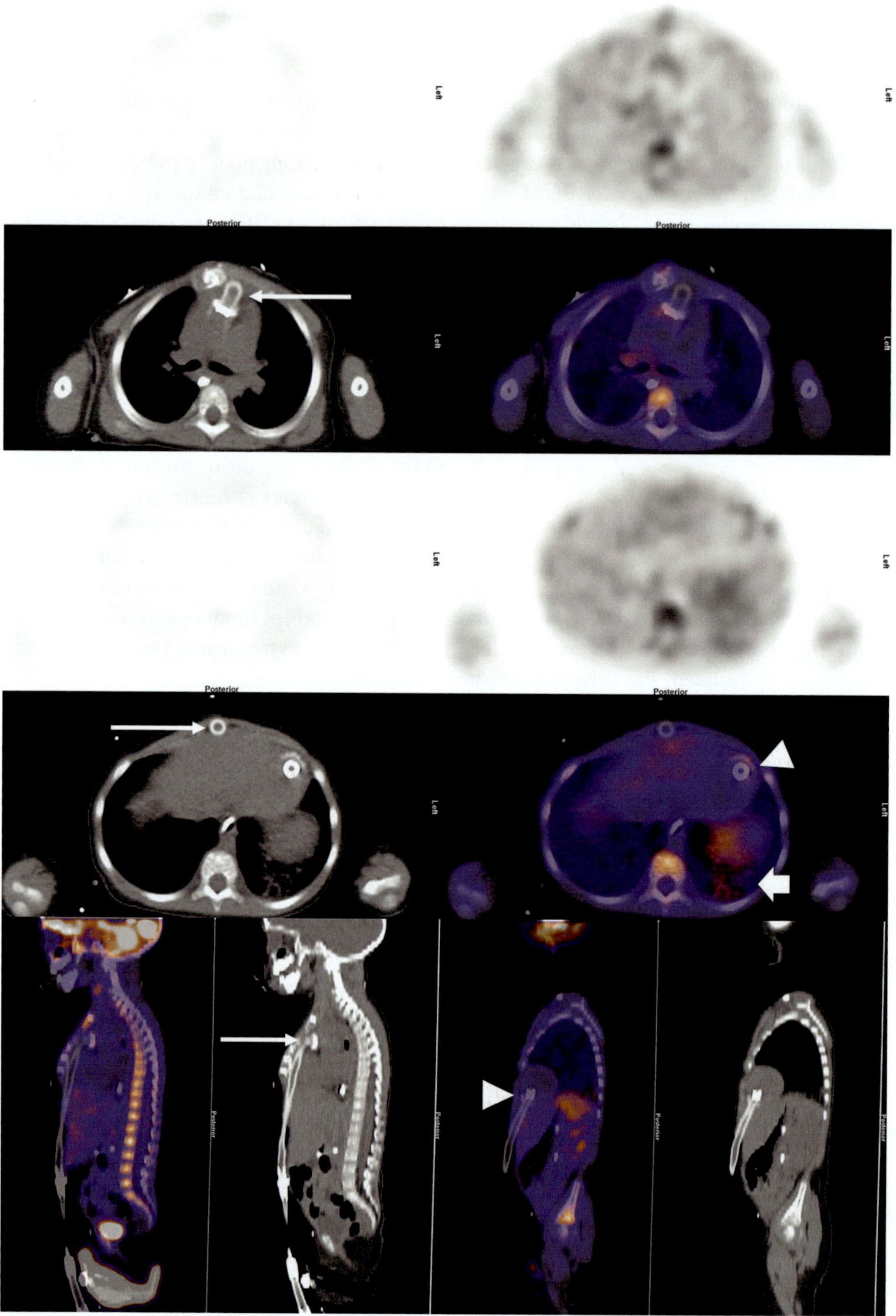

Fig. 21.7 ^{18}F-FDG PET/CT was performed in a 1.5-year-old girl with a history of recurrent fever and known Berlin Heart, a left ventricular assist device (LVAD). There was evidence of pneumonia in the left lung base (open arrow). There was physiologic radiotracer distribution associated with arterial cannula in the ascending aorta (long arrow) and atrial cannula in the left ventricle (short arrow), without evidence of material infection

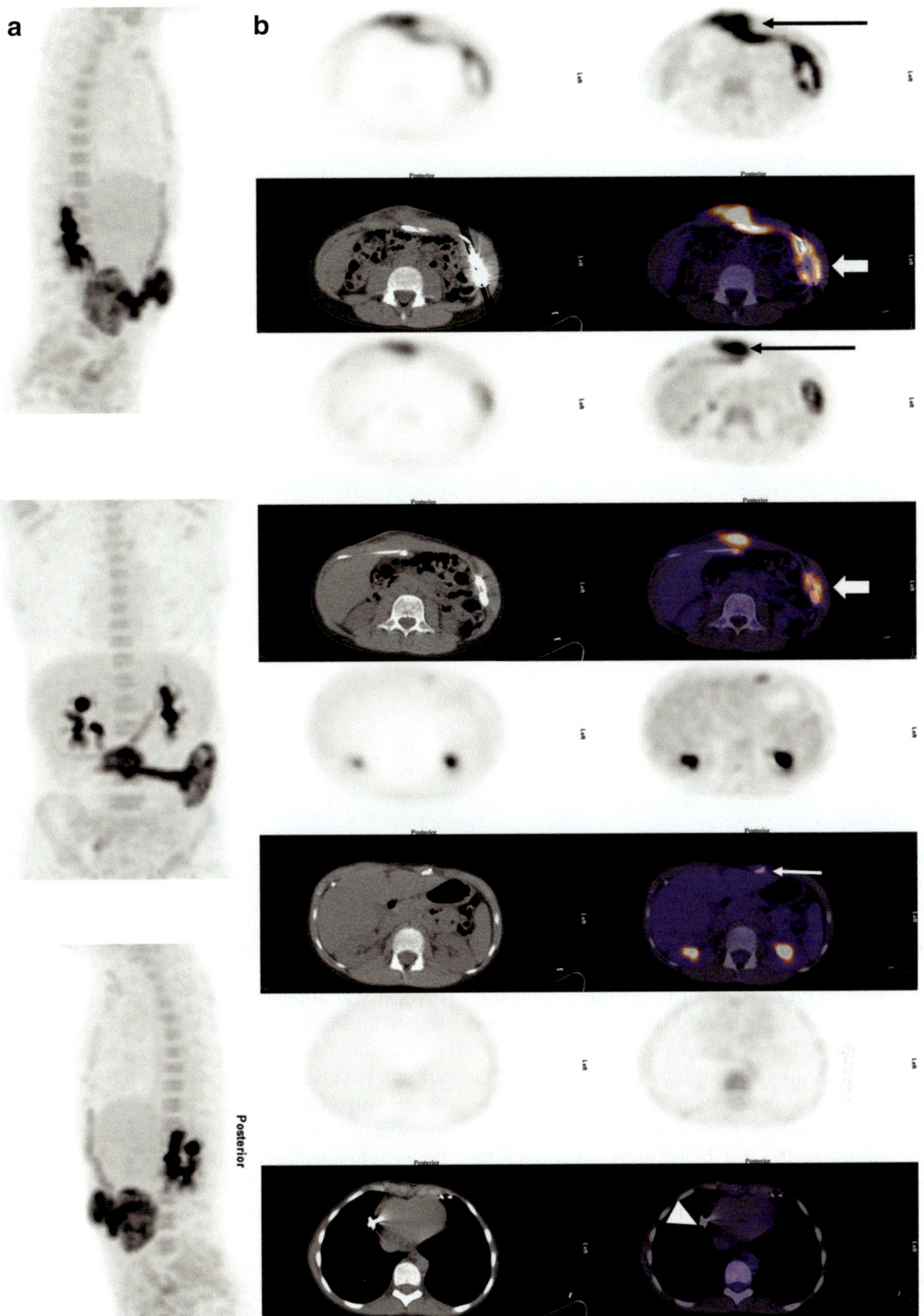

Fig. 21.8 ^{18}F-FDG PET/CT of a 9-year-old patient hospitalized for low-grade fever and induration in the epigastric region. The patient had multiple cardiac surgeries for congenital heart disease (double outlet right ventricle) including an epicardial dual chamber pacemaker implantation with implantable pulse generator in the left upper abdominal quadrant for third-degree atrioventricular block. After an inconclusive ultrasound of the latter region, ^{18}F-FDG PET/CT was performed: Maximum Intensity Projections (**a**) and selected axial images (**b**).

Increased activity was found on both the non–attenuation-corrected (NAC) and CT attenuation-corrected (CTAC) images around the pacemaker casing (open arrow) and along the tunneled wires (long thin arrow). However, there was no supradiaphragmatic extension to the wires (thin short arrow) or to the epicardial leads (arrowhead). The pacemaker was removed and infection was confirmed. After a course of antibiotics with the patient under external pacing, a new pacemaker was installed, with no further complications

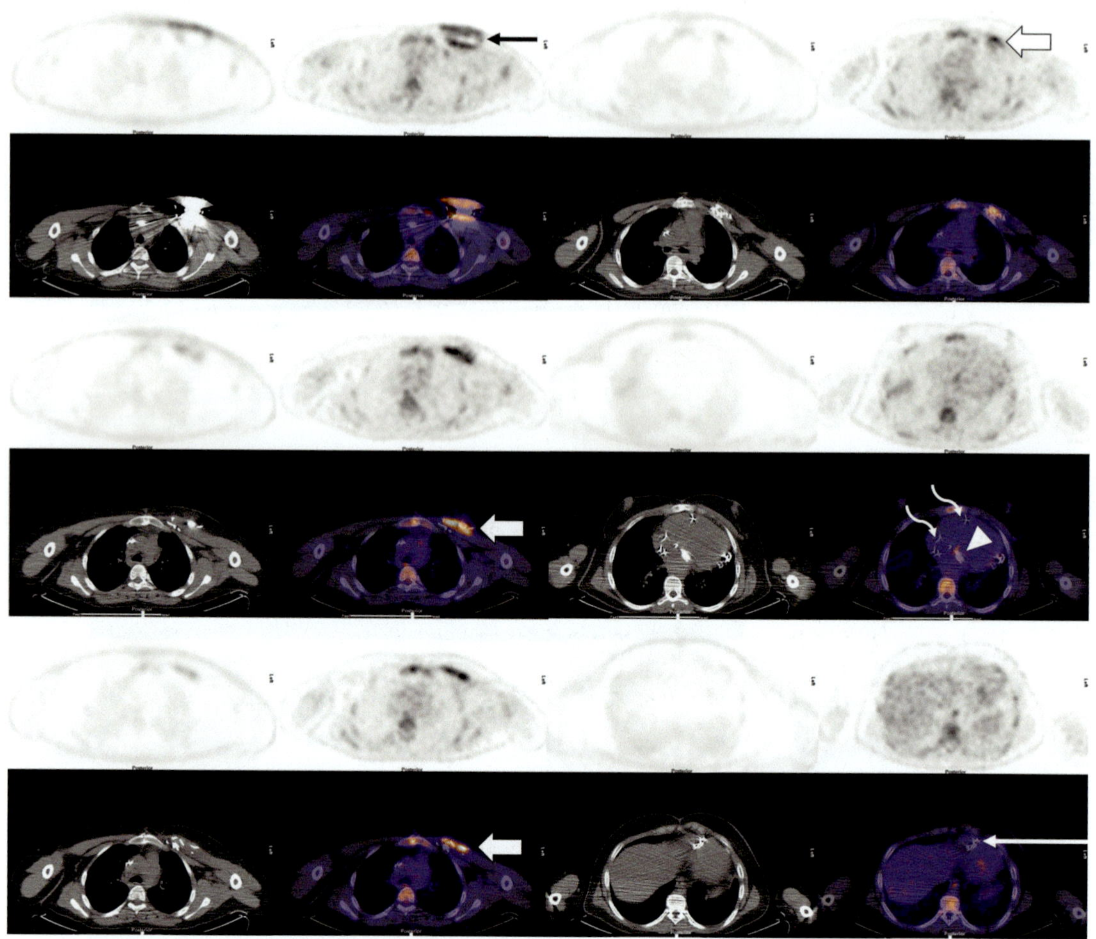

Fig. 21.9 ^{18}F-FDG PET/CT of a 15-year-old patient status post atrioventricular defect and coarctation of the aorta repair, post epicardial dual chamber pacemaker (ICD) implantation, and artificial mitral valve insertion. ICD replacement with three endovascular leads and one epicardial lead. There was a known superficial infection around the casing in the left hemithorax secondary to *Staphylococcus hominis*. As leads could not be properly visualized on echocardiogram, ^{18}F-FDG PET/CT with myocardial suppression protocol was performed. An active infectious process was demonstrated around the ICD casing (short thin arrow) and superficial wires (open arrow). No abnormal uptake was found at the level of the mitral valve (arrow head), endocardial leads (curvilinear arrows) or epicardial lead (long thin arrow). The patient underwent pacemaker extraction. After a course of antibiotics under external pacing, a new pacemaker was installed, without further complication

Pericardial Disease

Pericardial disease can be categorized as infectious versus noninfectious, and malignant versus nonmalignant. Etiologies include infectious, neoplastic, autoimmune, metabolic, iatrogenic, and traumatic causes. More often than not, the cause remains elusive [61]. The standard workup for pericarditis includes a thorough history, physical examination and additional investigations such as electrocardiogram, transthoracic echocardiography, and dosage or serum inflammatory biomarkers. ^{18}F-FDG PET/CT can play a role by assessing the activity of the pericardium and/or pericardial effusion (Fig. 21.10). In addition, whole body ^{18}F-FDG PET/CT can identify patterns of uptake suggestive of either infection, collagen vascular disease or neoplasm [62, 63]. Optimal imaging using myocardial suppression protocols should always be used.

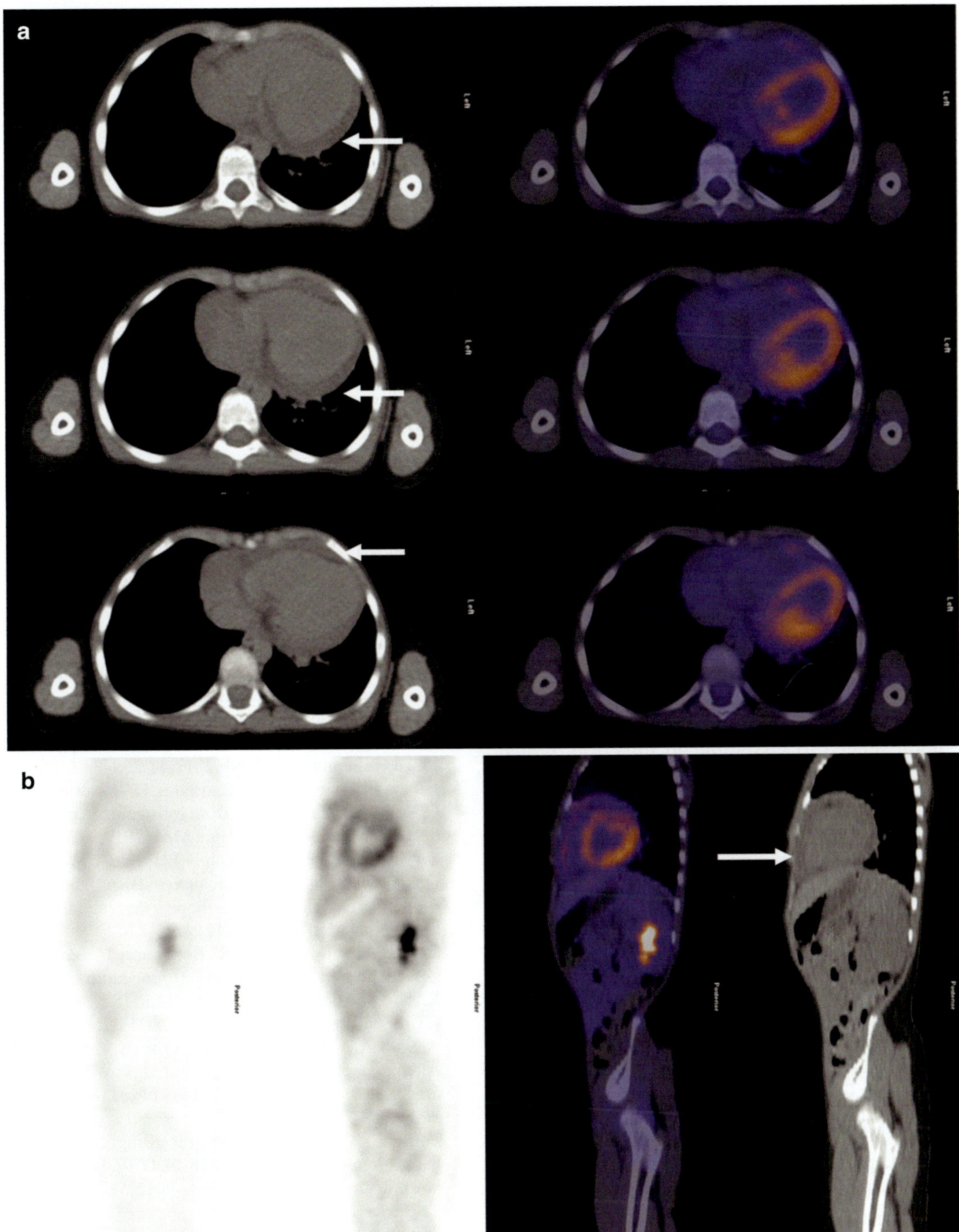

Fig. 21.10 ^{18}F-FDG PET/CT of a 5-year-old patient with a history of Kawasaki disease who presented with acute chest pain and heart palpitations. An echocardiogram demonstrated a pericardial effusion. ^{18}F-FDG PET/CT was requested to rule out collagen vascular disease as a clinical cause. Axial (**a**) and sagittal (**b**) images show significant pericardial effusion (arrow) with mild and diffuse uptake. The remaining study was normal. Biomarkers were negative. The final diagnosis was idiopathic pericarditis, which responded well to steroids

In neoplastic pericardial disease, ^{18}F-FDG PET/CT can help differentiate primary involvement of the pericardium from a paraneoplastic syndrome. Whereas direct involvement can originate from primary or metastatic malignancy, the most common underlying causes are different in children compared to adults. Hodgkin's lymphoma, especially bulky mediastinal disease, remains a frequent cause [63, 64]. Less frequently, other primary pericardial neoplasms such as sarcomas can be encountered [63]. Pericardial disease, especially when effusion is present, justifies investigation for an underlying malignancy.

Infectious pericardial disease etiologies include viral, bacterial, fungal, and rarely parasitic, with viral pericarditis being most frequent and often isolated. Apart from a viral prodrome, it resembles idiopathic pericarditis. It is usually not severe and has a good prognosis, although can be associated with a higher risk of myocardial damage [65]. ^{18}F-FDG PET/CT remains helpful for local evaluation of disease, along with cardiac MRI for the assessment of myocardial inflammation. It can also help detect septic emboli related to disseminated infection, which can change clinical management.

^{18}F-FDG PET/CT can be especially helpful for the investigation of tuberculous pericarditis. If left untreated, this condition can be associated with high morbidity and mortality. ^{18}F-FDG PET/CT can be helpful for the identification of pulmonary, bone, or colic foci, which can suggest the presence of underlying tuberculous infection and provide guidance for biopsy sampling [66, 67]. ^{18}F-FDG PET/CT can also help characterize constrictive pericarditis, associated with irreversible chronic inflammation and fibrosis of pericardium. Underlying causes can be idiopathic, postsurgical, postinfectious, or related to connective tissue diseases. Documenting active pericardial inflammation is helpful in the management of transient constrictive pericarditis [68].

Conclusion

Cardiac ^{18}F-FDG PET/CT in children has emerged as a useful tool allowing investigation of different pathologies affecting specific pediatric populations, such as those with congenital heart disease. Adapting nuclear medicine imaging and tailoring existing protocols to pediatric needs and adequate patient preparation depending on specific clinical indications ensures efficient and safe use of ^{18}F-FDG PET/CT in children, with minimization of adverse effects.

References

1. Edwards KW. Preparation and logistic considerations in performing PET and PET/computed tomography in pediatric patients. PET Clin. 2020;15(3):285–92.
2. Fahey FH, Goodkind A, MacDougall RD, Oberg L, Ziniel SI, Cappock R, et al. Operational and dosimetric aspects of pediatric PET/CT. J Nucl Med. 2017;58(9):1360–6.
3. Paiva FG, do Carmo Santana P, Mourao AP. Dosimetric study of pediatric PET/CT scan using different phantoms. Radiat Phys Chem. 2020;173:108887.
4. Parisi MT, Bermo MS, Alessio AM, Sharp SE, Gelfand MJ, Shulkin BL. Optimization of pediatric PET/CT. Semin Nucl Med. 2017;47:258–74.
5. Fahey FH, Goodkind AB, Plyku D, Khamwan K, O'Reilly SE, Cao X, et al. Dose estimation in pediatric nuclear medicine. Semin Nucl Med. 2017;47:118–25.
6. Treves ST, Gelfand MJ, Fahey FH, Parisi MT. 2016 update of the north American consensus guidelines for pediatric administered radiopharmaceutical activities. J Nucl Med. 2016;57(12):15N–8N.
7. Vali R, Alessio A, Balza R, Borgwardt L, Bar-Sever Z, Czachowski M, et al. SNMMI procedure standard/EANM practice guideline on pediatric 18F-FDG PET/CT for oncology 1.0. J Nucl Med. 2021;62(1):99–110.
8. Alessio AM, Kinahan PE, Manchanda V, Ghioni V, Aldape L, Parisi MT. Weight-based, low-dose pediatric whole-body PET/CT protocols. J Nucl Med. 2009;50(10):1570–8.
9. Turpin S, Abikhzer G, Lambert R. Simplified weight-based, low dose pediatric F18-FDG PET/CT protocols: dosimetry. J Nucl Med. 2011;52(supplement 1):1389.
10. McQuattie S. Pediatric PET/CT imaging: tips and techniques. J Nucl Med Technol. 2008;36(4):171–8.

11. Knuuti MJ, Nuutila P, Ruotsalainen U, Saraste M, Härkönen R, Ahonen A, et al. Euglycemic hyperinsulinemic clamp and oral glucose load in stimulating myocardial glucose utilization during positron emission tomography. J Nucl Med. 1992;33(7):1255–62.

12. Osborne MT, Hulten EA, Murthy VL, Skali H, Taqueti VR, Dorbala S, et al. Patient preparation for cardiac fluorine-18 fluorodeoxyglucose positron emission tomography imaging of inflammation. J Nucl Cardiol. 2017;24(1):86–99.

13. Schultz ML, Niescierenko M. Guidance for implementing pediatric procedural sedation in resource-limited settings. Clin Pediatr Emerg Med. 2019;20(2):116–22.

14. Mandell GA, Majd M, Shalaby-Rana E, Gordon I. Society of nuclear medicine procedure guideline for pediatric sedation in nuclear medicine. J Nucl Med. 2003;44:173–4.

15. Rosen D, Gamble J, Matava C. Canadian pediatric anesthesia society statement on clear fluid fasting for elective pediatric anesthesia. Can J Anesth. 2019;66(8):991–2.

16. Toney M, Pattishall S, Garber M. The time is now: standardized sedation training for pediatric hospitalists. Pediatrics. 2020;145(5):e20200446.

17. Sivaramakrishnan G, Sridharan K. Nitrous oxide and midazolam sedation: a systematic review and meta-analysis. Anesth Prog. 2017;64(2):59–65.

18. Eberson CP, Hsu RY, Borenstein TR. Procedural sedation in the emergency department. J Am Acad Orthop Surg. 2015;23(4):233–42.

19. Franco A. Current perspectives of pediatric PET/MRI. Clin Pediatr. 2019;2:1016.

20. Mannheim JG, Schmid AM, Schwenck J, Katiyar P, Herfert K, Pichler BJ, et al. PET/MRI hybrid systems. Semin Nucl Med. 2018;48:332–47.

21. Bezrukov I, Schmidt H, Gatidis S, Mantlik F, Schäfer JF, Schwenzer N, et al. Quantitative evaluation of segmentation-and atlas-based attenuation correction for PET/MR on pediatric patients. J Nucl Med. 2015;56(7):1067–74.

22. Boxt LM. Magnetic resonance and computed tomographic evaluation of congenital heart disease. J Magn Reson Imaging. 2004;19(6):827–47.

23. Boechat MI, Ratib O, Williams PL, Gomes AS, Child JS, Allada V. Cardiac MR imaging and MR angiography for assessment of complex tetralogy of Fallot and pulmonary atresia. Radiographics. 2005;25(6):1535–46.

24. Purz S, Sabri O, Viehweger A, Barthel H, Kluge R, Sorge I, et al. Potential pediatric applications of PET/MR. J Nucl Med. 2014;55(Supplement 2):32S–9S.

25. Hirsch FW, Sattler B, Sorge I, Kurch L, Viehweger A, Ritter L, et al. PET/MR in children. Initial clinical experience in paediatric oncology using an integrated PET/MR scanner. Pediatr Radiol. 2013;43(7):860–75.

26. Takalkar A, Chen W, Desjardins B, Alavi A, Torigian DA. Cardiovascular imaging with PET, CT, and MR imaging. PET Clin. 2008;3(3):411–34.

27. Rischpler C, Nekolla SG, Dregely I, Schwaiger M. Hybrid PET/MR imaging of the heart: potential, initial experiences, and future prospects. J Nucl Med. 2013;54(3):402–15.

28. Rife E, Gedalia A. Kawasaki disease: an update. Curr Rheumatol Rep. 2020;22(10):75.

29. Friedman KG, Gauvreau K, Hamaoka-Okamoto A, Tang A, Berry E, Tremoulet AH, et al. Coronary artery aneurysms in Kawasaki disease: risk factors for progressive disease and adverse cardiac events in the US population. J Am Heart Assoc. 2016;5(9):e003289.

30. Hernandez-Pampaloni M, Allada V, Fishbein MC, Schelbert HR. Myocardial perfusion and viability by positron emission tomography in infants and children with coronary abnormalities: correlation with echocardiography, coronary angiography, and histopathology. J Am Coll Cardiol. 2003;41(4):618–26.

31. Frommelt PC, Frommelt MA. Congenital coronary artery anomalies. Pediatr Clin North Am. 2004;51(5):1273–88.

32. Gittenberger-de Groot AC, Koenraadt WMC, Bartelings MM, Bökenkamp R, DeRuiter MC, Hazekamp MG, et al. Coding of coronary arterial origin and branching in congenital heart disease: the modified Leiden convention. J Thorac Cardiovasc Surg. 2018;156(6):2260–9.

33. Sithamparanathan S, Padley SPG, Rubens MB, Gatzoulis MA, Ho SY, Nicol ED. Great vessel and coronary artery anatomy in transposition and other coronary anomalies: a universal descriptive and alpha-numerical sequential classification. JACC Cardiovasc Imaging. 2013;6(5):624–30.

34. Click RL, Holmes DR, Vlietstra RE, Kosinski AS, Kronmal RA. Anomalous coronary arteries: location, degree of atherosclerosis and effect on survival—a report from the Coronary Artery Surgery Study. J Am Coll Cardiol. 1989;13(3):531–7.

35. Davis JA, Cecchin F, Jones TK, Portman MA. Major coronary artery anomalies in a pediatric population: incidence and clinical importance. J Am Coll Cardiol. 2001;37(2):593–7.

36. Dodge-Khatami A, Mavroudis C, Backer CL. Anomalous origin of the left coronary artery from the pulmonary artery: collective review of surgical therapy. Ann Thorac Surg. 2002;74(3):946–55.

37. Backer CL, Stout MJ, Zales VR, Muster AJ, Weigel TJ, Idriss FS, et al. Anomalous origin of the left coronary artery. A twenty-year review of surgical management. J Thorac Cardiovasc Surg. 1992;103(6):1049–57; discussion 1057-1058.

38. Azour L, Jacobi AH, Alpert JB, Uppu S, Latson L, Mason D, et al. Congenital coronary artery anomalies and implications. J Thorac Imaging. 2018;33(5):W30–8.

39. Walsh R, Nielsen JC, Ko HH, Sanz J, Srivastava S, Parness IA, et al. Imaging of congenital coronary artery anomalies. Pediatr Radiol. 2011;41(12):1526–35.

40. Hoffman JIE, Kaplan S. The incidence of congenital heart disease. J Am Coll Cardiol. 2002;39(12):1890–900.

41. McElhinney DB, Reddy VM, Silverman NH, Hanley FL. Modified Damus-Kaye-Stansel procedure for single ventricle, subaortic stenosis, and arch obstruction in neonates and infants: midterm results and techniques for avoiding circulatory arrest. J Thorac Cardiovasc Surg. 1997;114(5):718–25; discussion 725-726.

42. Jamar F, Buscombe J, Chiti A, Christian PE, Delbeke D, Donohoe KJ, et al. EANM/SNMMI guideline for 18F-FDG use in inflammation and infection. J Nucl Med. 2013;54(4):647–58.

43. Slart RHJA, Glaudemans AWJM, Gheysens O, Lubberink M, Kero T, Dweck MR, et al. Procedural recommendations of cardiac PET/CT imaging: standardization in inflammatory-, infective-, infiltrative-, and innervation- (4Is) related cardiovascular diseases: a joint collaboration of the EACVI and the EANM: summary. Eur Heart J Cardiovasc Imaging. 2020;21(12):1320–30.

44. Yabrodi M, Hermann JL, Brown JW, Rodefeld MD, Turrentine MW, Mastropietro CW. Minimization of surgical site infections in patients with delayed sternal closure after pediatric cardiac surgery. World J Pediatr Congenit Heart Surg. 2019;10(4):400–6.

45. Jha P, Woodward CS, Gardner H, Pietz C, Husain SA. A quality improvement initiative to reduce surgical site infections in patients undergoing delayed sternal closure after pediatric cardiac surgery. Pediatr Cardiol. 2020;41(7):1402–7.

46. Hariri H, Tan S, Martineau P, Lamarche Y, Carrier M, Finnerty V, et al. Utility of FDG-PET/CT for the detection and characterization of sternal wound infection following sternotomy. Nucl Med Mol Imaging. 2019;53(4):253–62.

47. Pelletier-Galarneau M, Abikhzer G, Harel F, Dilsizian V. Detection of native and prosthetic valve endocarditis: incremental attributes of functional FDG PET/CT over morphologic imaging. Curr Cardiol Rep. 2020;22(9):93.

48. Pizzi MN, Dos-Subirà L, Roque A, Fernández-Hidalgo N, Cuéllar-Calabria H, Pijuan Domènech A, et al. 18F-FDG-PET/CT angiography in the diagnosis of infective endocarditis and cardiac device infection in adult patients with congenital heart disease and prosthetic material. Int J Cardiol. 2017;248:396–402.

49. Partington SL, Valente AM, Landzberg M, Grant F, Di Carli MF, Dorbala S. Clinical applications of radionuclide imaging in the evaluation and management of patients with congenital heart disease. J Nucl Cardiol. 2016;23(1):45–63.

50. Zhang Y, Williams H, Pucar D. FDG-PET identification of infected pulmonary artery conduit following tetralogy of Fallot (TOF) repair. Nucl Med Mol Imaging. 2017;51(1):86–7.

51. Meyer Z, Fischer M, Koerfer J, Laser KT, Kececioglu D, Burchert W, et al. The role of FDG-PET-CT in pediatric cardiac patients and patients with congenital heart defects. Int J Cardiol. 2016;220:656–60.

52. Kouijzer IJE, Mulders-Manders CM, Bleeker-Rovers CP, Oyen WJG. Fever of unknown origin: the value of FDG-PET/CT. Semin Nucl Med. 2018;48(2):100–7.

53. Pijl JP, Kwee TC, Legger GE, Peters HJH, Armbrust W, Schölvinck EH, et al. Role of FDG-PET/CT in children with fever of unknown origin. Eur J Nucl Med Mol Imaging. 2020;47(6):1596–604.

54. Blokhuis GJ, Bleeker-Rovers CP, Diender MG, Oyen WJG, Draaisma JMT, de Geus-Oei L-F. Diagnostic value of FDG-PET/(CT) in children with fever of unknown origin and unexplained fever during immune suppression. Eur J Nucl Med Mol Imaging. 2014;41(10):1916–23.

55. Jeewa A, Imamura M, Canter C, Niebler RA, VanderPluym C, Rosenthal DN, et al. Long-term outcomes after transplantation after support with a pulsatile pediatric ventricular assist device. J Heart Lung Transplant. 2019;38(4):449–55.

56. Absi M, Bocchini C, Price JF, Adachi I. F-fluorodeoxyglucose-positive emission tomography/CT imaging for left ventricular assist device-associated infections in children. Cardiol Young. 2018;28(10):1157–9.

57. Burki S, Adachi I. Pediatric ventricular assist devices: current challenges and future prospects. Vasc Health Risk Manag. 2017;13:177–85.

58. Dell'Aquila AM, Mastrobuoni S, Alles S, Wenning C, Henryk W, Schneider SRB, et al. Contributory role of fluorine 18-Fluorodeoxyglucose positron emission tomography/computed tomography in the diagnosis and clinical Management of Infections in patients supported with a continuous-flow left ventricular assist device. Ann Thorac Surg. 2016;101(1):87–94. discussion 94

59. Mahmood M, Kendi AT, Ajmal S, Farid S, O'Horo JC, Chareonthaitawee P, et al. Meta-analysis of 18F-FDG PET/CT in the diagnosis of infective endocarditis. J Nucl Cardiol. 2019;26(3):922–35.

60. Turpin S, Lambert R, Poirier N. An unusual looking pacemaker infection imaged with 18F-FDG PET/CT. Eur J Nucl Med Mol Imaging. 2010;37(7):1438.

61. Chiabrando JG, Bonaventura A, Vecchié A, Wohlford GF, Mauro AG, Jordan JH, et al. Management of acute and recurrent pericarditis: JACC state-of-the-art review. J Am Coll Cardiol. 2020;75(1):76–92.

62. Kim M-S, Kim E-K, Choi JY, Oh JK, Chang S-A. Clinical utility of [18F]FDG-PET/CT in pericardial disease. Curr Cardiol Rep. 2019;21(9):107.

63. Martineau P, Dilsizian V, Pelletier-Galarneau M. Incremental value of FDG-PET in the evaluation of cardiac masses. Curr Cardiol Rep. 2021;23(7):78.

64. Bligh MP, Borgaonkar JN, Burrell SC, MacDonald DA, Manos D. Spectrum of CT findings in thoracic extranodal non-Hodgkin lymphoma. Radiographics. 2017;37(2):439–61.

65. Gerardin C, Mageau A, Benali K, Jouan F, Ducrocq G, Alexandra J-F, et al. Increased FDG-PET/CT peri-

cardial uptake identifies acute pericarditis patients at high risk for relapse. Int J Cardiol. 2018;271: 192–4.

66. Dong A, Dong H, Wang Y, Cheng C, Zuo C, Lu J. (18) F-FDG PET/CT in differentiating acute tuberculous from idiopathic pericarditis: preliminary study. Clin Nucl Med. 2013;38(4):e160–5.

67. Pelletier-Galarneau M, Martineau P, Zuckier LS, Pham X, Lambert R, Turpin S. 18F-FDG-PET/CT imaging of thoracic and extrathoracic tuberculosis in children. Semin Nucl Med. 2017;47:304–18.

68. Chang SA, Oh JK. Constrictive pericarditis: a medical or surgical disease? J Cardiovasc Imaging. 2019;27(3):178–86.

Johan Van Cleemput, Daan Dierickx,
and Olivier Gheysens

Introduction

Since the first heart transplantation was performed more than 50 years ago in Cape Town, South Africa, more than 200,000 patients have received a donor heart almost exclusively provided by donation after brain death. Currently more than 6000 heart transplantations are registered annually to the International Society of Heart and Lung Transplantation (ISHLT) [1]. This number is estimated to reflect about 80% of the actual heart transplant activity performed worldwide. Despite good outcome results, improved preservation techniques of the donor hearts and the recent use of donor hearts after

J. Van Cleemput
Department of Cardiology, University Hospitals
Leuven, Leuven, Belgium

Department of Cardiovascular Sciences, KU Leuven,
Leuven, Belgium
e-mail: johan.vancleemput@uzleuven.be

D. Dierickx
Laboratory for Experimental Hematology,
Department of Hematology, KU Leuven, University
Hospitals Leuven, Leuven, Belgium
e-mail: daan.dierickx@uzleuven.be

O. Gheysens (✉)
Department of Nuclear Medicine, Cliniques
Universitaires Saint-Luc and Institute of Clinical and
Experimental Research (IREC), Université
Catholique de Louvain (UC Louvain),
Brussels, Belgium
e-mail: olivier.gheysens@saintluc.uclouvain.be

circulatory death, it is unlikely that the number of heart transplantations will increase in the near future. In Europe, a decrease in the number of heart transplantations has been observed during the last decade, resulting in acceptance of older and so-called marginal donor hearts. North America seems to escape from this evolution, probably due to a higher incidence of young people dying accidentally and due to the opiate crisis [1]. The imbalance between candidate recipients and donor hearts has led to an increase in the average waiting time which in turn has resulted in a growing number of patients that need to be bridged by mechanical circulatory support (MCS) devices until a donor heart becomes available. Initially, these devices were temporary such as venoarterial extracorporeal membrane oxygenation (VA-ECMO) and extracorporeal life support (ECLS) devices, allowing to bridge for a couple of weeks in the intensive care unit. Nowadays, due to continuous improvements in intracorporeal left ventricular assist devices (LVAD), patients can be bridged and remain ambulatory for years and currently almost half of the candidates on the waiting list have a LVAD [1].

Once a daring experimental therapy, heart transplantation has evolved into a feasible treatment option in highly selected patients with end-stage heart failure in whom all other therapies have failed. Survival has gradually increased over the last decades with a median survival of

© The Author(s), under exclusive license to Springer Nature Switzerland AG 2022
M. Pelletier-Galarneau, P. Martineau (eds.), *FDG-PET/CT and PET/MR in Cardiovascular
Diseases*, https://doi.org/10.1007/978-3-031-09807-9_22

8.6 years in the 1980s over 10.5 years in the 1990s and an overall median survival of 12.5 years for patients transplanted between 2002 and 2009 according to the latest ISHLT report [1]. Single centers have even reported 1, 5, 10, and 15-years survival rates of 92, 87, 76, and 58%, resulting in a median survival of more than 18 years [2]. Unfortunately, heart transplant is not a definite cure and patients are at risk to develop mild to potentially fatal complications. The 5% 30-day mortality rate is mainly driven by primary graft failure (PGF) and multiple organ failure. The former mostly due to technical reasons often related to preservation difficulties and rarely as a consequence of hyperacute rejection. During the rest of the first postoperative year, the main causes of death are infection (<6 months) and graft failure due to acute cellular (ACR) or antibody-mediated rejection (AMR). Therefore, endomyocardial biopsies (EMB) are performed per protocol in the first postoperative year aiming at early diagnosis and treatment of rejection, before serious graft damage occurs. During long-term follow-up, late graft failure (LGF) and malignancies with increasing incidence after transplantation become the main threats for heart recipients.

This chapter summarizes the current evidence of FDG-PET/CT imaging in heart transplant candidates focusing on LVAD infections and its role in posttransplant complications such as infections, graft rejection, and malignancies.

Pretransplant Screening

Patients with ischemic cardiomyopathy constitute almost 30% of transplant candidates and, due to the scarcity of donor hearts, all other therapies must have been exhausted before considering heart transplantation [1]. Ischemic heart disease remains the only cause of left ventricular dysfunction that is amenable to the benefit of coronary artery bypass grafting (CABG). The assessment of myocardial viability, with an improvement in systolic function as reference standard, to identify patients who will most likely benefit from surgical revascularization remains a topic of debate. The formerly accepted concept, based on retrospective studies, that assessing myocardial viability using, for example, FDG PET is important to identify patients who might benefit from revascularization has been challenged by the myocardial viability substudy of the STICH trial and the PARR-2 trial [3, 4]. The initial report of this prospective myocardial viability substudy of the STICH trial did not show an association between the presence of myocardial viability and survival benefit from CABG after a median follow-up of 5.1 years [5]. The recent results after a median follow-up of 10.4 years showed an association between viable myocardium and improvement of LV systolic function irrespective of treatment but did not confirm a reduction in mortality by revascularizing patients with myocardial viability assessed with single-photon-emission computed tomography (SPECT) and/or stress echocardiography [6]. However, viability assessment was not performed with FDG-PET or cardiac magnetic resonance imaging considered as reference test to evaluate myocardial scarring. The role of FDG-PET/CT to assess myocardial viability and guide revascularization in patients with ischemic cardiomyopathy is discussed in detail in Chap. 20.

Probably one of the most important indications for FDG-PET/CT in the pretransplant setting, lies in the diagnosis of LVAD infections [7]. Owing to the shortage of donor hearts and increased waiting times, more patients need a LVAD as a bridge to transplantation or even as destination therapy [1, 8]. Recent improvements in assist device technology have resulted in better survival and less complications. The initial large pulsatile devices have been replaced by smaller nonpulsatile axial flow pumps still residing in the abdominal cavity. There is nowadays a shift toward fully magnetically levitated centrifugal continuous flow (CF) pumps, implanted within the pericardial sac. One and 2-year survival rates of 82% and 73% in patients with these CF devices are slowly approaching the results of heart transplantation [9]. Complications such as stroke and bleeding have significantly decreased, but infections of the LVAD remain a problem with increasing incidence over time and are associated with a high rate of hospitalization [10]. This is unlikely to change as long as the pump depends on energy transferred by a driveline that connects the implanted LVAD with the batteries outside the patient. The MOMENTUM-3 trial did not show any difference in infectious complications between axial flow and centrifugal flow devices: 22% developed a driveline infection, 14% had at least one episode of sepsis and 18% of the mortality in the first 2 years after implantation was related to infection [11, 12]. These prospective trial data largely confirm recent INTERMACS registry results [13]. In this registry, standardized definitions of VAD infections (VAD-specific, VAD-related, and non–VAD-related infections) have been used as proposed by the International Society of Heart and Lung Transplantation (ISHLT [14]. VAD-specific infections can affect the superficial or the deeper portion of the driveline, the pump, and/or the inflow and outflow cannulas or the pocket. VAD-related infections include infective endocarditis, blood stream infections, mediastinitis and sternal wound infections [14]. In the registry, 18% of the patients with a CF LVAD developed a VAD-specific infection, more than 19% suffered a VAD-related infection and 6% of the mortality was related to major infections [13]. Therefore, early and accurate diagnosis of LVAD infections is of the utmost importance.

Establishing the presence, extent, and severity of LVAD infections, especially deep and central infections, can be challenging since conventional imaging techniques such as echocardiography and CT are hampered by device-related artefacts. Aspiration of suspected fluid collections is not without risk and obtaining samples from tissue surrounding the driveline, pump, or cannulas requires major surgery. Therefore, several studies assessed the diagnostic performance of FDG-PET/CT for diagnosing VAD-specific infections and two recent meta-analyses reported a good diagnostic accuracy with overall high sensitivity but variable specificity [15, 16]. In the analysis by Ten Hove et al., visual analysis yielded a pooled sensitivity of 0.95 (95% confidence interval (CI) 0.89–0.97) and pooled specificity of 0.91 (95% CI 0.54–0.99) [16]. These results were quite similar when focusing on either pump/pocket infections or driveline infections. The wide CIs for specificity reflected the heterogeneity across different included studies that was attributed to differences in patient selection, scan procedures and interpretation, suboptimal dietary preparation or concurrent blood stream infection. Nevertheless, FDG-PET/CT is a powerful tool to exclude VAD-specific infections given the consistently high sensitivity and high negative predictive value [17]. On top of helping the clinician to diagnose VAD infections, FDG-PET/CT provides information on the exact location and extent of the infectious process that might influence the therapeutic strategy as was shown in different studies [18–21]. Representative FDG-PET/CT images of a VAD infection are shown in Fig 22.1. A localized infection at the exit or distal site of the driveline can be treated with antibiotics, while prolonged antibiotic therapy is needed once the infection extends along the tract toward the proximal portion. As a pump infection may upgrade the status on the waiting list of a transplant candidate in many allocation systems, an undisputable diagnosis is mandatory. Semi-quantitative measures such as standard uptake volume and metabolic volume might be helpful in estimating the severity of the infection and the effect of antibiotic therapy [21–24]. Since FDG-PET/CT is a whole-body imaging modality, it also allows detecting extracardiac infections and septic embolisms with high accuracy as was shown in several studies [23, 25, 26]. The diagnostic value of FDG-PET/CT for detecting VAD infections outperforms the yield of white blood cell scintigraphy and CT. In the only study comparing FDG-PET/CT with ^{99m}Tc-labeled white blood cell scintigraphy in 22 patients, a significantly lower sensitivity was observed for the latter [26]. Similarly, CT-scan only identified 4 of the 28 patients with a peripheral or central VAD-infection as detected by FDG-PET/CT [20]. A further improvement in diagnostic accuracy could be obtained by performing a baseline FDG-PET/CT scan to which the results of a subsequent scan could be compared. This strategy resulted in 100% sensitivity and 100% specificity to detect driveline infections [24]. Finally, one study

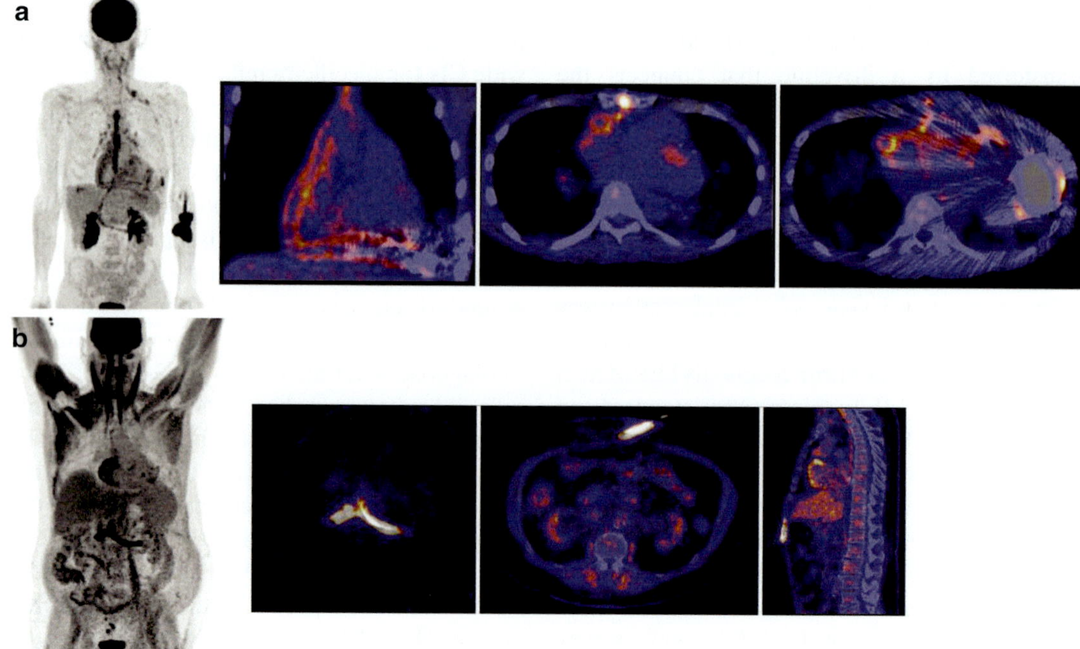

Fig. 22.1 VAD-specific infection. FDG maximum intensity projection (MIP) image, coronal and transaxial fused PET-CT images show heterogeneous uptake around the outflow tract corresponding to an infection. Note the reactive diffuse homogeneous driveline uptake shortly after LVAD implantation (~1 month) (**a**). FDG MIP image, coronal, transaxial and sagittal fused PET-CT images show intense FDG uptake around the driveline with a subcutaneous abscess without pathological FDG uptake at the pump or cannulas compatible with an isolated driveline infection. (**b**). (Image courtesy of D. ten Hove, UMCGroningen)

reported unexpectedly 3 peripheral and 3 central positive FDG-PET/CT scans among 11 patients without any clinical evidence of infection. Because of a similar increase in all-cause mortality in FDG-PET/CT positive patients irrespective of clinical evidence of infection, the authors suggest that these positive scans should be considered as markers of early infection where antibiotic treatment might prevent spreading the infection toward the pump and the cannulas [20].

Even though there is increasing evidence to perform FDG-PET/CT in patients with suspected VAD-specific infections as outlined above, the 2019 European Association of Cardio Thoracic Surgeons (EACTS) Expert Consensus on long-term Mechanical Circulatory Support paper, does not mention FDG-PET/CT, but states that white blood cell scintigraphy should be considered for the detection and location of infection and infected emboli (class IIA with level of evidence C). It is noteworthy to mention that both references supporting this recommendation refer to FDG-PET/CT [27]. VAD infections are discussed in greater details in Chap. 16.

Posttransplantation Graft-Related Complications

Similar to other solid-organ transplantations, acute rejection (AR) remains a feared complication after heart transplantation. Especially in the first postoperative year(s), AR still remains an important potential cause of mortality even though the incidence and impact on graft survival have decreased over the years due to improved immunosuppressive regimens [1]. The pathogenesis of rejection is linked to various pathways and two distinct mechanisms responsible for graft injury during acute rejection are nowadays recognized: acute cellular rejection (ACR) and antibody-mediated rejection (AMR). Initially the focus was on ACR, characterized by activation of T-lymphocytes infiltrating the interstitial space and finally leading to T-cell mediated damage of cardiomyocytes. This process has been defined and classified according to the amount and location of the inflammatory infiltrate and myocardial cell death, as described in the revision of the 1990 working formulation for the standardization of nomenclature in the diagnosis of heart rejection [28, 29]. Together with improvements in immunosuppressive therapy, the incidence of ACR has decreased and attention has shifted from ACR toward antibody-mediated rejection. This form of AR is driven by circulating human leucocyte antigen (HLA) and non-HLA antibodies directed against antigens expressed on endothelial cells which subsequently affects the vascular tree from the coronary arteries along the microvasculature to the venous structures of the entire donor heart [30–32]. As EMB is the gold standard for the diagnosis, AMR is primarily defined by pathological changes in the microvasculature [30]. Depending on the presence of intravascular activated mononuclear cells (mainly CD68 positive macrophages), capillary endothelial cell changes, deposition of fibrin, immunoglobulins and complement factors (mainly C4d) and interstitial edema, different grades of AMR have been defined [33, 34]. AMR can result in acute heart failure with reduced ejection fraction, but can also remain asymptomatic. Cardiac allograft vasculopathy (CAV) is one of the main long-term complications after heart transplantation. CAV is the arterial equivalent of AMR in the microvasculature and mainly affects the epicardial and intramyocardial muscular arteries and is characterized by a diffuse intimal proliferation of smooth muscle cells of the epicardial and intramyocardial arteries, hereby narrowing and

eventually completely occluding the arterial lumen [35]. The assessment of CAV is challenging due to the typical diffuse coronary epicardial and microvascular involvement [36]. Invasive angiography and intracoronary imaging are recommended for CAV surveillance but these techniques do not allow a detailed evaluation of distal vessels and microvasculature [37]. Moreover, surveillance by invasive strategies is not very practical and is associated with procedural risks. Therefore, evidence is accumulating to utilize noninvasive strategies for CAV surveillance and cardiac perfusion assessed by PET perfusion imaging is now included in imaging and transplantation guidelines [37, 38]. Although FDG-PET/CT does not play a role in detection of CAV, PET perfusion imaging may overcome the limitations of other techniques by providing absolute quantitative global and regional myocardial perfusion values and flow reserve, leading to increased sensitivity to detect diffuse epicardial and microvascular disease.

Chronic rejection (CR) remains ill-defined and late graft failure (LGF) is probably a more appropriate term, as CR is an endpoint rather than an active process. Clinically it presents as heart failure, often with preserved ejection fraction, developing insidiously many years after transplantation. It is characterized by diffuse interstitial fibrosis, with microinfarcts and a severely damaged vascular tree with narrowed arteries and a substantial reduction in the capillary density, the so-called capillary rarefaction on histology [33, 34]. The exact pathogenesis of LGF is incompletely understood, but it is likely the result of a combination of perioperative ischemic damage to the coronary arteries and the microvasculature with several episodes of postoperative clinical or subclinical ACR and AMR. Heart failure treatment is reinitiated, but to date retransplantation is the only curative therapy for LGF [32].

As both ACR and AMR are inflammatory processes, FDG-PET/CT might play a role to diagnose or even more importantly to monitor acute rejection, but few groups have investigated the role of FDG-PET/CT in this setting. Two animal experiments shed some light on the potential role of FDG-PET/CT in the diagnosis of AR [39, 40]. Both used heterotopic transplant rodent models with the heart implanted in the abdominal cavity and compared metabolism and perfusion, assessed by respectively FDG- and NH_3-PET, between the native hearts, the isografts and the allografts. In isograft models, donors and recipients are genetically identical, resulting in surgical insult without rejection. In allograft models the presence of major histocompatibility complex (MHC) mismatches, inevitably induces rejection on top of the surgical insult. The first report was published in 1992 by Hoff et al. using a heterotopic rat transplant model without immunosuppressive treatment in which FDG uptake and histology was analyzed at a single time point either 4 or 8 days postoperatively [39]. Histology showed mild ACR (inflammatory cell infiltration) at day 4 and severe ACR (myocyte necrosis) at day 8 in the allografts with a significantly increased FDG uptake both during mild and severe ACR compared to nonrejected isografts. There was no significant difference in FDG uptake between the mild and severe rejection groups. In addition to FDG uptake, NH_3 uptake tended to be higher in allografts than in isografts during mild ACR, but NH_3 uptake was significantly reduced during severe ACR suggesting the latter could be attributed to microvascular destruction and/or graft vasculopathy. Another preclinical study, more relevant from a clinical perspective given the longitudinal assessment, was performed by the group of Daly [40]. Between day 7 and day 42 after transplantation, FDG- and NH_3-PET imaging and histology were performed weekly in iso- and allografted mice. Some mice received no immunosuppressive therapy, some were treated with the costimulatory antagonist anti-CD40L and some received rapamycin. The FDG uptake in the isografts was not different from the uptake in the native hearts at day 7 but

decreased significantly thereafter. The reduction in metabolism was attributed to the fact that heterotopically implanted hearts do not actually work as the left ventricle remains empty. In the allografts implanted in mice without immunosuppression, the FDG uptake increased from day 7 onward and became significantly higher than the uptake in isografts at day 21 and day 28. This difference coincided with increasing degrees of rejection. Treatment with anti-CD40L completely abolished both the increase in FDG uptake over time and the histology of rejection in allografted mice. In mice treated with rapamycin, FDG uptake was lower than in mice not receiving immunosuppression but the difference was not significant and histology showed incomplete inhibition. Finally on day 28 the ratio of NH_3 uptake in the allograft to the uptake in the native heart was significantly reduced in the untreated allograft recipients. On histology, the former had significantly more CAV (expressed as average % vessel occlusion) and fewer vessels per area in biopsy sections, suggesting that the reduction in perfusion was due to micro- and macrovascular destruction. Although the authors conclude that their work might pave the way for PET/CT imaging into the clinical arena of heart transplantation, no follow-up studies are available. Cost, radiation exposure and limited availability should not be major concerns, considering the fact that most heart recipients are followed in tertiary centers and that the alternative of regular EMB biopsies is expensive as well and does also expose patients and personal to radiation. Probably the dietary preparation protocols, limited experience and lack of standardization and interpretation criteria form the major obstacles before utilization of FDG-PET/CT in this clinical scenario. To date, no FDG data are available to evaluate transplant rejection but two studies have investigated FDG uptake in heart transplant patients. The first publication by the group of London and Harefield compared myocardial FDG uptake in

10 heart recipients versus 9 healthy controls [41]. The recipients were 34 months after transplantation, had normal coronary angiographic findings and no clinical or histological evidence of graft rejection. The main finding of the study was a 2.5-fold increase in regional cardiac FDG uptake in the recipients compared to controls, a statistically significant difference that could not be explained by the increased regional myocardial blood flow, measured by ^{15}O-labeled water, or the increased rate pressure product. It was hypothesized that transplanted hearts shift their metabolism from free fatty acids to glucose and probably suffer a chronic imbalance between limited supply and increased demand. As none of the recipients was rejecting at the moment of the study, no conclusions could be drawn about a potential role of FDG-PET/CT in rejection. Another publication was entirely focused on patient preparation protocols to suppress physiological FDG uptake in the heart [42, 43]. Felix and colleagues compared 3 different protocols in patients that were scheduled for per protocol EMB in their first postoperative year. Images were analyzed visually and by measuring the relative ratio of cardiac uptake in regions of interest (RRCU) as compared to the uptake in the liver and the mediastinum. FDG uptake was considered adequately suppressed in 55 to 62% of the examinations. There was no significant difference between the 3 dietary protocols. None of the patients had an ACR necessitating therapy at the time of the FDG PET/CT scan. In 66% of the EMBs there was no abnormal infiltration of lymphocytes (grade 0R) whereas a minimal interstitial lymphocyte infiltration (grade 1R) was present in 34%. No significant difference was found in FDG uptake between patients with 0R of 1R biopsies, but the lack of microscopically significant rejection does not allow to make any conclusions on FDG imaging to identify patients with significant rejection. This clinical study might fuel new initiatives in this clinical setting.

Posttransplantation Non–Graft-Related Complications

Infections

Infectious complications remain a major hazard after heart transplant and are associated with significant morbidity and mortality. Due to alterations in their cellular and humoral immune system, solid-organ transplant patients are prone to opportunistic and complicated infections [44, 45]. The initial postoperative phase is the most critical period because of high immunosuppression and frailty of transplant recipients. The likelihood for a particular pathogen changes during the postoperative course with wound, fungal, and opportunistic infections being most prevalent in the early phase while community-based pathogens are more prevalent after the first year. In contrast to immunocompetent patients, infections in immunocompromised patients often have a clinically silent course or can be associated with atypical signs and symptoms making timely diagnosis very challenging. It is well known that FDG PET/CT is a powerful noninvasive technique to early detect various types of infectious processes wit high diagnostic accuracy [46]. Several studies assessing the diagnostic value of FDG PET/CT to detect infections after solid-organ transplantation reported excellent performance with overall high sensitivity and negative predictive value [47–50]. Fever of unknown origin (FUO), especially in immunocompromised patients, remains a diagnostic challenge and FDG PET/CT has been shown clinically useful in the majority of the cases with high negative predictive value [51, 52] (Fig. 22.2). The study by Wareham et al. confirmed that similar results were obtained in patients after solid-organ transplantation [47]. Several studies have demonstrated that FDG-PET/CT performed early during onset of symptoms in patients suspected for bacteremia can ensure timely diagnosis and treatment, minimize hospital admission time, and improve survival [53, 54]. These findings can

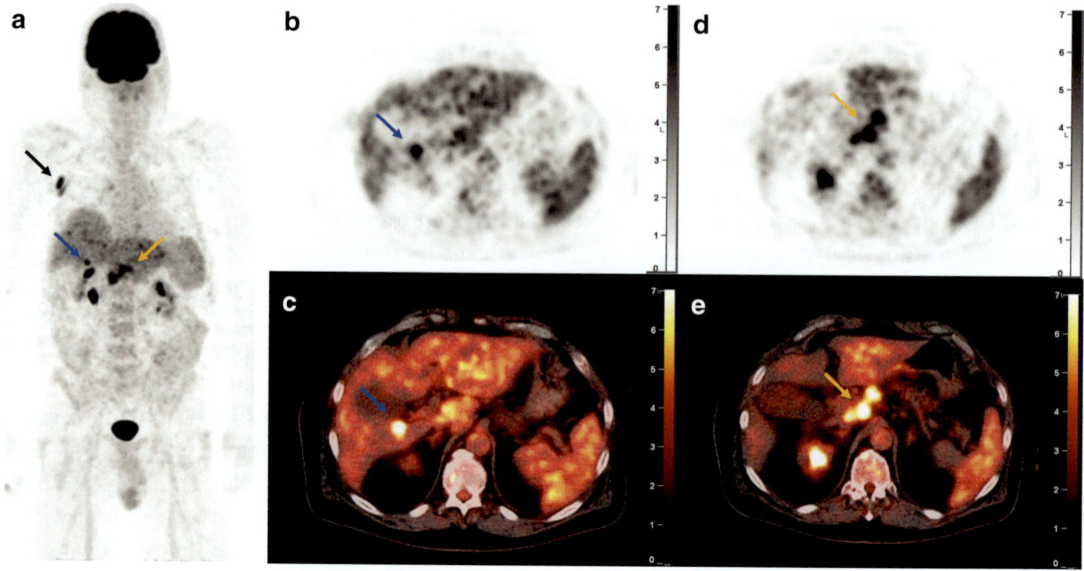

Fig. 22.2 A 59-year-old male who had undergone a heart transplantation for hyperthrophic cardiomyopathy 5 years ago presented with fever for 3 weeks and liver function abnormalities. MRI of the liver was suspicious for liver abscesses and a FDG-PET/CT was performed. The maximum intensity projection (MIP) image shows hypermetabolic axillary lymph nodes (black arrow), focal intense uptake in the liver (blue arrow) and multiple intensely FDG-avid gastrohepatic lymph nodes (orange arrow) (**a**). Transverse PET and fused images show the hypermetabolic lesion in the liver, compatible with an abscess (**b** and **c**) and the hypermetabolic lymph nodes (**d** and **e**). An excision biopsy of the axillary lymph node demonstrated focal necrotizing granulomatous lymphadenitis. Serology results and clinical presentation were compatible with a Bartonella henselae infection, complicated with liver abscesses and reactive lymph nodes

most likely be extrapolated to solid-organ transplant recipients.

Malignancies

Due to improved survival of both allograft and patient, development of posttransplant malignancies has emerged as important long-term complications together with cardiovascular disorders. The 10-year incidence of malignancies in patients treated with chronic immunosuppressive therapy after solid-organ transplant (SOT) is estimated to be as high as 20–30% [55, 56]. Although skin cancer is the most frequent malignancy, incidence of several other neoplasms has been shown to be increased compared to the nontransplant population [57]. In most cases, posttransplant malignan-cies occur de novo, but they can also be due to an underlying condition or, rarely, transmitted by the donor [58]. In this way, screening, early detection and adequate staging have gained much interest during follow-up of SOT patients [59].

Large population-based cohort studies have shown that standardized incidence ratios (SIR), which reflect the ratio between observed and expected cases, are increased for many cancers following SOT in general and heart transplantation in particular. A striking observation derived from these data is the substantial proportion of cases associated with a well known or suspected relation with infectious agents [60]. Nonmelanoma skin cancer, Kaposi sarcoma, and posttransplant lymphoproliferative disorders (PTLD) have the highest SIRs, exceeding up to 50-fold [61]. The overall risk for developing a malignancy after heart transplantation is estimated to be increased by two to fourfold in comparison with the general population [62, 63].

The pathogenesis of cancer following heart transplantation is multifactorial and complex, and a detailed description is beyond the scope of this chapter. Similar to the nontransplant population, environmental factors play an important role in the development of cancer. In particular, sun exposure and smoking largely contribute to the increased risk observed for skin and lung cancer respectively. These observations have led to intensive prevention and screening programs in transplant recipients. Chronic immunosuppressive therapy also plays a major role in carcinogenesis, not only by directly reducing the surveillance capacities of the immune system but also through direct oncogenic effects. Examples include (a) calcineurin inhibitor-induced enhanced production of transforming growth factor β1 (TGFβ-1) and impaired DNA repair and (b) synergism between azathioprine and ultraviolet radiation in carcinogenesis, resulting in increased skin cancer risk [58]. A third major mechanism is viral-induced oncogenesis, as exemplified by the role of Epstein–Barr virus (EBV) in up to 65% of the PTLD cases. Immune suppressive therapy leads to a deficient EBV-specific cellular immune response, not able anymore to control expansion and proliferation of EBV-infected B cells. As most EBV-latent antigens have oncogenic potential, this will lead to the development of EBV-related PTLD [64].

For symptomatic SOT recipients with a strong clinical suspicion for malignancy or infection, FDG PET/CT or FDG PET/MRI has shown excellent accuracy for diagnosing cancer or infection, as recently illustrated by a German analysis of 79 cases [49]. However, similar to the general population, it is of utmost importance to stress that suspicion of cancer in heart transplant recipients should always be confirmed by cytology and/or histopathology, allowing for subtyping according to the World Health Organization (WHO) classification.

Role of FDG-PET/CT in Detection, Staging, and Response Assessment of PTLD

All available literature on the use of FDG-PET/CT in PTLD include SOT recipients, with only one recent study exclusively including PTLD after heart transplantation [65]. The role of FDG-PET/CT in other cancer subtypes is not different from identical malignancies in immunocompetent patients.

Role of FDG-PET/CT in Detection and Staging of PTLD

FDG-PET/CT has emerged as an important diagnostic tool to detect several (in particular aggressive) lymphoma subtypes, including PTLD [66]. Hybrid FDG-PET/CT or MRI has several advantages compared to CT only, especially in this context. In contrast to other lymphomas, PTLD is associated with a high incidence of extranodal involvement, making CT scan alone not an appropriate imaging tool for detection and staging of PTLD [64]. A representative exemple with extranodal involvement is shown in Fig. 22.3. This has also been demonstrated in a small monocentric study in which 83% of patients had extranodal involvement and FDG-PET/CT detected occult lesions not identified on other imaging modalities in 57% of cases [67]. In addition, FDG-PET/CT has a significantly higher sensitivity to detect bone marrow involvement compared to bone marrow biopsy (100% vs. 17%), the latter being prone to sampling errors in cases with limited marrow involvement [68]. Finally, frequent administration of intravenous contrast agents is a major hurdle in transplant recipients due to the occurrence of (calcineurin inhibitor-induced) renal impairment. Even though FDG-PET/CT has an excellent performance, no single imaging modality reaches a sensitivity and specificity of 100%. Allograft and central nervous system involvement are observed in a substantial number

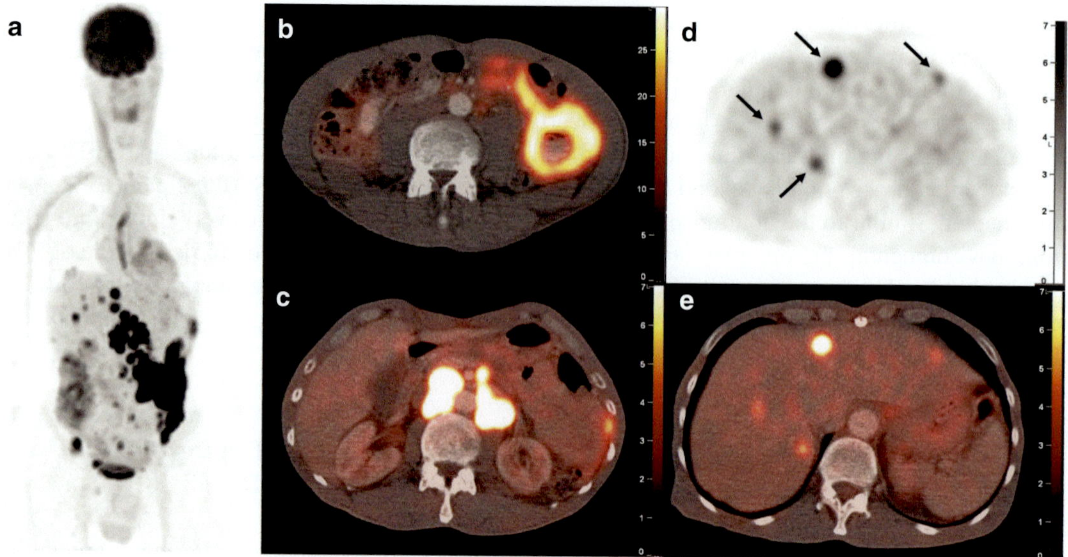

Fig. 22.3 PTLD staging and treatment follow-up. A 50-year-old male presented with reduced kidney function 7 1/2 years after heart transplantation for ischemic cardiomyopathy. CT showed abdominal lymphadenopathies and a FDG-PET/CT was performed. Maximum-intensity projection (MIP) image shows multiple foci with intense FDG avidity in the abdomen (**a**). Fused images show concentric hypermetabolism in a jejunal loop, with intraluminal iodinated oral CT contrast agent and air (**b**). Intensely hypermetabolic lymphadenopathies in the retroperitoneum (**c**). Native PET images (**d**) and fused images (**e**) show 4 liver lesions (arrows on **d**); with only the most intense lesion clearly visible on contrast-enhanced CT. Pathological analysis of a retroperitoneal lymph node revealed a monomorphic PTLD, diffuse large B-cell lymphoma type. PET images are displayed in standardized uptake values ranging from 0 to 7

of cases, increasing the risk for false-negative results with FDG-PET/CT due to high physiological background activity in central nervous system and urinary tracer elimination. On the other hand, false positive scans can be observed due to a variety of infectious or inflammatory conditions or other malignancies, hence underscoring the importance to obtain histological confirmation of the underlying pathology [69, 70].

The largest monocentric retrospective study by Dierickx et al. analyzing 125 FDG PET scans reported a sensitivity, specificity, positive predictive value and negative predictive value of 90%, 89%, 85%, and 93%, respectively [71]. Three recent meta-analyses including more than 300 patients who underwent FDG-PET/CT for suspicion of PTLD after SOT reported a pooled sensitivity, specificity, positive predictive value, and negative predictive value of 85–93%, 86–94%, 85–91%, and 87–93%, respectively [69, 72, 73]. In patients already diagnosed with PTLD (biopsy proven) before staging, FDG PET yielded a sensitivity of 89% [71]. One of the major drawbacks of all these retrospective studies is the huge heterogeneity in population size and methodology.

Whether quantitative FDG PET derived parameters can improve diagnostic accuracy for patients with suspected PTLD remains a matter of debate. In immunocompetent patients, maximum standardized uptake value (SUV_{max}) > 10 has been shown to predict an aggressive lymphoma subtype in immune competent patients [74]. Smaller retrospective studies have suggested an association between higher SUV_{max} and more aggressive PTLD subtypes [67, 75]. A recently published retrospective two-center study including 96 patients with biopsy-proven PTLD confirmed these findings, with significantly higher median SUV_{peak} at the biopsy site in cases with monomorphic PTLD compared to nondestructive and polymorphic subtypes. However, it was concluded that SUV-based parameters cannot be used as a noninvasive tool for PTLD subtyping, hence replacing histological classification, given the significant overlap in SUV values between the subtypes [76].

Role of FDG-PET/CT in Response Assessment of PTLD

Treatment response assessment using end-of-treatment PET (EOT) or interim PET (iPET) has been proven highly predictive for disease remission in both Hodgkin lymphoma (EOT-PET and iPET) and non-Hodgkin lymphoma (EOT-PET) [77, 78]. Despite the fact that evidence for FDG-PET/CT to assess treatment response in PTLD is less well established with only few studies reported so far, the clinical importance is high. Indeed, early identification of patients who are at high or low risk for recurrence would allow to adapt treatment early or to avoid unnecessary toxic treatment, respectively. Zimmermann et al. performed a retrospective study including 37 patients diagnosed with CD20-positive SOT-related PTLD treated with uniform rituximab-based protocols. Most importantly, negative predictive value of EOT-PET for disease relapse was 92%, identifying a group with low risk of recurrence and with excellent prognosis. On the other hand, the low positive predictive value of only 38% emphasizes the importance of additional diagnostic investigations before proceeding to new treatment [79]. Similar findings were observed in a retrospective study by Van Keerberghen et al., including 41 patients with CD20-positive PTLD following SOT, treated also with a uniform risk-stratified sequential treatment protocol (according to the Phase II PTLD-1 trial) [80, 81]. Positive and negative predictive values for EOT-PET were 33% and 87% respectively, confirming the identification of a subgroup of patients with low risk of disease recurrence. In addition, negative iPET scan yielded a negative predictive value of 85%, but a poor positive predictive value was observed (13%) [80]. In a small retrospective study in pediatric patients with SOT-related PTLD, the role of PET in response assessment seemed less clear due to the higher incidence of false positive cases both at interim and EOT PET; however,

these results should be interpreted with caution given the small sample size (n = 15) [82]. The value of FDG-PET/CT for treatment response assessment in pediatric PTLD warrants further investigation.

Prognostic Role of Baseline FDG PET/CT in PTLD

Although several PTLD-specific prognostic scores have been proposed, none of these have been confirmed or validated. In contrast, the International Prognostic Index (IPI)—consisting of 5 clinical/biochemical parameters: age, lactate dehydrogenase (LDH) level, Eastern Cooperative Oncology Group (ECOG) performance state, Ann Arbor stage and number of extranodal sites involved—which has been developed for aggressive lymphomas, seems to have prognostic relevance in PTLD patients [83–85]. In addition, the type of organ transplantation and the response to rituximab were additional prognostic markers in the prospective PTLD-1 trial [83]. In a recently published two-center trial including 88 patients, Montes de Jesus et al. explored the prognostic role of volumetric FDG-PET derived parameters, in particular metabolic tumor volume (MTV) and total lesion glycolysis (TLG) in patients diagnosed with PTLD [86]. In contrast to prognostic value of MTV/TLG in other lymphomas and compared to the IPI score, these volumetric quantitative parameters were not predictive of overall survival in their PTLD cohort [87, 88].

Several retrospective studies have shown that FDG-PET/CT is a valuable technique with high sensitivity and specificity to diagnose, stage and assess treatment response in PTLD patients. However, since large prospective studies are lacking, the level of evidence remains rather low. This is illustrated by several guidelines and recommendations, in which classical CT scans are recommended with FDG-PET/CT being considered a useful addition [70]. Prospective and multicenter trials including larger patient populations and well-designed methodologies are urgently needed to establish the exact role of FDG-PET/

CT in PTLD at baseline as well as during and after treatment. New hybrid imaging techniques such as FDG-PET/MRI may help reduce radiation exposure, which is extremely important in the pediatric transplant population.

Conclusion

All heart transplant recipients will suffer some form of complication and FDG-PET/CT has been proven a valuable tool to detect infectious complications as well as to stage and assess treatment response in PTLD patients. Even though the role of FDG-PET/CT to detect rejection of cardiac allografts has not been well investigated, preclinical data suggest its potential usefulness in this setting.

References

1. Khush KK, Cherikh WS, Chambers DC, Harhay MO, Hayes D, Hsich E, et al. The International Thoracic Organ Transplant Registry of the International Society for Heart and Lung Transplantation: thirty-sixth adult heart transplantation report—2019; focus theme: donor and recipient size match. J Heart Lung Transplant. 2019;38(10):1056–66.
2. Van Cleemput JJA, Verbelen TOM, Van Aelst LNL, Rega FRL. How to obtain and maintain favorable results after heart transplantation: keys to success? Ann Cardiothorac Surg. 2018;7(1):106–17.
3. Camici PG, Prasad SK, Rimoldi OE. Stunning, hibernation, and assessment of myocardial viability. Circulation. 2008;117(1):103–14.
4. Beanlands RSB, Nichol G, Huszti E, Humen D, Racine N, Freeman M, et al. F-18-Fluorodeoxyglucose positron emission tomography imaging-assisted management of patients with severe left ventricular dysfunction and suspected coronary disease. J Am Coll Cardiol. 2007;50(20):2002–12.
5. Bonow RO, Maurer G, Lee KL, Holly TA, Binkley PF, Desvigne-Nickens P, et al. Myocardial viability and survival in ischemic left ventricular dysfunction. N Engl J Med. 2011;364(17):1617–25.
6. Panza JA, Ellis AM, Al-Khalidi HR, Holly TA, Berman DS, Oh JK, et al. Myocardial viability and long-term outcomes in ischemic cardiomyopathy. N Engl J Med. 2019;381(8):739–48.
7. Chen W, Dilsizian V. Diagnosis and image-guided therapy of cardiac left ventricular assist device infections. Semin Nucl Med. 2021;51(4):357–63.
8. Kormos RL, Cowger J, Pagani FD, Teuteberg JJ, Goldstein DJ, Jacobs JP, et al. The society of thoracic surgeons intermacs database annual report: evolving indications, outcomes, and scientific partnerships. J Heart Lung Transplant. 2019;38(2):114–26.
9. Goldstein DJ, Meyns B, Xie R, Cowger J, Pettit S, Nakatani T, et al. Third annual report from the ISHLT mechanically assisted circulatory support registry: a comparison of centrifugal and axial continuous-flow left ventricular assist devices. J Heart Lung Transplant. 2019;38(4):352–63.
10. Siméon S, Flécher E, Revest M, Niculescu M, Roussel J-C, Michel M, et al. Left ventricular assist device-related infections: a multicentric study. Clin Microbiol Infect. 2017;23(10):748–51.
11. Mehra MR, Goldstein DJ, Uriel N, Cleveland JC, Yuzefpolskaya M, Salerno C, et al. Two-year outcomes with a magnetically levitated cardiac pump in heart failure. N Engl J Med. 2018;378(15):1386–95.
12. Mehra MR, Uriel N, Naka Y, Cleveland JC, Yuzefpolskaya M, Salerno CT, et al. A fully magnetically levitated left ventricular assist device—final report. N Engl J Med. 2019;380(17):1618–27.
13. Molina EJ, Shah P, Kiernan MS, Cornwell WK, Copeland H, Takeda K, et al. The society of thoracic surgeons intermacs 2020 annual report. Ann Thorac Surg. 2021;111(3):778–92.
14. Hannan MM, Husain S, Mattner F, Danziger-Isakov L, Drew RJ, Corey GR, et al. Working formulation for the standardization of definitions of infections in patients using ventricular assist devices. J Heart Lung Transplant. 2011;30(4):375–84.
15. Tam MC, Patel VN, Weinberg RL, Hulten EA, Aaronson KD, Pagani FD, et al. Diagnostic accuracy of FDG PET/CT in suspected LVAD infections. JACC Cardiovasc Imaging. 2020;13(5):1191–202.
16. ten Hove D, Treglia G, Slart RHJA, Damman K, Wouthuyzen-Bakker M, Postma DF, et al. The value of 18F-FDG PET/CT for the diagnosis of device-related infections in patients with a left ventricular assist device: a systematic review and meta-analysis. Eur J Nucl Med Mol Imaging. 2021;48(1):241–53.
17. ten Hove D, Treglia G, Slart RHJA, Damman K, Wouthuyzen-Bakker M, Postma DF, et al. The value of ^{18}F-FDG PET/CT for the diagnosis of device-related infections in patients with a left ventricular assist device: a systematic review and meta-analysis. Eur J Nucl Med Mol Imaging. 2020;48(1):241–53.
18. Dell'Aquila AM, Mastrobuoni S, Alles S, Wenning C, Henryk W, Schneider SRB, et al. Contributory role of fluorine 18-fluorodeoxyglucose positron emission tomography/computed tomography in the diagnosis and clinical management of infections in patients supported with a continuous-flow left ventricular assist device. Ann Thorac Surg. 2016;101(1):87–94.
19. Bernhardt AM, Pamirsad MA, Brand C, Reichart D, Tienken M, Barten MJ, et al. The value of fluorine-18 deoxyglucose positron emission tomography scans in patients with ventricular assist device specific infections. Eur J Cardiothorac Surg. 2017;51(6):1072–7.

20. Kim J, Feller ED, Chen W, Liang Y, Dilsizian V. FDG PET/CT for early detection and localization of left ventricular assist device infection. JACC Cardiovasc Imaging. 2019;12(4):722–9.

21. Sommerlath Sohns JM, Kröhn H, Schöde A, Derlin T, Haverich A, Schmitto JD, et al. 18 F-FDG PET/CT in left-ventricular assist device infection: initial results supporting the usefulness of image-guided therapy. J Nucl Med. 2020;61(7):971–6.

22. Avramovic N, Dell'Aquila AM, Weckesser M, Milankovic D, Vrachimis A, Sindermann JR, et al. Metabolic volume performs better than SUVmax in the detection of left ventricular assist device driveline infection. Eur J Nucl Med Mol Imaging. 2017;44(11):1870–7.

23. Dell'Aquila AM, Avramovic N, Mastrobuoni S, Motekallemi A, Wisniewski K, Scherer M, et al. Fluorine-18 fluorodeoxyglucose positron emission tomography/computed tomography for improving diagnosis of infection in patients on CF-LVAD: longing for more insights. Eur Heart J Cardiovasc Imaging. 2018;19(5):532–43.

24. Kanapinn P, Burchert W, Körperich H, Körfer J. 18F-FDG PET/CT-imaging of left ventricular assist device infection: a retrospective quantitative intrapatient analysis. J Nucl Cardiol. 2019;26(4):1212–21.

25. Akin S, Muslem R, Constantinescu AA, Manintveld OC, Birim O, Brugts JJ, et al. 18F-FDG PET/CT in the diagnosis and management of continuous flow left ventricular assist device infections: a case series and review of the literature. ASAIO J. 2018;64(2):e11–9.

26. de Vaugelade C, Mesguich C, Nubret K, Camou F, Greib C, Dournes G, et al. Infections in patients using ventricular-assist devices: comparison of the diagnostic performance of 18F-FDG PET/CT scan and leucocyte-labeled scintigraphy. J Nucl Cardiol. 2019;26(1):42–55.

27. Potapov EV, Antonides C, Crespo-Leiro MG, Combes A, Färber G, Hannan MM, et al. 2019 EACTS expert consensus on long-term mechanical circulatory support. Eur J Cardiothorac Surg. 2019;56(2):230–70.

28. Stewart S, Winters GL, Fishbein MC, Tazelaar HD, Kobashigawa J, Abrams J, et al. Revision of the 1990 working formulation for the standardization of nomenclature in the diagnosis of heart rejection. J Heart Lung Transplant. 2005;24(11):1710–20.

29. Crespo-Leiro MG, Zuckermann A, Bara C, Mohacsi P, Schulz U, Boyle A, et al. Concordance among pathologists in the second cardiac allograft rejection gene expression observational Study (CARGO II). Transplantation. 2012;94(11):1172 7.

30. Berry GJ, Burke MM, Andersen C, Bruneval P, Fedrigo M, Fishbein MC, et al. The 2013 International society for heart and lung transplantation working formulation for the standardization of nomenclature in the pathologic diagnosis of antibody-mediated rejection in heart transplantation. J Heart Lung Transplant. 2013;32(12):1147–62.

31. Kobashigawa J, Crespo-Leiro MG, Ensminger SM, Reichenspurner H, Angelini A, Berry G, et al. Report from a consensus conference on antibody-mediated rejection in heart transplantation. J Heart Lung Transplant. 2011;30(3):252–69.

32. Loupy A, Lefaucheur C. Antibody-mediated rejection of solid-organ allografts. N Engl J Med. 2018;379(12):1150–60.

33. Bruneval P, Angelini A, Miller D, Potena L, Loupy A, Zeevi A, et al. The XIIIth Banff conference on allograft pathology: the Banff 2015 heart meeting report: improving antibody-mediated rejection diagnostics: strengths, unmet needs, and future directions. Am J Transplant. 2017;17(1):42–53.

34. Fedrigo M, Leone O, Burke MM, Rice A, Toquet C, Vernerey D, et al. Inflammatory cell burden and phenotype in endomyocardial biopsies with antibody-mediated rejection (AMR): a multicenter pilot study from the AECVP. Am J Transplant. 2015;15(2):526–34.

35. Van Keer JM, Van Aelst LNL, Rega F, Droogne W, Voros G, Meyns B, et al. Long-term outcome of cardiac allograft vasculopathy: importance of the international society for heart and lung transplantation angiographic grading scale. J Heart Lung Transplant. 2019;38(11):1189–96.

36. Chih S, Chong AY, Mielniczuk LM, Bhatt DL, Beanlands RSB. Allograft vasculopathy. J Am Coll Cardiol. 2016;68(1):80–91.

37. Chih S, McDonald M, Dipchand A, Kim D, Ducharme A, Kaan A, et al. Canadian cardiovascular society/canadian cardiac transplant network position statement on heart transplantation: patient eligibility, selection, and post-transplantation care. Can J Cardiol. 2020;36(3):335–56.

38. Dilsizian V, Bacharach SL, Beanlands RS, Bergmann SR, Delbeke D, Dorbala S, et al. ASNC imaging guidelines/SNMMI procedure standard for positron emission tomography (PET) nuclear cardiology procedures. J Nucl Cardiol. 2016;23(5):1187–226.

39. Hoff SJ, Stewart JR, Frist WH, Kessler RM, Sandler MP, Atkinson JB, et al. Noninvasive detection of heart transplant rejection with positron emission scintigraphy. Ann Thorac Surg. 1992;53(4):572–7.

40. Daly KP, Dearling JLJ, Seto T, Dunning P, Fahey F, Packard AB, et al. Use of [18F]FDG positron emission tomography to monitor the development of cardiac allograft rejection. Transplantation. 2015;99(9):e132–9.

41. Rechavia E, de Silva R, Kushwaha SS, Rhodes CG, Araujo LI, Jones T, et al. Enhanced myocardial 18F-2-Fluoro-2-Deoxyglucose uptake after orthotopic heart transplantation assessed by positron emission tomography. J Am Coll Cardiol. 1997;30(2):533–8.

42. Felix RCM, Gouvea CM, Reis CCW, dos Santos Miranda JS, Schtruk LBCE, Colafranceschi AS, et al. 18F-fluorodeoxyglucose use after cardiac transplant: a comparative study of suppression of

physiological myocardial uptake. J Nucl Cardiol. 2020;27(1):173–81.

43. Jayadeva PS, Better N. Opening the door to noninvasive assessment of cardiac transplant rejection: It's all in the preparation. J Nucl Cardiol. 2020;27(1):182–5.

44. Fishman JA. Infection in organ transplantation. Am J Transplant. 2017;17(4):856–79.

45. San Juan R, Aguado JM, Lumbreras C, Díaz-Pedroche C, López-Medrano F, Lizasoain M, et al. Incidence, clinical characteristics and risk factors of late infection in solid organ transplant recipients: data from the RESITRA study group. Am J Transplant. 2007;7(4):964–71.

46. Jamar F, Buscombe J, Chiti A, Christian PE, Delbeke D, Donohoe KJ, et al. EANM/SNMMI guideline for 18 F-FDG use in inflammation and infection. J Nucl Med. 2013;54(4):647–58.

47. Wareham NE, Lundgren JD, Da Cunha-Bang C, Gustafsson F, Iversen M, Johannesen HH, et al. The clinical utility of FDG PET/CT among solid organ transplant recipients suspected of malignancy or infection. Eur J Nucl Med Mol Imaging. 2017;44(3):421–31.

48. Muller N, Kessler R, Caillard S, Epailly E, Hubelé F, Heimburger C, et al. 18F-FDG PET/CT for the diagnosis of malignant and infectious complications after solid organ transplantation. Nucl Med Mol Imaging. 2017;51(1):58–68.

49. Guberina N, Gäckler A, Grueneisen J, Wetter A, Witzke O, Herrmann K, et al. Assessment of suspected malignancy or infection in immunocompromised patients after solid organ transplantation by [18F]FDG PET/CT and [18F]FDG PET/MRI. Nucl Med Mol Imaging. 2020;54(4):183–91.

50. Graute V, Jansen N, Sohn H-Y, Becker A, Klein B, Schmid I, et al. Diagnostic role of whole-body [18F]-FDG positron emission tomography in patients with symptoms suspicious for malignancy after heart transplantation. J Heart Lung Transplant. 2012;31(9):958–66.

51. Bleeker-Rovers CP, van der Meer JWM, Oyen WJG. Fever of unknown origin. Semin Nucl Med. 2009;39(2):81–7.

52. Keidar Z, Gurman-Balbir A, Gaitini D, Israel O. Fever of unknown origin: the role of 18 F-FDG PET/CT. J Nucl Med. 2008;49(12):1980–5.

53. Vos FJ, Bleeker-Rovers CP, Sturm PD, Krabbe PFM, van Dijk APJ, Cuijpers MLH, et al. 18 F-FDG PET/CT for detection of metastatic infection in Gram-positive bacteremia. J Nucl Med. 2010;51(8):1234–40.

54. Vos FJ, Bleeker-Rovers CP, Kullberg BJ, Adang EMM, Oyen WJG. Cost-effectiveness of routine 18 F-FDG PET/CT in high-risk patients with Gram-positive Bacteremia. J Nucl Med. 2011;52(11):1673–8.

55. Buell JF, Gross TG, Woodle ES. Malignancy after transplantation. Transplantation. 2005;80(2 Supplement):S254–64.

56. Potena L, Zuckermann A, Barberini F, Aliabadi-Zuckermann A. Complications of cardiac transplantation. Curr Cardiol Rep. 2018;20(9):73.

57. Gutierrez-Dalmau A, Campistol JM. Immunosuppressive therapy and malignancy in organ transplant recipients. Drugs. 2007;67(8):1167–98.

58. Ajithkumar TV, Parkinson CA, Butler A, Hatcher HM. Management of solid tumours in organ-transplant recipients. Lancet Oncol. 2007;8(10):921–32.

59. Acuna SA, Huang JW, Scott AL, Micic S, Daly C, Brezden-Masley C, et al. Cancer screening recommendations for solid organ transplant recipients: a systematic review of clinical practice guidelines. Am J Transplant. 2017;17(1):103–14.

60. Grulich AE, van Leeuwen MT, Falster MO, Vajdic CM. Incidence of cancers in people with HIV/AIDS compared with immunosuppressed transplant recipients: a meta-analysis. Lancet. 2007;370(9581):59–67.

61. de Fijter JW. Cancer and mTOR inhibitors in transplant recipients. Transplantation. 2017;101(1):45–55.

62. Engels EA, Pfeiffer RM, Fraumeni JF, Kasiske BL, Israni AK, Snyder JJ, et al. Spectrum of cancer risk among us solid organ transplant recipients. JAMA. 2011;306(17):1891.

63. Van Keer J, Droogné W, Van Cleemput J, Vörös G, Rega F, Meyns B, et al. Cancer after heart transplantation: a 25-year single-center perspective. Transplant Proc. 2016;48(6):2172–7.

64. Dierickx D, Habermann TM. Post-transplantation lymphoproliferative disorders in adults. N Engl J Med. 2018;378(6):549–62.

65. Sica A, De Rimini ML, Sagnelli C, Casale B, Spada A, Reginelli A, et al. Post-heart transplantation lymphoproliferative diseases (PTLDs) and the diagnostic role of [18f] FDG-PET/CT. Minerva Med. 2021;112(3):338–45.

66. Weiler-Sagie M, Bushelev O, Epelbaum R, Dann EJ, Haim N, Avivi I, et al. 18 F-FDG avidity in lymphoma readdressed: a study of 766 patients. J Nucl Med. 2010;51(1):25–30.

67. Takehana CS, Twist CJ, Mosci C, Quon A, Mittra E, Iagaru A. 18F-FDG PET/CT in the management of patients with post-transplant lymphoproliferative disorder. Nucl Med Commun. 2014;35(3):276–81.

68. Gheysens O, Thielemans S, Morscio J, Boeckx N, Goffin KE, Deroose CM, et al. Detection of bone marrow involvement in newly diagnosed post-transplant lymphoproliferative disorder: 18F-Fluorodeoxyglucose positron emission tomography/computed tomography versus bone marrow biopsy. Leuk Lymphoma. 2016;57(10):2382–8.

69. Montes de Jesus FM, Kwee TC, Nijland M, Kahle XU, Huls G, Dierckx RAJO, et al. Performance of advanced imaging modalities at diagnosis and treatment response evaluation of patients with post-transplant lymphoproliferative disorder: a systematic review and meta-analysis. Crit Rev Oncol Hematol. 2018;132:27–38.

70. Song H, Guja KE, Iagaru A. 18F-FDG PET/CT for evaluation of post-transplant lymphoproliferative disorder (PTLD). Semin Nucl Med. 2021;51(4):392–403.

71. Dierickx D, Tousseyn T, Requile A, Verscuren R, Sagaert X, Morscio J, et al. The accuracy of positron emission tomography in the detection of posttransplant lymphoproliferative disorder. Haematologica. 2013;98(5):771–5.

72. Kim K, Kim S-J. Diagnostic performance of F-18 fluorodeoxyglucose PET/computed tomography for diagnosis of polymyalgia rheumatica. Nucl Med Commun. 2020;41(12):1313–21.

73. Ballova V, Muoio B, Albano D, Bertagna F, Canziani L, Ghielmini M, et al. Diagnostic performance of 18F-FDG PET or PET/CT for detection of post-transplant lymphoproliferative disorder: a systematic review and a bivariate meta-analysis. Diagnostics (Basel). 2020;10(2):101.

74. Ngeow JYY, Quek RHH, Ng DCE, Hee SW, Tao M, Lim LC, et al. High SUV uptake on FDG–PET/CT predicts for an aggressive B-cell lymphoma in a prospective study of primary FDG–PET/CT staging in lymphoma. Ann Oncol. 2009;20(9):1543–7.

75. Vali R, Punnett A, Bajno L, Moineddin R, Shammas A. The value of 18 F-FDG PET in pediatric patients with post-transplant lymphoproliferative disorder at initial diagnosis. Pediatr Transplant. 2015;19(8):932–9.

76. Montes de Jesus F, Vergote V, Noordzij W, Dierickx D, Dierckx R, Diepstra A, et al. Semi-quantitative characterization of post-transplant lymphoproliferative disorder morphological subtypes with [18F]FDG PET/CT. J Clin Med. 2021;10(2):361.

77. Barrington SF, Trotman J. The role of PET in the first-line treatment of the most common subtypes of non-Hodgkin lymphoma. Lancet Haematol. 2021;8(1):e80–93.

78. Trotman J, Barrington SF. The role of PET in first-line treatment of Hodgkin lymphoma. Lancet Haematol. 2021;8(1):e67–79.

79. Zimmermann H, Denecke T, Dreyling MH, Franzius C, Reinke P, Subklewe M, et al. End-of-treatment positron emission tomography after uniform first-line therapy of B-cell posttransplant lymphoproliferative disorder identifies patients at low risk of relapse in the prospective German PTLD Registry. Transplantation. 2018;102(5):868–75.

80. Van Keerberghen C-A, Goffin K, Vergote V, Tousseyn T, Verhoef G, Laenen A, et al. Role of interim and end of treatment positron emission tomography for response assessment and prediction of relapse in post-transplant lymphoproliferative disorder. Acta Oncol. 2019;58(7):1041–7.

81. Trappe R, Oertel S, Leblond V, Mollee P, Sender M, Reinke P, et al. Sequential treatment with rituximab followed by CHOP chemotherapy in adult B-cell post-transplant lymphoproliferative disorder (PTLD): the prospective international multicentre phase 2 PTLD-1 trial. Lancet Oncol. 2012;13(2):196–206.

82. Montes de Jesus FM, Glaudemans AWJM, Tissing WJ, Dierckx RAJO, Rosati S, Diepstra A, et al. 18 F-FDG PET/CT in the diagnostic and treatment evaluation of pediatric posttransplant lymphoproliferative disorders. J Nucl Med. 2020;61(9):1307–13.

83. Trappe RU, Choquet S, Dierickx D, Mollee P, Zaucha JM, Dreyling MH, et al. International prognostic index, type of transplant and response to rituximab are key parameters to tailor treatment in adults with CD20-positive B cell PTLD: clues from the PTLD-1 trial. Am J Transplant. 2015;15(4):1091–100.

84. Dierickx D, Tousseyn T, Morscio J, Fieuws S, Verhoef G. Validation of prognostic scores in post-transplantation lymphoproliferative disorders. J Clin Oncol. 2013;31(27):3443–4.

85. International Non-Hodgkin's Lymphoma Prognostic Factors Project. A predictive model for aggressive non-Hodgkin's lymphoma. N Engl J Med. 1993;329(14):987–94.

86. Montes de Jesus F, Dierickx D, Vergote V, Noordzij W, Dierckx RAJO, Deroose CM, et al. Prognostic superiority of international prognostic index over [18F]FDG PET/CT volumetric parameters in post-transplant lymphoproliferative disorder. EJNMMI Res. 2021;11(1):29.

87. Cottereau A-S, Versari A, Loft A, Casasnovas O, Bellei M, Ricci R, et al. Prognostic value of baseline metabolic tumor volume in early-stage Hodgkin lymphoma in the standard arm of the H10 trial. Blood. 2018;131(13):1456–63.

88. Meignan M, Cottereau AS, Versari A, Chartier L, Dupuis J, Boussetta S, et al. Baseline metabolic tumor volume predicts outcome in high–tumor-burden follicular lymphoma: a pooled analysis of three multicenter studies. J Clin Oncol. 2016;34(30):3618–26.

Part VI

Variants and Cases

Normal Variants, Not-So-Normal Variants, and Pitfalls of FDG-PET in Cardiovascular Imaging

Ingrid Bloise, Matthieu Pelletier-Galarneau, and Patrick Martineau

Introduction

Positron emission tomography (PET) is emerging as an increasingly valuable tool for assessing cardiovascular pathology. Increases in camera and radiotracer availability, as well as its technical superiority over single photon emission computed tomography (SPECT), have resulted in an increased use of PET for cardiac imaging [1]. Over the last few decades, cardiac PET imaging has evolved from a specialized research tool contributing to the understanding of cardiac pathophysiology, to being firmly established in clinical practice for the diagnosis and prognostication of various cardiac pathologies [2].

Even though the last few years have seen a push in the development and use of novel radiotracers, ^{18}F-fluorodeoxyglucose (FDG) remains the workhorse of PET imaging, including for cardiovascular PET imaging. This can be accounted for by several factors. First, FDG benefits from being well established due to widespread use in oncological imaging. Second, a growing body of literature supports the use of FDG PET in several cardiovascular indications, such as for the evaluation of cardiovascular infection and inflammation. Third, the physical properties of ^{18}F, including its relatively long half life of 110 min and short positron range makes it ideal for the purposes of cardiovascular imaging.

As previously discussed in Chap. 3, the myocardium is a metabolic omnivore which can use multiple different sources of energy, but preferentially uses free fatty acids and carbohydrates; however, subject to availability and hormonal conditions, cardiomyocytes can alter their preferred substrate. For example, in the fasted state, fatty acids constitute the preferred source of energy. Following a meal, blood insulin levels increase and carbohydrates again become the dominant source of adenosine triphosphate (ATP) [3, 4]. The variability in the use of glucose (and by extension, FDG) results in the variable patterns of normal FDG uptake in the heart encountered in clinical practice. Despite the variability, the patterns of uptake seen in normal myocardium are finite and can easily be recognized by the trained physician.

In this chapter, we review the normal patterns of myocardial FDG uptake. We also discuss commonly seen variants which can occasionally be associated with pathology, as well as review potential pitfalls which are occasionally encountered.

I. Bloise
Department of Radiology, University of British Columbia, Vancouver, BC, Canada

M. Pelletier-Galarneau
Montreal Heart Institute, Montréal, QC, Canada
e-mail: Matthieu.pelletier-galarneau@icm-mhi.org

P. Martineau (✉)
BC Cancer, Vancouver, BC, Canada
e-mail: patrick.martineau@bccancer.bc.ca

Patterns of Myocardial Uptake

Left Ventricular Uptake

It is well established that, even after careful patient preparation with fasting for at least 4–6 h prior to imaging, physiological cardiac FDG uptake may occur inhomogeneously in the left ventricle. Furthermore, cardiac segments in the same subjects may have significant variations when compared in serial studies [5], with either an increase or decrease in tracer accumulation in specific segments, or demonstrating an altogether different pattern of uptake (Fig. 23.1). In cases in which the patient has not been prepared using a specific myocardial suppression protocol, myocardial uptake is usually considered nonspecific regardless of the uptake distribution.

The most commonly described patterns of physiologic myocardial FDG uptake are (a) *none* when the activity in the myocardium is the same or less than in the blood pool in the ventricular cavity, (b) *diffuse* with intense uptake seeing diffusely throughout all walls of the left ventricle, and (c) *lateral free wall* when there is diffusely increased FDG uptake in the lateral free wall of the left ventricle. Also described is regional FDG uptake in the basal segments of all four walls assuming a ring figure, known as a basal-ring pattern (Fig. 23.2).

In 1990, Gropler et al. evaluated healthy patients with no history of cardiovascular disease and no significant risk factors for coronary artery disease, and were able to show that the mean activity in the septum and anterior walls was 20% less than the mean activity in the inferior and lateral walls [6]. This was later confirmed by other authors [5, 7, 8]. Reduced septal uptake has been reported in patients with complete left bundle branch block with this finding unrelated to changes in perfusion [9, 10]. The mechanism responsible for this is unclear but may be related to mechanical dysynchrony. Finally, Gropler et al. also demonstrated that there was no significant difference in activity between the inferior and lateral walls [6].

A focal area of increased metabolic activity has been reported as the least common pattern of uptake following myocardial suppression preparation [11]. When this pattern is present, uptake is considered pathological unless it is related to FDG accumulation in the papillary muscles, nor-

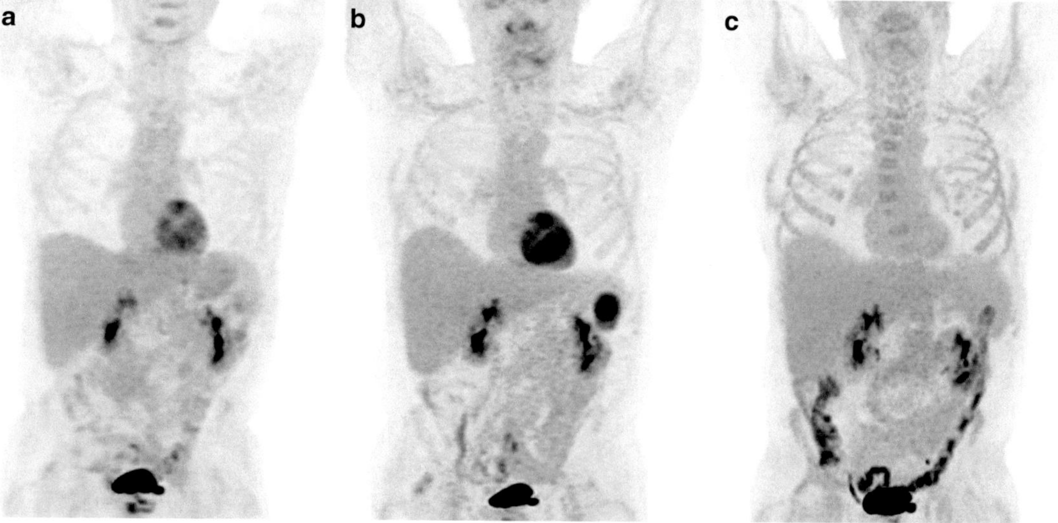

Fig. 23.1 Sequential MIP images of a 63-year-old man following 6-h fasting shows variations in both the pattern and intensity of myocardial uptake: on the earliest scan (**a**) there is mild FDG uptake in a basal-ring pattern, which increases in intensity on the following study (**b**), but which shows no myocardial activity on the subsequent study (**c**)

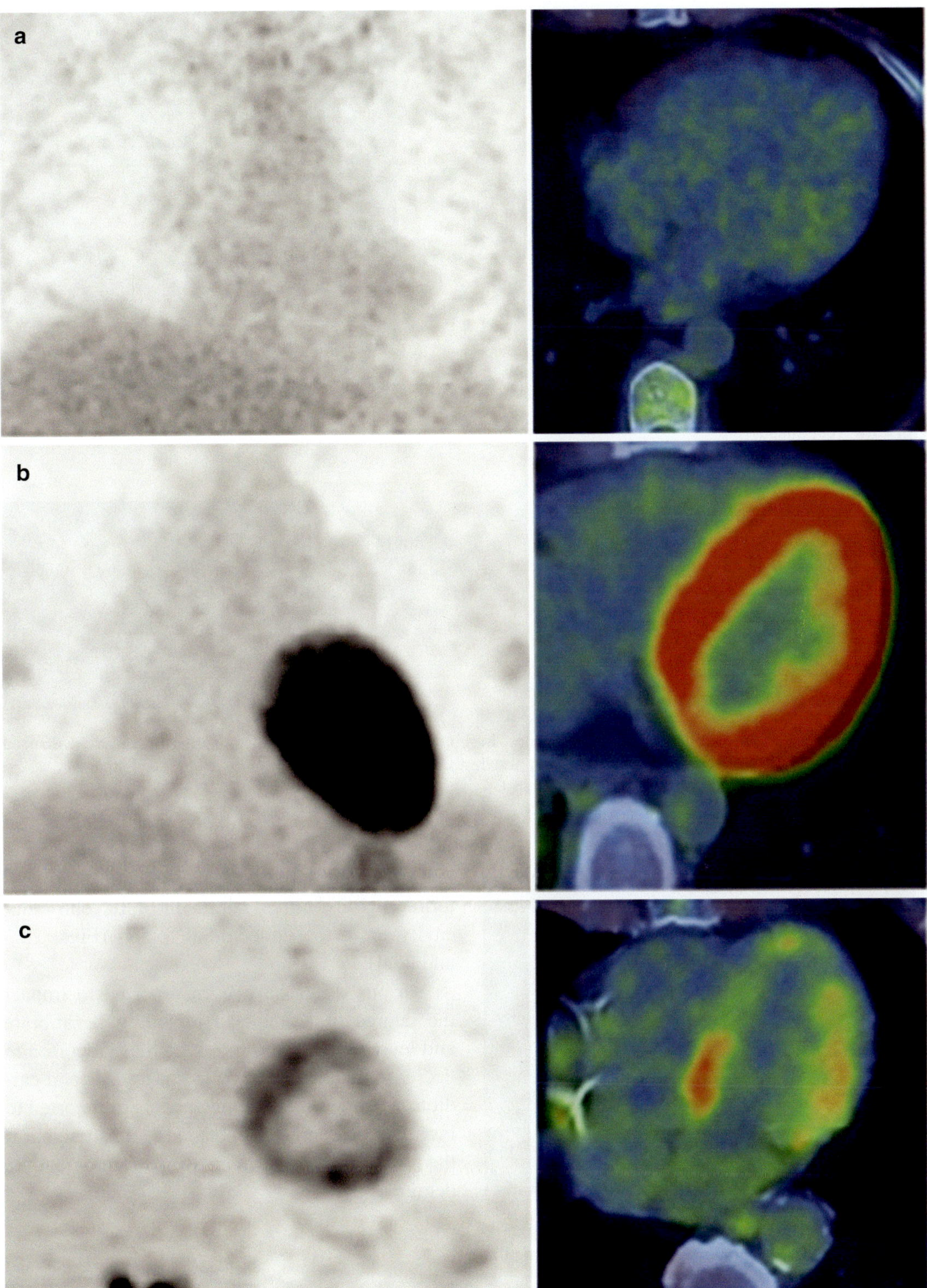

Fig. 23.2 Examples of the various patterns of normal myocardial distribution encountered in clinical practice. The column on the left demonstrates maximum intensity projection images viewed anteriorly while the column on the right shows transaxial fused PET-CT images through the left ventricle. The various patterns are (**a**) absent uptake, (**b**) diffuse left ventricular uptake, (**c**) basal ring, and (**d**) lateral free wall uptake

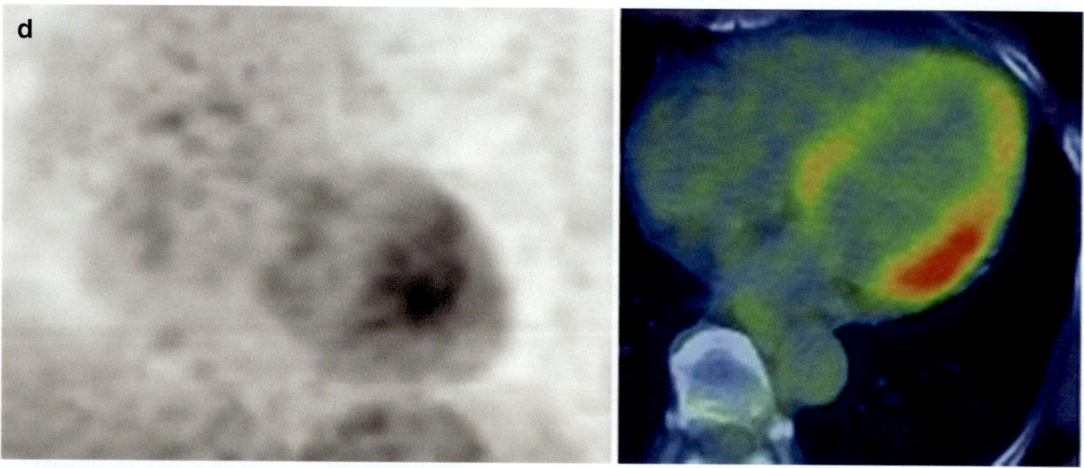

Fig. 23.2 (continued)

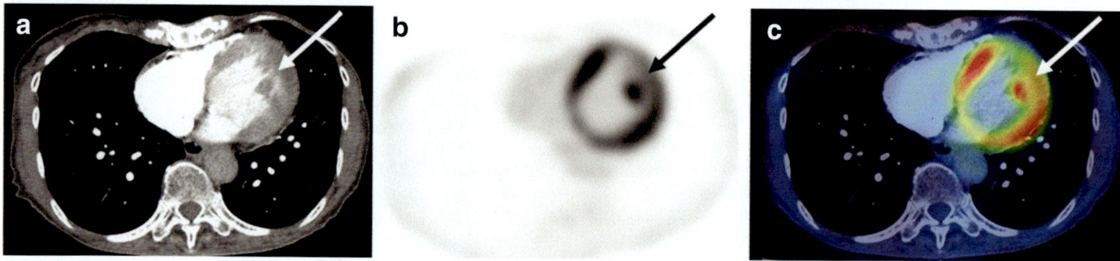

Fig. 23.3 Focal uptake within the papillary muscles. In this patient with diffuse left ventricular activity, focal activity is clearly seen to localize within the left anterolateral papillary muscle (arrow) on (**a**) contrast-enhanced CT, (**b**) axial PET, and (**c**) Fused PET/CT images

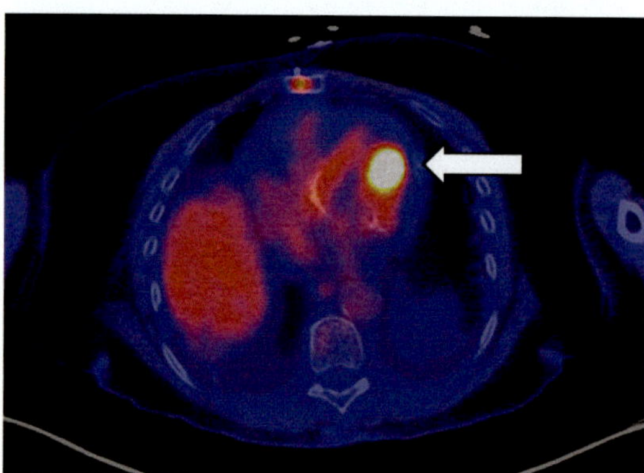

Fig. 23.4 Less commonly seen is intense papillary muscle activity in the absence of significant left ventricular uptake such as in this case

mally located in the anterolateral and inferoposterior regions, either within the left ventricular cavity or in the endocardial region (Figs. 23.3 and 23.4).

Various drugs have been reported to impact the degree of LV uptake including bezafibrate and levothyroxine, both of which are reported to decrease uptake, while benzodiazepines and cardiotoxic chemotherapeutic agents are reported to increase the degree of uptake [12]. It is unclear if the use of these drugs alters the pattern or just the degree of uptake.

Right Ventricular Uptake

Abnormal myocardial glucose metabolism in the right ventricle (RV) in the form of diffuse tracer uptake within the ventricular wall has been reported in multiple previous studies and is often related to a shift in metabolism related to increased RV pressures and/or hypertrophy caused by pulmonary artery hypertension, either idiopathic or secondary to underlying pulmonary disease [13, 14]. Compared to the LV, FDG uptake in the RV walls is usually much less conspicuous [8] (Figs. 23.5 and 23.6).

Some studies have shown a causal relationship between FDG uptake in the RV and RV dysfunction, with increased RV uptake correlating with a decrease in systolic function [15–17]. Mehmet et al. confirmed that patients with higher RV glucose metabolic rate tend to have higher RV loads and worse function [13]. Mielniczuk et al. have shown a significant relation between increased uptake in the RV and a decrease in RV ejection fraction, even after applying partial-volume correction owing to differences in wall thickness [18]. In patients with idiopathic pulmonary artery hypertension, the degree of RV uptake has been shown to be elevated at baseline and decreased after treatment [13, 19]. Studies have also shown that the degree of FDG uptake within the RV wall correlates with serum levels of N-terminal pro-brain natriuretic peptide (NT-proBNP) in patients with idiopathic pulmonary arterial hypertension [20, 21]. Furthermore, in a study examining patients with coronary artery disease and ischemic cardiomyopathy, the degree of FDG uptake in the RV was associated with RV pressure overload, with higher ventricular uptake (both left and right) associated with poor outcomes [22]. Additional studies have confirmed the prognostic significance of increased RV uptake in patients with pulmonary hypertension [23–25]. As such, the presence of diffuse RV wall uptake should be considered a "not-so-normal" variant; however, the degree of clinical significance of this finding and its interpretation in routine clinical practice requires additional study.

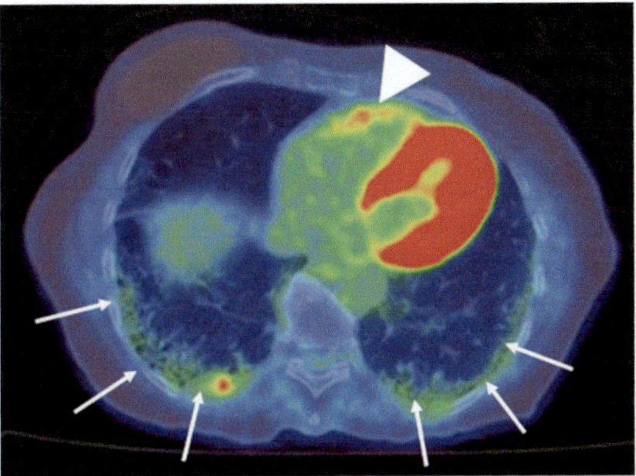

Fig. 23.6 Axial PET image of the chest of a 79-year-old female patient with interstitial lung disease (arrows). There is physiological FDG uptake in the right ventricular wall (arrowhead), well above the blood pool activity. There is also intense diffuse accumulation of the radiotracer in the left ventricular walls and papillary muscle

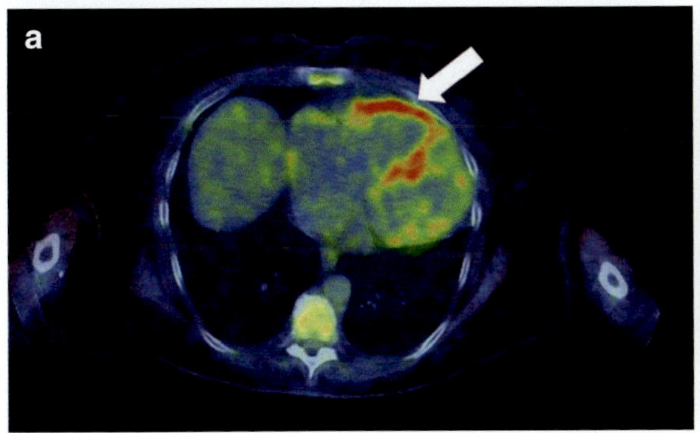

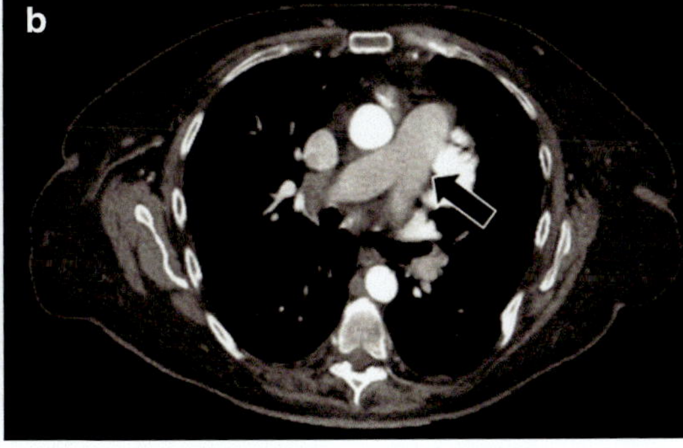

Fig. 23.5 Axial PET images of the chest of a 54-year-old woman with pulmonary hypertension demonstrating relatively intense but diffuse uptake through the right ventricular wall (**a**, arrow). Note the dilation of the pulmonary trunk (**b**, arrow), in keeping with elevated pulmonary arterial pressure

Atrial Uptake

In the majority of patients, atria are devoid of significant FDG activity. Atrial activity has been studied since the late 1990s when Fujii et al. reported FDG uptake in the walls of the right atrium in 10 of 2367 (0.4%) patients being assessed for oncological indications [26]. These authors found that patients with atrial uptake suffered from cardiac disorders, with atrial fibrillation particularly prevalent in their subjects. They also noted that right atrial activity was much more conspicuous than left atrial uptake. A recent study showed that 30% of patients with atrial fibrillation (AF) presented with diffuse atrial FDG uptake involving at least the right atrial wall (Fig. 23.7) and, of these, approximately one third also had activity in the left atrial wall [27].

A predilection for right atrial uptake (when compared to the left) in patients with AF was also confirmed in the study by Xie et al. [28]. Interestingly, these authors compared the atrial uptake to the activity seen in epicardial adipose tissue (EAT). They found that atrial and atrial appendage uptake was linearly correlated with activity in the EAT. In a subsequent prospective study, the same group demonstrated an association between atrial uptake and levels of NT-proBNP, in addition to an association between increased right atrial levels and successful termination of AF by radiofrequency catheter ablation [29]. These findings, together with the known association between EAT activity and inflammation, suggest that FDG PET may provide a new lens by which to observe the known relationship between inflammation and atrial fibrillation [30, 31].

A recent study by Sinigaglia et al. further confirmed the association between atrial uptake and atrial fibrillation, while also finding an association with an increased risk of cardioembolic stroke [27]. In fact, the authors report that, on multivariate analysis, right atrial uptake had a greater odds ratio for stroke than conventional risk factors (including current smoking, hypertension, diabetes, and dyslipidemia).

In summary, atrial activity should be considered "not-so-normal" as it most likely reflects an element of underlying cardiovascular pathology; however, further research is required before the implications of incidental atrial activity on FDG PET translate to routine clinical practice.

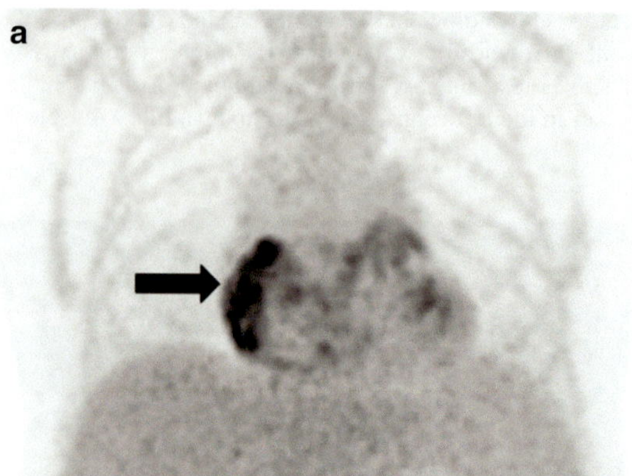
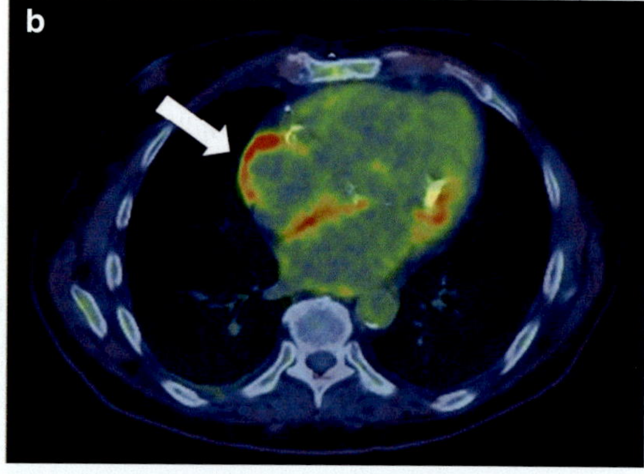

Fig. 23.7 PET images showing intense diffuse right atrial uptake in this patient with atrial fibrillation on MIP (**a**) and axial images (**b**). Left ventricular basal lateral uptake is nonspecific and represents incomplete myocardial suppression

Pitfalls

Knowledge of the physiological FDG distribution and glucose metabolism in every cardiac chamber, as well as the normal variants, is imperative in order to avoid misinterpretation and misdiagnoses. Most pitfalls take the form of focal, occasionally intense, uptake localizing within the various cardiac chambers or walls. Such findings can be highly suggestive of pathology, particularly masses, but frequently correspond to benign processes; however, with knowledge of the imaging and clinical features, physiological distribution, and a careful eye, these can be recognized and misdiagnosis avoided.

Focal uptake in the left ventricular wall is a common pattern of physiologic FDG uptake and typically attributable to physiological uptake in papillary muscles, although rarely displayed in isolation [32]. When not related to the papillary muscles (Figs. 23.3 and 23.4), the patient history should be carefully evaluated as focal uptake can also be related to hibernating myocardium [2, 33–35], cardiac sarcoidosis, and increase stress on papillary

muscles (dilated cardiomyopathy, valvular insufficiency, valvular stenosis, chordal failure, etc.).

A relatively common finding is increased FDG accumulation associated with fatty deposition within the interatrial septum—a condition typically referred to as lipomatous hypertrophy of the interatrial septum (LHIAS)—seen in approximately 3% of patients [36, 37]. In these cases, image reconstruction with proper CT fusion to ensure anatomical correlation is of utmost importance. The CT findings in LHIAS typically consist of a "dumbbell" shape fat density lesion localizing to the interatrial septum— this is due to fat accumulation cephalad and caudal to the fossa ovalis, with the fossa itself typically spared. While the mechanism of uptake is generally considered to be the same as that of brown fat, some authors have suggested that the FDG uptake in LHIAS may represent inflammation [38]. Irrespective of the mechanism of uptake, LHIAS can be easily recognized due to a pathognomonic appearance on CT (Fig. 23.8). The presence of hypermetabolic brown adipose tissue in the mediastinum, although uncommon,

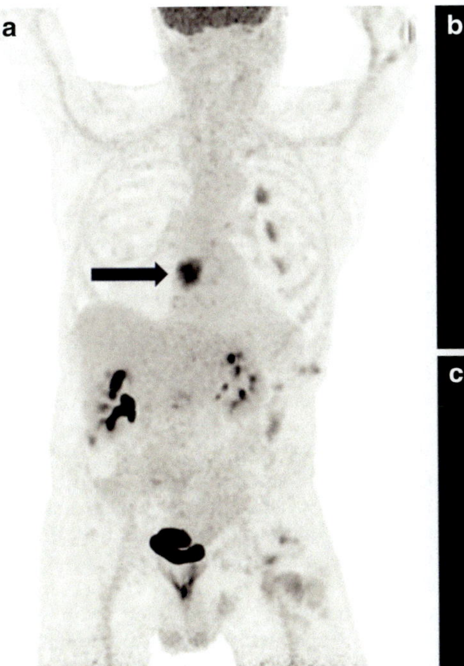
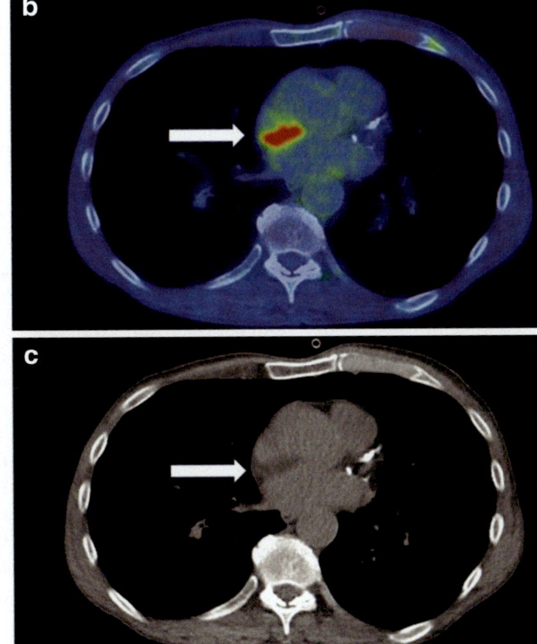

Fig. 23.8 Lipomatous hypertrophy of the interatrial septum (LHIAS) is a potential pitfall in cardiac imaging but can be easily recognized by correlating with the CT images. In this 52-year-old man, unusually avid focal cardiac uptake can be seen on the MIP images (**a**, arrow), localizing to the interatrial septum on axial fused images (**b**, arrow). Comparison to the unenhanced CT images (**c**, arrow) reveals corresponding fat density, diagnostic of LHIAS

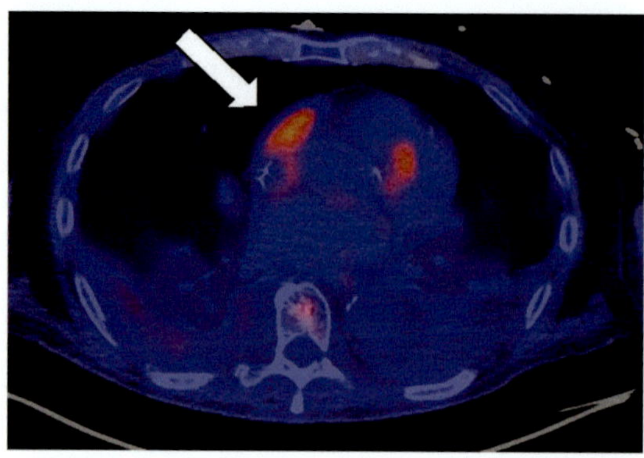

Fig. 23.9 Diffuse uptake can occasionally be seen in the atrial appendage. The significance of this finding remains uncertain

is another potential pitfall, especially in patients that do not present it in other usual regions such as in the cervical and paravertebral soft tissues [39].

Focal activity can also be seen within the atrial appendages. Although often associated with cardiac disease, this finding can also be present in patients without cardiac pathology [40, 41]. In addition, focal activity has been reported within the crista terminalis, which is the muscular band at the junction of the right atrium and appendage, and which contains the sinoatrial node [42]. The reason for uptake in these structures remains uncertain (Fig. 23.9).

Conclusion

In order to confidently identify pathological patterns of FDG uptake in the heart, one must first be cognizant of the normal patterns of myocardial activity, as well as of the potential pitfalls that are frequently seen during cardiac imaging.

References

1. Davidson CQ, Phenix CP, Tai T, Khaper N, Lees SJ. Searching for novel PET radiotracers: imaging cardiac perfusion, metabolism and inflammation. Am J Nucl Med Mol Imaging. 2018;8(3):200–27.
2. Santos BS, Ferreira MJ. Positron emission tomography in ischemic heart disease. Rev Port Cardiol. 2021;38(8):599–608.
3. Tamaki N, Morita K, Kuge Y, Tsukamoto E. The role of fatty acids in cardiac imaging. J Nucl Med. 2000;41(9):1525–34.
4. Yoshinaga K, Tamaki N. Imaging myocardial metabolism. Curr Opin Biotechnol. 2007;18:52–8.
5. Inglese E, Leva L, Matheoud R, Sacchetti G, Secco C, Gandolfo P, et al. Spatial and temporal heterogeneity of regional myocardial uptake in patients without heart disease under fasting conditions on repeated whole-body 18F-FDG PET/CT. J Nucl Med. 2007;48(10):1662–9.
6. Gropler RJ, Siegel BA, Lee KJ, Moerlein SM, Perry DJ, Bergmann SR, et al. Nonuniformity in myocardial accumulation of fluorine-18-Fluorodeoxyglucose in normal fasted humans. J Nucl Med. 1990;31(11):1749–56.
7. Maurer AH, Burshteyn M, Adler LP, Steiner RM. How to differentiate benign versus malignant cardiac and paracardiac 18F FDG uptake at oncologic PET/CT. Radiographics. 2011;31(5):1287–305.
8. Lobert P, Brown RKJ, Dvorak RA, Corbett JR, Kazerooni EA, Wong KK. Spectrum of physiological and pathological cardiac and pericardial uptake of FDG in oncology PET-CT. Clin Radiol. 2013;68(1):e59–71.
9. Zanco P, Desideri A, Mobilia G, Cargnel S, Milan E, Celegon L, et al. Effects of left bundle branch block on myocardial FDG PET in patients without significant coronary artery stenoses. J Nucl Med. 2000;41(6):973–7.
10. Nowak B, Sinha AM, Schaefer WM, Koch K-C, Kaiser H-J, Hanrath P, et al. Cardiac resynchronization therapyhomogenizes myocardial glucosemetabolism and perfusion in dilatedcardiomyopathy and left bundle branch block. J Am Coll Cardiol. 2003;41(9):1523–8.
11. Nose H, Otsuka H, Otomi Y, Terazawa K, Takao S, Iwamoto S, et al. The physiological uptake pattern of 18F-FDG in the left ventricular myocardium of patients without heart disease. J Med Invest. 2014;61:55–8.
12. Israel O, Weiler-Sagie M, Rispler S, Bar-Shalom R, Frenkel A, Keidar Z, et al. PET/CT quantitation of the effect of patient-related factors on cardiac 18F-FDG uptake. J Nucl Med. 2007;48(2):234–9.
13. Wang L, Li W, Yang Y, Wu W, Cai Q, Ma X, et al. Quantitative assessment of right ventricular glucose metabolism in idiopathic pulmonary arterial hypertension patients: a longitudinal study. Eur Heart J Cardiovasc Imaging. 2016;17(10):1161–8.
14. Basu S, Alzeair S, Li G, Dadparvar S, Alavi A. Etiopathologies associated with intercostal muscle Hypermetabolism and prominent right ventricle visualization on 2-Deoxy-2[F-18]fluoro-d-glucose-positron emission tomography: signifi-

cance of an incidental finding and in the setting of a known pulmonary disease. Mol Imaging Biol. 2007;9(6):333–9.

15. Ohira H, deKemp R, Pena E, Davies RA, Stewart DJ, Chandy G, et al. Shifts in myocardial fatty acid and glucose metabolism in pulmonary arterial hypertension: a potential mechanism for a maladaptive right ventricular response. Eur Heart J Cardiovasc Imaging. 2016;17(12):1424–31.

16. Lundgrin EL, Park MM, Sharp J, Tang WHW, Thomas JD, Asosingh K, et al. Fasting 2-Deoxy-2-[^{18}F]fluoro-D-glucose positron emission tomography to detect metabolic changes in pulmonary arterial hypertension hearts over 1 year. Ann Am Thorac Soc. 2013;10(1):1–9.

17. Yang T, Wang L, Xiong C-M, He J-G, Zhang Y, Gu Q, et al. The ratio of 18F-FDG activity uptake between the right and left ventricle in patients with pulmonary hypertension correlates with the right ventricular function. Clin Nucl Med. 2014;39(5):426–30.

18. Mielniczuk LM, Birnie D, Ziadi MC, deKemp RA, DaSilva JN, Burwash I, et al. Relation between right ventricular function and increased right ventricular [^{18}F]Fluorodeoxyglucose accumulation in patients with heart failure. Circ Cardiovasc Imaging. 2011;4(1):59–66.

19. Oikawa M, Kagaya Y, Otani H, Sakuma M, Demachi J, Suzuki J, et al. Increased [18F] Fluorodeoxyglucose accumulation in right ventricular free wall in patients with pulmonary hypertension and the effect of Epoprostenol. J Am Coll Cardiol. 2005;45(11):1849–55.

20. Hagan G, Southwood M, Treacy C, Ross RM, Soon E, Coulson J, et al. 18FDG PET imaging can quantify increased cellular metabolism in pulmonary arterial hypertension: a proof-of-principle study. Pulm Circ. 2011;1(4):448–55.

21. Can MM, Kaymaz C, Tanboga IH, Tokgoz HC, Canpolat N, Turkyilmaz E, et al. Increased right ventricular glucose metabolism in patients with pulmonary arterial hypertension. Clin Nucl Med. 2011;36(9):743–8.

22. Tsai S-Y, Wu Y-W, Wang S-Y, Shiau Y-C, Chiu K-M, Tsai H-Y, et al. Clinical significance of quantitative assessment of right ventricular glucose metabolism in patients with heart failure with reduced ejection fraction. Eur J Nucl Med Mol Imaging. 2019;46(12):2601–9.

23. Kluge R, Barthel H, Pankau H, Seese A, Schauer J, Wirtz H, et al. Different mechanisms for changes in glucose uptake of the right and left ventricular myocardium in pulmonary hypertension. J Nucl Med. 2005;46(1):25–31.

24. Tatebe S, Fukumoto Y, Oikawa-Wakayama M, Sugimura K, Satoh K, Miura Y, et al. Enhanced [18F] fluorodeoxyglucose accumulation in the right ventricular free wall predicts long-term prognosis of patients with pulmonary hypertension: a preliminary observational study. Eur Heart J Cardiovasc Imaging. 2014;15(6):666–72.

25. Li W, Wang L, Xiong C-M, Yang T, Zhang Y, Gu Q, et al. The prognostic value of 18F-FDG uptake ratio between the right and left ventricles in idiopathic pulmonary arterial hypertension. Clin Nucl Med. 2015;40(11):859–63.

26. Fujii H, Ide M, Yasuda S, Takahashi W, Shohtsu A, Kubo A. Increased FDG uptake in the wall of the right atrium in people who participated in a cancer screening program with whole-body PET. Ann Nucl Med. 1999;13(1):55–9.

27. Sinigaglia M, Mahida B, Piekarski E, Chequer R, Mikail N, Benali K, et al. FDG atrial uptake is associated with an increased prevalence of stroke in patients with atrial fibrillation. Eur J Nucl Med Mol Imaging. 2019;46(6):1268–75.

28. Xie B, Chen B-X, Wu J-Y, Liu X, Yang M-F. Factors relevant to atrial 18F-fluorodeoxyglucose uptake in atrial fibrillation. J Nucl Cardiol. 2018;27(5):1501–12.

29. Xie B, Chen B-X, Nanna M, Wu J-Y, Zhou Y, Shi L, et al. 18F-fluorodeoxyglucose positron emission tomography/computed tomography imaging in atrial fibrillation: a pilot prospective study. Eur Heart J Cardiovasc Imaging. 2022;23(1):102–12.

30. Mazurek T, Zhang L, Zalewski A, Mannion JD, Diehl JT, Arafat H, et al. Human Epicardial adipose tissue is a source of inflammatory mediators. Circulation. 2003;108(20):2460–6.

31. Hu Y-F, Chen Y-J, Lin Y-J, Chen S-A. Inflammation and the pathogenesis of atrial fibrillation. Nat Rev Cardiol. 2015;12(4):230–43.

32. Betancourt Cuellar SL, Palacio D, Benveniste MF, Carter BW, Gladish G. Pitfalls and misinterpretations of cardiac findings on PET/CT imaging: a careful look at the heart in oncology patients. Curr Probl Diagn Radiol. 2019;48(2):172–83.

33. Haider A, Bengs S, Schade K, Wijnen WJ, Portmann A, Etter D, et al. Myocardial 18F-FDG uptake pattern for cardiovascular risk stratification in patients undergoing oncologic PET/CT. J Clin Med. 2020;9(7):2279.

34. Ando V, Koestner S, Pruvot E, Kamani C-H, Ganiere V. Cardiac sarcoidosis involving the papillary muscle: a case report. Heart Rhythm Case Rep. 2021;7(12):801–5.

35. Duchenne J, Turco A, Bézy S, Ünlü S, Pagourelias ED, Beela AS, et al. Papillary muscles contribute significantly more to left ventricular work in dilated hearts. Eur Heart J Cardiovasc Imaging. 2019;20(1):84–91.

36. Laura DM, Donnino R, Kim EE, Benenstein R, Freedberg RS, Saric M. Lipomatous atrial septal hypertrophy: a review of its anatomy, pathophysiology, multimodality imaging, and relevance to percutaneous interventions. J Am Soc Echocardiogr. 2016;29(8):717–23.

37. Kuester LB, Fischman AJ, Fan C-M, Halpern EF, Aquino SL. Lipomatous hypertrophy of the interatrial septum: prevalence and features on fusion 18F

fluorodeoxyglucose positron emission tomography/CT. Chest. 2005;128(6):3888–93.

38. Zukotynski KA, Israel DA, Kim CK. FDG uptake in lipomatous hypertrophy of the interatrial septum is not likely related to brown adipose tissue. Clin Nucl Med. 2011;36(9):767–9.

39. Truong MT, Erasmus JJ, Munden RF, Marom EM, Sabloff BS, Gladish GW, et al. Focal FDG uptake in mediastinal Brown fat mimicking malignancy: a potential pitfall resolved on PET/CT. Am J Roentgenol. 2004;183(4):1127–32.

40. Nguyen BD. PET demonstration of left atrial appendage in chronic atrial fibrillation. Clin Nucl Med. 2005;30(3):177.

41. Okura K, Maeno K, Hirazawa M, Takemori H, Toya D, Tanaka N, et al. Fluorodeoxyglucose accumulation in the left atrial appendage of a patient with paroxysmal atrial fibrillation. J Cardiol Cases. 2012;5(1):e32–5.

42. Minamimoto R. Series of myocardial FDG uptake requiring considerations of myocardial abnormalities in FDG-PET/CT. Jpn J Radiol. 2021;39(6):540–57.

Cardiovascular FDG-PET Atlas of Cases

Yousif A. Lucinian, Patrick Martineau, and Matthieu Pelletier-Galarneau

Acronyms

AF	Atrial fibrillation
AFB	Acid-fast bacillus
AV block	Atrioventricular block
CAD	Coronary artery disease
CCTA	Coronary computed tomography angiography
CIED	Cardiac implantable electronic device
CIED-LI	Cardiac implantable electronic device lead infection
COPD	Chronic obstructive pulmonary
CRP	C-reactive protein
CS	Cardiac sarcoidosis
CT	Computed tomography
CTA	Computed tomography angiography
CTPA	Computed tomography pulmonary angiography
DES	Drug-eluting stent
DSWI	Deep sternal wound infection
ECMO	Extracorporeal membrane oxygenation
ER	Emergency room
FDG	^{18}F-fluorodeoxyglucose
GCA	Giant-cell arteritis
GPI	Generator pocket infection
HRS	Heart and Rhythm Society
hs-cTnT	High-sensitivity cardiac troponin T
ICD	Implantable cardioverter-defibrillator
IE	Infective endocarditis
JCS	Japan Circulation Society
LAD	Left anterior descending coronary artery
LDCT	Low-dose CT scan
LVEF	Left ventricular ejection fraction
LVV	Large-vessel
MPA	Main pulmonary artery
MPI	Myocardial perfusion imaging
MRI	Magnetic resonance imaging
MSSA	Methicillin-susceptible Staphylococcus aureus
NVE	Native valve infective endocarditis
PAS	Pulmonary artery sarcoma
PE	Pulmonary emboli
PET	Positron emission tomography
PICC	Peripherally inserted central catheter
PVE	Prosthetic valve infective endocarditis
82Rb	Rubidium-82
RCA	Right coronary artery
RHS	Right heart strain
RUL	Right upper lobe
SSWI	Superficial sternal wound infection
STEMI	ST-elevation myocardial infarction

Y. A. Lucinian · M. Pelletier-Galarneau (✉)
Montreal Heart Institute, Montréal, QC, Canada
e-mail: yousif.al-ali@umontreal.ca;
Matthieu.pelletier-galarneau@icm-mhi.org

P. Martineau
BC Cancer Agency, Vancouver, BC, Canada
e-mail: patrick.martineau@bccancer.bc.ca

M. Pelletier-Galarneau, P. Martineau (eds.), *FDG-PET/CT and PET/MR in Cardiovascular Diseases*, https://doi.org/10.1007/978-3-031-09807-9_24

SUV	Standardized uptake value
SWI	Sternal wound infection
TAK	Takayasu arteritis
TAVR	Transcatheter aortic valve replacement
TEE	Transoesophageal echocardiogram
TTE	Transthoracic echocardiogram
VG	Vascular graft
VGI	Vascular graft infection
VSD	Ventricular septal defect
WBC	White blood cell

Case 1

Initial Evaluation

An 85-year-old male had a history of type 2 diabetes mellitus, polycystic kidney disease, hypertension, atrial fibrillation (AF), and nonischemic cardiomyopathy with a left ventricular ejection fraction (LVEF) of 25% and a biventricular pacemaker (CRT-D) presented to the ER in septic shock with an infection of unknown origin. He reported coughing with worsening dyspnea and new-onset back pain in the preceding weeks. Blood cultures were positive for *Salmonella* group D. Chest radiographs showed a left perihilar infiltration. Transoesophageal echocardiogram (TEE) demonstrated thickening of the right atrium lead with a mobile millimetric mass, suggesting either a thrombus or a vegetation (Fig. 24.1).

Follow-Up

Despite clinical improvement under antibiotics, bacteremia persisted. A chest radiograph was repeated, showing regression of the previously noted left lung opacities. A pacemaker lead infec-

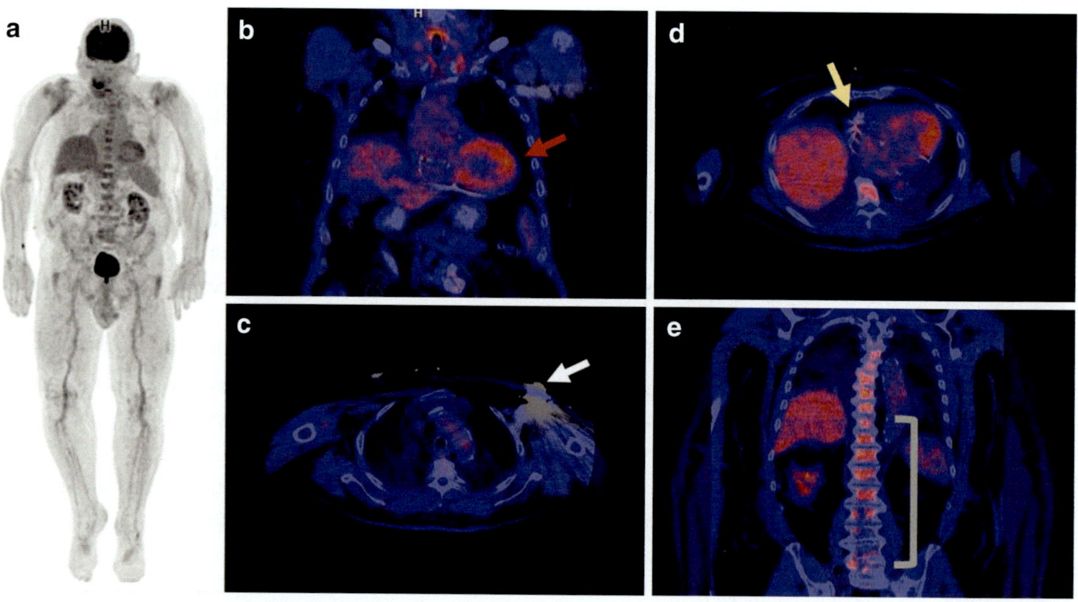

Fig. 24.1 PET 1 Interpretation. Whole-body FDG-PET/CT (**a**) was performed following a myocardial suppression protocol consisting of a low-carbohydrate diet, 12 h fasting, and intravenous heparin in order to exclude endocarditis or pacemaker lead infection. Of note, the patient had already undergone 7 days of treatment with large spectrum antibiotics. Myocardial suppression was suboptimal with diffuse left ventricular myocardial uptake (**b**). No abnormal uptake was seen at the levels of the pacemaker generator pocket and leads, including the right atrium lead (**c**, **d**). Slightly heterogeneous FDG distribution was noted at the thoracolumbar spine, but without evidence of spondylodiscitis (**e**)

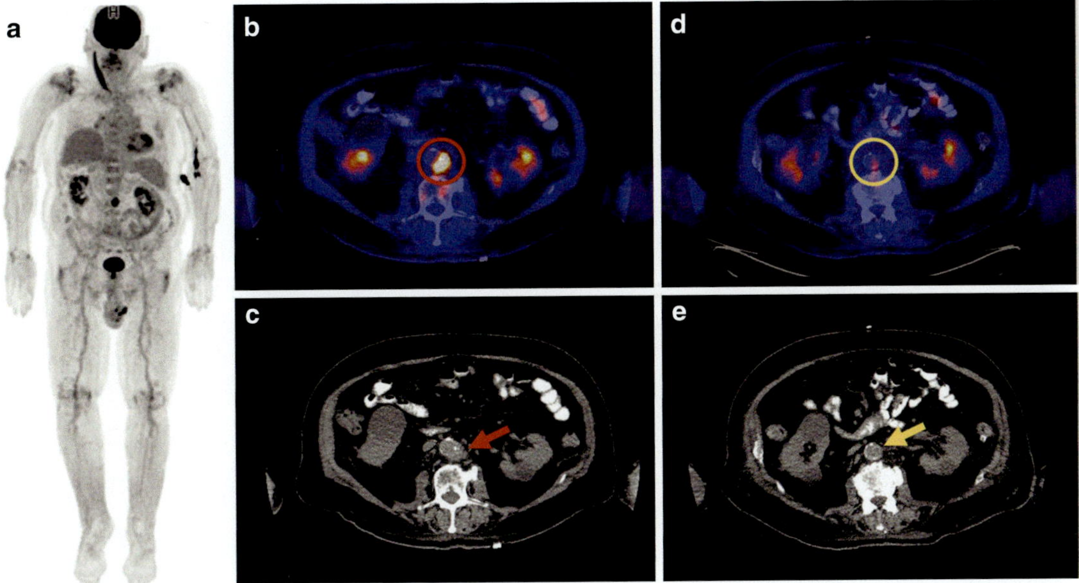

Fig. 24.2 PET 2 Interpretation. A second whole-body FDG-PET/CT (**a**) was performed 17 days following the initial evaluation. Myocardial suppression was again suboptimal despite adherence to the preparation protocol, limiting evaluation of valvular areas. However, there was still no evidence of pacemaker-related infection. At the level of the infrarenal aorta, a new intense hypermetabolic lesion was noted on the left posterolateral side (**b**) (SUV_{max} = 9.5). A probable saccular dilatation was demonstrated on concomitant unenhanced CT (**c**). A diagnosis of mycotic aneurysm was made. In retrospect, on the initial FDG-PET, a nonspecific slight increase in uptake (**d**) (SUV_{max} = 2.9) was seen at approximately the same level with an otherwise normal appearing aorta on CT (**e**)

tion was again suspected, prompting consideration of device removal (Fig. 24.2).

Teaching Point

The patient's initial clinical evaluation was ambiguous, as no clear source of bacteremia was evident. Both initial and follow-up FDG-PET/CT accurately excluded a pacemaker-related infectious process, minimizing unnecessary interventions. The abdominal aorta appeared grossly normal on initial FDG-PET/CT other than nonspecific FDG uptake, most likely a result of an early disease process combined with ongoing antibiotic treatment. A follow-up FDG-PET/CT performed because of persistent bacteremia evidenced an aortic mycotic aneurysm, possibly causing the patient's back pain. As the great majority of aortic mycotic aneurysms are metabolically active, the sensitivity of FDG-PET in the detection of infected aortic aneurysms is very high (>90%), while its specificity is lowered by similar imaging findings in inflammatory aneurysms [1–3]. Contrast enhanced CT remains the most commonly employed imaging modality to assess aortic infections [4]. However, FDG-PET has been shown to have higher diagnostic accuracy while also providing supplemental useful information for reaching a conclusive diagnosis in patients without infection [1].

Case 2

Initial Evaluation

An 81-year-old-male, known for AF, a permanent pacemaker (implanted 5 years prior) and severe aortic stenosis, presented to the ER 6 weeks after transcatheter aortic valve replacement (TAVR) with fever and chills. Multiple blood cultures were positive for *Staphylococcus epidermidis*. No clear source of infection was evident. Gallium-67 scintigraphy was normal. Both initial and repeat transoesophageal echocar-

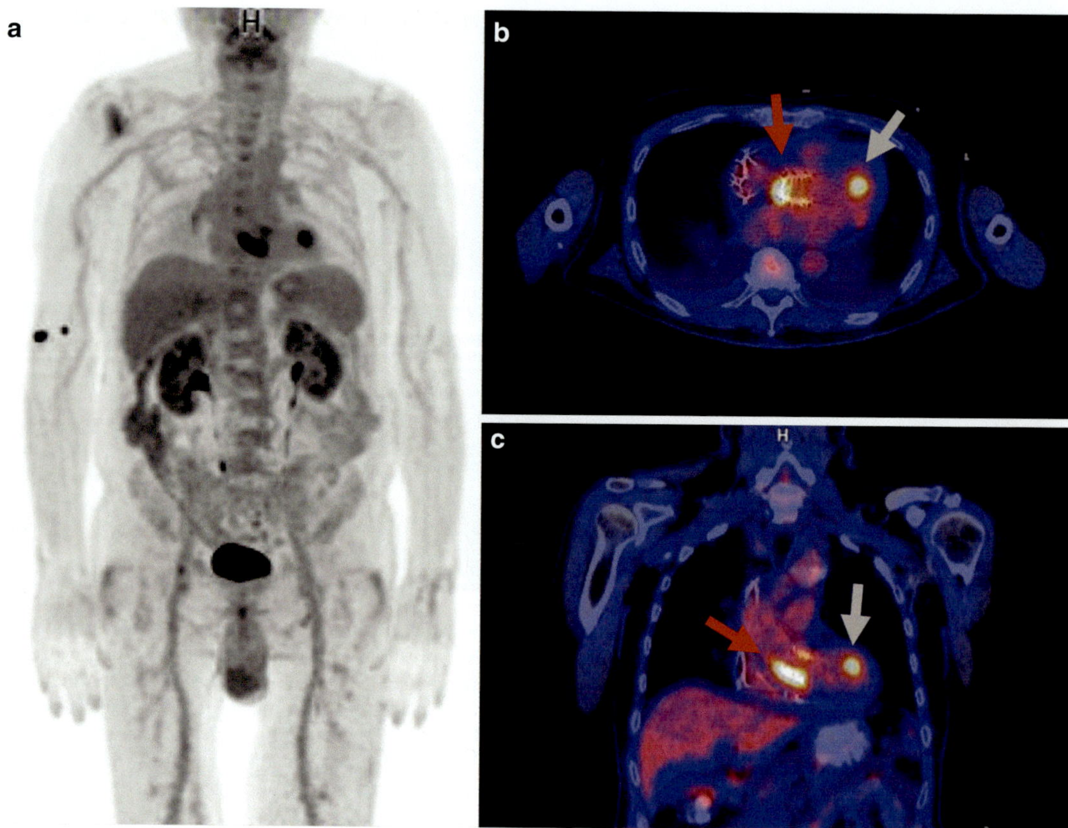

Fig. 24.3 PET Interpretation. Whole-body FDG-PET/CT (**a**) was performed following a myocardial suppression protocol consisting of a low-carbohydrate diet, 12 h fasting, and intravenous heparin. Myocardial suppression was adequate. No abnormal uptake was seen at the levels of the pacemaker generator pocket and leads. Intense, heterogeneous, and asymmetric uptake ($SUV_{max} = 10.8$) extending inferiorly was noted at the level of the TAVR prosthesis (**b**, **c**, red arrows). Increased uptake was also seen at the level of a left ventricle papillary muscle, a non-specific finding (**b**, **c**, gray arrows). The remainder of the study was unremarkable

diogram (TEE) were negative for endocarditis, with a reported transprosthetic pressure gradient of 10 mmHg. Pacemaker-related infection was strongly suspected (Fig. 24.3).

Teaching Point

The patient's clinical presentation was strongly suggestive of infective endocarditis after TAVR (TAVR-IE). Because TEE was inconclusive, a pacemaker-related infection was initially suspected. FDG-PET correctly identified TAVR-IE and was crucial in guiding subsequent manage-ment. FDG-PET's usefulness in imaging prosthetic valve infective endocarditis (PVE) is well established, making it a major criterion in the European Society of Cardiology diagnostic criteria for PVE [5, 6]. FDG-PET/CT also offers the possibility of treatment response monitoring [7]. However, data about the diagnostic performance of FDG-PET in TAVR-IE remains limited [8–10]. A recent retrospective analysis by Wahadat et al. involving 30 patients showed promising results, as FDG-PET/CT helped reclassify 8 patients from the initial possible TAVR-IE group to either the definite or the rejected TAVR-IE groups [11].

Case 3

Initial Evaluation

A 66-year-old woman, known for type 2 diabetes and AF, underwent cardiac transplantation 7 years prior for hypertrophic cardiomyopathy. She presented with worsening dyspnea over the course of several months. Transplant rejection was suspected. CT pulmonary angiography (CTPA) was remarkable for a right atrial filling defect measuring 24 × 18 × 29 mm. Transthoracic echocardiogram (TTE) showed a normal left ventricle with a systolic ejection fraction of 60%. However, a mobile, lobulated mass measuring 25 × 22 mm was reported alongside the anterior wall of the dilated right atrium. The differential diagnosis included a thrombus, myxoma, or metastasis (Fig. 24.4).

Follow-Up

The patient underwent surgery for mass resection. Histopathologic analysis confirmed the diagnosis of myxoma. Follow-up TTE showed no residual mass.

Teaching Point

Right atrial location of cardiac masses increases the likelihood of malignancy [12]. In this case, however, the associated low intensity uptake seen on FDG-PET accurately predicted a benign lesion. There is a broad differential for cardiac masses, from pseudotumors (e.g., thrombus, vegetation, abscess, aneurysm) to neoplasms [4, 13]. Most cardiac lesions are benign, while primary malignant tumors of the heart are mainly sarco-

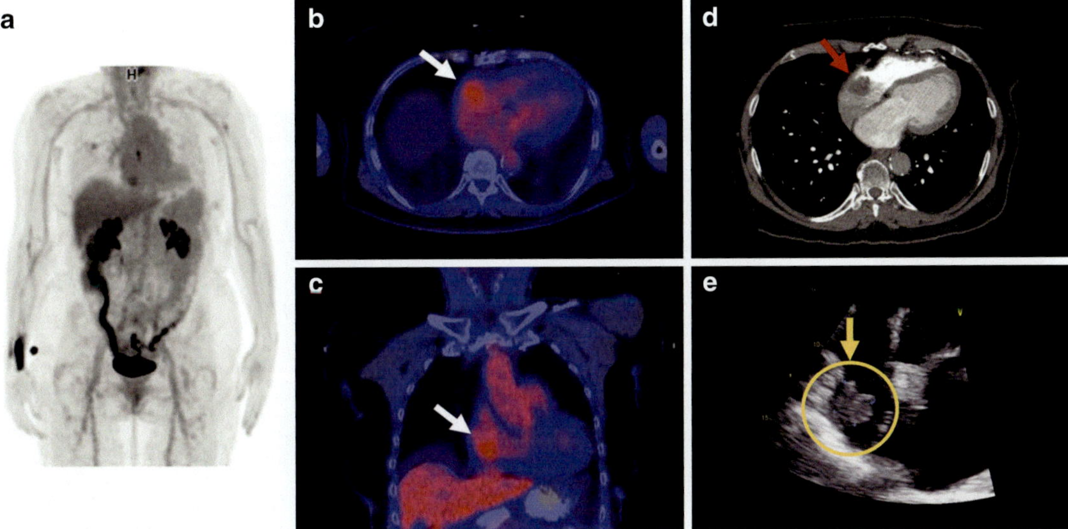

Fig. 24.4 PET Interpretation. Whole-body FDG-PET/CT (**a**) was performed following a myocardial suppression protocol consisting of a low-carbohydrate diet, 12 h fasting, and intravenous heparin in order to further characterize the right atrial mass. Myocardial suppression was excellent. A low intensity (SUV$_{max}$ = 3.5) and homogeneous focus of uptake was visualized within the right atrium (**b**, transaxial plane) (**c**, coronal plane). The corre-sponding right atrium filling defect seen on CTPA and mass visualized on TTE are shown in images (**d**) and (**e**), respectively. No pericardial or pleural effusions were seen. Diffuse low grade uptake at the site of the previous sternotomy was seen, without evidence of infection. A diagnosis of myxoma was favored. No extracardiac hypermetabolic lesions were seen on whole-body FDG-PET images

matous [4, 13, 14]. Although echocardiography is frequently employed, magnetic resonance imaging (MRI) is usually considered the gold standard for the characterization of cardiac masses [12, 13, 15]. FDG-PET's role in the diagnostic work up of cardiac masses continues to develop. However, many studies suggest its potential usefulness and high diagnostic accuracy for distinguishing malignant from benign lesions [16].

Case 4

Initial Evaluation

An 89-year-old woman, known for type 2 diabetes, hypertension and end stage chronic kidney disease (CKD), presented with acute pleuritic chest pain and shortness of breath. Review of systems revealed hematochezia accompanied by weight loss and night sweats in the preceding months. Both white blood cell count (WBC) and C-reactive protein (CRP) levels were elevated.

High-sensitivity cardiac troponin T (hs-cTnT) levels were slightly elevated at 39 ng/L (normal <14 ng/L), without significant change on serial measurements. D-dimer levels were highly elevated at 3952 ng/mL (normal <250 ng/mL). ECG showed a sinus rhythm with widespread concave up ST elevation. Ventilation/perfusion lung scan with ^{99m}Tc-technegas and ^{99m}Tc-MAA performed to exclude pulmonary embolism was normal. Transthoracic echocardiogram (TTE) showed a small (2 mm thick) anterior pericardial effusion that was not present on TTE performed a year prior. A diagnosis of acute pericarditis was strongly suspected (Fig. 24.5).

Follow-Up

Pericardiocentesis was not performed. A diagnosis of idiopathic/viral pericarditis was retained. The patient underwent a 3 months treatment course with oral prednisone. Her symptoms quickly resolved, with follow-up TTE showing

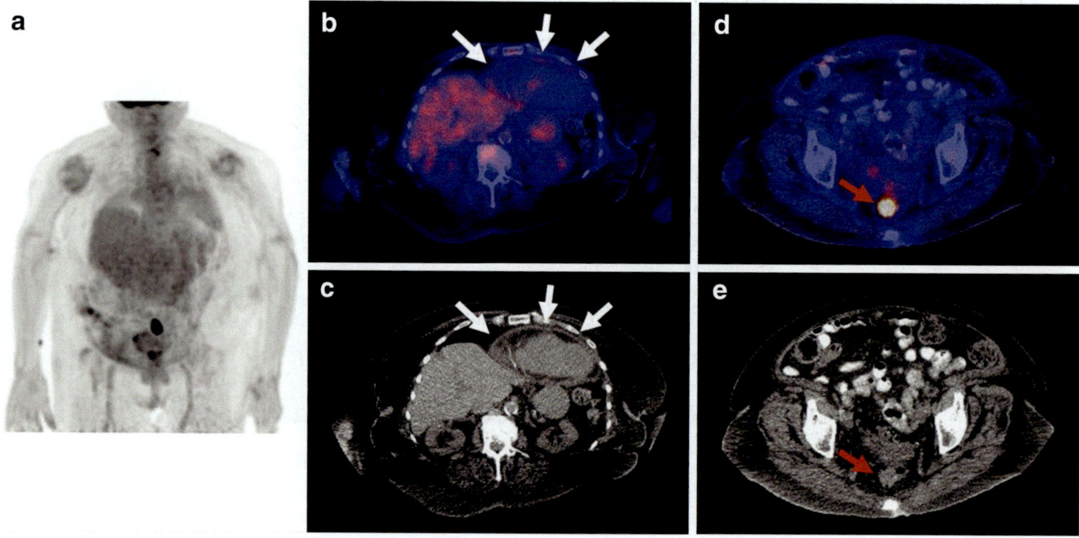

Fig. 24.5 PET Interpretation. Whole-body FDG-PET/CT (**a**) was performed in order to help determine an etiology for pericardial effusion. The pericardial effusion associated with circumferential, low intensity uptake (SUV$_{max}$ = 2.5), compatible with the diagnosis of pericarditis (**b**, **c**). No signs suggestive of pericardial malignancy were seen. A hypermetabolic lesion (SUV$_{max}$ = 14.2) measuring approximately 30 × 20 × 20 mm at the level of the rectosigmoid colon was visualized (**d**, **e**). No hypermetabolic lymph nodes or lesions suggestive of a metastatic process were seen

no residual pericardial effusion. Colonoscopy discovered 2 polyps, a 5 mm sessile polyp and a 30 mm subpedunculated polyp, both localized in the rectum.

Teaching Point

Although most pericarditis cases are considered benign and attributed to viral infection, a nonnegligible proportion have an underlying neoplastic process (5–23%), especially in the presence of pericardial effusion [17]. As primary malignant tumors of the heart are rare, most cases of cancer-related pericarditis are caused by metastatic or locally infiltrating tumors [17–20]. However, other mechanisms have been described, including radiotherapy, chemotherapy, and paraneoplastic syndrome [17–20]. In this context, FDG-PET/CT may be clinically helpful in the diagnostic workup of pericarditis, especially when malignancy is suspected and pericardiocentesis is non-diagnostic or technically difficult to perform [21].

Other potential roles of FDG-PET/CT include determining the extent of tuberculous pericarditis and predicting treatment response in constrictive pericarditis [21, 22].

Case 5

Initial Evaluation

A 55-year-old male, known for type 2 diabetes mellitus, hypertension, AF, ischemic cardiomyopathy with a LVEF of 25% and a dual chamber implantable cardioverter-defibrillator (ICD), presented with fatigue and fever. Blood cultures were positive for methicillin-susceptible *Staphylococcus aureus* (MSSA). Multiple pulmonary opacities were seen on chest radiograph. TEE demonstrated thickening of the right atrium ICD lead with partial mobility, suspicious for vegetation. An indeterminate filament-like structure attached to the aortic valve was also visualized (Fig. 24.6).

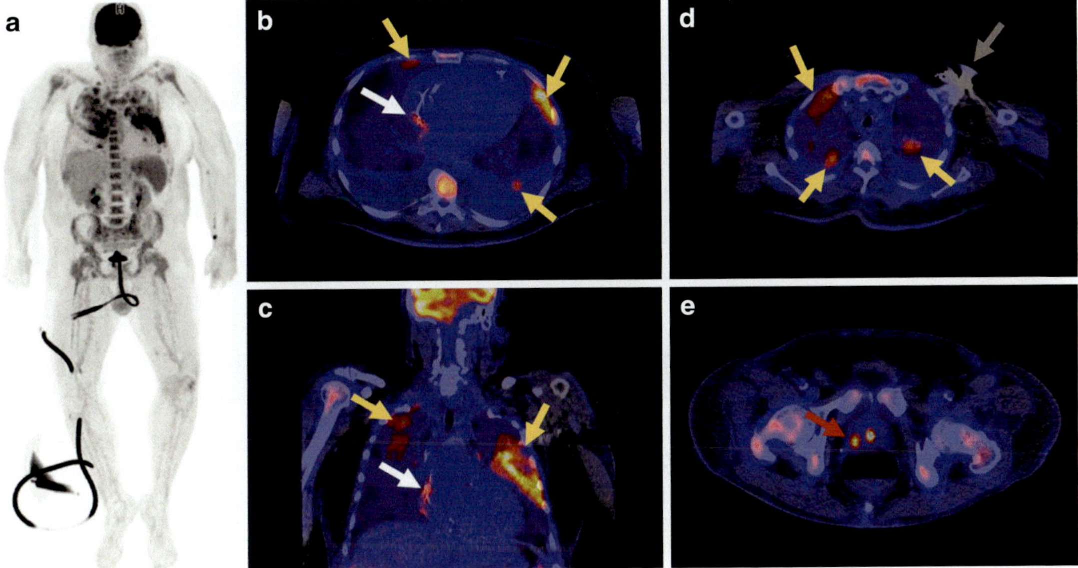

Fig. 24.6 PET 1 interpretation. Whole-body FDG-PET/CT (**a**) was performed following a myocardial suppression protocol (low-carbohydrate diet, 12 h fasting, and intravenous heparin) in order to further characterize TEE findings. Of note, the patient had undergone 4 days of antibiotic treatment. Myocardial suppression was adequate. Focal increased uptake (SUV_max = 3.7) was visualized on the ICD lead (**b**, **c**, white arrows) at the cavoatrial junction. Uptake was also present on non–attenuation-correction images (not shown). Increased uptake within bilateral lung consolidations was seen (**b**, **c**, **d**, yellow arrows). No abnormal uptake was seen within the generator pocket (**d**, gray arrow) and valvular areas. An incidental focus of uptake (SUV_max = 6.0) was noted within the prostate (**e**, red arrow)

Follow-Up

A diagnosis of ICD lead infection with septic pulmonary emboli (PE) was made on the basis of the PET findings. The aortic valve findings on initial TEE were considered possibly degenerative due to the lack of FDG uptake, although absence of uptake does not exclude endocarditis of native valve. The ICD was removed. Microbiological analysis of the lead samples was positive for MSSA (Fig. 24.7).

Teaching Point

On the initial PET, FDG-PET/CT accurately identified ICD lead infection with septic PE. The absence of abnormal uptake within the tricuspid valve area is reassuring, but FDG-PET has suboptimal sensitivity for the detection of ICD-IE [23]. Cardiac implantable electronic device (CIED) infection can arise at any level, from the generator pocket to the intracardiac leads. Echocardiographic evaluation of CIED lead infection (LI) can be challenging due to considerable artifacts. The accuracy of the Modified Duke's Criteria has also been shown to be reduced in this context [24, 25]. FDG-PET/CT can be especially useful when CIED-LI is clinically suspected in the presence of indeterminate diagnostic findings [26, 27]. Moreover, extracardiac findings such as septic emboli can provide crucial information for diagnosis and optimal management [28, 29].

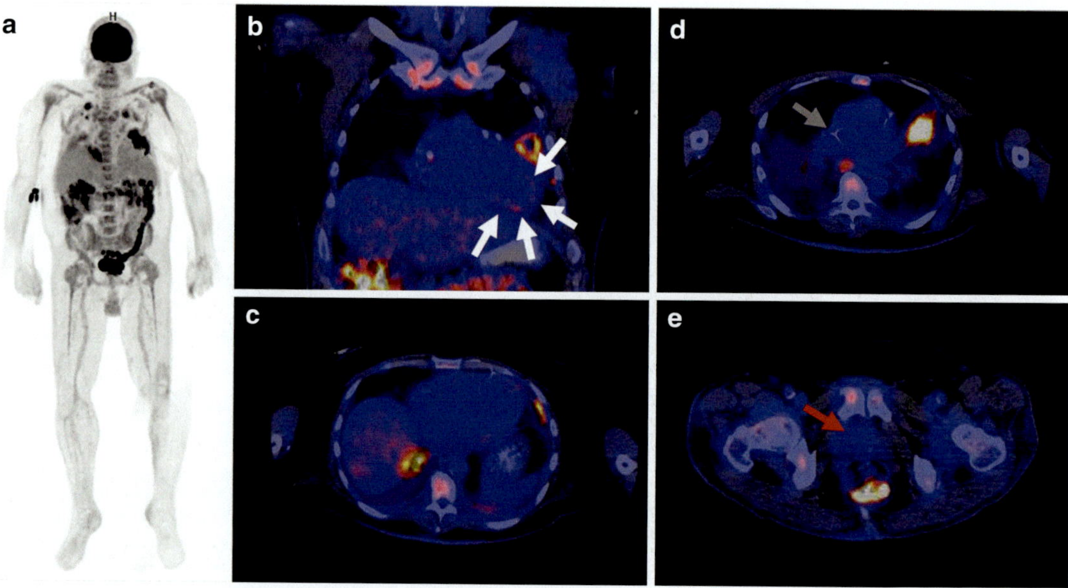

Fig. 24.7 PET 2 interpretation. A second whole-body FDG-PET/CT (**a**) was performed 14 days following the initial evaluation. The quality of myocardial suppression was slightly suboptimal as there was low-intensity diffuse uptake within the left ventricular walls (**b**, white arrows). Again, no abnormal uptake was seen at the levels of the valves (**c**). A PICC line had been placed in the interval (**d**, gray arrow). The previously visualized lung consolidations had partly resolved. The hypermetabolic focus of uptake within the prostate had resolved in the interval (**e**, red arrow)

Case 6

Initial Evaluation

A 73-year-old man was known for obstructive sleep apnea and hypertension. On a routine chest radiograph, a right apical opacity was noted. Review of systems was unremarkable other than nonspecific fatigue. Noncontrast chest CT scan revealed a possible right apical centimetric nodule within fibrotic changes (Fig. 24.8).

Follow-Up (1)

Large-vessel vasculitis (LVV) was strongly suspected, presumed to be giant-cell arteritis (GCA) given the patient's age. Rest ECG was unremarkable. Computed tomography angiography (CTA) performed from the carotids down to the lower extremities showed arterial wall thickening at the levels of the distal ascending aorta, the brachiocephalic trunk, the circumflex artery, the abdominal aorta, and both common iliac arteries, but no stenosis or dilation. In the absence of symptoms, a multidisciplinary team opted for a wait-and-see approach rather than initiating pharmacologic treatment. Temporal artery biopsy was not pursued (Fig. 24.9).

Follow-Up (2)

As the patient remained asymptomatic, treatment was not initiated. Five months later, the patient started experiencing increased fatigue and dyspnea on exertion. During exercise ECG stress testing, the patient's dyspnea was elicited alongside inferolateral horizontal ST depressions. Flare-up of LVV was suspected (Fig. 24.10).

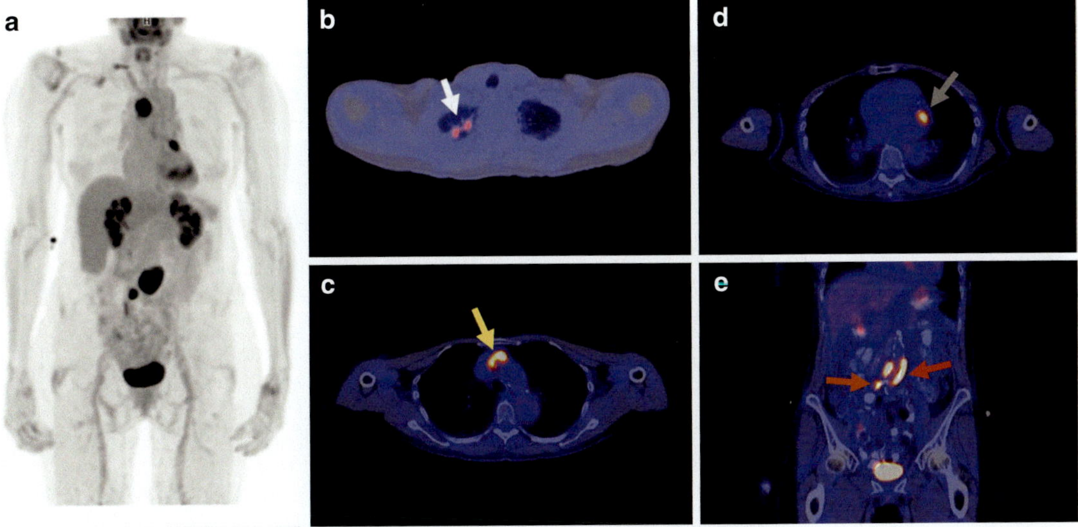

Fig. 24.8 PET 1 interpretation. Whole-body FDG-PET/CT (**a**) was performed for further assessment. Slight hypermetabolism was seen within the lung nodule and fibrotic changes in the right lung apex (**b**, white arrow, $SUV_{max} = 3.5$). Multiple vascular abnormalities were visualized. Intense uptake was seen at the origin of the brachiocephalic trunk and the distal ascending aorta (**c**, yellow arrow, $SUV_{max} = 9.2$), the circumflex coronary artery (**d**, gray arrow, $SUV_{max} = 6.3$) and the abdominal aorta (**e**, red arrow, $SUV_{max} = 12.9$) with extension to the right common iliac artery (**e**, orange arrow, $SUV_{max} = 6.8$)

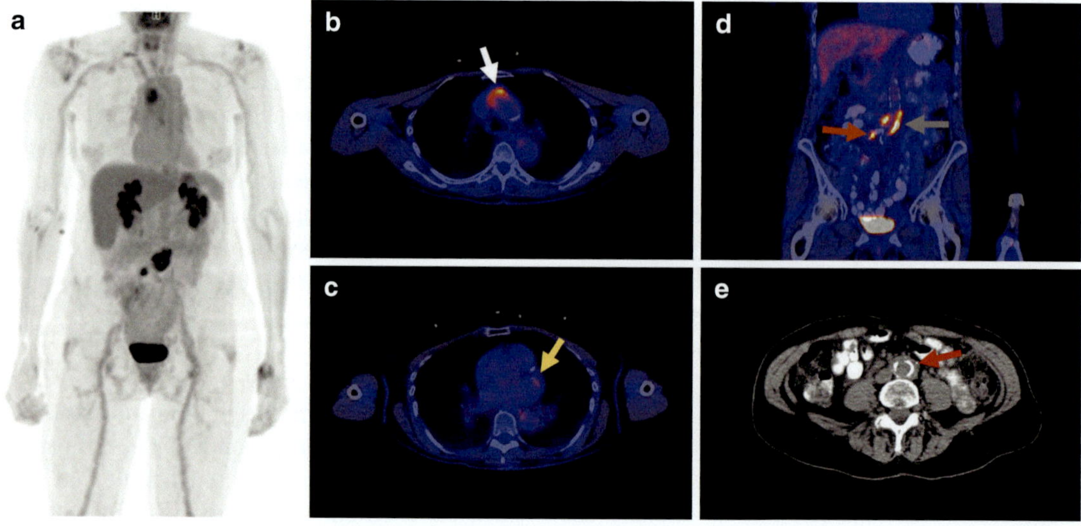

Fig. 24.9 PET 2 interpretation. Whole-body FDG-PET/CT (**a**) following a myocardial suppression protocol was performed 10 months later. Myocardial suppression was excellent. No significant change was seen within the right lung apex. Uptake within the origin of the brachiocephalic trunk and the distal ascending aorta (**b**, white arrow, SUV_{max} = 4.9), the circumflex coronary artery (**c**, gray arrow, SUV_{max} = 2.5) and the abdominal aorta (**d**, gray arrow, SUV_{max} = 7.2) showed partial interval regression. Uptake within the right common iliac artery was stable (**d**, orange arrow, SUV_{max} = 6.4). Arterial wall thickening at the level of the abdominal aorta is seen (**e**, red arrow, 6.7 mm) without significant progression compared to CTA performed 4 months prior (6.4 mm)

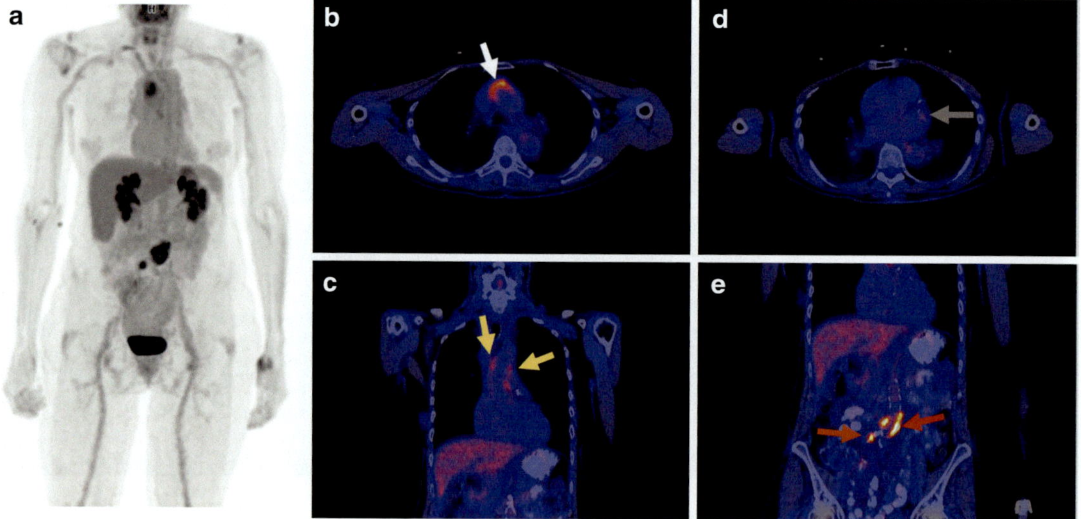

Fig. 24.10 PET 3 interpretation. Whole-body FDG-PET/CT (**a**) following a myocardial suppression protocol was performed. Myocardial suppression was excellent. Uptake within the origin of the brachiocephalic trunk (**b**, white arrow) and the distal ascending aorta (**c**, yellow arrows) was slightly decreased from prior (SUV_{max} = 3.9). Uptake at the level of the circumflex coronary artery was stable (**d**, gray arrow, SUV_{max} = 2.4). Uptake at the level of the abdominal aorta (**e**, red arrow, SUV_{max} = 6.2) and the right common iliac artery (**e**, orange arrow, SUV_{max} = 4.8) was also partially regressed. Uptake in the iliac arteries corresponded to residual blood pool activity

Follow-Up (3)

Coronary CT angiography (CCTA) was remarkable for proximal circumflex artery mural thickening alongside atherosclerotic plaque luminal narrowing of 70%. Coronary angiogram showed luminal narrowing of 70% at the level of the second left marginal artery which was successfully stented. Minimal/nonobstructive coronary artery disease (CAD) was seen within the right coronary artery (RCA) and the left anterior descending coronary artery (LAD).

Teaching Point

The two major categories of LVV are GCA and Takayasu arteritis (TAK) [30]. Although large vessel involvement is grossly similar in both entities, coronary arteries are more frequently affected in TAK [31]. Serious complications of coronary arteritis include stenosis, aneurysm and thrombosis, but may also manifest as accelerated atherosclerosis [31–34]. When interpreting LVV on FDG-PET/CT, a standardized approach using a 4 point-scale system (comparing vascular uptake to liver uptake) is recommended [35]. FDG-PET/CT is also useful for treatment monitoring, as uptake is typically decreased within 4–12 weeks following effective treatment initiation [35]. Of note, faint uptake can persist for several months despite successful therapy [35–37]. This case illustrates the unique ability of FDG-PET/CT to detect LVV in the early phase of the disease before significant morphological changes have occurred. The regression of FDG uptake between initial and subsequent PETs possibly represents a transition from an acute inflammatory phase to a chronic phase in which morphological changes predominate [35].

Case 7

Initial Evaluation

A 45-year-old male, known for type 2 diabetes mellitus and active smoking, presented to the emergency department with new-onset epigastric pain. ECG demonstrated ST-elevation myocardial infarction (STEMI) in the anterolateral territories. Cardiac catheterization showed a proximally occluded LAD and a severely diseased RCA while the circumflex artery had minimal/nonobstructive CAD. Two drug-eluting stents (DES) were successfully deployed within the LAD. Shortly after the procedure, the patient progressed to cardiogenic shock and required extracorporeal membrane oxygenation (ECMO) for the subsequent 4 days. TTE showed a severely reduced LVEF (25%) with apical akinesia (Fig. 24.11).

Follow-Up

Standard heart failure treatment was initiated. Medical treatment was chosen for the RCA instead of revascularization. Follow-up TTE performed 6 months later showed slight improvement in LVEF (35%), but severe hypokinesis within the LAD myocardial territories persisted.

Teaching Point

FDG-PET combined with MPI has been considered the gold standard for determining myocardial viability. Myocardial viability as determined by FDG-PET predicts improvement in regional function after revascularization with a pooled sensitivity of 88–93% and specificity of 58–73% [38–41]. In this case, the presence of hibernating myocardium in the RCA territory may suggest a benefit for revascularization of this territory, especially in the presence of reduced LVEF. On the other hand, the presence of a resting perfusion defect with preserved FDG uptake in the LAD territory, despite successful revascularization, could be due to inflammation in the recent post infarct period. It has been reported that PET performed up to 1 week in the post infarct period can overestimate the potential for recovery [41–44]. As well, in the days following successful revascularization, fixed perfusion defects may persist despite preserved viability.

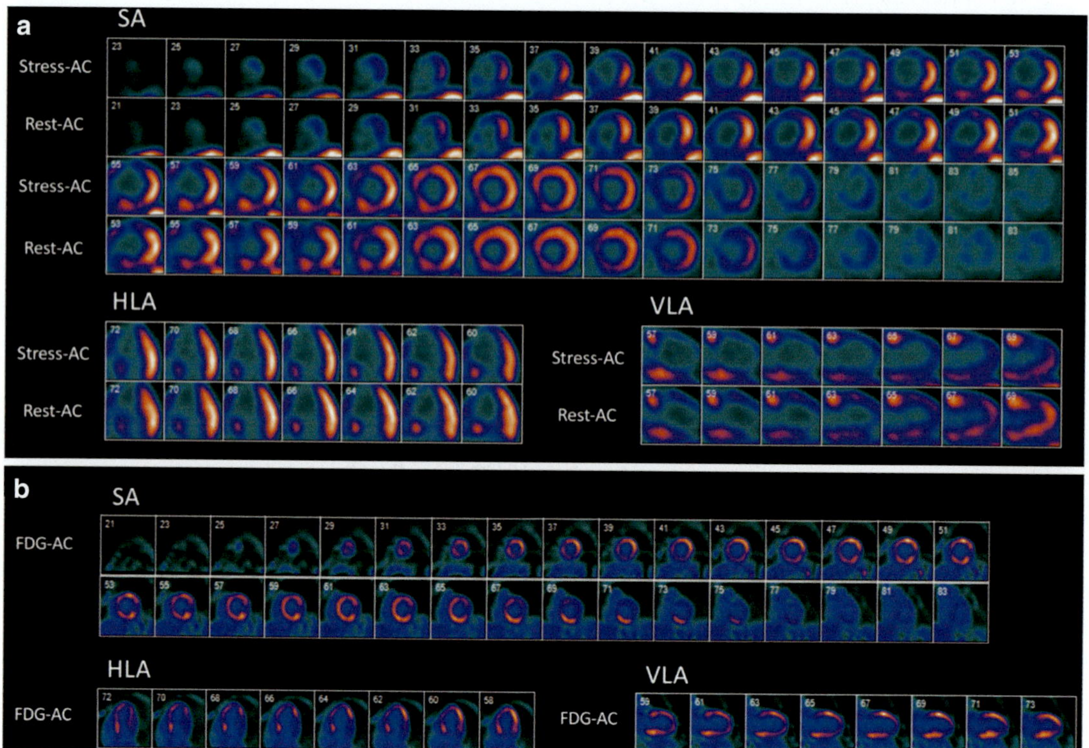

Fig. 24.11 PET Interpretation. Dipyridamole stress rubidium-82 positron emission tomography myocardial perfusion imaging (^{82}Rb PET-MPI) (**a**) was performed alongside an FDG-PET myocardial viability study (**b**). Imaging was performed 5 days post-infarct. A large and severe fixed perfusion defect was seen in the anterior wall with extension to anterolateral and septal territories. A moderate fixed perfusion defect was seen in the inferior wall. The lateral wall was free of perfusion defects. On FDG-PET, significant FDG uptake was seen within the majority of the anterior, septal, anterolateral, and inferior territories. The mismatched perfusion defect with preserved metabolism in the LAD territory could be related to inflammation or stunned myocardium in the setting of recent STEMI and revascularization. Viability within the myocardial territory supplied by the chronically diseased RCA was compatible with hibernating myocardium

Case 8

Initial Evaluation

An 85-year-old man, known for AF, ischemic cardiomyopathy and ICD implantation for secondary prevention, presented with fever and generalized malaise 5 weeks after undergoing generator replacement. No obvious signs of generator pocket infection were present. Blood cultures were positive for MSSA. TEE did not evidence any signs of lead infection (Fig. 24.12).

Follow-Up

On the basis of these findings, a diagnosis of CIED generator pocket infection (CIED-GPI) was made. A procedure to completely remove the ICD was performed. Microbiological analysis of

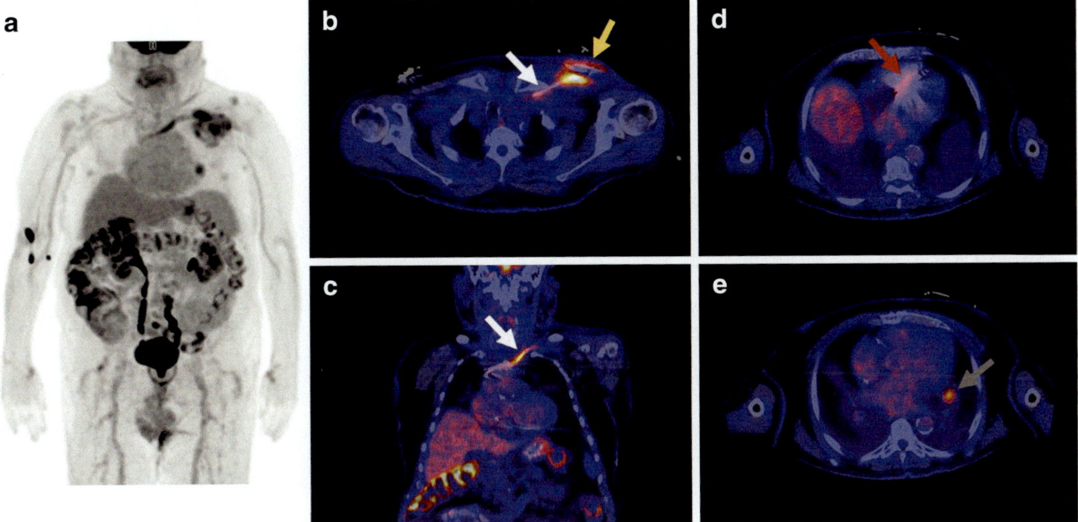

Fig. 24.12 PET Interpretation. Whole-body FDG-PET/ CT (**a**) was performed following a myocardial suppression protocol for further assessment of ICD infection. The patient had undergone 2 days of antibiotic treatment prior to imaging. Myocardial suppression was adequate. Intense and heterogeneous uptake was visualized posterior to the generator pocket (**b**, yellow arrow, $SUV_{max} = 7.9$), extending along the lead up to the origin of the superior vena cava (**b**, **c**, white arrows, $SUV_{max} = 5.1$). There was no evidence of infection at the level of the intracardiac lead (**d**, red arrow). A hypermetabolic pulmonary nodule near the left hilar region was incidentally found (**e**, gray arrow, $SUV_{max} = 4.5$). These findings are compatible with deep generator pocket infection and lead infection. Lung uptake could represent a septic embolus in this context but should be followed on imaging as malignancy cannot be entirely excluded

generator pocket and lead sample were both positive for MSSA.

Teaching Point

In this case, FDG-PET/CT accurately identified CIED-GPI with extension into the intravascular portion of the lead. FDG-PET/CT has the ability of being able to evaluate the presence of CIED infection, from the generator pocket up to the intracardiac leads [45]. The diagnostic accuracy of FDG-PET/CT in evaluating CIED-GPI is very high with a sensitivity of 96% and a specificity of 97% [26, 27, 45–47]. It can also detect GPI before obvious clinical signs such as purulent discharge are present [45].

Case 9

Initial Evaluation

A 55-year-old woman, known for type 2 diabetes mellitus and hypertension, presented with dyspnea and peripheral edema a month after experiencing an episode of profuse diaphoresis and weakness. Typical features of recent anterolateral STEMI were seen on ECG. TTE showed severe left ventricular dysfunction with a LVEF of 23%. Cardiac catheterization demonstrated chronic total occlusion of the proximal LAD. Both the RCA and circumflex artery had minimal/nonobstructive epicardial lesions. Revascularization was not performed and aggressive medical treatment was initiated instead (Fig. 24.13).

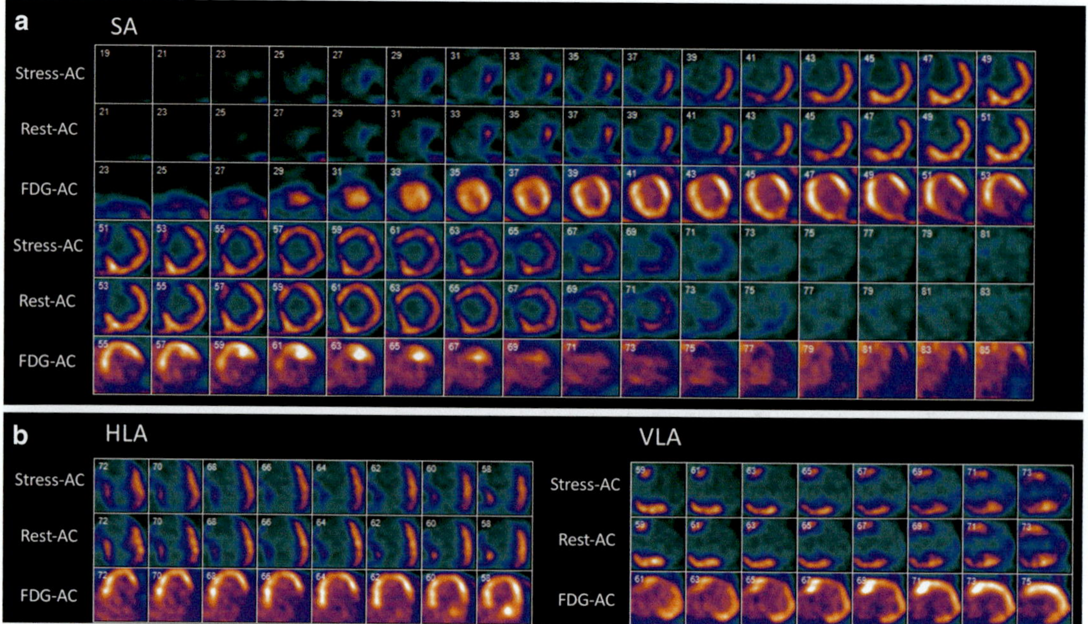

Fig. 24.13 PET Interpretation. Dipyridamole stress ^{82}Rb PET-MPI was performed alongside FDG-PET myocardial viability study (**a**, **b**) approximately 2 months post-infarct. An extensive and severe fixed perfusion defect was seen in the anterior, anteroseptal, septal and apical territories (**a**). On FDG-PET, FDG uptake was preserved within those territories (mismatched), compatible with the presence of hibernating myocardium (**b**). As such, the myocardial territory supplied by the LAD was deemed viable

Follow-Up

Despite optimization of medical therapy, the patient remained severely symptomatic. Six months later, the patient underwent successful revascularization following the placement of 3 DES within the LAD.

Teaching Point

In this case, significant improvement in left ventricular function should be expected during follow-up. Multiple studies have shown that the extent of perfusion–metabolic mismatch correlates linearly with the improvement of both LVEF and functional status following revascularization [48–50]. For instance, Di Carli et al. reported that patients with mismatches totaling ≥18% of myocardium achieved significantly higher functional status compared to those with minimal mismatch [48].

Case 10

Initial Evaluation

A 56 year-old man, known for hypertension and chronic obstructive pulmonary disease (COPD), presented with shortness of breath, chest pain and syncope. ECG was remarkable for sinus tachycardia, right axis deviation and T-wave inversions in leads V1, V2 and V3. TTE showed a dilated right ventricle with signs of pressure overload. CTPA showed multiple bilateral segmental and subsegmental pulmonary embolisms (PE) accompanied by a focal opacity of 11 mm within the right upper lobe (RUL) attributed to probable alveolar hemorrhage (Fig. 24.14).

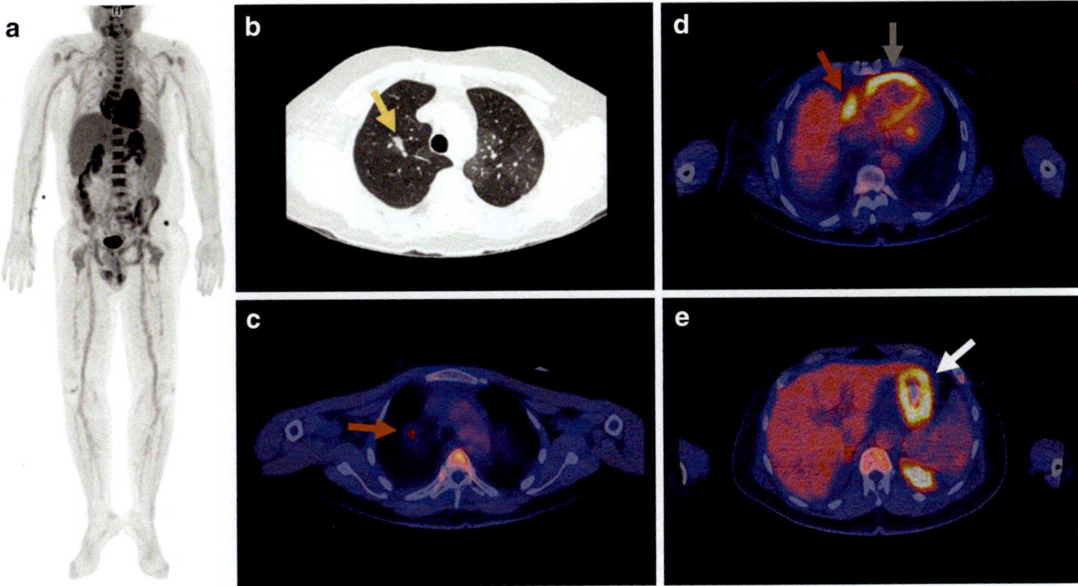

Fig. 24.14 PET 1 Interpretation. Whole-body FDG-PET/CT (**a**) was performed in order to exclude an underlying neoplastic process given the important extent of PE. The RUL opacity seen on CTPA (**b**, yellow arrow) was associated with slightly increased uptake (**c**, orange arrow, $SUV_{max} = 3.4$). Alveolar hemorrhage remained the most probable diagnosis. Diffuse increased uptake is seen within the right atrium (**d**, red arrow, $SUV_{max} = 6.2$) and right ventricle (**d**, gray arrow, $SUV_{max} = 7.5$), compatible with right heart strain (RHS). Isolated uptake in the posterolateral papillary muscle of the left ventricle is seen (**d**, green arrow, $SUV_{max} = 4.7$), a nonspecific finding. Diffuse increased uptake is visualized at the level of the stomach (**e**, white arrow), suggestive of gastritis. No clear underlying neoplastic process was evidenced

Follow-Up

Oral anticoagulation was initiated, with indeterminate duration of therapy. A follow-up TTE performed 4 months later showed improvement of the right ventricle dilation and pressure overload (Fig. 24.15).

Teaching Point

As FDG-PET/CT scans are often performed without contrast, a diagnosis of PE is mostly suggested by the presence of indirect signs [51]. The "rim sign" (slight FDG uptake around the area of subpleural consolidation) is strongly suggestive of pulmonary infarction which can be secondary to PE or tumoral arterial obstruction [51]. An additional secondary sign is the presence of increased FDG uptake within the right heart chambers, suggestive of RHS [52–54]. However, RHS is not specific to PE as there exists multiple causes of increased pulmonary arterial pressure [52]. In this case, intense uptake was seen within both the right atrium and right ventricle, while the left heart chambers were spared. Multiple patterns of RHS secondary to PE have been reported, including four-chamber increase in cardiac uptake, isolated right ventricular uptake, and moderate right atrial uptake with very subtle right ventricular uptake [52–54].

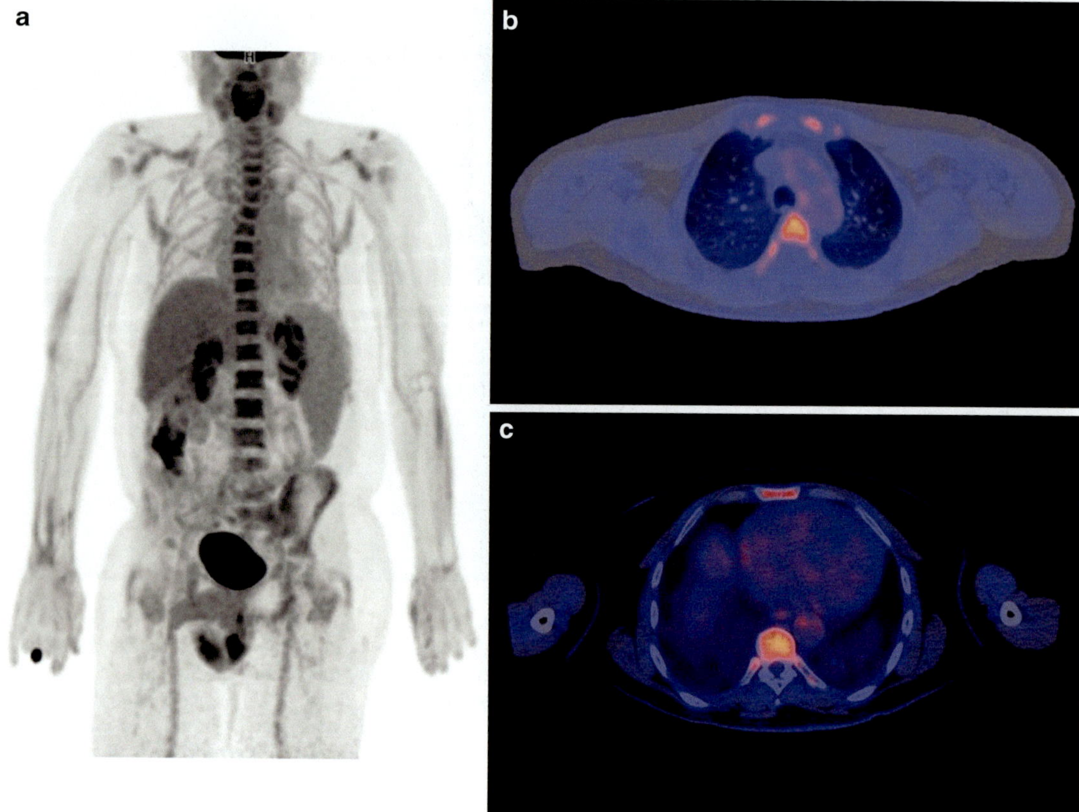

Fig. 24.15 PET 2 Interpretation. Follow-up whole-body FDG-PET/CT (**a**) performed 6 months following the initiation of anticoagulant therapy showed resolution of the hypermetabolic RUL opacity (**b**). Increased uptake was not seen within the right atrium and right ventricle (**c**), suggesting resolution of the RHS

Case 11

Initial Evaluation

A 59-year-old, known for hypertension, presented with frequent palpitations and a feeling of chest "heaviness." Physical examination revealed a systolic ejection murmur best heard in the left upper sternal border, which increased with inspiration. Holter monitoring showed frequent premature ventricular contractions. CTPA performed to exclude PE showed a multilobulated anterior mediastinal mass measuring 3.9 × 6.2 cm invading the main pulmonary artery (MPA). Proximal MPA thrombosis could not be excluded. On TTE, the mass was shown to cause severe supravalvular pulmonary stenosis (Fig. 24.16).

Follow-Up

As thrombosis within the MPA was strongly suspected, low molecular weight heparin was initiated in order to prevent embolism. The patient subsequently underwent surgery for mass resection with pulmonary homograft implantation. Histopathologic analysis confirmed the diagnosis of undifferentiated sarcoma with central necrosis. The surgeon described a mass originating from within the anterolateral wall of the MPA. The final diagnosis was pulmonary artery sarcoma (PAS).

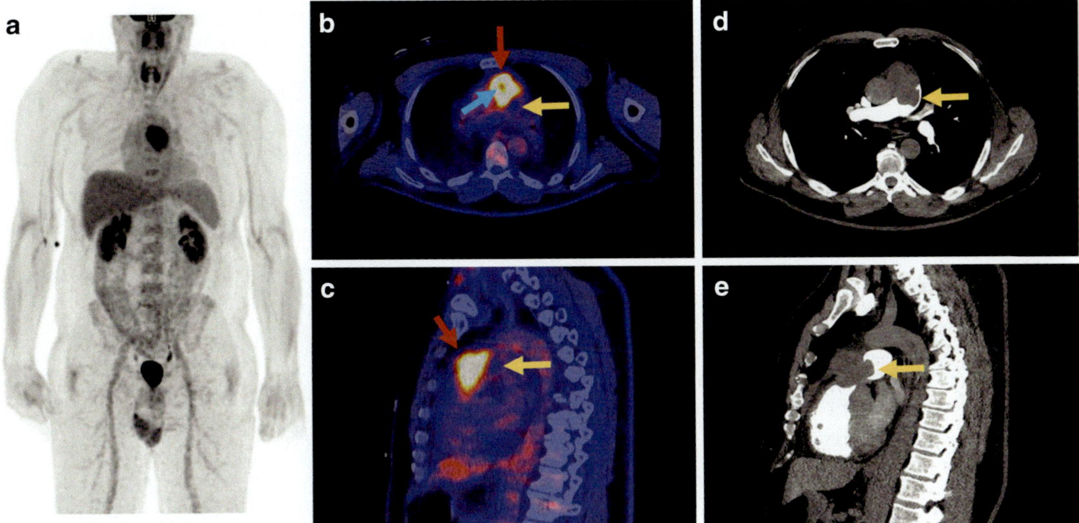

Fig. 24.16 PET Interpretation. Whole-body FDG-PET/CT (**a**) was performed to further characterize the mediastinal mass and assess the extent of disease involvement. Intense FDG uptake (SUV_{max} = 8.0) within the mass of interest was visualized (**b**, transaxial view, red arrow) (**c**, sagittal view, red arrow). Hypometabolism within the center of the mass was seen (**b**, blue arrow) consistent with central necrosis. A focus of hypometabolism was also noted posterolaterally to the mass (**b**, **c**, yellow arrows), corresponding to a filling defect on CTPA (**d**, **e**, yellow arrows) and most likely representing an associated thrombus in the MPA. No hypermetabolic pulmonary nodules or lymphadenopathy were seen. In the absence of other associated lesions and given the lesion uptake intensity, the diagnosis of a primary malignant tumor such as a sarcoma was strongly favored

Teaching Point

In this case, FDG-PET complemented CTPA findings by identifying thrombosis within the MPA. Indeed, hypometabolic filling defects in the pulmonary arteries can be suggestive of PE [51, 55]. Intense FDG uptake confirmed the malignant nature of the mass. PET also played an integral role in the preoperative workup by excluding metastases and another primary neoplastic lesion. The value of FDG-PET in the detection of soft tissue and bone sarcomas is well documented, with a reported pooled sensitivity of 91% and specificity of 85% [56]. However, as PAS are excessively rare, only a few cases have been reported in the literature [57–59]. Tueller et al. described a series of patients with PAS in which FDG-PET played an integral role in the preoperative workup, including tumor staging [59].

Case 12

Initial Evaluation

A 45-year-old man, known for COPD, hypertension, repaired ventricular septal defect (VSD) and thoracic aortic aneurysmal dilatation with dissection, underwent vascular graft replacement of both ascending and descending aorta, as well as endovascular stent placement within the transverse and descending aorta. At the time of presentation, he had not undergone any invasive procedure in the preceding 2 years. A week after being treated for pneumonia, the patient presented with fatigue, fever, chills and diaphoresis. Blood cultures were positive for *Haemophilus influenzae*. TTE showed a mobile structure within the left ventricle that was suggestive of either vegetation or surgical material from his VSD

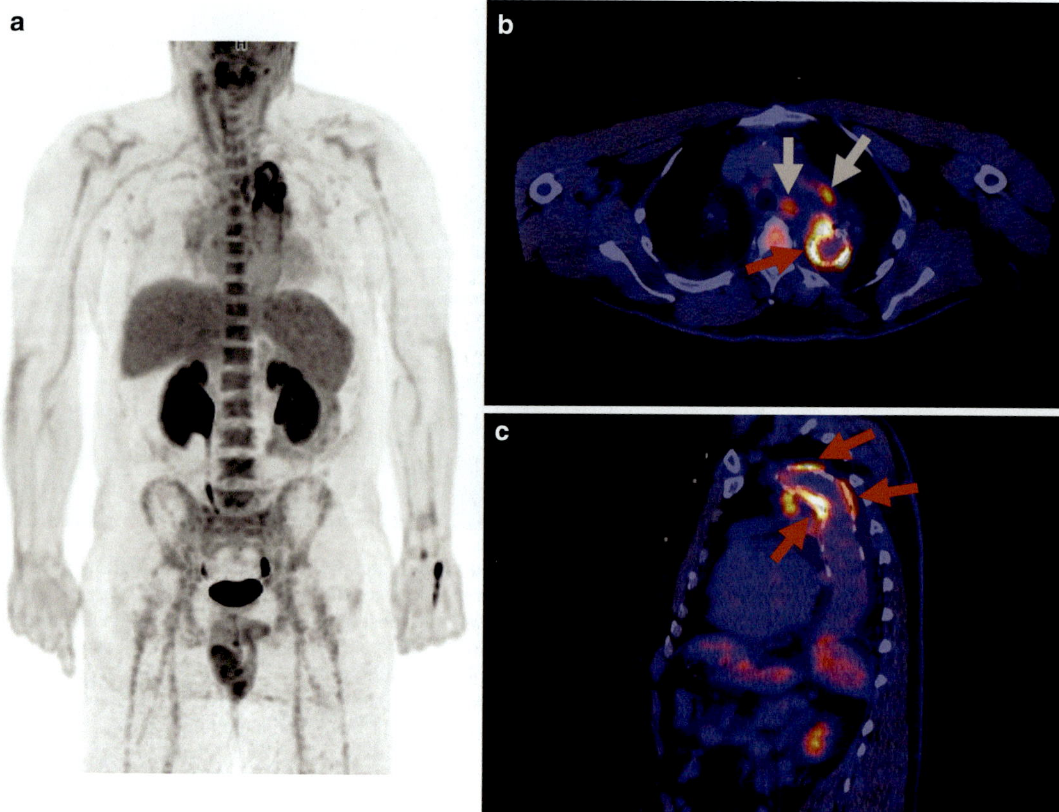

Fig. 24.17 PET 1 Interpretation. Whole-body FDG-PET/CT (**a**) was performed following a myocardial suppression protocol. Myocardial suppression was adequate. Intense and heterogeneous FDG uptake ($SUV_{max} = 10.7$) was seen within the endovascular stent (**b**, **c**, red arrows). The areas involved extended from the mid-portion of the aortic arch to the beginning of the descending thoracic aorta. Adjacent hypermetabolic lymph nodes were noted (**b**, gray arrows, $SUV_{max} = 5.3$). Valvular areas were free of abnormal FDG uptake. These findings were compatible with vascular graft infection (VGI)

repair. CTPA showed a very small perigraft air bubble at the level of the aortic arch (Fig. 24.17).

Follow-Up

As the patient had already undergone multiple cardiovascular interventions, conservative medical treatment with antibiotics was chosen (Fig. 24.18).

Teaching Point

In this case, FDG-PET was helpful in confirming the diagnosis of VGI in light of nondefinitive TTE and CTPA findings, as well as assessing treatment efficacy. VGI is associated with significant morbidity and mortality, with early and accurate diagnosis critical for optimal management. However, diagnosis remains challenging despite the introduction of standardized diagnostic criteria [60, 61]. FDG-

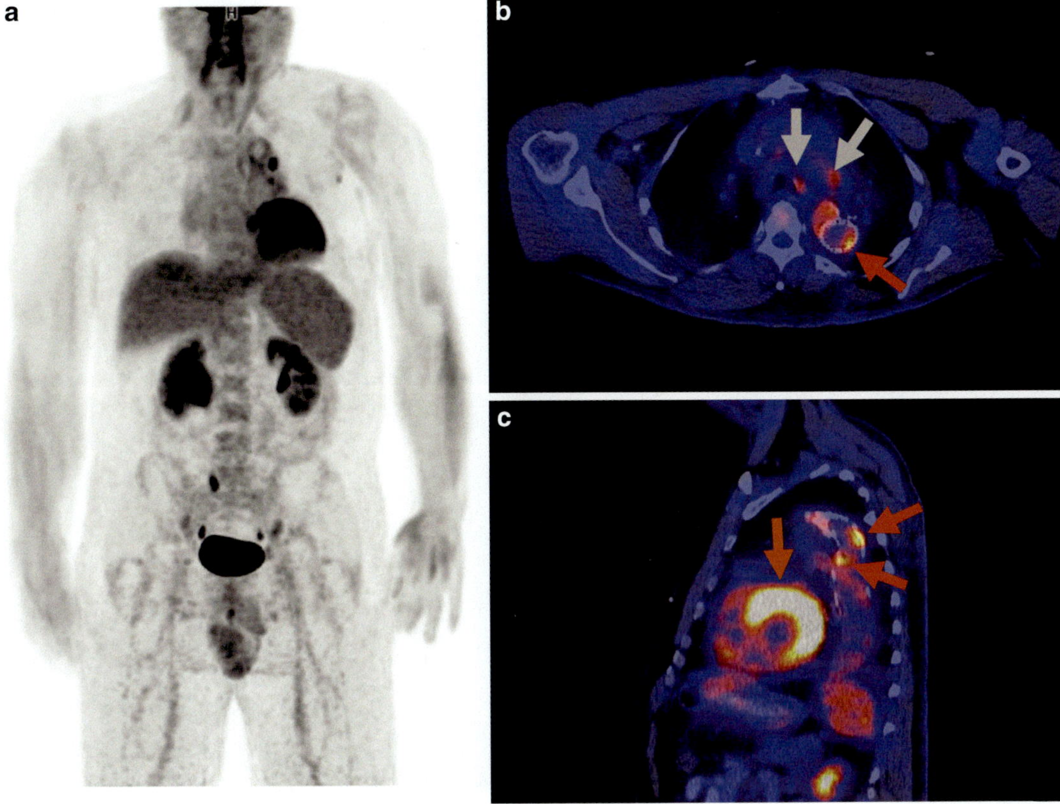

Fig. 24.18 PET 2 Interpretation. Follow-up whole-body FDG-PET/CT (**a**) was performed following 5 weeks of antibiotic treatment. A significant decrease in FDG uptake within the aortic endovascular stent was noted (**b, c**, red arrows), and SUV_{max} reduced from 10.7 to 6.5. Adjacent lymphadenopathy persisted on CT, but their associated uptake was significantly decreased (**b**, gray arrows, $SUV_{max} = 3.7$) from the prior study. Myocardial suppression was inadequate, with relatively intense uptake seen within both the left and right ventricular walls (**c**, orange arrow)

PET/CT is increasingly used for both imaging and treatment monitoring of VGI [7, 62–64]. Reported diagnostic accuracy is excellent, with pooled sensitivity of 93–96% and specificity of 74–80% [62, 65, 66]. Specificity of FDG-PET/CT in this setting is mainly hampered by postoperative inflammation, which can be observed several months following intervention. In the meta-analysis by Folmer et al., FDG-PET/CT was shown to outperform CT angiography (CTA) which had a reported pooled sensitivity of 67% and specificity of 63% [66].

Case 13

Initial Evaluation

A 40-year-old man noticed discharge at the level of his sternotomy wound. He underwent heart transplantation 2 years ago for restrictive cardiomyopathy. Discharge culture was positive for *Staphylococcus epidermidis*, but there was doubt about skin contamination. Blood cultures were negative (Fig. 24.19).

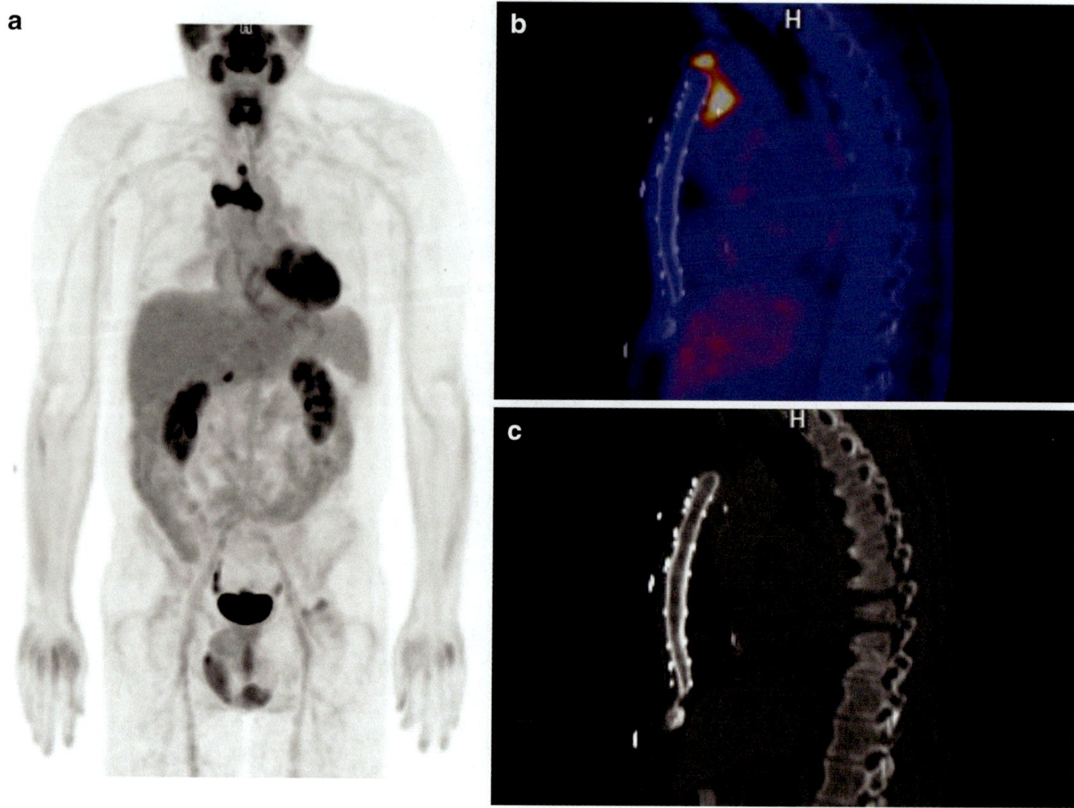

Fig. 24.19 PET 1 Interpretation. Whole-body FDG-PET/CT (**a**) was performed following a myocardial suppression protocol in order to evaluate for the presence of a sternal wound infection (SWI). Myocardial suppression was sub-optimal. A small retrosternal collection associated with intense FDG uptake (SUV$_{max}$ = 11.7) affecting the anterior portion of the superior mediastinum was seen (**b**), extending superiorly above the manubrium and reaching the skin. On the low-dose CT scan (LDCT), no bone abnormalities at the level of the sternum were noted (**c**). These findings were compatible with deep SWI (DSWI)

Follow-Up (1)

A diagnosis of DSWI with sternocutaneous fistula was made. A 3 week course of antibiotic treatment was initiated. Despite initial improvement, suprasternal discharge relapsed 3 months later (Fig. 24.20).

Follow-Up (2)

In light of the FDG-PET/CT results compatible with progression of the infectious process, a second course of antibiotic treatment was initiated alongside surgical debridement. Clinical improvement occurred rapidly and was sustained (Fig. 24.21).

Follow-Up (3)

Residual FDG uptake was deemed secondary to a chronic quiescent infection. As the patient was clinically stable and no discharge was apparent, further treatment was not pursued.

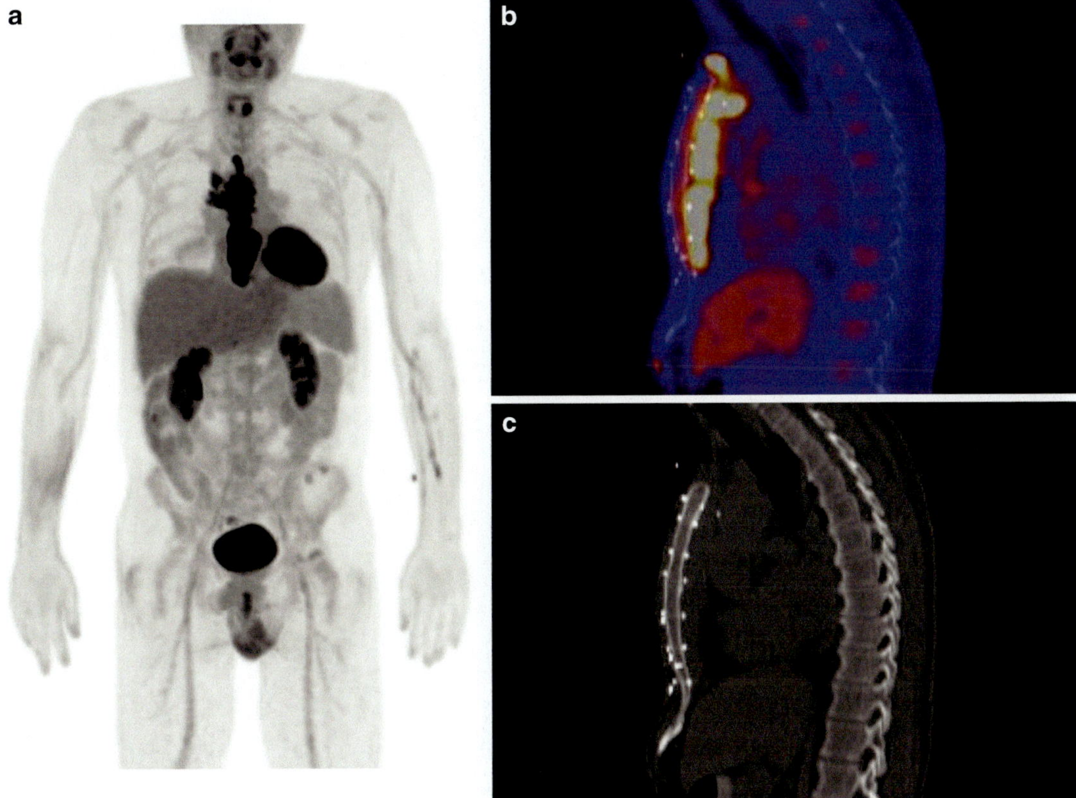

Fig. 24.20 PET 2 Interpretation. A second whole-body FDG-PET/CT (**a**) was performed. Myocardial suppression failed despite adherence to the preparation protocol. Marked progression of the retrosternal collection was noted, now extending from the manubrium to the xiphoid process. The FDG uptake intensity slightly increased from an SUV_{max} value of 11.7 to 13.6 (**b**). Hypermetabolic lymph nodes were noted in the anterior mediastinum. Again, no obvious bone abnormalities were seen on LDCT (**c**)

Teaching Point

In this case, FDG-PET was helpful in confirming diagnosis of DSWI, assessing its extent, and monitoring treatment efficacy. SWIs represent a rare but dangerous complication following cardiac surgery [67, 68]. Management depends on the depth of the infection [67]. CT is usually the initial imaging modality employed to evaluate SWI [68]. Its reported sensitivity is very high, but its specificity is hampered by postsurgical changes which can be indistinguishable from infection. Although literature on FDG-PET assessment of SWI is limited, published case reports and retrospective studies suggest its utility in this setting [69–71]. Hariri et al. reported an excellent diagnostic accuracy of 94%, with a sensitivity of 91% and a specificity of 97%, with qualitative analysis employing uptake patterns (diffuse low-grade, diffuse high-grade, focal, sternal wire, soft-tissue extension) outperforming quantitative analysis [69].

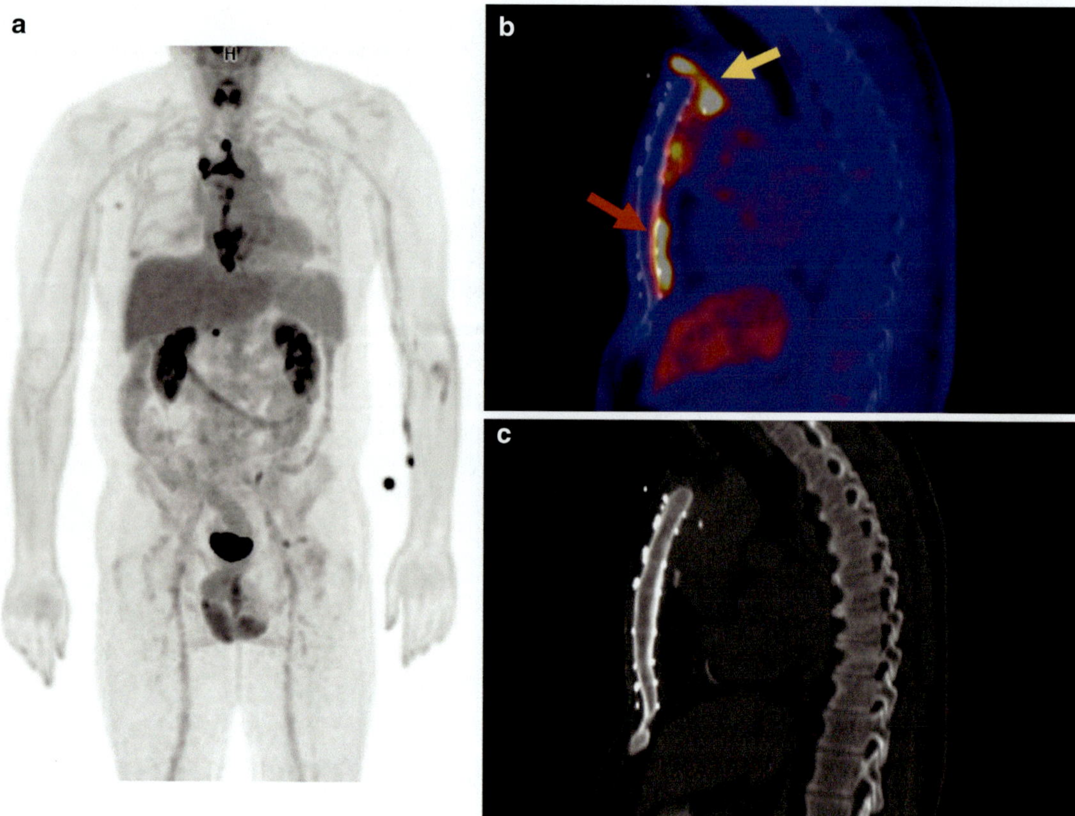

Fig. 24.21 PET 3 Interpretation. Follow-up whole-body FDG-PET/CT (**a**) was performed a year later. Overall, the extent of the retrosternal hypermetabolic activity regressed significantly (**b**); however, two residual foci of FDG uptake persisted, one involving the mediastinum anterior to the aortic arch with extension to the skin above the manubrium (**b**, yellow arrow) and the other involving the lower portion of the retrosternal region (**b**, red arrow). FDG uptake intensity did not vary significantly ($SUV_{max} = 14.5$). No musculoskeletal abnormalities were noted on LDCT (**c**)

Case 14

Initial Evaluation

A 61-year-old woman, known for liver hemangioma and colorectal polyps, presented with palpitations and fatigue. Blood cultures were negative. CTPA showed a nodular lesion with lobulated contours attached to the leaflets of the pulmonary valve. TEE showed a lobulated mass of 18 × 10 mm alongside the anterior wall of the MPA superior to the pulmonary valve accompanied by a filament-like structure of 3 × 12 mm attached to the pulmonary valve. Suspected diagnoses included marantic endocarditis, thrombosis at the level of the pulmonary valve, and a neoplastic process (Fig. 24.22).

Follow-Up

The patient underwent surgical resection of the mass. Histopathologic analysis confirmed the diagnosis of fibroelastoma. Follow-up TTE showed no residual mass.

Teaching Point

Multiple studies have suggested FDG-PET's utility in distinguishing malignant from benign cardiac lesions, primarily using semiquantitative analysis [16]. In this case, the absence of significant FDG uptake within the lesion was compatible with a benign process. Although papillary fibroelastomas represent the second most common pri-

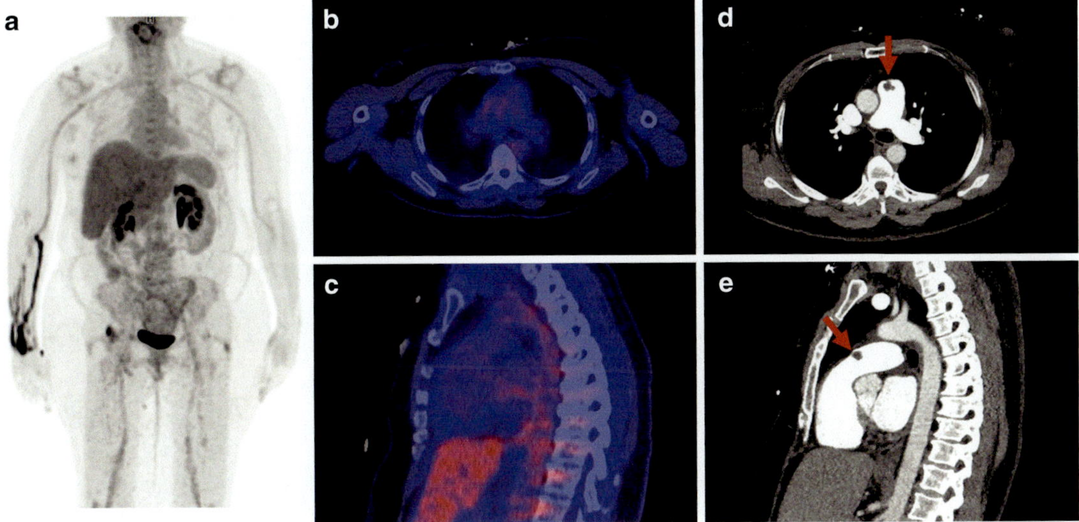

Fig. 24.22 PET Interpretation. Whole-body FDG-PET/CT (**a**) was performed following a myocardial suppression protocol. Myocardial suppression was excellent. No abnormal uptake was seen at the level of the myocardium, valvular areas (including the pulmonary valve) and the MPA (**b**, transaxial view) (**c**, sagittal view), suggestive of a benign etiology. There were no hypermetabolic lesions on whole-body FDG-PET/CT images. The lesion seen on CTPA is shown in images (**d**) (transaxial view, red arrow) and (**e**) (sagittal view, red arrow)

mary cardiac tumor in adults, reports of associated FDG-PET findings are very scarce [72, 73]. Nensa et al. reported the case of a patient with aortic valve fibroelastoma associated with low FDG uptake (SUV_{max} = 2.1) [72]. Similarly, Ibrahim et al. reported the case of a pulmonary valve fibroelastoma without associated focal uptake [74].

Case 15

Initial Evaluation

A 57-year-old man, with no relevant medical history, presented with shortness of breath and generalized weakness. Physical exam only revealed bradycardia. High-sensitivity cardiac troponin T (hs-cTnT) levels were normal. ECG showed third degree (complete) atrioventricular (AV) block. A chest radiograph was normal. TTE was normal, with a reported LVEF of 65%. As the patient was relatively young with a seemingly unexplained AV block, cardiac sarcoidosis (CS) was suspected (Fig. 24.23).

Follow-Up (1)

The patient underwent dual chamber permanent pacemaker implantation as well as endobronchial ultrasound guided biopsy of the hilar lymph nodes. Histopathologic analysis showed the presence of noncaseating granulomas, compatible with a diagnosis of sarcoidosis. As such, the patient was diagnosed with CS according to both the Heart and Rhythm Society (HRS) and Japan Circulation Society (JCS) proposed diagnostic criteria [82, 83]. Oral prednisone treatment was initiated at a dose of 60 mg per day (Fig. 24.24).

Follow-Up (2)

Tapering of prednisone was pursued. Pacemaker interrogation revealed that ventricular pacing dropped from 100% to <1%, suggesting improvement of complete heart block.

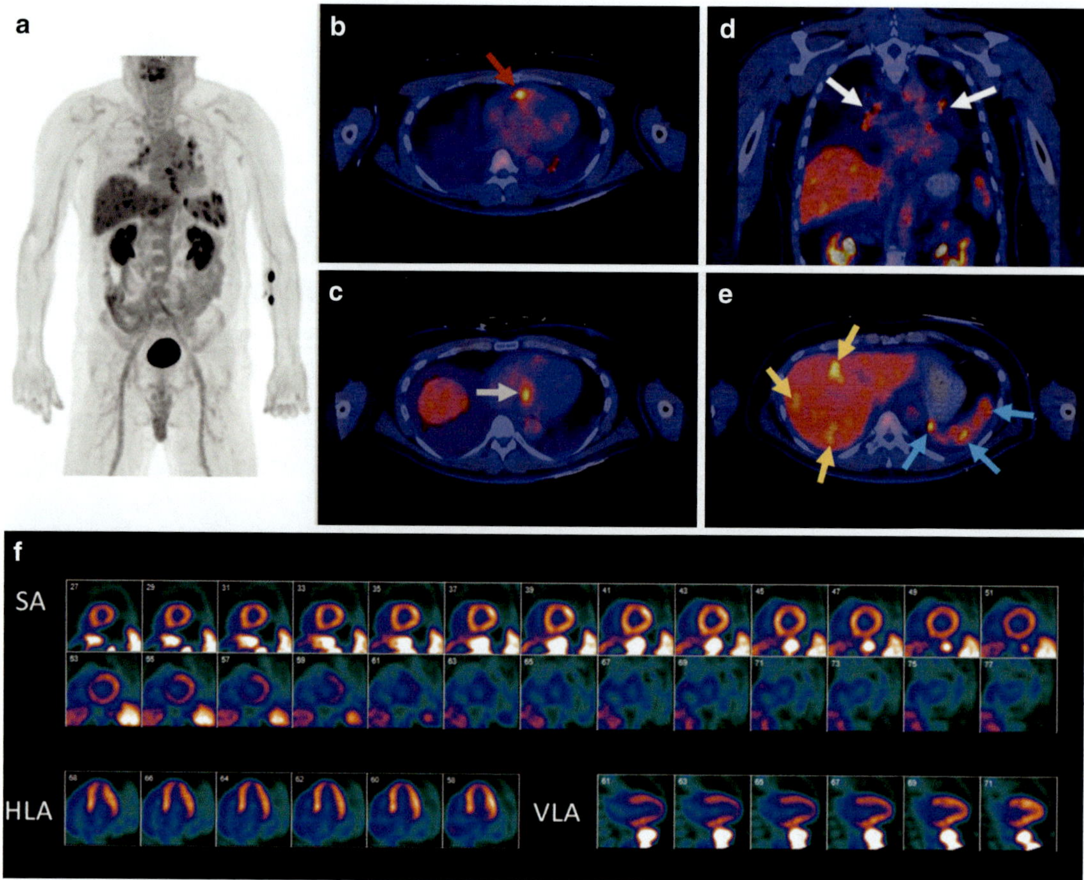

Fig. 24.23 PET 1 Interpretation. Whole-body FDG-PET/CT was performed following a myocardial suppression protocol consisting of low-carbohydrate diet, 12 h fasting, and intravenous heparin in order to exclude cardiac sarcoidosis (**a**). Myocardial suppression was excellent. Focal myocardial uptake was visualized at the level of the right ventricle free wall (**b**, red arrow, $SUV_{max} = 5.3$) and the basal inferoseptal wall (**c**, gray arrow, $SUV_{max} = 5.2$). Hypermetabolic bilateral hilar lymphadenopathy was seen (**d**, white arrows, $SUV_{max} = 4.8$). No other abnormal uptake was noted at the thoracic level. Multiple hypermetabolic foci were visualized within the liver (**e**, yellow arrows, $SUV_{max} = 5.5$) and spleen (**e**, blue arrows, $SUV_{max} = 5.4$). Rest [82]Rb PET-MPI performed concomitantly showed homogeneous perfusion throughout the left ventricle (**f**). In light of PET findings, sarcoidosis with hilar, myocardial, splenic and hepatic involvement was strongly suspected, although a lymphoproliferative disorder was not completely excluded

Teaching Point

In this case, FDG-PET/CT was crucial for the initial diagnosis of CS, identifying extra-cardiac involvement, guiding biopsy, and monitoring treatment efficacy. As focal FDG uptake was present in the absence of perfusion defects, early-stage CS was most likely [75]. FDG-PET also showed good anatomic correlation between the suspected cause of the ECG abnormality (i.e., involvement of the bundle of His in the basal interventricular septum) and the location of FDG uptake. As reported by Manabe et al., interventricular septum FDG uptake is associated with AV block [76]. Multiple studies have shown FDG-PET to be an accurate and useful imaging modality in the evaluation of CS [77]. As such, the two main consensus guidelines to propose diagnostic criteria for CS, the 2014 HRS expert consensus statement and the 2016 JCS guidelines for the diagnosis and treatment of cardiac sarcoidosis, include PET imaging [78–79].

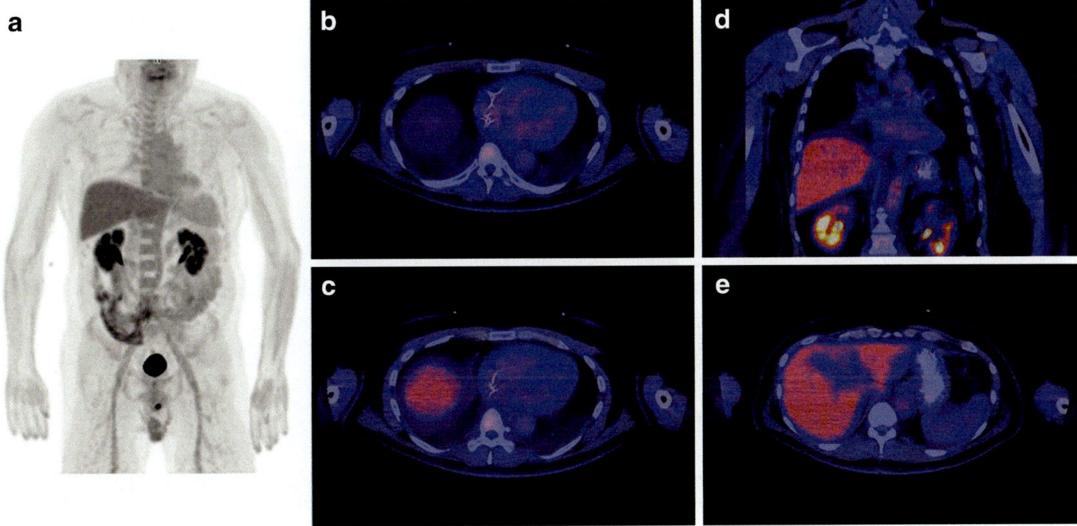

Fig. 24.24 PET 2 Interpretation. A second whole-body FDG-PET/CT (**a**) was performed 3 months following initiation of corticosteroids. Prednisone dosage had been tapered down to 40 mg. Myocardial suppression was again excellent. There was complete resolution of the pre- viously seen FDG uptake at the level of the myocardium (**b**) (**c**), hila (**d**), liver (**e**), and spleen (**e**). Rest ^{82}Rb PET-MPI still showed no perfusion defect throughout the left ventricle (not shown)

Moreover, multiple suggested treatment algorithms for CS include PET imaging to guide immunosuppressive therapy [78, 80–85].

Case 16

Initial Evaluation

A 72-year-old woman, known for hypertension, type 2 diabetes mellitus and rheumatoid arthritis, presented to the ER with sinus tachycardia, fever, and lower back pain. Blood cultures were positive for MSSA. TEE showed the presence of two vegetations (9 mm and 5 mm) at the level of the mitral valve (Fig. 24.25).

Follow-Up

A coronary CT angiogram was subsequently performed. Although assessment was limited due to the presence of diffuse calcifications, occlusion of the middle RCA was seen, corresponding to the zone of hypermetabolism visualized on the FDG-PET. A diagnosis of an RCA mycotic aneurysm complicated by thrombosis was suggested, but the presence of an abscess could not be excluded. The patient underwent standard medical treatment with antibiotics.

Teaching Point

Although FDG-PET's role in imaging PVE is well established, the literature for native valve infective endocarditis (NVE) is limited but suggests a lower sensitivity than for PVE [5, 6]. Adequate myocardial suppression, initiation of antibiotic treatment prior to imaging, and vegetation size all represent important factors to consider when evaluating NVE on FDG-PET [23, 86]. In this case, FDG-PET helped confirm the presence of spondylodiscitis while also identifying the presence of unsuspected RCA aneurysm. Antibiotic treatment prior to PET imaging and smaller vegetation size on TEE may have contributed to the lower FDG uptake observed within the mitral valve area.

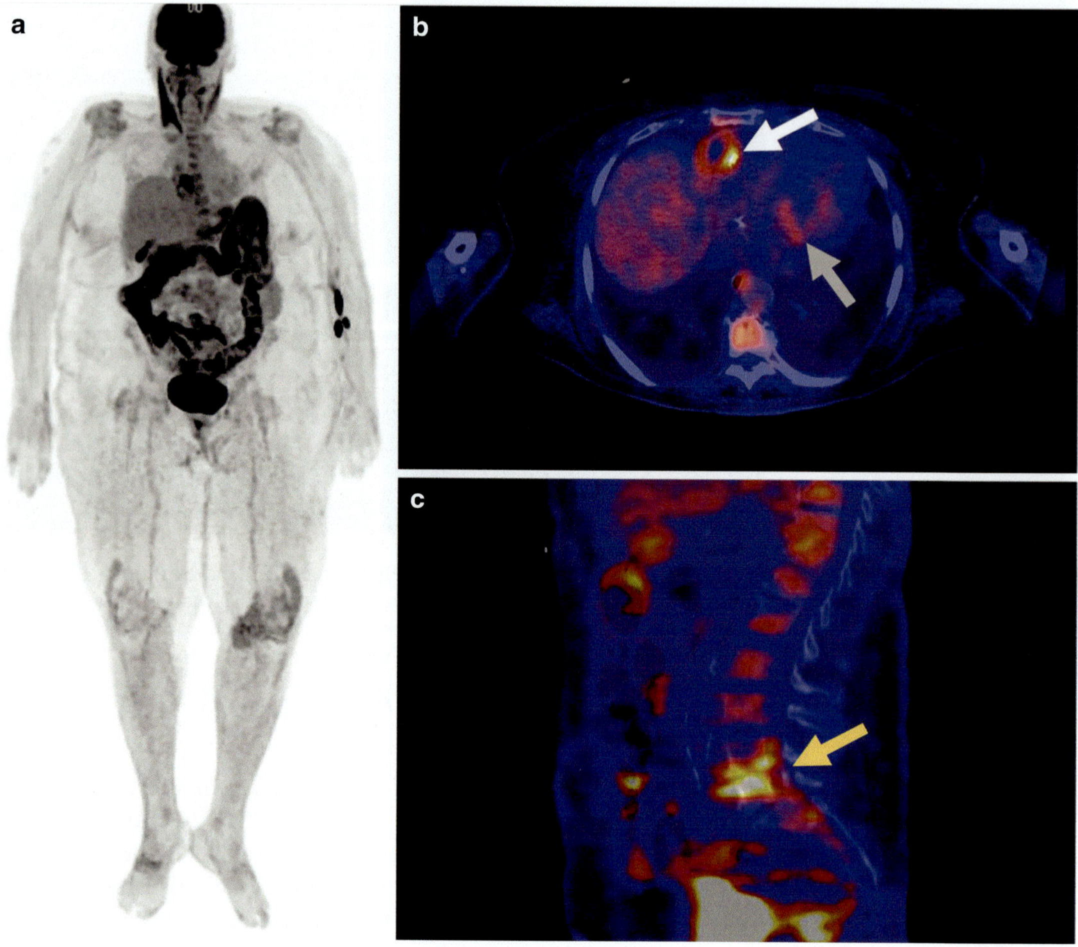

Fig. 24.25 PET Interpretation. Whole-body FDG-PET/ CT (**a**) was performed following a myocardial suppression protocol to further characterize TEE findings and assess for possible spondylodiscitis. At the time of imaging, the patient had undergone 5 days of antibiotic treatment. Myocardial suppression was excellent. Faint FDG uptake was seen within the mitral valve area (**b**, gray arrow). Increased uptake was also seen within a hypodensity at the level of the atrioventricular sulcus (**b**, white arrow, $SUV_{max} = 9.2$). The differential diagnosis included a RCA mycotic aneurysm or an abscess. Findings consistent with spondylodiscitis at the level of the L4-L5 vertebral bodies was seen (**c**, yellow arrow, $SUV_{max} = 9.7$)

Case 17

Initial Evaluation

A 73-year-old woman originally from Cambodia presented with shortness of breath and coughing. She had no relevant medical history. A CTPA performed to exclude PE instead revealed pericardial and pleural effusions, in addition to mediastinal and hilar lymphadenopathy which were deemed reactive. An organized fibrous pericardial effusion was visualized on TTE. Differential considerations included a chronic infectious process as well as a neoplastic origin. Early microbiological and histopathological analysis of both pleural and pericardial effusions were inconclusive (Fig. 24.26).

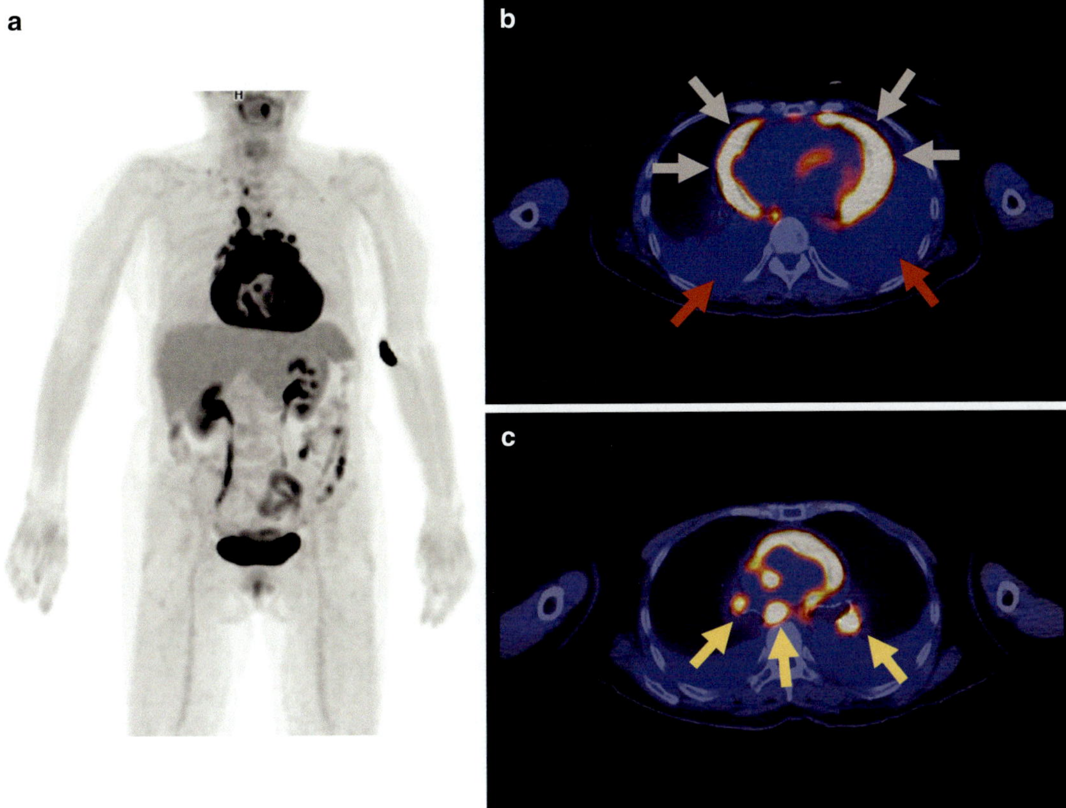

Fig. 24.26 PET Interpretation. Whole-body FDG-PET/CT (**a**) was performed in order to exclude a neoplastic process. Circumferential pericardial effusion associated with high intensity uptake (SUV_{max} = 14.4) was seen (**b**, gray arrows). The bilateral pleural effusions previously noted on CTPA were not associated with increased uptake (**b**, red arrows). Markedly hypermetabolic mediastinal and hilar lymphadenopathy (up to an SUV_{max} of 11.4) were present (**c**, yellow arrows). No other abnormalities were noted. On the basis of these findings, the differential diagnosis remained broad, and included lymphoproliferative and infectious processes

Follow-Up

Pericardial biopsy culture subsequently showed the presence of *Mycobacterium tuberculosis*, confirming the diagnosis of tuberculous pericarditis, and appropriate medical treatment was initiated.

Teaching Point

The diagnosis of tuberculous pericarditis can be challenging as the diagnostic yield of both pericardial biopsy and AFB staining are poor [87, 88]. Lung and lymph node involvement are common in the presence of tuberculous pericarditis and can be accurately identified by FDG-PET/CT [21, 89–92]. Moreover, FDG uptake intensity in both the pericardium and lymph nodes is typically much higher in tuberculous pericarditis when compared to idiopathic pericarditis [21, 89–91, 93–95]. The number of hypermetabolic lymph nodes was also shown to be higher in patients with tuberculous pericarditis [89]. FDG-PET/CT has also been reported to be useful in assessing treatment response [90].

References

1. Husmann L, Huellner MW, Ledergerber B, Eberhard N, Kaelin MB, Anagnostopoulos A, et al. Diagnostic accuracy of PET/CT and contrast enhanced CT in patients with suspected infected aortic aneurysms. Eur J Vasc Endovasc Surg. 2020;59(6):972–81.
2. Macedo TA, Stanson AW, Oderich GS, Johnson CM, Panneton JM, Tie ML. Infected aortic aneurysms: imaging findings. Radiology. 2004;231(1):250–7.
3. Murakami M, Morikage N, Samura M, Yamashita O, Suehiro K, Hamano K. Fluorine-18-fluorodeoxyglucose positron emission tomography–computed tomography for diagnosis of infected aortic aneurysms. Ann Vasc Surg. 2014;28(3):575–8.
4. Murphy DJ, Keraliya AR, Agrawal MD, Aghayev A, Steigner ML. Cross-sectional imaging of aortic infections. Insights Imaging. 2016;7(6):801–18.
5. Habib G, Lancellotti P, Antunes MJ, Bongiorni MG, Casalta J-P, Del Zotti F, et al. 2015 ESC guidelines for the management of infective endocarditis: the task force for the management of infective Endocarditis of the European Society of Cardiology (ESC). Endorsed by: European Association for Cardio-Thoracic Surgery (EACTS), the European Association of Nuclear Medicine (EANM). Eur Heart J. 2015;36(44):3075–128.
6. Saby L, Laas O, Habib G, Cammilleri S, Mancini J, Tessonnier L, et al. Positron emission tomography/computed tomography for diagnosis of prosthetic valve endocarditis: increased valvular 18F-fluorodeoxyglucose uptake as a novel major criterion. J Am Coll Cardiol. 2013;61(23):2374–82.
7. Erba PA, Sollini M, Lazzeri E, Mariani G. FDG-PET in cardiac infections. Semin Nucl Med. 2013;43(5):377–95.
8. Salaun E, Sportouch L, Barral P-A, Hubert S, Lavoute C, Casalta A-C, et al. Diagnosis of infective endocarditis after TAVR: value of a multimodality imaging approach. JACC Cardiovasc Imaging. 2018;11(1):143–6.
9. Swart LE, Scholtens AM, Liesting C, van Mieghem NMDA, Krestin GP, Roos-Hesselink JW, et al. Serial 18F-fluorodeoxyglucose positron emission tomography/CT angiography in transcatheter-implanted aortic valve endocarditis. Eur Heart J. 2016;37(39):3059.
10. Roque A, Pizzi MN. 18F-FDG PET/CT and cardiac CTA in transcatheter aortic valve implanted endocarditis: still at the beginning of a long road. J Nucl Cardiol. 2021;28(5):2083–5.
11. Wahadat AR, Tanis W, Swart LE, Scholtens A, Krestin GP, van Mieghem NMDA, et al. Added value of 18F-FDG-PET/CT and cardiac CTA in suspected transcatheter aortic valve endocarditis. J Nucl Cardiol. 2021;28(5):2072–82.
12. Randhawa K, Ganeshan A, Hoey ETD. Magnetic resonance imaging of cardiac tumors: part 2, malignant tumors and tumor-like conditions. Curr Probl Diagn Radiol. 2011;40(4):169–79.
13. Saponara M, Ambrosini V, Nannini M, Gatto L, Astolfi A, Urbini M, et al. 18F-FDG-PET/CT imaging in cardiac tumors: illustrative clinical cases and review of the literature. Ther Adv Med Oncol. 2018;10:1758835918793569.
14. Silvestri F, Bussani R, Pavletic N, Mannone T. Metastases of the heart and pericardium. G Ital Cardiol. 1997;27(12):1252–5.
15. Hoffmann U, Globits S, Schima W, Loewe C, Puig S, Oberhuber G, et al. Usefulness of magnetic resonance imaging of cardiac and paracardiac masses. Am J Cardiol. 2003;92(7):890–5.
16. Martineau P, Dilsizian V, Pelletier-Galarneau M. Incremental value of FDG-PET in the evaluation of cardiac masses. Curr Cardiol Rep. 2021;23(7):78.
17. Søgaard KK, Farkas DK, Ehrenstein V, Bhaskaran K, Bøtker HE, Sørensen HT. Pericarditis as a marker of occult cancer and a prognostic factor for cancer mortality. Circulation. 2017;136(11):996–1006.
18. Burazor I, Imazio M, Markel G, Adler Y. Malignant pericardial effusion. Cardiology. 2013;124(4):224–32.
19. Quint LE. Thoracic complications and emergencies in oncologic patients. Cancer Imaging. 2009;9(Special issue A):S75–82.
20. Mainzer G, Zaidman I, Hatib I, Lorber A. Intrapericardial steroid treatment for recurrent pericardial effusion in a patient with acute lymphoblastic leukaemia. Hematol Oncol. 2011;29(4):220–1.
21. Kim M-S, Kim E-K, Choi JY, Oh JK, Chang S-A. Clinical utility of [18F]FDG-PET/CT in pericardial disease. Curr Cardiol Rep. 2019;21(9):107.
22. Chang S-A, Choi JY, Kim EK, Hyun SH, Jang SY, Choi J-O, et al. [18F]Fluorodeoxyglucose PET/CT predicts response to steroid therapy in constrictive pericarditis. J Am Coll Cardiol. 2017;69(6):750–2.
23. Pelletier-Galarneau M, Abikhzer G, Harel F, Dilsizian V. Detection of native and prosthetic valve endocarditis: incremental attributes of functional FDG PET/CT over morphologic imaging. Curr Cardiol Rep. 2020;22(9):93.
24. Li JS, Sexton DJ, Mick N, Nettles R, Fowler VG, Ryan T, et al. Proposed modifications to the duke criteria for the diagnosis of infective endocarditis. Clin Infect Dis. 2000;30(4):633–8.
25. Habib G, Hoen B, Tornos P, Thuny F, Prendergast B, Vilacosta I, et al. Guidelines on the prevention, diagnosis, and treatment of infective endocarditis (new version 2009): the task force on the prevention, diagnosis, and treatment of infective endocarditis of the European Society of Cardiology (ESC). Endorsed by the European Society of Clinical Microbiology and Infectious Diseases (ESCMID) and the International Society of Chemotherapy (ISC) for infection and cancer. Eur Heart J. 2009;30(19):2369–413.
26. Bensimhon L, Lavergne T, Hugonnet F, Mainardi J-L, Latremouille C, Maunoury C, et al. Whole body [18F]fluorodeoxyglucose positron emission tomography imaging for the diagnosis of pacemaker or implantable cardioverter defibrillator infection: a

preliminary prospective study. Clin Microbiol Infect. 2011;17(6):836–44.

27. Ploux S, Riviere A, Amraoui S, Whinnett Z, Barandon L, Lafitte S, et al. Positron emission tomography in patients with suspected pacing system infections may play a critical role in difficult cases. Heart Rhythm. 2011;8(9):1478–81.

28. Pizzi MN, Roque A, Fernández-Hidalgo N, Cuéllar-Calabria H, Ferreira-González I, Gonzàlez-Alujas MT, et al. Improving the diagnosis of infective endocarditis in prosthetic valves and intracardiac devices with 18F-Fluordeoxyglucose positron emission tomography/computed tomography angiography. Circulation. 2015;132(12):1113–26.

29. Bonfiglioli R, Nanni C, Morigi JJ, Graziosi M, Trapani F, Bartoletti M, et al. 18F-FDG PET/CT diagnosis of unexpected extracardiac septic embolisms in patients with suspected cardiac endocarditis. Eur J Nucl Med Mol Imaging. 2013;40(8):1190–6.

30. Stamatis P. Giant cell arteritis versus takayasu arteritis: an update. Mediterr J Rheumatol. 2020;31(2):174–82.

31. Pelletier-Galarneau M, Ruddy TD. Molecular imaging of coronary inflammation. Trends Cardiovasc Med. 2019;29(4):191–7.

32. Cohen Tervaert JW. Cardiovascular disease due to accelerated atherosclerosis in systemic vasculitides. Best Pract Res Clin Rheumatol. 2013;27(1):33–44.

33. Matthew J. Koster, Kenneth J. Warrington. Vasculitis of the coronary arteries. Am Coll Cardiol. 2022. https://www.acc.org/latest-in-cardiology/articles/2019/03/13/06/50/http%3a%2f%2fwww.acc.org%2flatest-in-cardiology%2farticles%2f2019%2f03%2f13%2f06%2f50%2fvasculitis-of-the-coronary-arteries.

34. Mukhtyar C, Brogan P, Luqmani R. Cardiovascular involvement in primary systemic vasculitis. Best Pract Res Clin Rheumatol. 2009;23(3):419–28.

35. Pelletier-Galarneau M, Ruddy TD. PET/CT for diagnosis and management of large-vessel vasculitis. Curr Cardiol Rep. 2019;21(5):34.

36. Lensen KDF, Comans EFI, Voskuyl AE, van der Laken CJ, Brouwer E, Zwijnenburg AT, et al. Large-vessel vasculitis: interobserver agreement and diagnostic accuracy of 18F-FDG-PET/CT. Biomed Res Int. 2015;2015:e914692.

37. de Boysson H, et al. Repetitive 18F-FDG-PET/CT in patients with large-vessel giant-cell arteritis and controlled disease. Eur J Intern Med. 2022;46:66–70. https://www.ejinme.com/article/S0953-6205(17)30315-1/fulltext.

38. Bax JJ, Cornel JH, Visser FC, Fioretti PM, van Lingen A, Huitink JM, et al. Comparison of fluorine-18-FDG with rest-redistribution thallium-201 SPECT to delineate viable myocardium and predict functional recovery after revascularization. J Nucl Med. 1998;39(9):1481–6.

39. Bax JJ, Patton JA, Poldermans D, Elhendy A, Sandler MP. 18-Fluorodeoxyglucose imaging with positron emission tomography and single photon emission computed tomography: cardiac applications. Semin Nucl Med. 2000;30(4):281–98.

40. Schinkel AFL, Poldermans D, Elhendy A, Bax JJ. Assessment of myocardial viability in patients with heart failure. J Nucl Med. 2007;48(7):1135–46.

41. Grandin C, Wijns W, Melin JA, Bol A, Robert AR, Heyndrickx GR, et al. Delineation of myocardial viability with PET. J Nucl Med. 1995;36(9):1543–52.

42. Gropler RJ, Siegel BA, Sampathkumaran K, Pérez JE, Sobel BE, Bergmann SR, et al. Dependence of recovery of contractile function on maintenance of oxidative metabolism after myocardial infarction. J Am Coll Cardiol. 1992;19(5):989–97.

43. Schwaiger M, Brunken R, Grover-McKay M, Krivokapich J, Child J, Tillisch JH, et al. Regional myocardial metabolism in patients with acute myocardial infarction assessed by positron emission tomography. J Am Coll Cardiol. 1986;8(4):800–8.

44. Habib G, Erba PA, Iung B, Donal E, Cosyns B, Laroche C, et al. Clinical presentation, aetiology and outcome of infective endocarditis. Results of the ESC-EORP EURO-ENDO (European infective endocarditis) registry: a prospective cohort study. Eur Heart J. 2019;40(39):3222–32.

45. Ahmed FZ, Arumugam P. 18F-FDG PET/CT now endorsed by guidelines across all types of CIED infection: evidence limited but growing. J Nucl Cardiol. 2019;26(3):971–4.

46. Juneau D, Golfam M, Hazra S, Zuckier LS, Garas S, Redpath C, et al. Positron emission tomography and single-photon emission computed tomography imaging in the diagnosis of cardiac implantable electronic device infection. Circ Cardiovasc Imaging. 2017;10(4):e005772.

47. Mahmood M, Kendi AT, Farid S, Ajmal S, Johnson GB, Baddour LM, et al. Role of 18F-FDG PET/CT in the diagnosis of cardiovascular implantable electronic device infections: a meta-analysis. J Nucl Cardiol. 2019;26(3):958 70.

48. Di Carli MF, Asgarzadie F, Schelbert HR, Brunken RC, Laks H, Phelps ME, et al. Quantitative relation between myocardial viability and improvement in heart failure symptoms after revascularization in patients with ischemic cardiomyopathy. Circulation. 1995;92(12):3436–44.

49. Maddahi J. Factors influencing predictive value of fdg imaging for evaluating myocardial viability. J Nucl Cardiol. 2004;11(5):524–6.

50. Schöder H, Campisi R, Ohtake T, Hoh CK, Moon DH, Czernin J, et al. Blood flow–metabolism imaging with positron emission tomography in patients with diabetes mellitus for the assessment of reversible left ventricular contractile dysfunction. The Laboratory of Structural Biology and Molecular Medicine is operated for the U.S. Department of Energy by the University of California under Contract #DE-FC03-87ER60615. J Am Coll Cardiol. 1999;33(5):1328–37.

51. Singh D, Foessel R, Nagra N, Lau P, Brauchli D. Acute saddle pulmonary embolism on 18F-FDG

PET/CT: diagnosis by functional imaging. Respirol Case Rep. 2019;7(8):e00476.

52. Franceschi AM, Matthews R, Mankes S, Safaie E, Franceschi D. Four chamber FDG uptake in the heart: an indirect sign of pulmonary embolism. Clin Nucl Med. 2012;37(7):687–91.

53. Flavell RR, Behr SC, Brunsing RL, Naeger DM, Pampaloni MH. The incidence of pulmonary embolism and associated FDG-PET findings in IV contrast-enhanced PET/CT. Acad Radiol. 2014;21(6):718–25.

54. Soussan M, Rust E, Pop G, Morère J-F, Brillet P-Y, Eder V. The rim sign: FDG-PET/CT pattern of pulmonary infarction. Insights Imaging. 2012;3(6):629–33.

55. Wittram C, Scott JA. 18F-FDG PET of pulmonary embolism. Am J Roentgenol. 2007;189(1):171–6.

56. Bastiaannet E, Groen H, Jager PL, Cobben DCP, van der Graaf WTA, Vaalburg W, et al. The value of FDG-PET in the detection, grading and response to therapy of soft tissue and bone sarcomas; a systematic review and meta-analysis. Cancer Treat Rev. 2004;30(1):83–101.

57. Thurer RL, Thorsen A, Parker JA, Karp DD. FDG imaging of a pulmonary artery sarcoma. Ann Thorac Surg. 2000;70(4):1414–5.

58. Chong S, Kim TS, Kim B-T, Cho EY, Kim J. Pulmonary Artery Sarcoma mimicking pulmonary thromboembolism: integrated FDG PET/CT. Am J Roentgenol. 2007;188(6):1691–3.

59. Tueller C, Fischer Biner R, Minder S, Gugger M, Stoupis C, Krause TM, et al. FDG-PET in diagnostic work-up of pulmonary artery sarcomas. Eur Respir J. 2010;35(2):444–6.

60. Pelletier-Galarneau M, Juneau D. Vascular graft infection: improving diagnosis with functional imaging. J Nucl Cardiol. 2020. https://doi.org/10.1007/s12350-020-02269-z.

61. Lyons OTA, Baguneid M, Barwick TD, Bell RE, Foster N, Homer-Vanniasinkam S, et al. Diagnosis of aortic graft infection: a case definition by the Management of Aortic Graft Infection Collaboration (MAGIC). Eur J Vasc Endovasc Surg. 2016;52(6):758–63.

62. Rojoa D, Kontopodis N, Antoniou SA, Ioannou CV, Antoniou GA. 18F-FDG PET in the diagnosis of vascular prosthetic graft infection: a diagnostic test accuracy meta-analysis. Eur J Vasc Endovasc Surg. 2019;57(2):292–301.

63. Sarrazin J-F, Trottier M, Tessier M. How useful is 18F-FDG PET/CT in patients with suspected vascular graft infection? J Nucl Cardiol. 2020;27(1):303–4.

64. Lucinian YA, Lamarche Y, Demers P, Martineau P, Harel F, Pelletier-Galarneau M. FDG-PET/CT for the detection of infection following aortic root replacement surgery. JACC Cardiovasc Imaging. 2020;13(6):1447–9.

65. Kim S-J, Lee S-W, Jeong SY, Pak K, Kim K. A systematic review and meta-analysis of 18F-fluorodeoxyglucose positron emission tomography or positron emission tomography/computed tomography for detection of infected prosthetic vascular grafts. J Vasc Surg. 2019;70(1):307–13.

66. Reinders Folmer EI, Von Meijenfeldt GCI, Van der Laan MJ, Glaudemans AWJM, Slart RHJA, Saleem BR, et al. Diagnostic imaging in vascular graft infection: a systematic review and meta-analysis. Eur J Vasc Endovasc Surg. 2018;56(5):719–29.

67. Lazar HL, Salm TV, Engelman R, Orgill D, Gordon S. Prevention and management of sternal wound infections. J Thorac Cardiovasc Surg. 2016;152(4):962–72.

68. Hever P, Singh P, Eiben I, Eiben P, Nikkhah D. The management of deep sternal wound infection: literature review and reconstructive algorithm. JPRAS Open. 2021;28:77–89.

69. Hariri H, Tan S, Martineau P, Lamarche Y, Carrier M, Finnerty V, et al. FDG-PET/CT for the assessment of sternal wound infection following sternotomy. J Nucl Med. 2019;60(supplement 1):223.

70. Zhang R, Feng Z, Zhang Y, Tan H, Wang J, Qi F. Diagnostic value of fluorine-18 deoxyglucose positron emission tomography/computed tomography in deep sternal wound infection. J Plast Reconstr Aesthet Surg. 2018;71(12):1768–76.

71. Liu S, Zhang J, Yin H, Pang L, Wu B, Shi H. The value of ^{18}F-FDG PET/CT in diagnosing and localising deep sternal wound infection to guide surgical debridement. Int Wound J. 2020;17(4):1019–27.

72. Nensa F, Tezgah E, Poeppel TD, Jensen CJ, Schelhorn J, Köhler J, et al. Integrated ^{18}F-FDG PET/MR Imaging in the assessment of cardiac masses: a pilot study. J Nucl Med. 2015;56(2):255–60.

73. Gowda RM, Khan IA, Nair CK, Mehta NJ, Vasavada BC, Sacchi TJ. Cardiac papillary fibroelastoma: a comprehensive analysis of 725 cases. Am Heart J. 2003;146(3):404–10.

74. Ibrahim M, Masters RG, Hynes M, Veinot JP, Davies RA. Papillary fibroelastoma of the pulmonary valve. Can J Cardiol. 2006;22(6):509–10.

75. Skali H, Schulman AR, Dorbala S. 18F-FDG PET/CT for the assessment of myocardial sarcoidosis. Curr Cardiol Rep. 2013;15(4):352.

76. Manabe O, Ohira H, Yoshinaga K, Sato T, Klaipetch A, Oyama-Manabe N, et al. Elevated 18F-fluorodeoxyglucose uptake in the interventricular septum is associated with atrioventricular block in patients with suspected cardiac involvement sarcoidosis. Eur J Nucl Med Mol Imaging. 2013;40(10):1558–66.

77. Martineau P, Pelletier-Galarneau M, Juneau D, Leung E, Birnie D, Beanlands RSB. Molecular imaging of cardiac sarcoidosis. Curr Cardiovasc Imaging Rep. 2018;11(3):6.

78. Terasaki F, Azuma A, Anzai T, Ishizaka N, Ishida Y, Isobe M, et al. JCS 2016 guideline on diagnosis and treatment of cardiac sarcoidosis-digest version. Circ J. 2019;83(11):2329–88.

79. Birnie DH, Sauer WH, Bogun F, Cooper JM, Culver DA, Duvernoy CS, et al. HRS expert consensus statement on the diagnosis and management of arrhythmias associated with cardiac sarcoidosis. Heart Rhythm. 2014;11(7):1305–23.

80. Birnie DH, Nery PB, Ha AC, Beanlands RSB. Cardiac sarcoidosis. J Am Coll Cardiol. 2016;68(4):411–21.

81. Shelke AB, Aurangabadkar HU, Bradfield JS, Ali Z, Kumar KS, Narasimhan C. Serial FDG-PET scans help to identify steroid resistance in cardiac sarcoidosis. Int J Cardiol. 2017;228:717–22.

82. Lee P-I, Cheng G, Alavi A. The role of serial FDG PET for assessing therapeutic response in patients with cardiac sarcoidosis. J Nucl Cardiol. 2017;24(1):19–28.

83. Ning N, Guo HH, Iagaru A, Mittra E, Fowler M, Witteles R. Serial cardiac FDG-PET for the diagnosis and therapeutic guidance of patients with cardiac sarcoidosis. J Card Fail. 2019;25(4):307–11.

84. Ahmadian A, Pawar S, Govender P, Berman J, Ruberg FL, Miller EJ. The response of FDG uptake to immunosuppressive treatment on FDG PET/CT imaging for cardiac sarcoidosis. J Nucl Cardiol. 2017;24(2):413–24.

85. Ishiyama M, Soine LA, Vesselle HJ. Semi-quantitative metabolic values on FDG PET/CT including extracardiac sites of disease as a predictor of treatment course in patients with cardiac sarcoidosis. EJNMMI Res. 2017;7(1):67.

86. Abikhzer G, Martineau P, Grégoire J, Finnerty V, Harel F, Pelletier-Galarneau M. [18F]FDG-PET CT for the evaluation of native valve endocarditis. J Nucl Cardiol. 2020;29(1):158–65. https://doi.org/10.1007/s12350-020-02092-6.

87. Chang S-A. Tuberculous and infectious pericarditis. Cardiol Clin. 2017;35(4):615–22.

88. Sagristà-Sauleda J, Permanyer-Miralda G, Soler-Soler J. Tuberculous pericarditis: ten year experience with a prospective protocol for diagnosis and treatment. J Am Coll Cardiol. 1988;11(4):724–8.

89. Dong A, Dong H, Wang Y, Cheng C, Zuo C, Lu J. (18)F-FDG PET/CT in differentiating acute tuberculous from idiopathic pericarditis: preliminary study. Clin Nucl Med. 2013;38(4):e160–5.

90. Vorster M, Sathekge MM, Bomanji J. Advances in imaging of tuberculosis: the role of ^{18}F-FDG PET and PET/CT. Curr Opin Pulm Med. 2014;20(3):287–93.

91. Sathekge MM, Maes A, Pottel H, Stoltz A, van de Wiele C. Dual time-point FDG PET-CT for differentiating benign from malignant solitary pulmonary nodules in a TB endemic area. South Afr Med J. 2010;100(9):598–601.

92. Pelletier-Galarneau M, Martineau P, Zuckier LS, Pham X, Lambert R, Turpin S. 18F-FDG-PET/CT imaging of thoracic and extrathoracic tuberculosis in children. Semin Nucl Med. 2017;47(3):304–18.

93. Ha J-W, Lee J-D, Ko Y-G, Yun M, Rim S-J, Chung N, et al. Assessment of pericardial inflammation in a patient with tuberculous effusive constrictive pericarditis with ^{18}F-2-deoxyglucose positron emission tomography. Circulation. 2006;113(1):e4–5.

94. Testempassi E, Kubota K, Morooka M, Ito K, Masuda-Miyata Y, Yamashita H, et al. Constrictive tuberculous pericarditis diagnosed using 18F-fluorodeoxyglucose positron emission tomography: a report of two cases. Ann Nucl Med. 2010;24(5):421–5.

95. Kim SM, Park S-J, Park JR, Choi JH, Yang JH, Noh HJ, et al. A newly developed pericardial tuberculoma during antituberculous therapy. Korean Circ J. 2011;41(12):750–3.

Index

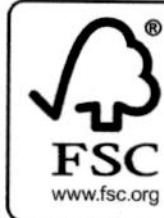